Integrating Physical Agents in Rehabilitation
SECOND EDITION

Bernadette Hecox, PT, MA
Associate Professor in Clinical Physical Therapy, Retired
Program in Physical Therapy
Columbia University
New York, New York

Tsega Andemicael Mehreteab, PT, MS
Clinical Professor
Department of Physical Therapy
New York University
New York, New York

Joseph Weisberg, PT, PhD
Dean
Barry Z. Levine School of Health Sciences
Touro College
Dix Hills, New York

John Sanko, PT, EdD
Associate Professor
Program in Physical Therapy
University of Scranton
Scranton, Pennsylvania

Consulting Editors:
Thomas Holland PhD, PT
Assistant Professor
Physical Therapy Program
School of Health Sciences
City University of New York - Hunter College
New York, New York

Gary Krasilovsky, PhD, PT
Associate Professor and Director
Physical Therapy Program
School of Health Sciences
City University of New York - Hunter College
New York, New York

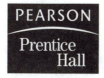

Upper Saddle River, New Jersey 07458

Library of Congress Cataloging-in-Publication Data

Integrating physical agents in rehabilitation / [edited by] Bernadette Hecox ... [et al.].-- 2nd ed.
  p. ; cm.
  Rev. ed of: Physical agents / Bernadette Hecox, Tsega Andemicael Mehreteab, Joseph Weisberg. c1994.
  Includes bibliographical references and index.
  ISBN 0-8385-8132-3
 1. Physical therapy.
  [DNLM: 1. Physical Therapy Techniques. WB 460 I59 2006] I. Hecox, Bernadette. II. Hecox,
Bernadette. Physical agents.
  RM700.H43 2006
  615.8'2--dc22

                                                                    2004028729

Notice: The authors and the publisher of this volume have taken care that the information and technical recommendations contained herein are based on research and expert consultation, and are accurate and compatible with the standards generally accepted at the time of publication. Nevertheless, as new information becomes available, changes in clinical and technical practices become necessary. The reader is advised to carefully consult manufacturers' instructions and information material for all supplies and equipment before use, and to consult with a healthcare professional as necessary. This advice is especially important when using new supplies or equipment for clinical purposes. The authors and publisher disclaim all responsibility for any liability, loss, injury, or damage incurred as a consequence, directly or indirectly, of the use and application of any of the contents of this volume.

Publisher: Julie Levin Alexander
Assistant to Publisher: Regina Bruno
Senior Acquisitions Editor: Mark Cohen
Associate Editor: Melissa Kerian
Editorial Assistant: Jaquay Felix
Media Editor: John J. Jordan
Development Editor: Judith Johnstone
Director of Production and Manufacturing: Bruce Johnson
Managing Production Editor: Patrick Walsh
Production Liaison: Christina Zingone
Production Editor: Patty Donovan, Pine Tree Composition

Manufacturing Manager: Ilene Sanford
Manufacturing Buyer: Pat Brown
Design Director: Cheryl Asherman
Design Coordinator: Christopher Weigand
Cover Designer: Christopher Weigand
Director of Marketing: Karen Allman
Channel Marketing Manager: Rachele Strober
Manager of Media Production: Amy Peltier
New Media Project Manager: Stephen Hartner
Composition: Pine Tree Composition, Inc.
Printer/Binder: Courier Companies
Cover Printer: Phoenix Color Corp.

Pearson Prentice Hall™ is a trademark of Pearson Education, Inc.
Pearson® is a registered trademark of Pearson plc.
Prentice Hall® is a registered trademark of Pearson Education, Inc.

Pearson Education Ltd., *London*
Pearson Education Australia Pty. Limited, *Sydney*
Pearson Education Singapore, Pte. Ltd.
Pearson Education North Asia Ltd., *Hong Kong*
Pearson Education Canada, Ltd., *Toronto*

Pearson Educación de Mexico, S.A. de C.V.
Pearson Education—Japan, *Tokyo*
Pearson Education Malaysia, Pte. Ltd.
Pearson Education, Upper Saddle River, New Jersey

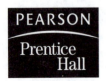

10 9 8 7 6 5 4 3 2 1
ISBN 0-8385-8132-3

Contents

Preface

The new edition of this text is designed to provide both the theoretical and practical information in a single text, required for today's entry-level education related to the physical agents. Current evidence-based information and trends in clinical practice have been added throughout the text. Normal and abnormal anatomy and physiology is presented in the early chapters as the foundation for selection and application of the appropriate physical agents. Emphasis on the "why" as well as the "how" is presented when using the physical agents for therapeutic interventions.

The authors of this text, each with extensive experience teaching physical agents courses, selected the depth and extent of information they considered appropriate for basic courses of professional instruction. This approach was taken to assist instructors, students and practitioners in focusing on and clarifying the essential content required for integrating the physical agents in rehabilitation.

Advancements in scientific research and clinical studies now authenticate the value of some physical agents and tend to disprove others. As popularity of treatments that are not as scientifically based continues to increase, so does the need to be able to intelligently distinguish valid treatment options from those that lack legitimacy. The profession recognizes the increasing need for physical therapists to be selective and to make intelligent judgments. This text includes modalities ranging from those for which there is much supportive research to those that require further clinical research. Each modality discussed is accompanied by extensive citations in the rehabilitation literature related to specific modality indication, rationale, precautions and contraindications.

With the current constraints in the health care delivery system, the role of the physical therapist and physical therapy assistant is also changing. This text honestly strives to present the pros and cons regarding the quality, effects, and value of each modality while considering the constraints on personnel, time, etc. of therapists and patients. With the advancement in their education and clinical skills, physical therapists are assuming more specialty roles. We have added information regarding the integration of physical agents in the management of wounds and pelvic floor dysfunction. In addition, physical therapy assistants, now perform more hands-on interventions formerly given exclusively by physical therapists. This requires that both branches of the profession be prepared to assume more responsibility. The physical therapy assistants must have a higher level of knowledge and understanding as well as skill, to safely and efficiently perform the skilled treatments now expected of them.

This book is divided into six parts. Part I is a review of basic information of how the human body responds to the various modalities. Part II presents thermal agent information with inclusion of pertinent physics as well as normal and abnormal physiological responses to heat and cold. Part III covers the uses of therapeutic electricity and electrophysiologic testing procedures. Part IV reviews the mechanical agents; traction, external compression and hydrotherapy, a modality used for its thermal and mechanical effects. Part V presents current information on the two photochemical modalities; ultraviolet and low level laser. Part VI includes different forms of biofeedback used in rehabilitation and kinesiological electromyography clinical applications. In addition, normal and abnormal pelvic floor function and integration of the physical agents for pelvic floor rehabilitation is presented in Part VI.

Clinical cases and lab experiments for the different physical agents are presented in the Appendix. Instructors and students are encouraged to use these cases and experiments in the lecture and laboratory components of their physical agents coursework. For quick reference, indication and contraindication boxes with applicable rationale are situated throughout the text. The emphasis and focus in this text continues to be safe and effective physical agent application with sound rationale as part of the overall rehabilitation intervention.

Contributors

Donna Adams, MA, PT, OCS
Chapter 28
Assistant Professor
Academic Coordinator of Clinical Education
Physical Therapy Program
Touro College
The School of Health Sciences
Bay Shore, New York

Joseph A. Balogun, PT, Ph.D, FACSM
Chapter 27
Professor and Dean
College of Health Sciences
Chicago State University
Chicago, Illinois

William E. DeTurk, PT, PhD
Chapter 6
Clinical Associate Professor
Doctor of Physical Therapy Program
School of Health Technology & Management
Stony Brook University
Stony Brook, New York

Marilyn Freedman, PT, BCIA-C, PMDB
Chapter 30
Director of Physical Therapy
Essential Physical Therapy, PLLC
Great Neck, New York

Bernadette Hecox, PT, MA
Chapters 3, 5, 8, 9, 10, 11, 12, 13, 14, 17, 25, 26
Associate Professor in Clinical Physical Therapy,
    Retired
Program in Physical Therapy
Columbia University
New York, New York

Thomas Holland, PT, Ph.D.
Chapters 18, 19, 20, 22
Assistant Professor
Physical Therapy Program
City University of New York—Hunter
New York, New York

Laura F. Jacobs, MD, Ph.D
Chapter 25
President
International Society of Pneumatic Medicine

Mary Jane Day, PT, MS
Chapter 16
Assistant Professor of Clinical Physical Therapy
Program in Physical Therapy
Columbia University
New York, New York

Joanne S. Katz, PT, Ph.D
Chapter 16
Assistant Professor
Interim Chairperson
Physical Therapy Program
State University of New York—Downstate
    Medical Center
Brooklyn, New York

Gary Krasilovsky, PT, Ph.D.
Chapter 29
Associate Professor and Director
Physical Therapy Program
City University of New York—Hunter
New York, New York

Peter M. Leininger, MSPT, OCS, CSCS
Chapter 26
Assistant Professor
Department of Physical Therapy
University of Scranton
Scranton, Pennsylvania

**Louise E. Marks, MS, OTR, BCIA-C
    Biofeedback, EEG, PMDB**
Chapter 30
Owner, Occupational Therapist, Educator, Consultant
Boulder Neuro Training Center
2300 Broadway
Boulder, CO

Andrew L. McDonough, PT, Ed.D
Chapter 2
Associate Professor of Physical Therapy
New York University
The Steinhardt School of Education
New York, New York

Tsega Andemicael Mehreteab, PT, MS
Chapter 18, 19, 20, 22
Clinical Professor
Department of Physical Therapy
New York University
New York, New York

Michael Moran, PT, ScD.
Chapter 1
Professor
Physical Therapy Department
College Misericordia
Dallas, Pennsylvania

Arthur Nelson, Jr., PT, Ph.D, FAPTA
Chapter 23
Professor and Director of Research
Physical Therapy Department
College of Staten Island
Staten Island, New York

John Sanko, PT, EdD
Chapters 3, 5, 8, 9, 10, 11, 12, 13, 14, 17
Associate Professor
Program in Physical Therapy
University of Scranton
Scranton, Pennsylvania

Theresa A. Schmidt, MS, PT, OCS, LMT
Chapter 24
Professor and Chair
Physical Therapy Assistant Programs
Touro College
New York, New York

Leslie Schonbrun, MS, PT, MBA, DABFE
Chapter 7
Assistant Professor
Physical Therapy Program
Touro College
School of Health Sciences
New York, New York

Elise Stettner MPS, PT, BCIA-C Biofeedback, PMDB
Chapter 30
Partner, Physical Therapist
Manhasset Physical Therapy Associates
Manhasset, New York

Robert Troiano, MA, PT, CHT
Chapter 21
Chairperson of Physical Therapy
Touro College
Bay Shore, New York

Mary Walsh
Chapter 30
Administrative Director
Advantage Physical Therapy

R. Scott Ward, PT, Ph.D
Chapter 4
Professor and Department Chair
Dean of The College of Health
University of Utah
Salt Lake City, Utah

Joseph Weisberg, PT, PhD
Chapters 6, 7, 21, 24, 27, 28
Dean
Barry Z. Levine School of Health Sciences
Touro College
Dix Hills, New York

Ronald W. Sweitzer
Chapter 15
Director
Pleasantville Physical Therapy & Sport Care PC
Lecturer
Program in Physical Therapy
Pleasantville, New York

Reviewers

Cheryl Adams, PT, MHS, OCS
Assistant Professor
Department of Physical Therapy
Husson College
Bangor, Maine

Wendy Bircher, PT, MS
Program Director
Physical Therapist Assistant Program
San Juan College
Farmington, New Mexico

Barbara Bradford, MPH, PT
Program Director
Physical Therapist Assistant Program
Bishop State Community College
Mobile, Alabama

Mary DeNotto, MS, PT
Program Chair
Physical Therapist Assistant Program
Oakton Community College
Des Plaines, Illinois

Elaine Eckel, PT, MA
Program Chair
Physical Therapist Assistant Program
Fayetteville Technical Community College
Fayetteville, North Carolina

Ruth Freeman, PT, M.Ed
Program Manager
Physical Therapist Assistant Program
Daytona Beach Community College
Daytona Beach, Florida

Burke Gurney, PT, Ph.D.
Assistant Professor
Physical Therapy Department
University of New Mexico
Albuquerque, New Mexico

Aimee Klein
Clinical Assistant Professor
Physical Therapy Program
MGH Institute of Health Professions
Boston, Massachusetts

David Levine, PT, Ph.D., OCS
Professor
Department of Physical Therapy
University of Tennessee at Chattanooga
Chattanooga, Tennessee

Winifred Mauser, PT, Ed.D.
Associate Professor
Ithaca College
Department of Physical Therapy
Ithaca, New York

Janice Pollock, PT, MHS
Program Director
Physical Therapist Assistant Program
Manatee Community College
Bradenton, Florida

Martha Zimmerman, PT, MA
Program Director
Physical Therapist Assistant Program
Caldwell Community College and Technical Institute
Hudson, North Carolina

Approaching Physical Agents

Everyone who responsibly includes physical agents as part of a treatment program must have an understanding of related physical, biological and psychological information. Prerequisite courses required for any students entering physical therapy programs include general courses containing this information.

This section includes an Introduction (Chapter One) followed by a few topics selected from these general courses that are especially meaningful to clinicians who include physical agents in their treatment programs. Each chapter reviews information on one topic focusing on factors related to physical therapy treatments in general and to physical agents in particular.

The topic of Chapter Two is The Skin. Biological factors pertaining to the skin and its accessory organs, and the wound healing processes are reviewed. Skin conditions which are commonly observed when applying physical agents are described. The normal stages of wound healing (Chapter 4) are presented to provide rationale for using the various physical agents.

Chapter Three is a brief review of peripheral vascular and lymphatic circulations. Emphasis is on the role these systems play in controlling the temperature of local body tissues and general body temperature, and on the mechanisms which control the flow of blood and lymphatics through the body. The last part of the chapter gives examples of how this information can be applied when considering physical therapy procedures.

Chapter Five discusses *edema*, a condition frequently seen in patients receiving physical agents treatments. It includes information about the causes and various types of edema, and considerations concerning physical therapy intervention.

Chapter Six discusses *pain/spasms*, both the physical and psychological components. These signs and symptoms are perhaps seen more than any others in physical therapy. Former pain theories are reviewed briefly to help the reader relate to the theories presently being considered, which are discussed in more detail. Information concerning the conditions called "spasms" is given as well as the relationship between pain and spasms.

Chapter Seven reviews the *electro-magnetic spectrum* and electro-magnetic theories. Frequencies, wave lengths and depth of penetration into the body must be considered for many physical agents, especially the radiation therapies and Short Wave Diathermy. The basic laws of radiated energy included in this chapter will be referred to in future chapters, especially the Infrared, Ultraviolet and Diathermy chapters.

The intention of including these background information chapters is to avoid redundancy in future chapters. The many chapters which would otherwise need to include this information may only summarize and refer the reader to the chapter in this section that contains more detailed information.

The use of physical energies have and continue to be a valuable adjunct in the rehabilitation of individuals with physical dysfunction. Thermal, electrical, mechanical, and photochemical modalities are used to enhance the benefits of the primary parts of the physical therapy intervention. Interventions such as: manual therapy, therapeutic exercise, patient education, pain management, and wound management and prevention are often preceded or followed by one of the physical agents.

1

Introduction

MICHAEL MORAN PT, SCD

The *Guide to Physical Therapist Practice* lists many procedural interventions used by practicing physical therapists. Three categories of those interventions are discussed in this text: *electrotherapeutic modalities, physical agents*, and *mechanical modalities*.

The *Guide*[1] defines those categories as the following:

Electrotherapeutic modalities are a broad group of agents that use electricity and are intended to assist functional training; assist muscle force generation and contraction; decrease unwanted muscular activity; increase the rate of healing of open wounds and soft tissue; maintain strength after injury or surgery; modulate or decrease pain; or reduce or eliminate soft tissue swelling, inflammation, or restriction.

Physical Agents are a broad group of procedures using various forms of energy that are applied to tissues in a systematic manner and that are intended to increase connective tissue extensibility; increase the healing rate of open wounds and soft tissue; modulate pain; reduce or eliminate soft tissue swelling, inflammation, or restriction associated with musculoskeletal injury or circulatory dysfunction; remodel scar tissue; or treat skin conditions.

Mechanical modalities are a group of devices that use forces such as approximation, compression, and distraction and that are intended to improve circulation, increase range of motion, modulate pain, or stabilize an area that requires temporary support.

For the sake of simplicity, this chapter will group *electrotherapeutic modalities, physical agents*, and *mechanical modalities* into the term "physical agents."

REASONS FOR USING PHYSICAL AGENTS

Overall, the reasons for using physical agents are as follows:

1. Decrease pain, edema, and swelling
2. Decrease neural compression
3. Improve
   a. activity and task performance
   b. health, wellness or fitness
   c. movement performance
   d. physical performance
   e. wound healing
   f. airway clearance
4. Increase joint mobility, muscle performance, and neuromuscular performance
5. Increase tissue perfusion and decrease soft tissue and circulatory disorders
6. Prevent or remediate impairments, functional limitations, or disabilities to improve physical function
7. Reduce risk factors and complications

Physical agents are not typically used in isolation but are used as part of an overall intervention strategy.

Decision Making and Physical Agents

The various chapters in this text will help the reader explore and understand the uses of physical agents in selected patient conditions and pathologies. Of primary concern is that the reader understands that selection of a physical agent depends upon the following:

1. Examination findings
2. Diagnosis
3. Prognosis
4. Efficacy and safety considerations

There are many textbooks available to assist students and practitioners to develop the skills necessary to perform an examination and arrive at a diagnosis and prognosis. This text will not attempt to duplicate that information. Rather, this chapter will focus on the decision making process of selecting and applying physical agents. This text stresses the integration of physical agents in the total intervention program.

The clinical application of physical agents largely depends upon the following:

1. Patient selection
2. Goals and outcomes (ie, tissue, system, and body responses)
3. Therapist expertise
4. Risk management and legal considerations, including documentation

Patient Selection

Patient selection includes several factors. Those factors are as follows:

1. *Age:* Tissue, system, and body responses to physical agents can vary tremendously according to patient age. For example, an older individual's thermoregulation can be hampered, compared with that of a younger person. Therefore, administering heat or cold may yield less predictable responses from a geriatric patient. Another good example draws upon the pediatric population: comprehension of instructions or precautions may be impossible for a very young child. In this example, educating the pertinent caregivers may be a necessary component of the intervention.

2. *Gender:* A patient's gender can, at times, be a specific consideration when selecting a physical agent. For example, use of therapeutic ultrasound over a pregnant uterus is considered a contraindication.

3. *Culture:* Some patients will resist or object to the use of physical agents on the basis of cultural considerations. For example, a husband may find it culturally unacceptable that a male therapist is administering a physical agent to the husband's wife. Although the male therapist may be competent, it may be necessary to recognize and be sensitive to the cultural beliefs of patients and their significant others.

4. *Lifestyle:* Patients' lifestyles may range considerably. One patient may have an unchanging daily schedule, whereas another's routine will vacillate. Administration of a physical agent may be affected by a patient's schedule. For instance, whereas one patient may be able to receive clinic-based intervention, another may need to have an extensive home program established. In other words, the latter patient may need to be instructed in the use of a physical agent (eg, traction) in a home setting.

5. *Environment:* Many people work or live in settings where the use of physical agents may involve patient safety. Perhaps the patient is a construction worker who must be freely mobile to climb ladders. If transcutaneous electrical nerve stimulation (TENS) is being used for pain control, the required electrodes and wires must not hamper the patient's movements.

Goals and Outcomes

It is always important to have clear goals and objectives for physical therapy intervention. The chapters of this text will explain the selection and use of various physical agents. Readers are reminded that selection and use are goal driven. Establishing goals begins with the examination process and includes re-examinations. Specific procedures for each physical agent will not be discussed here. However, this section of this chapter will briefly address two issues pertinent to all uses of physical agents: physical agent application and patient positioning.

Physical Agent Application

Regardless of the specific physical agent chosen, it must be applied correctly. The physical agent will be used to affect human tissues and as such can cause either beneficial effects or harm. Appropriate cleansing procedures of both the physical agent and the tissues must be used. Inappropriate cleaning of equipment or tissues may result in undesired effects such as tissue irritation or infection.

In addition, the areas to which the physical agent will be applied should be inspected first. Clothing or other materials may hide the true appearance of tissues and impair the identification of contraindications or precautions for physical agent use.

A physical agent should itself be inspected, prior to use, for indications of incorrect or nonfunctioning components. For example, if a hot pack is leaking material, it should be discarded. Further, the temperature of the water bath for the hot packs should also be monitored to ensure that an appropriate amount of heat is being delivered.

The actual application of the physical agent should follow accepted clinical standards. For example, when using ultrasound, a coupling media is required. Commercially available warming units help prevent patient discomfort from the application of cold gel. It is unadvisable to use a hydrocollator unit to warm the tube of ultrasound gel, since the gel may become hot and may burn the patient upon application.

Sufficient explanation regarding the physical agent and its effects should be given to the patient. Signs and symptoms of both desired and undesired effects should be included so that the patient can inform the therapist of potential complications. If left unattended, the patient should be given a means of calling for assistance, such as a bell or other signaling device.

The patient should be appropriately monitored while the physical agent is being used. Of importance is that some patients may fall asleep or become otherwise inattentive during interventions using physical agents. Frequent inspection of the patient's tissues and close observation of the patient are considered good clinical practice.

Following the removal of the physical agent, the patient's tissues and patient responses to the intervention should be assessed.

Patient Positioning

Appropriate patient positioning for the application of physical agents should, at the least, include the following:

1. *Safety:* The patient should be positioned and monitored so that the patient is free from harm. For example, a patient receiving hydrotherapy should be securely positioned and monitored to ensure that airway obstruction from the water does not occur.
2. *Comfort:* Patients typically are asked to remain in a somewhat limited position while a physical agent is applied. If the purpose of the intervention is to cause muscular relaxation, that body part must be correctly supported so that tissues are slack. Consideration should be given to the use of measures such as pillows and other padding materials to reduce or eliminate patient discomfort from staying in one position for a relatively lengthy period of time.
3. *Dignity:* Patients should be appropriately draped and cared for in a manner to ensure adequate privacy.

THERAPIST EXPERTISE

The educational preparation of United States–trained physical therapists has long included physical agents. However, the relative extent and emphasis placed on that training can vary by educational program. Also, clinical practice is a factor to consider when discussing individual therapists' expertise in physical agents.

For instance, some therapists may have practiced for many years but not used one or more physical agents since school. Perhaps the practice setting is not always conducive to using physical agents (eg, using shortwave diathermy in home health), or perhaps a therapist has chosen not to use them. In any event, the subsequent chapters of this text will help new and experienced therapists select and use physical agents.

A reader may wish to use a physical agent but not feel competent to do so. If a student, the reader may wish to ask for assistance from a professor or clinical instructor. For a practicing therapist, however, it may be more difficult to locate someone for instructional assistance. Therefore, it may be appropriate to refer the patient to another physical therapist with the necessary expertise. An example of such a situation includes referring a patient with psoriasis to a therapist with expertise in using ultraviolet light.[2]

RISK MANAGEMENT AND LEGAL CONSIDERATIONS, INCLUDING DOCUMENTATION

Risk management includes identifying, analyzing, and addressing areas of existing and potential risk. One known risk of using physical agents is burns.[3] Of course, many other potential injuries are possible when applying physical agents to patients. The first step to avoiding risk was mentioned earlier: perform an examination and arrive at a diagnosis and prognosis. Doing so helps identify precautions and contraindications for using physical agents. The second step is selecting and correctly applying an appropriate physical agent. The subsequent chapters are a useful resource for that step. The third step is to properly monitor the patient and make changes to the intervention accordingly. The fourth step is to reexamine the patient to determine whether goals and objectives were accomplished. The fifth and final step (but as important as all the others) is to document the physical agent intervention.

In today's health care arena, legal considerations abound. It is important to know the legal responsibilities of physical therapy practice. In the United States, each state has a physical therapy practice act. The language in the state acts can vary in terms of what physical agents are used and who may apply them (ie, delegation issues). Therefore, it is imperative that physical therapists know and practice according to state law.

One example of using physical agents in accordance with state law is iontophoresis of prescription medication. Physical therapists do not typically have the legal right to prescribe medication. To administer a prescription medication via iontophoresis, a practitioner licensed to prescribe the medication must first do so. Then, once the medication has been legally dispensed, a physical therapist may administer the iontophoresis.

Documentation of the use of physical agents is required by professional standards of practice and legality. The *Guide to Physical Therapist Practice* contains documentation guidelines.[4] In addition to those guidelines, documentation of physical agents must also meet requirements of third-party payers.[5]

SUMMARY

The chapters of this text will help readers select, apply, and assess the efficacy of physical agents. That knowledge becomes more valuable when combined with information from the *Guide to Physical Therapist Practice*. The combined information value is the safe, effective, and contemporary practice of physical therapy.

REFERENCES

1. *Guide to Physical Therapist Practice*. 2nd ed. *Physical Therapy;* January 2001; 81(1):126–29.

2. Brimer M, Moran M (eds.): *Clinical Cases in Physical Therapy.* Butterworth-Heinemann, Philadelphia, PA; 2004; 135–41.

3. Thut C: *A Risky Business*. HPA Resource, American Physical Therapy Association, Alexandria, VA, August 2003; 3(2):4–5.

4. *Guide to Physical Therapist Practice*. 2nd ed. *Physical Therapy*, January 2001; 81(1):703–05.

5. Baeten A, Moran M, Phillippi L: *Documenting Physical Therapy—The Reviewer Perspective*. Butterworth-Heinemann, Philadelphia, PA; 1999.

2

The Skin

ANDREW L. MCDONOUGH, PT, EDD

Chapter Outline

Skin is the largest organ of the body, representing approximately 15 to 20 percent of its total mass.[1] Skin consists of two layers of tissue, through which underlying structures can be treated with various modalities. This chapter describes the structural and functional aspects of the skin and related structures, and it discusses some common skin conditions and diseases about which physical therapists should be aware when designing interventions for patients with physical agents. Knowledge of the structure and function of the skin and the effects of physical agents upon it will help therapists determine the efficacy of various modalities and permit the modification of regimens if skin changes are observed.

STRUCTURE AND FUNCTION

The basic structure of the skin includes a thin layer of epithelial cells (epidermis) overlying a mesh of connective tissue (dermis) (**Fig. 2–1**). The average thickness of the epidermis is 0.06 to 0.6 mm;[1] however, its thickness can range from 0.5 mm in the eyelids to as much as 5 mm in the interscapular region.[2] Thicker

skin (eg, calluses) may develop over areas that are subjected to excessive mechanical stresses. Accessory organs (eg, hair follicles, sweat glands, receptors) are supported and protected by the enveloping skin.

Skin has a number of interrelated physiologic and mechanical functions, including protection (physical and immunologic), sensation, secretion, and regulation:

- *Protection.* The skin protects against infection by acting as an important intermediary between the environment and the other organs. In addition, it retains or excludes fluid, primarily water, by a layer of waterproof keratin, a proteinaceous (waxlike) substance located in the most superficial layer of the epidermis. The barrier function of the skin can be appreciated when some or all of the skin is lost through burn injury. In such instances, fluid lost to the outside environment may lead to significant, sometimes life-threatening, alterations in concentrations of electrolytes called burn shock.[1] Langerhans cells appear to function as antigen-presenting (immunologic) cells when antigenic agents are present on the skin surface.[3]

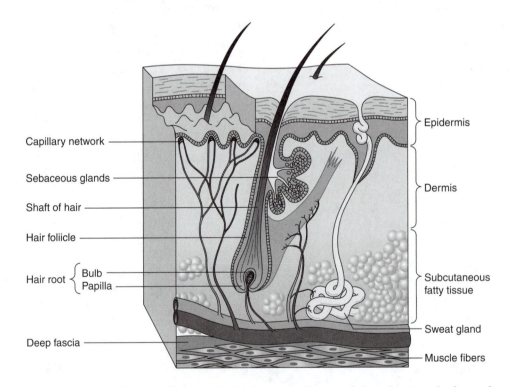

Capillary network

Sebaceous glands

Shaft of hair

Hair foliicle

Hair root { Bulb / Papilla

Deep fascia

Epidermis

Dermis

Subcutaneous fatty tissue

Sweat gland

Muscle fibers

FIGURE 2–1   Schematic drawing of the skin and its appendages, showing the layered arrangement of the body's covering and the hairs and glands embedded within the skin and subcutaneous tissue.

- *Sensation.* Sensory function can be attributed to the skin because it serves as the interface between the outside environment and the afferent nervous system. Several types of receptors that react to physical stimuli are embedded in the skin. These provide the patient with information regarding thermal, mechanical, or electrical stimuli applied to the surface; they are thus important factors in determining modality tolerance.

- *Secretion and regulation.* The skin regulates body temperature and fluid balance by working in conjunction with the circulatory system. Fat aids the skin in temperature regulation by acting as an insulating layer to prevent heat loss. When excess heat must be removed to avoid a potentially catastrophic rise in core temperature, sweat glands are activated to liberate heat.

General Appearance

The general appearance of the skin yields important information about its health and the function of the underlying organs. For example, increased amounts of hair may suggest an endocrine disturbance;[4] thick, coarse hair situated over the spine may indicate the failure of the vertebral column to close during development, as in spina bifida.[5]

Many pathologies can cause atrophy of the skin (loss of substance). The most common cause of skin atrophy is the occlusion of small arteries. The degree of atrophy depends on the amount of oxygen deprivation relative to the oxygen requirements of the tissue. Sweat glands, hair follicles, and neurons cannot tolerate low oxygen concentration and will atrophy first. Fibroblasts, the primary cells of connective tissue, can tolerate relatively low concentrations of oxygen and will be affected the least. Oxygen deprivation causes skin to be shiny, dry, and hairless. Oxygen-deprived skin is easily damaged and heals very slowly; its manifestations are often seen in the lower limbs of patients with diabetes and related peripheral vascular diseases.[6]

The color and texture of the skin suggests the following metabolic or mechanical disorders:

- **Jaundice** (yellow skin) is often associated with liver or gallbladder disease, whereas bronze skin may be symptomatic of glandular disorders.[2]
- **Cyanosis** (bluish skin) is associated with diminished or absent circulation or decreased concentrations of oxygen in the blood, whereas the blackened, apparently charred, skin associated

with gangrenous lesions indicates a total absence of blood supply.

- **Erythema** (reddened skin) secondary to dilation and congestion of superficial vessels may be a response to a heightened emotional state (eg, blushing) or to thermal injury (eg, mild sunburn).
- **Mottled erythema** refers to harmful reactions to infrared radiation; white patches interspersed with vivid red blotches warn that a burn is likely to occur.[7] Mottling is the result of a vasomotor response caused by dilation of capillaries in the dermis.
- **Erythema ab igne** is a persistent erythema and pigmentation produced by long-term exposure to excessive nonburning heat.[8] This type of erythema begins as a mottling caused by local hemostasis and becomes a meshlike erythema that leaves pinkish-rose or dark purplish-brown patches.
- **Blisters,** vesicles of fluid that collect between the layers of skin, or smaller vesicles called **blebs,** may indicate damage caused by burns. For example, blistering of the skin, among other factors, distinguishes first- from second-degree bums. Blisters also may suggest increased mechanical stress (eg, when skin rubs against poorly fitting shoes).
- **Decubitus ulcers** (sores) indicate compression or shear stress to skin over bony prominences resulting from prolonged periods of immobilization, especially when cutaneous sensation is impaired or absent.
- **Wheals,** or **hives,** also known as urticaria, are localized pruritic (itchy) skin eruptions caused by a histaminic reaction usually brought on by allergic responses to certain foods, insect bites, or inhaled substances such as pollen or mold spores. Minor irritations such as those caused by severe heat, intense itching, or rough massage may produce temporary local wheals.
- **Rashes** may be associated with primary disease of the skin or may be caused by local or systemic allergic or autoimmune responses. For example, the peculiar "butterfly" rash over the bridge of the nose caused by deposits of antibodies (immunoglobulins and other compounds) is common in systemic lupus erythematosus.[6]

Conversely, certain localized patches such as freckles, birthmarks, and "age spots" are usually physiologically inconsequential.[9]

GROSS AND MICROSCOPIC STRUCTURE

The skin consists of two layers: a multicellular epidermis and a dense, irregular, underlying layer of connective tissue called the dermis or corium (see **Fig. 2–1**). The *epidermis* is derived from ectoderm and may include two, or as many as five, cell strata, the thickness of which will vary over different body areas.[10] Different modalities have different effects on each stratum. For example, the primary effect of ultraviolet light occurs in the two deepest layers, whereas resistance to electrical current occurs primarily in the most superficial layers.

Epidermis

Most of the cells that make up the **epidermis** are cuboidal or squamous in shape. *Melanocytes* are a second cell type and are found principally in the deepest two layers of the epidermis, producing melanin. This pigment imparts a tannish to blackish color to the skin.[3] A third, less-numerous cell type is the *Langerhan* cell. This irregularly shaped cell with an indented nuclei is probably a form of macrophage (phagocyte) and thus a component of the immune system functioning as an antigen-presenting cell in certain forms of contact dermatitis.[3]

Five layers of cells may be present in the epidermis (listed in order from deepest to most superficial): basale, spinosum, granulosum, lucidum, and corneum (see **Figs. 2–1** and **2–2**). The two deepest layers, basale and spinosum, have well-developed nuclei and are the most viable layers. The remaining, more superficial layers show progressively less cellular vitality. This tendency is especially true of the most superficial layer, the stratum corneum.

Strata Basale and Spinosum.

The deepest layer, the **stratum basale,** also called the stratum germinativum, is a single layer of high-cuboidal to low-columnar epithelial cells that are anchored to a basement membrane (see **Figs. 2–2** and **2–3**). The nuclei of these cells tend to be oval and eccentrically located in the cytoplasm, usually close to the basement membrane. The mitotic figures seen in this layer indicate a reproductively active stratum. In addition to a well-defined nucleus, a large number of ribosomes are found, indicating an active capacity to synthesize proteins. The basal cells abut one another

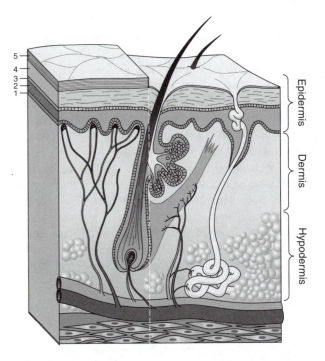

FIGURE 2–2 Oblique cross section of the skin demonstrating the epidermis, dermis and hypodermis. In thick skin there are 5 layers of cells including the stratum: 1 = basale; 2 = spinosum; 3 = granulosum; 4 = lucidum; 5 = cormneum. Three levels of blood vessels are also demonstrated: $Pl_{1–3}$.

and are connected to their neighbors by a series of interdigitating cytoplasmic processes.

The layer overlying the stratum basale, the **stratum spinosum,** is several cell layers thick and consists of cells that vary in shape from squat cuboidal, in the lower regions, to polygonal to squamous in more superficial layers (see **Fig. 2–3**). These cells are bound together by cytoplasmic processes that appear, under high magnification, as "spines" (spinosum), suggesting a layer of spiny or prickle cells.[3]

Stratum Granulosum.

The **stratum granulosum** is usually 2 to 5 cell layers thick. These cells begin to take on a more elongated and flattened (squamous) appearance (see **Fig. 2–3**). The fact that fewer interdigitating processes are found in this layer compared with the deeper two layers suggests reduced intercellular communication and, accordingly, less cellular vitality. Some dead cells also are found in this layer. Keratohyalin granules, produced in this stratum,

Stratum lucidum

Stratum corneum

Stratum granulosum

Stratum spinosum

Stratum basale

Dermis

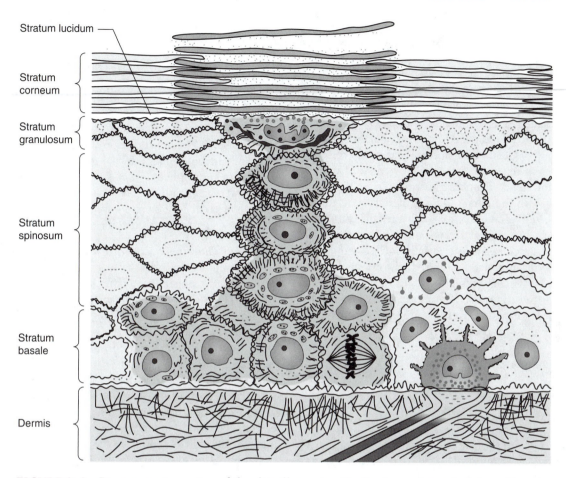

FIGURE 2–3   Diagrammatic section of the skin illustrating the five layers (strata) of the epidermis.

ascend to the stratum corneum (keratinization) and exclude or retain water.[2]

Stratum Lucidum.   The optically clear layer known as the **stratum lucidum** is typically 3 to 5 cell layers thick (see **Fig. 2–2**). Cells in this layer lack nuclei, and the cell borders are poorly defined. The cytoplasm has a semifluid consistency and contains the protein keratin, a compound believed to be a transformation product of keratohyalin.[2] This layer may be absent in "thin" skin (see below).

Stratum Corneum.   The most superficial cells comprise a translucent stratum, the **stratum corneum,** that consists of many dead cells that are periodically sloughed. Also known as the cornified layer, the cytoplasm in this layer of cells is replaced by "soft keratin," a product of the keratinization process that transforms epithelial cells into hardened scales and gives skin its characteristic waterproofing properties.

Subsequent hardening of and reduction of fluid in this layer, especially in "thick" skin, increases resistance to electrical currents.[11] This configuration of scales excludes foreign bodies that might lead to infection. It is also the layer that lends electrical resistance; if removed, it can significantly lower the resistance of the skin.

Dermis

The **dermis,** or *corium*, is derived from mesoderm and is composed of two layers of irregular connective tissue called papillary and reticular layers. No clear demarcating line is noted between these layers. Dermis is usually 2 to 4 mm thick (see **Fig, 2–2**).[4]

The uppermost layer, the **papillary layer,** which is usually thinner than the reticular layer, anchors the dermis to the overlying epidermis. It is essentially a layer of loose connective tissue composed primarily of collagen and elastic fibers. Accessory skin organs are supported and maintained by this layer and by the underlying reticular layer.

The **reticular layer,** as its name suggests, is a meshwork (reticulum) of denser connective tissue composed of coarse collagen fibers and some elastic and reticular fibers. Some deep accessory organs such as hair follicles are found in this layer, and the muscles that control facial expression are inserted here.

Lines of tension created by movement of underlying joints tend to orient the collagen of the dermis parallel with these lines. This preferential orientation of collagen establishes a "grain" to the skin called Langer's lines. Surgical incisions made parallel with Langer's lines result in a cleanly incised wound that heals with minimal scarring. Incisions made transversely across Langer's lines result in gaping wounds with ragged edges that heal more slowly and result in thick scar formation. **Keloids** are raised scars and appear to be more prevalent in darkly pigmented skin.[6] Thick scars tend to concentrate wave energy that, if sufficiently intense, can cause burns.[12]

THIN VERSUS THICK SKIN

In areas where the skin is subjected to substantial and repetitive mechanical stress, it is strengthened and referred to as "thick" skin. Specific sites of thick skin include the soles and palms, the pads of the fingers and toes, and parts of the external genitalia.[2] The remainder of the body is covered with "thin" skin.

Thick skin can be distinguished from thin skin in several ways. First, the epidermis of thick skin has five well-developed cell layers. The stratum corneum is usually fortified with as many as 50 layers of keratinized cells. In thin skin, situated in less mechanically stressed areas (eg, the dorsal surface of the hand), one or more cell layers are absent. The strata basale and spinosum are always intact; however, the thickness of the stratum spinosum may be reduced. The stratum lucidum is usually absent. Second, the dermis of thick skin, in section, appears to be corrugated. A downward protrusion of the epidermis toward the dermis is called an epidermal (rete) peg, whereas an upward extension of the papillary layer toward the epidermis is called a dermal papilla. This arrangement of layers serves to strengthen thick skin in a manner that is similar to the way that corrugated cardboard is stronger than a flat piece of cardboard.

ACCESSORY ORGANS

Hair Follicles.   Early in fetal development, a downward projection of epidermis invaginates the dermis. The space created by this action gives rise to a hair follicle (**Fig. 2–4**). In the deepest part of that cavity, a cluster of germinal matrix cells consolidates and gives rise to a hair.[3] Epithelial cells in the upper part of the follicle contribute to an external root sheath that connects with the surface of the skin. These cells nearest the surface are keratinized. Matrix cells also generate a tubular internal root sheath composed of soft keratin that extends partway up the follicle (see **Fig. 2–4**).

Sebaceous Glands.   Associated with the hair follicles are **sebaceous glands:** oil-producing glands that drain into the upper part of the follicle or, occasionally, directly onto the skin surface (see **Fig. 2–4**). **Sebum,** a fatty secretory product, is produced by the disintegration of cells lining the gland. This process is known as the holocrine mode of secretion.[3] Sebum coats and lubricates the hair shaft and the area adjacent to it as the shaft emerges from the skin. This protective coating prevents excess evaporation of water from the stratum corneum and probably acts to conserve heat. Prolonged exposure to water can reduce the amount of sebum on the skin.

Sebum is expressed from the gland onto the hair by contraction of the arrector pili muscle (see **Fig. 2–4**). This bundle of smooth-muscle fibers is attached to a sheath of connective tissue investing the hair shaft. After looping around the sebaceous gland, the arrector pili muscle inserts into the papillary layer of the dermis. When the muscle contracts, the gland is squeezed, and its contents (sebum) are expressed onto the hair shaft.[2] Excessive production of sebum, especially during puberty, leads to localized pockets of oil that are deposited on the skin. Subsequent bacterial infection may lead to acne.[4] Male hormones (in adolescent males and females) apparently lead to a rapid turnover of glandular cells and overproduction of sebum.

Concurrent with its action on the sebaceous gland, the arrector pili muscle pulls the hair shaft into an erect or semierect position. Known as "gooseflesh" or "goosepimples," this action represents an attempt to trap a thin layer of air against the skin to prevent loss of heat to the outside environment. Because hair is sparsely distributed over the human body, this mechanism is relatively ineffective. Arrector pili muscles are

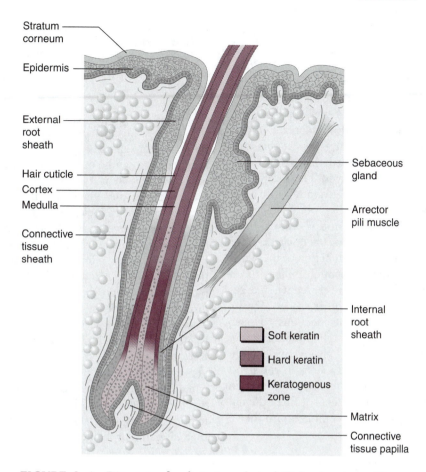

Stratum corneum

Epidermis

External root sheath

Hair cuticle

Cortex

Medulla

Connective tissue sheath

Sebaceous gland

Arrector pili muscle

Internal root sheath

Soft keratin

Hard keratin

Keratogenous zone

Matrix

Connective tissue papilla

FIGURE 2–4 Diagram of a hair in a hair follicle showing adjacent structures.

not associated with the hairs of the beard or pubic regions; they also are not found in the eyelids, eyebrows, or eyelashes.

Sweat Glands. (See **Fig. 2–1**.) Humans have two types of sweat glands: apocrine and eccrine. The apocrine glands are situated primarily in the axillary and genital regions. The eccrine (merocrine) glands are distributed throughout the body; large concentrations are found in the skin of the soles and palms.

Both the duct and the secretary parts of apocrine glands lie coiled in the dermis. Larger glands often extend deep into the hypodermis, subcutaneous connective tissue under the skin, also known as the superficial fascia.[12] The lumen is lined with a layer of cuboidal or low columnar cells that continuously secrete small amounts of sweat into the hair follicle and, occasionally, directly onto the surface of the skin. Apocrine

sweat glands, which are innervated by the autonomic nervous system, are activated primarily by emotional or painful stimuli.[2] At first, the sweat produced is odorless, but it is quickly contaminated and degraded by bacteria, thus causing its characteristic odor.

Eccrine sweat glands, excluding those found in the palms and soles, are activated by increased heat and are part of a thermoregulatory mechanism. The eccrine glands found in the palms and soles are activated primarily by changes in emotional state (eg, nervousness) rather than thermoregulation. The secretary part of the gland is situated in the subcutaneous tissue space immediately below the dermis (hypodermis). A tortuous duct courses through both layers of the skin, delivering sweat directly to the surface. Eccrine glands are innervated by the sympathetic division of the autonomic nervous system, and most are linked to and controlled by the hypothalamus.[3,4]

Vascular Supply

The epidermis is an avascular layer of cells that relies on diffusion of fluids for sustenance.[10] Unlike the epidermis, the dermis (especially the papillary layer) has an extensive vascular supply. Arteries supplying this region extend from the hypodermis and reach upward toward and through the reticular layer. At this level, an arterial network is established that gives rise to capillary beds in the papillary layer. These capillaries are especially numerous near the stratum basale of the epidermis (see **Fig. 2–2**).

The papillary layer of the dermis is drained of excess fluid by lymphatic capillaries lined with a single layer of endothelial cells. At the junction of these cells are fibrils that anchor the lymphatic capillary to enveloping connective tissue and are tensed when excess fluid accumulates in the intercellular spaces. Tension on the fibrils forces the cellular junctions to open, permitting fluid to enter the lymphatic capillary. Accumulated fluid moves through progressively larger lymphatic vessels that accompany veins in the hypodermis. These larger lymphatics become afferent ducts flowing toward lymph nodes that filter the collected fluid. Lymph eventually is emptied into the venous system by lymphatic ducts.

Tanning and Coloration

Skin color results from a combination of factors, including the relative abundance of melanocytes and the presence of blood. Melanocytes produce **melanin** (brown or black granules) in the strata basale and spinosum. Blood is found in networks of vessels in the reticular layer and deeper aspects of the papillary layer of the dermis (see **Fig. 2–1**).

Skin tanning is a protective mechanism against exposure to ultraviolet (UV) radiation, which stimulates the production of melanin in deeper strata. Melanin appears to ascend into the more superficial zones, causing a darkening of the skin as concentrations increase. Tanning partially blocks penetration of UV radiation, thus reducing injury secondary to sunburn or other damaging effects of UV radiation.

Caucasian skin has relatively small concentrations of melanin in the deeper strata. Interspersed blood vessels impart a pinkish tinge to the skin. Darker skin contains more melanin, which is distributed more homogeneously throughout the epidermis. Increased concentrations of carotene account for the orange or yellow skin tones characteristic of some populations. *Albinism* refers to skin that is unable to produce melanin and therefore is unable to block the harmful effect of UV radiation.

Neural Receptors

Because skin supports and maintains various types of **receptors,** it can be considered to be an integral part of the afferent (sensory) nervous system. Receptors in the epidermis, the dermis, and the hypodermis report sensory changes. **Nociceptors** transmit sensations of pain, **thermoreceptors** are sensitive to changes in temperature, and **mechanoreceptors** report changes in pressure, touch, vibration, or two-point discrimination (**Fig. 2–5**).[3] Although classification schemes for receptors vary, two general categories are commonly distinguished and are based in part on the status of encapsulation: free nerve endings, which are unencapsulated and unmyelinated as they approach the surface of the skin; and encapsulated (corpuscular) nerves, which have both myelinated and unmyelinated fibers (e.g., Meissner's corpuscles, which are mechanoreceptors).[13] **Table 2–1** summarizes the main receptors associated with the skin and indicates their sites and probable functions.

Wound Healing

Two types of wound healing can be distinguished. Simple incisions, which involve only minor loss of tissue and have edges that are closely approximated, heal by "primary intention." Surgical incisions typically heal in this manner. Large gaping wounds, which are characterized by substantial removal or loss of tissue and widely separated ragged edges, heal by "secondary intention." The main difference between the two types of wound healing is the type of wound created, not the ongoing physiologic processes, which are essentially the same.

Primary Intention Healing

Immediately after injury or incision, blood fills the space between the apposed edges of the wound, forming a small clot. An acute inflammatory response ensues, the end stage of which represents the beginning of a reparative process. Twenty-four to 36 hours after the injury, epithelial cells from the cut edges of the adjacent epidermis migrate into the small cavity

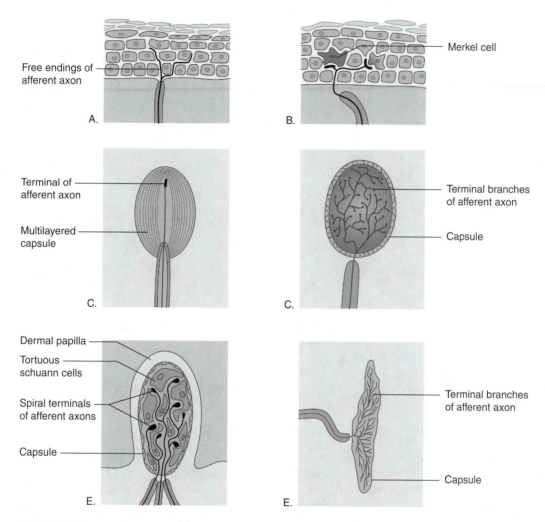

FIGURE 2–5 Nonencapsulated (A, B) and encapsulated (C–F) neural receptors embedded in the skin. A = free ending; B = Merkel ending; C = Pacinian corpuscle; D = Krause end bulb; E = Meissner's corpuscle; F = Ruffini corpuscle.

between the dermis and the previously formed clot to form a continuous sheet.[14,15] During the next 24 hours, epidermal cells migrate and invade the space where connective tissue will develop to complete the healing process. Next, rapid infiltration by capillary buds from the hypodermis and deposition of macrophages clear the area of debris. Vascularization of the wound facilitates the deposition of collagen fibers, which ultimately fill and repair the defect. The newly established tissue is strengthened through apparent bonding of adjacent collagen fibers. Eventually (within 6 to 12 months), the pinkish color imparted by vascularized tissue fades as vessels disintegrate and are reabsorbed. Over time the size of the scar decreases, in part because of remodeling forces gener-

ated by mechanical stresses created by muscular contractions and motion of the joints.[15]

Secondary Intention Healing

Healing by secondary intention initially involves an inflammatory period, followed by an ensuing reparative phase. First, a large clot fills the defect, consolidating and splinting the wound to cushion and protect it from further injury. Epidermal cells adjacent to the wound are then stimulated to migrate into the wound cavity between the clot above and the viable tissue below. Fibrolytic enzymes are apparently secreted by epidermal cells to break down necrotic tissue.[15] Debris is removed from the wound by an

TABLE 2–1 *Neural Receptors of the Skin*

Receptor	Encapsulation	Type[*]	Function	Location[†]	Distribution
Free nerve ending	No	T, M, N	Pain, temperature, pressure	Ep, Dr	Entire body[‡]
Meissner's corpuscles	Yes	M	Touch, 2-pt discrimination	Dr[ǁ]	Palms, soles,[§] fingers, toes (volar aspects), lips, eyelids, volar forearms, external genitalia
Pacinian corpuscles	Yes	M	Pressure, vibration	Hd	Hands, feet, penis, nipple
Ruffini organs	Yes	M	Proprioception	Dr?, HD	Entire body, tendons, ligaments, joint capsules, deep fascia

[*]T = thermoreceptor, M = mechanoreceptor, N = nociceptor.

[†]Ep = epidermis, Dr = dermis, Hd = hypodermis.

[‡]Nonglabrous (hair-covered) surfaces.

[§]Glabrous (without hair) surfaces.

[ǁ]Near epidermis.

More prevalent in visceral structures.

influx of phagocytes brought by capillaries that infiltrate the base of the wound from the hypodermis. The initial appearance of these cells as red dots or "granules" marks the emergence of granulation tissue.[1,15] The pinkish color of granulation tissue is the hallmark of a good healing outcome. Although granulation tissue also forms in wound healing by primary intention, considerably more is laid down in open wounds and thus quantitatively distinguishes secondary from primary intention healing. With the onset of granulation, the epidermis continues to migrate, ultimately covering the granulation tissue and establishing a line of demarcation between the scab and the new tissue below. Eventually, the scab is sloughed at this line. Through regenerative processes (mitosis), the epidermis gradually thickens and begins to organize into a multilayered covering. Because the new epidermis is typically thinner than the original tissue it replaced, it is less able to withstand mechanical stress, thus providing the possibility for reinjury.

The resultant scar, a consolidation of dense, randomly oriented collagen, is thicker and less compliant than the original tissue. Large, thick scars may become moderately or severely distorted. Skin contractures may develop and may restrict underlying structures, especially joints. Excessive collagen accumulates in a scar, especially after a burn, and may lead to the formation of hypertrophic scar tissue. The collagen of these raised nodular areas is initially deposited in an unorganized manner, which results in a cosmetically unsightly mass that may limit movement of the skin, joints, or both.[4]

Large scars, including keloids, are typically devoid of melanocytes and accessory skin organs, including hair follicles, sebaceous glands, sweat glands, and nerve receptors. Cutaneous receptors also may be absent. The loss of melanin in scar tissue makes these tissues sensitive to exposure to UV radiation, with greater heat buildup in the scar. Similarly, other forms of energy (e.g., electricity) conducted over or through a scar may be concentrated and cause thermal damage to adjacent tissues. Subsequent damage also may result from a lack of sensation in the affected area; thus, it is also necessary to take precautions when applying heat to an affected area. Because patients may be unaware of excessive accumulation of energy that can lead to burns in a denervated area, they need to limit their exposure to sunlight until scar thickness is reduced, cutaneous innervation regenerates, or both. Conversely, some physical agents may hasten wound healing and reduce or prevent adhesions and excessive scarring.

APPLICATION TO PHYSICAL THERAPY

Clinically, routine observation of the skin is an important element of physical examination. This chapter has described skin structure and related conditions that are either signs of health or signs of local or systemic disease. Preintervention observations may suggest that a particular physical agent is indicated, should be used cautiously, or should not be used at all. The following examples illustrate how some skin conditions might affect interventions with physical agents.

Breaks in the Skin.   Breaks in the skin may cause changes in the concentrations of electrolytes in body fluids or invite infections or cross-contamination. Such breaks may indicate that sterile techniques are necessary, especially if hydrotherapy is indicated. Areas with no skin (e.g., a decubitus ulcer) have markedly less electrical resistance. Thus, when electrical modalities are used, current should be applied carefully over such areas because far less voltage is needed than is required over intact skin.

Rough or Thick Skin.   Because the electrical resistance of rough or thick skin is greatly increased, such skin should be abraded. This procedure will reduce the voltage needed to permit the flow of an electrical current.

Thick Scars.   Because energy tends to concentrate in scarred areas, infrared, UV, and other radiation therapies should be used cautiously over these areas. If the areas are covered and protected, the intervention may be given to areas around, rather than over, the scar. Again, it is necessary to take precautions when applying heat to the area.

Sensory Receptors.   Intact sensory receptors and nerves may contribute to the relief of symptoms and enable the patient to report whether the selected intervention dosage is intense enough to cause pain or tissue damage. If the sensory receptors are not intact, most thermal and electrical modalities should be used cautiously or not at all because the patient cannot report the intensity of the dosage.

Glands.   Sebaceous glands lubricate the skin. Excessive use of water or radiation modalities tend to reduce the amount of sebum available and cause dryness. However, if the goal is to diminish the activity of the gland—for example, when treating acne—hydrotherapy or radiation may be useful. Overactive sweat glands can be treated with various unidirectional (galvanic) electrical modalities that may retard sweating.

Color.   Because bluish-black color of the skin indicates severe circulatory problems, heat therapies in that area are generally contraindicated. Sometimes, however, mild heat, if used cautiously, can be applied in an attempt to achieve a slight increase in blood flow to the area. Electrical stimulation that produces muscle contractions, thereby increasing blood flow, may also be used.

The patient's skin color must be carefully noted before interventions. When using UV radiation, both the potentially beneficial and potentially harmful effects are related to the color of the skin being irradiated. Remember that the skin color of both the patient and the treating clinician must be considered. Therapists or patients with albinism should not be exposed to UV radiation.

Skin that is highly pigmented requires special attention when determining the presence of erythema, cynanosis, or other change of skin color. The quantity and composition of melanin in the skin varies dramatically among ethnic groups.[16] Thong et al.[17] note that "Europeans, Chinese, and Mexicans have approximately half as much melanin as the most darkly pigmented (African and Indian) skin types." Further, skin that is typically exposed during the day is consistently darker in pigmentation than skin that is covered.[17] The research literature is lacking documentation on the best method of assessing changes in skin color in people with high pigmentation.[17] On the basis of an informal survey of clinicians, comparison to adjacent skin for erythema, temperature, turgor, and sensory integrity is presently the method of choice.

After intervention, the condition of the patient's skin should again be noted. Therapists must be able to recognize and distinguish between normal, acceptable changes and changes that indicate an overdose or abnormal reactions to intervention.

REVIEW QUESTIONS

1. What are the most important functions of the skin?
2. What is the significance of skin appearing shiny, dry, and hairless?
3. What is the significance of Langer's lines in regard to skin healing?
4. Describe the role of sebaceous and sweat glands.
5. Describe the role of melanin in skin protection.
6. List and describe the three types of neural receptors located in the skin.
7. Describe primary intention healing.
8. Describe secondary intention healing.

KEY TERMS

jaundice
cyanosis
erythema
blisters
blebs
wheals
hives
epidermis

stratum basal
stratum spinosum
stratum granulosum
stratum lucidum
stratum corneum
dermis (corium)
 papillary layer
 reticular layer

keloids
sebaceous glands
sebum
melanin
receptors
 nociceptors
 thermoreceptors
 mechanoreceptors

REFERENCES

1. Myers B: *Wound Management, Principles, and Practice.* Upper Saddle River, NJ: Prentice Hall; 2004.

2. Kelly DE, Wood RL, Enders, AC: *Bailey's Textbook of Histology.* 18th ed. Baltimore: Williams & Wilkins; 1984.

3. Ross MH, Romrell LJ, Gordon IK: *Histology: A Text and Atlas.* 3rd ed. Philadelphia: Lippincott Williams & Wilkins; 1995.

4. Fitzpatrick TB, Eizen AZ, Wollf K, Freidberg IM, Austin KF. eds: *Dermatology in General Medicine.* 3rd ed. New York: McGraw Hill; 1987.

5. Salter RB: *Textbook of Disorders and Injuries of the Musculoskeletal System: An Introduction to Orthopaedics, Fractures and Joint Injuries and Rheumatology.* 3rd ed. Baltimore: Williams & Wilkins; 1998.

6. Goodman CC, Boissonnault WG, Fuller KS: *Pathology: Implications for the Physical Therapist.* 2nd ed. Philadelphia: Saunders; 2003.

7. Griffin J: *Physical Agents for Physical Therapists.* 2nd ed. Springfield, IL: Charles C Thomas; 1982.

8. *Miller-Keane Encyclopedia and Dictionary of Medicine, Nursing, and Allied Health.* Philadelphia: Saunders; 1992; p. 514.

9. Cotran RS, Collins T, Robbins SL, Kumar V: *Robbins Pathologic Basis of Disease.* 6th ed. Philadelphia: WB Saunders; 1998.

10. Williams, PL, Bannister LH, Martin MB, Collins P, Dysan M, Dussek JE, Ferguson MWJ (eds): *Gray's Anatomy: The Anatomical Basis of Medicine and Surgery.* 38th ed. New York: Churchill Livingstone; 1995.

11. Nelson RM, Currier DP (eds): *Clinical Electrotherapy.* 2nd ed. Norwalk, CT: Appleton and Lange; 1991.

12. Montagna W, Carlisle KS, Kligman AM: *Atlas of Normal Human Skin.* Portland, OR: New Books, Inc.; 1992.

13. Kandel ER, Schwartz JH, Jessell TM: *Principles of Neural Science.* 3rd ed. New York: Elsevier; 1991.

14. Walter JB: *An Introduction to the Principles of Disease.* 3rd ed. Philadelphia: WB Saunders; 1992.

15. Walter JB: *An Introduction to the Principles of Disease.* 3rd ed. Philadelphia: WB Saunders; 1992.

16. Kloth LC, McCulloch JM: *Wound Healing: Alternatives in Management.* 3rd ed. Philadelphia: F.A. Davis Company; 2002.

17. Thong HY, Jee SH, Sun CC, Boissy RE: The Patterns of Melanosome Distribution in Keratinocytes of Human Skin as One Determining Factor of Skin Colour. *British Journal of Dermatology,* 2003; 149(3):498–505.

3

The Circulatory System

BERNADETTE HECOX, PT, MA
JOHN P. SANKO, PT, PhD

Chapter Outline

Many physical agents can affect the vascular and/or lymphatic systems of the peripheral circulation. Depending on the agent and the patient's status, the agent may be beneficial or harmful. This chapter reviews these systems as they apply to the use of the physical agents discussed in later chapters. It focuses on the circulation to skin, muscle, and bone.

PERIPHERAL VASCULAR SYSTEM

Blood leaves the heart through the arterial system and flows through arteries that continually branch and diminish in size. Eventually, the blood flows to the arterioles, the smallest arteries, and then to the capillary beds. At the capillary region, O_2 and other nutrients are dispersed to the tissues, and CO_2 and other wastes enter the blood stream. This deoxygenated blood returns to the heart through the venous system[*]: first through venules, the smallest veins; thence from smaller to larger veins; and eventually to the great veins, which carry the blood back to the heart. The blood flow continues through the pulmonary system to the lungs, where the wastes are exchanged for nutrients, then returns to the heart to repeat the cycle.

Control of Blood Flow

Control of blood flow is largely related to the circumference of the **lumen,** or hollow center, of blood vessels. The circumference can actively change through **vasoconstriction** and **vasodilation.** Narrowing or widening of the lumen can be the result of central nervous system control, local reactions, humoral control, or all of these mechanisms. The exact involvement of each is, as yet, not completely known.

Control by the Central Nervous System.   The sympathetic branch of the autonomic system carries both vasoconstricting and vasodilating fibers. Vasoconstriction occurs in the superficial blood vessels that supply the skin, whereas vasodilation generally occurs in the deep blood vessels that supply skeletal muscle when the sympathetic nervous system is activated. Chemical transmitters are released from the nerve endings at target areas. The adrenergic nerves release norepi-

nephrine, which acts directly on the receptors of smooth muscle within the vessels to cause vasoconstriction. Normal vascular motor tone represents a continuous mild vasoconstriction. Cholinergic nerves release acetylcholine (ACh), which causes vessels to dilate. The specific action of ACh is not known: ACh may act to diminish the release of norepinephrine, thereby inhibiting constriction, or it may produce dilation directly.

Control by Local Reactions.   Vasoactive agents released in local tissues, including histamine, bradykinin, and some of the prostaglandins, may act to dilate vessels or to affect the endothelial cells of the vessels directly. This activity of endothelial cells may leave gaps between cells, thereby increasing the permeability of the cell membrane. Histamine is released whenever tissues are damaged or are subjected to a noxious stimulus. Formation of bradykinin results from activation of precursor enzymes and may be related to the activity of sweat glands.

Humoral Control.   Humoral control of vasomotor tone refers to the effect of all the substances mentioned above as well as that of many other ions: these ions not only act locally but also travel in the bloodstream. The concentration of ions in the bloodstream affects vasomotor activity.[2,3]

Thermal Regulatory Function

The peripheral vascular system serves to regulate the temperature of both local tissues and the body. Two of the ways in which it accomplishes this are by transferring **heat** to and from vessels, other tissues, and the environment, and by transferring **blood** through the peripheral circulatory systems and between the peripheral and other circulatory systems.

Heat Transfer

The peripheral vascular system is one major means by which loss and gain of body heat are controlled. Heat is transported by the circulating blood, and heat exchange occurs between blood and other tissues and/or the environment. The location and the arrangement of the vessels also affect the distribution of body heat. Blood returns to the heart through both deep and superficial veins. The superficial veins located in the superficial fascia travel various courses before joining major veins. For example, the saphenous veins in the legs remain superficial until they join the deep

---

[*]Although venous blood is often called "deoxygenated" blood, this term is a misnomer in the purest sense because venous blood still contains O_2 but less of it than does arterial blood. For example, partial pressure of O_2 in arterial blood can be 95 mm Hg; in venous blood, it can be 40 mm Hg.[1]

femoral veins at the groin, and the cephalic veins in the arms are superficial until they join the axillary veins. In general, deep veins run parallel to the arteries (**Fig. 3–1**). The arrangement of two or more veins parallel to an artery is referred to as **venae comitantes.**[4] To some extent, this parallel position influences both core and tissue temperatures.

The blood leaving the heart is at approximately core temperature. Depending on the temperature of tissues, the environment, or both in the cutaneous capillary region, the incoming arterial blood may be warmer or cooler than the venous blood that is flowing in the opposite direction in veins adjacent to the arteries. For example, in a cold environment, in blood leaving the capillaries, venous blood will be cooler than arterial blood. Until the temperature of the parallel veins and arteries is in equilibrium, some heat will transfer to the arteries or veins carrying the cooler blood, thus contributing to the maintenance of a constant core temperature.

This conductive transfer of heat (not blood) is termed **countercurrent exchange (CCE).** In hotter environmental conditions, more venous blood appears to be directed through superficial veins; in colder environmental conditions, it appears to be directed through the deep-lying venae comitas.[5] **Figure 3–2** illustrates the CCE that might occur in the arm (1) if the room temperature is 50°F (10°C), with more blood flowing through the deeper veins, and (2) if the room temperature is 86°F (30°C), with more blood flowing through the superficial veins.

Heat transfer by conduction also occurs between the blood vessels and the tissues through which they pass. Usually, the deeper the tissues, the higher their temperature. Although the heat exchange with either adjacent vessels or other tissues is a factor in maintaining a constant core temperature, the exchange is limited because of the rapid velocity at which blood flows through any area. Heat exchange is especially limited in areas where the temperature gradient between either the adjacent vessels or other tissues is low.

Shunting Mechanisms. When the demand for blood to a particular area of the body is greater than the amount usually provided (eg, when the temperature of the tissues in that area is dangerously increased or decreased), the mechanism of *shunting* can occur. In general, **shunting** refers to the temporary closing or reduction of blood flow to one area of the body so

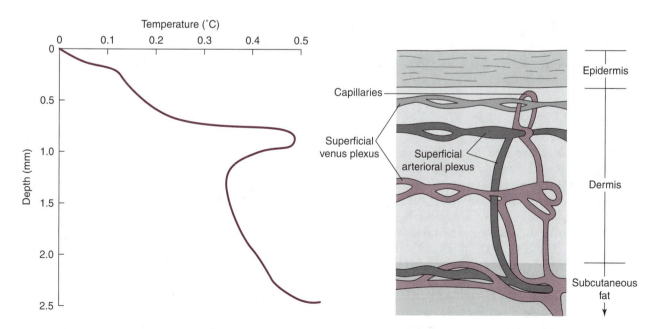

FIGURE 3–1   Diagrammatic rendering of the skin and subcutaneous circulation. On reaching the subcutaneous layer, the arteries and veins follow a similar course.

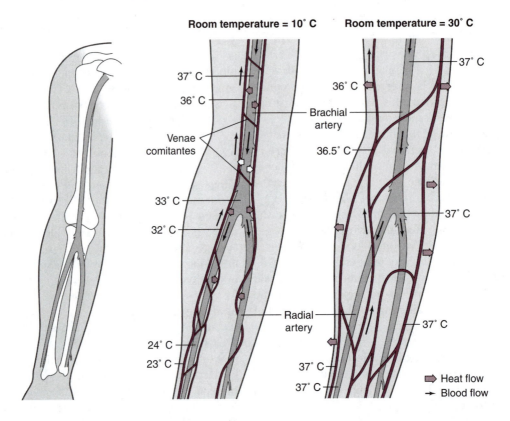

Room temperature = 10° C   Room temperature = 30° C

37° C

36° C

Venae comitantes

33° C

32° C

24° C

23° C

37° C

36° C

Brachial artery

36.5° C

Radial artery

37° C

37° C

37° C

37° C

37° C

➡ Heat flow
→ Blood flow

FIGURE 3–2   Countercurrent heat exchange in the human arm. Intravascular temperatures show that patterns of venous blood flow in the arm adjust to counteract thermal environmental stress. In the cold (10°C), venous blood flow is mainly through the deep venae comitantes, which receive heat from blood flowing out in the arteries and thereby minimize loss of body heat. In a warm environment (30°C), venous blood flow is mainly in superficial veins that, being close to the surface, increase the loss of body heat. Note the various courses of the veins situated in the superficial fascia and the parallel courses of the deep arteries and veins.

that more blood can flow to another area that is in danger of being damaged. Three shunt mechanisms can be activated by thermal agents, fevers, or environmental conditions: anteriovenous (A-V) shunts that are found in the skin of the nose, ears, tongue, erectile sexual tissue, hands, and feet; shunts from deeper systems to the cutaneous circulation; and shunts to and from different branches of the peripheral circulation. *A-V shunts (arteriovenous anastomosis)* involve specific vessels through which blood flows only under extremely hot or cold conditions. These shunts are described later in this chapter. The shunting of blood to the cutaneous circulation, while reducing the flow to deeper circulatory systems, brings more blood to the

surface for cooling when the internal temperature is elevated. The shunting of blood to and from various branches of the peripheral circulation is discussed more in Chapter 9.[6,7] In extremely hot weather, half of the total cardiac output is shunted from elsewhere to the skin.

Of interest to physical therapists is the evidence that branches to the superficial and deeper muscles are not derived from the same vessels. Vessels passing through superficial muscles are mainly the superficial capillaries and their terminal arterioles and venules, whereas the circulation to the underlying deep muscles is completely independent of the cutaneous circulation.[8] Thus, shunting does not occur between superficial and underlying muscles in a local area. Blood flow to deep muscles appears to be directly related to their metabolic demands. An extremely low percentage of total blood flows through muscles at rest, but the percentage can increase 15- to 25-fold with exercise.[3] The clinical implication is that active exercise is the best choice for increasing blood flow to muscle and is not necessarily a superficial thermal agent.

Determinants of Arterial and Capillary Flow

Arterial Flow.   The blood pressure and the amount of blood flow to the capillaries are determined by cardiac stroke volume and peripheral resistance. Factors controlling peripheral resistance include the size and pliability of arterial vessels and the integrity of the smooth muscles in these vessels. When the smooth muscles within the arteries and arterioles contract, the vessels constrict, which increases the peripheral resistance to blood flow, thus increasing the blood pressure. When these muscles relax, the vessels dilate, allowing more profuse flow and decreasing the blood pressure. When tissue metabolism increases, the vessels supplying those tissues dilate, thus increasing the amount of blood flow to the area necessary to meet its metabolic demands. Neural problems affecting the sympathetic nervous system or **peripheral vascular disease** may alter the normal processes of constriction and dilation. For example, **arteriosclerosis,** which narrows the lumen of the arteries and renders them less pliable, prevents normal flow to the capillaries.

Capillary Flow.   **Capillaries,** the vessels that connect the arterioles and venules, are composed of a single layer of endothelial cells surrounded by a more or less continuous basement membrane.[9] Metabolically, the endothelium is highly active and can synthesize or break down many chemical substances.[10] Variations in capillary structure are categorized according to the type of organs in which they are situated (ie, somatic or visceral) or by their histological appearance.[9] Because capillaries are microscopic in size, averaging 5 μm in diameter, blood cells must adapt in shape to pass through them.[10] One square inch of tissue may have as many as 1.5 million capillaries.[11] The diameter of each capillary is extremely small; however, if all the capillaries in one area were combined, their total area, taken in cross section, would be far greater than the cross

section of the large arteries and veins for which they are connecting channels.

The capillary membrane is semipermeable, allowing the O_2 and nutrients in arterial blood to be transported through this membrane to the interstitial fluid and hence to body cells. Carbon dioxide and wastes are transported in the opposite direction and return to the heart through venous and lymphatic vessels.

The transport of blood gases such as O_2 and CO_2 across capillary membranes occurs by diffusion. Water and small solutes such as glucose and amino acids pass through intercellular clefts between endothelial cells. Proteins, which are large water solutes, are transported either through wider clefts or by vesicles that enable them to move across the endothelium.[12] Fluids are transported via filtration caused by hydrostatic and osmotic pressure (see Chapter 5).

Precisely how transport occurs across the membrane is under investigation.[12] Although the structural basis determines the permeability of capillaries,[13] vasoactive substances, including bradykinin, histamine, and the prostaglandins, are believed to participate, either directly or by interaction, in altering the permeability of the capillary membrane.[12]

There is general agreement that transcapillary transport increases as the temperature increases. But how much is the result of the decreased viscosity of blood that occurs with a rise in temperature, alterations in the geometry of the transcapillary pathway, or other mechanisms has not been fully explained.[10,14]

Aterioventricular Shunts

A-V shunts (arteriovenous anastomosis) are anatomic channels that connect arterioles directly with venules. The function of these shunts is to protect cutaneous tissues from damage caused by excessive heat or cold, and possibly to prevent extremely high core temperatures.[15] When the temperature of peripheral tissue is within the normal range, these shunts are closed; however, they open when the temperature of tissues is high or low enough to endanger them. When shunts are open, a large amount of blood flows through them, increasing local blood flow. These shunts are coiled channels with thick musculature that is under the control of the sympathetic nervous system. This central control activates the shunts when the tissue temperature increases to approximately 104°F (40°C),[11] reducing the sympathetic vasoconstrictor tone[16] and thus increasing cutaneous blood flow and enhancing heat loss.

The shunting activity caused by cold appears to be a strictly local response with no need for central input. Evidence indicates that at specific cold temperatures, various neurotransmitters that control vasoconstriction and dilation are released and that these neurotransmitters may control the activity of the shunts.[16] Some authors have theorized that an "axon reflex" (see Chapter 9) may activate these shunts.[17] When shunts open as a result of tissue cooling, blood continues to flow through the area by bypassing the capillaries, thus rewarming the skin of the tissues. Although shunts are found throughout the skin, they are richly concentrated in the areas most susceptible to damage by cold: the fingers, toes, nail beds, face, lips, and ears.

Determinants of Venous Flow

In addition to its function of controlling both local tissue and core temperatures, the peripheral venous system is responsible for transporting deoxygenated blood and much of the metabolic waste away from local tissues. Removal of metabolic wastes can reduce pain and muscle spasms caused by excessive accumulation of acid in muscles or other tissues. The return of blood to the heart is controlled by (1) the blood pressure gradient, (2) the integrity of the valves and muscles of the veins, (3) "muscle pumps," and (4) the volume of flow.

Blood Pressure Gradient. The amount of pressure and the **pressure gradient** are crucial determinants of venous flow. Fluid always flows in the direction from higher to lower pressure. If no pressure gradient is present, no blood flows. The gradual decrease in blood pressure that occurs along the path of the vessels after blood leaves the heart dictates the direction of flow. Venous pressure, which is lower than arterial pressure, gradually declines to just a few mm Hg before entering the right atrium of the heart; thus, blood accumulates in the veins. Obviously, the pressure gradient factor alone cannot maintain a sufficient flow of blood to the heart (**Fig. 3–3**). The other three factors mentioned earlier help to increase the rate of venous return.

Integrity of the Veins. Although muscles in the walls of veins are not as numerous as they are in arterial vessels, they do contract and relax to assist the pumping of blood through the veins. As blood passes through the veins, with each stroke the pressure increases as the muscles contract, and decreases when the muscles relax. During each stroke the increase in pressure forces bicuspid valves in the veins to open; between strokes, as muscles relax, the valves close. The "one-way" valve mechanism prevents a backflow of blood between strokes. However, distended or **varicose veins** limit adequate closing of the valves, which makes the valves less effective and the flow of blood toward the heart more difficult (**Fig. 3–4**).

Muscle Pumps. Rhythmical contractions of skeletal muscle also help pump and maintain venous flow. Venous flow in the legs is assisted by the tricep surae

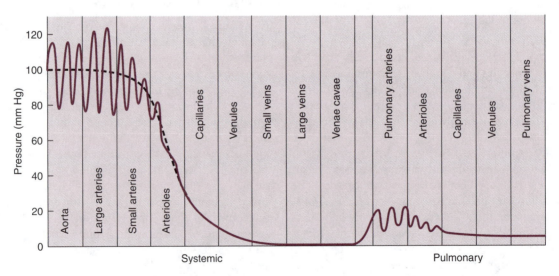

FIGURE 3–3   Blood pressures in the various portions of the circulatory system. *(Reproduced with permission from Guyton & Hall.* Textbook of Medical Physiology, *9/E. Elsevier, 1995.)*

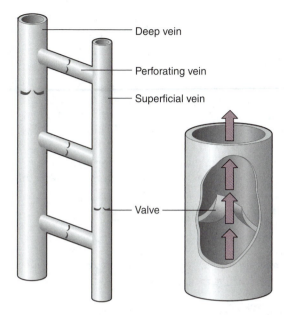

FIGURE 3–4 The venous valves of the legs. *(Reproduced with permission from Guyton & Hall.* Textbook of Medical Physiology, 9/E. *Elsevier, 1995.)*

muscles in particular, and in the trunk it is assisted primarily by the abdominal muscles. Actions of the muscles in the trunk are often called the abdominal and respiratory pumps. When these muscles are less active, as occurs in prolonged bed rest, fluids that are usually returned by veins and lymph vessels may accumulate in the distal extremities. To prevent this accumulation of fluid, *the legs of nonambulatory patients need to be positioned frequently at horizontal or elevated levels,* and external pressures such as elastic bandages or stockings should be applied.

Volume of Flow. Normally, two-thirds of the peripheral blood supply is on the venous side. Whenever a higher-than-normal percentage of blood remains on the venous side, the volume of blood returning to the heart is decreased. A reduction in cardiac filling ultimately results in less than normal cardiac output.

Any conditions that retard venous return to the heart create a condition called **venous pooling.** Wherever venous pooling occurs, more deoxygenated blood remains in tissues. This stagnant blood may cause stasis ulcers or other stasis dermatological conditions.

Venous pooling can also be caused by systemic problems such as congestive heart failure (CHF). If the heart is unable to pump enough blood through the pulmonary system, as is the case in CHF, blood may be dammed up on the venous side. The venous pressure gradient may reverse, becoming higher in veins near the heart than in those near the capillaries. Pooling of venous blood in the extremities would then indicate that excessive fluid already exists in the region of the lungs and heart. In such systemic conditions, the use of any physical agents that may force fluid back to the thoracic region is contraindicated.

LYMPHATIC SYSTEM

The lymphatic system begins in the capillary area. Lymph channels have openings that can expand enough to permit proteins as well as other large molecules to pass from the interstitium into the lymphatic system. The interstitial fluid, including large molecules, that passes through these channels is termed **lymph.**

Like veins, lymphatic channels contain valves; thus, the lymph can move in only one direction. Much like venous flow, any pressure from contraction of the walls of the lymphatic channels themselves or from outside pressure such as muscle contractions will squeeze these channels and cause the lymph to move toward the heart. The lymph flowing through the channels from the upper-right quadrant of the body empties into the right lymphatic duct. The rest of the body's channels drain into the thoracic duct. Ultimately, the lymph ducts join the great veins near the heart, where the lymph mixes with the venous blood returning to the heart.[9]

Lymph nodes are situated along the route of the lymphatic vessels and are arranged in clusters at various locations throughout the body. Much, but not all, of the lymph passes through and temporarily accumulates in these nodes. When the nodes must be surgically removed, some of the lymph flowing toward the great veins may be blocked.

The lymphatic process, as presented here, is based on the most commonly accepted theory. However, mounting evidence indicates that lymphatic return to venous blood may take place by somewhat different pathways (see **Chapter 5**).[12]

An understanding of the physiologic activities of all body systems and the way physical agents affect them is the basis for determining the indications, contraindications, and cautious use of physical agents in patient interventions.

APPLICATION TO PHYSICAL THERAPY

The peripheral circulatory systems must function properly to supply the body tissues with oxygen and other nutrients; remove excess fluids, CO_2, and metabolic wastes; and help maintain a constant body temperature. Malfunctioning of some parts of these systems can occur for a variety of reasons.

Because humans are bipedal, gravity is a powerful force in reducing blood flow from distal segments of the extremities—especially from the lower limbs—back to the heart. With increasing age, or with certain lifestyles, the risk of some type of peripheral vascular disease is relatively high.

Peripheral vascular disease (PVD) is a general name for any problems involving the peripheral circulatory systems. These problems range from mild to severe to even life-threatening. Peripheral vascular disease includes problems related to the arterial, venous, or lymphatic circulations. (The lymphatic dysfunctions are discussed in **Chapter 5.**)

Arterial Dysfunction

Factors preventing normal arterial function include the following: (1) cardiac problems, which *prevent* sufficient cardiac stroke volume; (2) dysfunction of the sympathetic nerves, which control constriction and dilation of the smooth muscles within the vessels or deficiencies in the arterial vessels; and (3) *arteriolosclerosis*, a thickening of the walls of the arterioles, which causes a loss of pliability that reduces the ability of the vessel to constrict and dilate. In turn, this decreases the flow of oxygenated blood.

Clinical Signs and Symptoms. The skin may be paler or cooler than normal. The pulse may be weak, which can be determined by palpating the radial pulse in the upper extremities and the dorsal pulse or posterior tibial pulses. Leg cramps are a common complaint.

Physical Therapy Interventions. Extremities can be alternately elevated and lowered to allow gravity to help the flow of blood through the arterial vessels. In addition, brief periods of walking should be encouraged, and patients with severe arterial dysfunction should stand for very brief periods throughout the day.

Whenever there is a lack of oxygenated blood flow, physical agents must be used cautiously. The affected extremity should be kept warm, but intense heat modalities must be avoided because they increase tissue metabolism. To prevent tissue damage, the circulation must meet metabolic demands for oxygen. Although intermittent pneumatic compression pumps are sometimes used, the specific recommended dosages must be followed carefully.

Details of intervention for arteriole insufficiency are beyond the scope of this chapter; however, clinicians are advised to become knowledgeable in this area before performing any aggressive therapies.

Venous Dysfunction

The common venous dysfunctions are varicose veins, local stasis ulcers, and phlebitis and thrombosis.

Varicose Veins. This condition refers to veins that are distended and often twisted. Whenever excessive amounts of blood are pooled in the veins for a prolonged period, the increase in venous pressure can cause the vessels to become permanently enlarged. This condition prevents the valves from closing. As a result, these valves become incompetent. Because gravitational forces tend to draw fluids downward, **varicose veins** often occur in the lower extremities, where varicosities can develop in superficial or deep veins.

Superficial varicosities are visible and can be diagnosed easily, but the diagnosis of varicosities of deeper veins requires specific testing. Skin in the involved area may be bluer or paler than normal because of the accumulation of deoxygenated blood. Patients commonly complain of pressure or pain in the affected extremity.

Stasis Ulcers. **Stasis ulcers** are caused by the lack of oxygen and decreased clearing of CO_2 and metabolites from a local area. They develop as the duration and severity of varicosities increases.

Clinical Signs and Symptoms. In the early stages, patients may complain of tenderness in the area, and rashes can be observed. If untreated, the condition can eventually progress to open (superficial) ulcers.

Phlebitis and Thrombosis. **Phlebitis** is an inflammation within the vein. **Venous thrombosis** involves formation of a crusty clot on the inside wall of the vein that usually occurs as a consequence of the phlebitis. Whenever these conditions exist, there is danger of the clot's detaching from the wall. A dislodged clot is called an *embolism*, which may travel through the bloodstream and lodge elsewhere in the veins or in the lungs or, rarely, the heart. The result may be local necrosis, a heart attack, or death.

Clinical Signs and Symptoms.   Areas of phlebitis are usually warm, pink, swollen, and tender. A superficial thrombosis can be palpated. The most common location is the lower leg, with pain/tenderness elicited upon stretching. Although therapists sometimes test for deep-vein thrombosis by applying deep pressure to an area to elicit pain, this test is not conclusive. Positive results serve as a warning that the patient should be seen by a cardiovascular specialist. Diagnostic tests that include a Doppler ultrasound can be used to detect obstructions in normal venous blood flow. The normal venous sounds that can be detected with the Doppler will be absent proximal to the thrombus formation. *Negative tests do not confirm the absence of a deep thrombus.* Whenever a thrombus is suspected, a cardiovascular specialist should be notified. Any PT intervention is contraindicated in the presence of deep vein thrombosis.

Physical Therapy Procedures.   Before any interventions are initiated, the patient must be thoroughly tested to determine the type and severity of the vascular problem. For less severe venous problems, the following therapeutic procedures are usually indicated to prevent more serious problems:

- Patients with problems in the lower extremities should be encouraged to walk, run, rise on their toes, and so forth to maximize muscle contrac-tions. Static standing should be discouraged because it may increase venous pooling.
- The involved extremity should be elevated at least to a horizontal position whenever possible.
- Gentle massage can be given to move the stagnant blood and relieve the pressure. If a thrombus is suspected, however, *massage is contraindicated.*
- Intermittent pneumatic compression interventions are commonly given, often followed by exercises with the involved extremities elevated to a near-vertical position to take advantage of the gravitational force. At the end of the intervention, an elasticized garment or ace bandage is applied immediately, while the extremity is in an elevated position.
- Electrical stimulation as well as active exercises are recommended for the intermittent pumping action of the muscles in the extremity.
- If extremities are cold, only mild local heat should be used.
- With any peripheral vascular disease, patients should be advised against wearing tight bands, such as garters, that may interfere with circulation.

The clinical considerations presented in this chapter are by no means complete. They represent a sample that will help the reader understand the relationship between the anatomy and the physiology of the peripheral circulation and the reasons that physical agents may or may not be indicated for patients with peripheral circulatory problems.

REVIEW QUESTIONS

1. Describe the way that the circulatory system responds with either heat conservation or heat dissipation when exposed to thermal stimuli.
2. Identify the vasoactive substances that influence transcapillary transport of vascular fluid.
3. Identify the factors that influence the return of blood to the heart from the venous system.
4. Provide the therapeutic rationale for use of external compression with socks or bandages for an individual who is nonambulatory.
5. Identify the factors that affect normal arterial blood flow.
6. Identify the clinical signs and symptoms associated with arterial dysfunction.
7. Identify the clinical signs and symptoms associated with venous dysfunction.
8. Describe the condition of phlebitis, and include the clinical signs and symptoms associated with it.
9. Describe the circulation of lymphatic fluid in the body.
10. Describe the differences in lower-leg positioning between individuals with arterial dysfunction and venous dysfunction.

KEY TERMS

heat	peripheral vascular disease	varicose veins
lumen	arteriosclerosis	venous pooling
vasoconstriction	capillaries	lymph
vasodilation	A-V shunts	stasis ulcers
venae comitantes	pressure gradient	phlebitis
countercurrent exchange (CCE)	blood	venous thrombosis

REFERENCES

1. Selkurt E, ed: *Basic Physiology for the Health Sciences*. 2nd ed. Boston: Little, Brown; 1982; 344.

2. Roddie IC, Shepherd JT, Abboud FM, eds: Circulation to skin and adipose tissue. In: *Handbook of Physiology*, 2nd ed. Bethesda, MD: American Physiological Society; 1984; 285–317.

3. Guyton AC: *Textbook of Medical Physiology*. 10th ed. Philadelphia: WB Saunders; 2000.

4. *Stedman's Medical Dictionary*. 25th ed. Baltimore: Williams & Wilkins; 1990.

5. Leithead C, Lind A: *Heat Stress and Heat Disorders*. Philadelphia: FA Davis; 1964; 10.

6. Rowell L: Human cardiovascular adjustments to exercise and thermal stress. *Physiol Rev*. 1974; 54:75–159.

7. Rowell L, Marx H, Bruce R, et al: Reductions in cardiac output, central blood volume, and stroke volume with thermal stress in normal men during exercise. *Clin Invest*. 1966; 45:1801–16.

8. Weinbaum S, Jiji LM, Lemons D: Theory and experiment for the effect of vascular microstructure on surface heat transfer. *Biomech Eng*. 1984; 106:337.

9. Carola R, Harley J, Noback C: *Human Anatomy & Physiology*, New York: McGraw-Hill; 1990.

10. Noring S: Dynamics of blood flow. *P & S J* (Columbia University College of Physicians & Surgeons). Fall 1983:4–13.

11. Lockhart R, Hamilton G, Fyfe F: *Anatomy of the Human Body*. Philadelphia: JB Lippincott; 1965: *Vascular System*. 586; 583.

12. Baez S, Knobel E, eds: Microcirculation. In: *Ann Rev Physiol*. Palo Alto, CA: Ann Rev Inc. 1977; 39:394, 400–407.

13. Mellander S, Hall VE, eds: Systemic circulation: Local control. In: *Ann Rev Physiol*. Palo Alto, CA: Ann Rev Inc. 1970; 32:313–344.

14. Wolf M, Watson P: Effects of temperature on transcapillary water movement in isolated cat hindlimb. *Am J Physiol*. 249(4):H792–H798.

15. Hales J, Iriki M, Tsuchiijak K, et al: Thermally induced cutaneous sympathetic activity related to blood flow through capillaries and arteriovenous anastomoses. *Pflug Arch*. 1978; 375:17–24.

16. Lehmann J, ed: Heat. In: *Therapeutic Heat and Cold*. 3rd ed. Baltimore: Williams & Wilkins; 1982; 418. Chap 10. Lehmann & DeLatteur: Therapeutic Heat 464–562.

17. Shepherd J, Vanhoutte P: Cold vasoconstriction and cold vasodilation in Vanhoutte P, Leusen I, eds: *Vasodilation*. New York: Raven Press; 1981; 263–71.

4

Wound Management

R. SCOTT WARD, PT, PhD

Chapter Outline

Injury to the skin is a significant problem, with possible complications including chronic inflammation, infection, and scarring. The damage must be remedied by all means available. Some physical agents are used as direct interventions for a variety of integumentary wounds. Wounds are often associated with other impairments such as pain and decreased mobility and motor function. Physical agents may also be useful direct interventions or adjuncts to the interventions with impairments associated with wounds. Knowledge of types of wounds and documentation of wounds will help the therapist not only determine potential uses of physical agents on some wounds but also determine the effectiveness of the application of selected physical agents to interventions with those wounds.

OVERVIEW OF WOUNDS

To be able to document the effectiveness of any physical agent in interventions with wounds, it is important to understand wound etiology and the impact of wound depth, size, location, inflammation, and scarring on expected prognosis.

Phases of Wound Healing

It is important to be aware that the phases of wound healing represent a continuum of the healing processes that overlap in time and are not separate, mutually exclusive episodes.

Inflammatory Phase. The **inflammatory phase** heralds the beginning of healing. This phase of healing consists of vascular responses to injury that include initial vascular constriction to decrease blood loss and to allow for more efficient clotting followed by vasodilatation to deliver chemicals, cells, nutrients, and oxygen to the injured tissue. Chemicals delivered to the site of injury promote capillary permeability, chemotaxis (cell movement along a chemical concentration gradient, positively or negatively), and cellular function, including the stimulation of fibroblast and macrophage activity. Among the cells delivered to the site are macrophages, leukocytes, and lymphocytes. Increased capillary permeability allows the conveyance of these cells to the tissue but also leads to formation of localized edema. Where the wound is indolent, the inflammatory phase may actually be induced by the use of physical agents to achieve better wound healing.

Proliferative Phase. The **proliferative phase** of wound healing is typified by the chemotactic convergence of fibroblasts to the site. The phase commences when fibroblasts arrive and begin to produce collagen to rebuild and strengthen the site of injury. The collagen scaffold supplied by the fibroblasts supports new vascular tissue. Re-epithelialization occurs during this phase of healing, either by regeneration of the epidermis from existing basal cells in the wound base or via migration from skin peripheral to the wound. In the case of some deep wounds that remain recalcitrant, surgical transplant (eg, grafting) may be required to re-epithelialize the wound.

Remodeling Phase. The **remodeling phase,** also referred to as the *maturation phase*, consists of continued fibroblastic activity and collagen deposition. The collagen undergoes both synthesis and lysis, and the balance between the two processes determines the eventual amount of scar formation at the wound site. This phase is characterized by scar contraction and may also include scar hypertrophy. During this phase, collagen is arranged along lines of tension and stress, and therefore requires insistent rehabilitative effort. Because of the effect of heat on collagen,[1,2] the application of thermal agents may be useful during this phase of healing if there are problems with severe scar contraction.

Wound Etiology

Trauma. Wounds caused by trauma may include lacerations, abrasions, avulsions, punctures, or burns. *Lacerations* represent a cutting or tearing of the skin and are most often caused by sharp objects or surface edges. *Abrasion wounds* result from skin being "scraped off" consequent to shearlike contact with a rough surface or object. *Avulsion injuries* are a consequence of the separation of the skin, or the skin and some subcutaneous tissue from underlying tissue (these injuries are sometimes referred to as *degloving injuries*). Skin damage from flame, chemicals, radiation, scalding, or electrical current are referred to as *burn injuries.*

Some traumatic skin injuries may result from a decrease or loss of sensation. Impaired ability to feel objects may inhibit normal withdrawal responses, decreasing ability to alter a potentially harmful circumstance. For example, if an individual is unaware of a stone in the shoe, the stone may cause an abrasion or laceration of the foot.

Vascular Insufficiency.   Many integumentary wounds result from an insufficient vascular network—either venous or arterial—at the site or in the area of the wound. This vascular compromise may be secondary to pathology of the vascular system or the local vascular network, or to disruption of vascular flow (ischemia), as might be seen with chronic pressure on a site.

Venous insufficiency can lead to breakdown of the skin. Although the exact cause of tissue damage is not known, fibrin-cuff formation and leukocyte trapping are theories that provide a possible explanation for the wound. Leakage of fibrinogen and other large molecules out of the capillaries secondary to venous hypertension leads to accumulation of fibrin (ie, fibrin-cuff formation) in the interstitium that inhibits transport of oxygen and nutrients to tissue.[3] Leukocyte trapping may occur with venous hypertension because of a decrease in capillary flow and the resultant removal of white cells. These trapped cells obstruct capillaries, thereby leading to local ischemia.[4] *Arterial insufficiency* leads to tissue death in the area that is deprived of requisite oxygen and nutrients.

Pressure ulcers are localized wounds caused by pressure-induced ischemia. These wounds commonly occur at sites over bony prominences, and tissue damage can arise after only a few hours of pressure.[5,6,7] Common sites for pressure ulcers include the ischial tuberosity, sacral/coccygeal area, lateral malleolus, posterior heel, and greater trochanter. They may also occur at other sites of bony prominence such as the occiput, olecranon process, and scapulae. Positioning for pressure relief is imperative as a preventive measure against the development of pressure ulcers.

A loss or decrease of sensory integrity may also lead to ischemic tissue damage. If an ulcer forms over an area where sensation is decreased, that wound is often referred to as a *neuropathic ulcer* or *neurotropic ulcer.*

Disease.   Benign skin diseases that may include associated skin breakdown include severe cases of *dermatitis*, an inflammatory skin disease. Patients with dermatitis may also experience itching and scaling of skin that, if scratched vigorously, may result in skin injury. Skin abscesses may result from plugged sebaceous glands, foreign bodies under the skin, or bacteria. If these abscesses rupture, there may be an ensuing wound created by the break in the skin. This is generally a wound care issue only if there are many abscesses or if the abscesses are large.

Wound Depth

As discussed in **Chapter 2** (The Skin), the skin layers, with their specific anatomical structures, help the skin to provide protection, sensation, and temperature regulation. The epidermis defends the internal tissues from the external environment. It further serves protective roles in the production of melanin (melanocytes) and in immune function (Langerhans cells). The junction between the epidermis and the dermis is not flat but is made of up epidermal and dermal ridges, and penetrates the dermis as invaginations of accessory organs including hair follicles, sebaceous glands, apocrine glands, and sweat (eccrine) glands. The basal layer of the epidermis, which can be found surrounding each of these epidermal invaginations, is made of cells that produce keratinocytes. Keratinocytes are the "skin" cells of the epidermis. Healthy basal-cell activity is important in normal regeneration of the epidermis.

The dermis consists of elastic and fibrous connective tissue wrapped in ground substances such as glycoaminoglycans and proteoglycans. Elastic connective tissue provides flexibility and helps restore the dermis to a resting orientation. Fibrous connective tissue provides tensile strength while still allowing movement. The **ground substance** affords a cushion for the skin to allow for some surmountable compression. The dermis supports the vascular and neural networks as well as the accessory skin organs. The vascular network in the dermis is dense and serves to nourish the skin; it is critical in the inflammatory process, which is necessary for proper wound healing. Additionally, the vascular network is an important contributor to thermal regulation. The nerves in the skin provide important afferent information about ambient temperature, pain, and various tactile stimuli (eg, light and deep touch, vibration). A healthy efferent cutaneous nervous system also affects the function of dermally located structures such as blood vessels and sweat glands.

Subcutaneous tissues, including loose connective tissue and adipose tissue, bind the dermis to the organ adjacent to it (eg, to fascia or muscle). The attachment to the subcutaneous organ(s) is sufficient for connectivity but is also pliable enough to allow for essential movement of the skin over the organ without displacement of the skin or damage to the organ.

Wound depth is described in terms of the integumentary structures involved in the wound.[8] Depth may have the most likely impact on wound repair and must be considered when determining a prognosis for healing. It can be stated generally that the deeper the wound, the longer it will take to heal, and the longer it takes a wound to heal, the greater is the risk for infection.

Superficial Wounds. **Superficial wounds** spare most, if not all, of the basal-cell layer of the epidermis with no associated disruption of the skin. This basal-cell preservation allows for regeneration of normal skin within 3 to 7 days with no scarring in the absence of skin disease or further skin trauma. Superficial wounds are painful because the pain fibers remain intact and are stimulated by the activated inflammatory response. Because there is no disruption of the epidermis, the chances for infection are minimal.

Partial-Thickness Wounds. Disruption of the integument and exposure of the dermis characterize **partial-thickness wounds.** Healing time of partial-thickness wounds will vary depending on the actual depth of the wound. Partial-thickness wounds may be described as being superficial partial-thickness, partial-thickness, or deep partial-thickness. *Superficial partial-thickness* wounds involve the very upper layers of the dermis, where preservation of basal cells is evident in regions of uncompromised epidermal ridges and accessory skin organs. These wounds heal within 7 to 14 days with minimal or no scarring. *Partial-thickness* wounds under this classification include damage through the mid-dermis with preservation of some basal cells. In most cases, sufficient numbers of basal cells exist to allow these wounds to heal within 14 to 21 days with little or no scarring. *Deep partial-thickness* wounds extend deep into the dermis and generally leave few, if any, viable basal cells. These wounds often take longer than 21 days to heal, and they commonly scar. Partial-thickness wounds are very painful, moist and weepy, and red or pink. Because of the disruption of the integument, there is an ever-present risk of infection (**Table 4–1**).

Full-Thickness Wounds. **Full-thickness wounds** represent a destruction of the epidermis, dermis, and all of the associated organs, nerves, and vascular tissue in those skin layers (see **Table 4–1**). No true regeneration of the skin will occur in these wounds. These wounds can take many weeks to heal, and scarring is associated with the healing. Full-thickness wounds are generally not painful because of the destruction of the dermal nerves, but there may be pain associated with the wounds secondary to inflammation that activates nerves in adjacent tissue. The risk for infection in full-thickness wounds is high (**Fig. 4–1**).

Subcutaneous Tissue Wounds. These wounds result in exposure to the deep subcutaneous tissue such as fascia, muscle, and bone (see **Table 4–1**). Healing time for **subcutaneous tissue wounds** can be weeks to months. Other concerns about problems associated with the damaged tissue must also be addressed, such as loss of strength or mobility secondary to muscle damage. These wounds are at great jeopardy for infection. Pain is typically associated with the damaged and inflamed tissue. Care must taken to protect exposed structures such as bone, tendon, and nerve.

TABLE 4–1   *Partial-Thickness and Full-Thickness Skin Loss*

Thickness of Skin Loss	Definition	Clinical Examples/Healing Process
Partial-thickness skin loss	Extends through the epidermis, into but not through the dermis	Skin tears, abrasions, tape damage, blisters, perineal dermatitis from incontinence; heal by epidermal resurfacing or epithelialization
Full-thickness skin loss	Extends through the epidermis and the dermis, extending into subcutaneous fat and deeper structures	Donor sites, venous ulcers, surgical wounds; heal by granulation tissue formation and contraction
Subcutaneous tissue wounds	Additional classification level for full-thickness wounds, extending into or beyond the subcutaneous tissue	Surgical wounds, arterial/ischemic wounds; heal by granulation tissue formation and contraction

Source: Sussman C and Bates-Jensen BM: *Wound Care.* 2nd ed. Lippincott, Williams, and Wilkins; 2001:90.

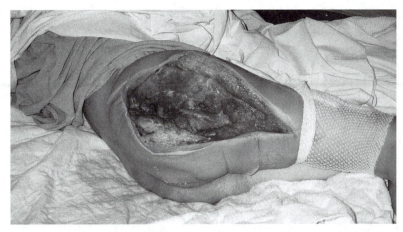

FIGURE 4–1   A lateral thigh pressure ulcer illustrating a full-thickness wound extending into subcutaneous tissue. (*Myers, Betsy,* Wound Management: Principles and Practice, *1st Edition,* © 2004. *Reprinted by permission of Pearson Education, Inc., Upper Saddle River, NJ.*)

Wound Size

The size of the wound has a great impact on the rate of healing and must be considered along with wound depth. The amount of body surface area involved (in association with wound depth) will also have an impact on the physiologic response to the wound. The most recognizable physiologic response is the local inflammatory response including pain. Large wounds also increase basal metabolic rate secondary to healing, affect temperature regulation, and can stress the cardiovascular and pulmonary systems. Also, large wounds can increase the basal metabolic rate such that nutritional demands induce catabolism of body proteins that may lead to muscle wasting. Any of these physiologic demands will increase as wound size increases, and will increase further if the wound becomes infected.

Wound Location

The location of an integumentary injury is important both for diagnostic reasons and for planning care. Diagnostically, the location of the wound may provide some indication of its etiology. Lower-leg ulcers commonly are of venous etiology, whereas foot and ankle wounds are more commonly of arterial origin. Wounds over sites of bony prominence may be ulcers created by pressure. Plan of care will be influenced by the location of the wound as it relates to joint mobility, function, or cosmesis. For example, wounds on the hands may affect several activities of daily living (ADLs), wounds on the feet may affect gait, and wounds over joints may impair motion. Wounds on visible sites, particularly wounds that heal with scarring, may cosmetically affect the appearance of the individual.

Inflammation

With any injury to the skin, an inflammatory process is initiated that signals the beginning of tissue repair. Early, confined vascular and cellular reactions include clotting of blood vessels (aided by an initial vasoconstriction), subsequent vascular dilatation, and leukocyte and macrophage migration to the problem site.

Repair of damaged blood vessels begins quickly after clotting. Leukocytes, macrophages, and lymphocytes are recruited chemotactically to the area and can be delivered in large numbers secondary to the increased blood flow associated with vasodilatation. Neutrophils fight early bacterial infection.[9,10] Macrophages serve to phagocytose (ingest) cellular debris and necrotic tissue while also releasing cytokines, growth factors, and collagenases to promote healing.[11] Lymphocytes perform many important functions in wound healing, including support of the immune response and the release of physiologic factors such as those that stimulate macrophages and fibroblasts.[12,13,14]

Increased capillary permeability that occurs during the vasodilatation phase of inflammation often leads to the development of local edema. Healing is compromised by the presence of edema because of the reduction in arterial delivery to tissue and the decrease in venous and lymphatic uptake, all of which lead to improper tissue nutrition, oxygenation, and waste disposal.

These factors also contribute to an increased risk for infection in the swollen tissue, particularly if an open skin wound is present. Edema often leads to limited motion, which can lead to more chronic tissue fibrosis.

A normal acute inflammatory response persists for about 2 weeks. An extended period of inflammation, which is commonly associated with the presence of infection or a foreign body in the tissue, is referred to as *chronic inflammation*.

Scar Tissue

If the depth of the wound is enough to compromise normal regeneration (ie, deep partial-thickness, full-thickness, and full-thickness extending into fascia muscle and bone), these wounds primarily heal by scarring. As the wound **scars,** collagen fibers are deposited to fill in the tissue defect left by the wound. These fibers are variably oriented in whorllike patterns, unlike normal connective tissue collagen, which is oriented along lines of tissue tension. If the collagen production exceeds collagen lysis, a scar forms.[15]

During the time that scar tissue is actively forming (possibly several months), the scar contracts. This process is referred to as *scar contraction*. Scar contraction that leads to a fixed loss of mobility of a joint is labeled a *scar contracture*. Active and passive stretching and the application of certain modalities may be useful in decreasing the chances of the formation of scar contractures.

EXAMINATION OF THE WOUND AND SKIN

An examination of a wound should include a conscientious history plus a physical assessment of the etiology, depth, and size of the wound. The examination should include assessment of inflammation and screening for signs of infection. Skin that is associated with or adjacent to the wound is also examined for normal functions, including temperature, sensation, mobility, pliability, and hair growth. It is also important to establish the adjacent skin's color (eg, blue or pallor for poor perfusion, red for inflammation) and texture. *This examination of adjacent, unwounded skin is even more critical if physical agents will be a part of the intervention with the wound or its related impairments.*

Wound size can be determined by several techniques, including calculating **total body surface area (TBSA),** diagramming the wound by tracing it, and using photography. Wound depth can be measured by injecting known volumes of fluid (usually normal saline) into the wound opening, subtracting the amount of remaining saline from the total amount to give a volumetric measure of wound size. A wound filler (eg, dental alginate) may also be used in the wound and then transferred to a volumeter with the amount of displaced fluid representing the wound volume. The type of tissue exposed may also reflect wound depth. Partial-thickness wounds expose a moist pink or red, very painful tissue. Full-thickness wounds permit recognition of adipose tissue and/or fascia, whereas wounds that penetrate the subcutaneous tissue expose muscle, tendon, nerve, or bone.

Trauma

The etiology, location, size, and depth of a traumatic wound are documented. Any traumatic wound of concern is referred for primary medical care. Associated skin and tissue injury must also be assessed in preparation for the possible use of physical agents, either to assist wound healing or for treating other impairments related to the trauma in general.

Vascular Insufficiency

Venous Ulcers.   **Venous ulcers** are commonly found on the lower leg (**Fig. 4–2**). These wounds are generally irregularly shaped with a shallow red or pink wound base. The wounds will exhibit exudate (weeping) and will have associated edema. The edema is secondary to delayed wound healing. There may be some pain coupled with the ulcer, but the pain predictably decreases with elevation of the extremity. Adjacent skin is characterized by abnormal pigmentation, inflammation, dilated veins, and induration (hardness), and the skin may be dry and scaly. Pulses in the affected extremity should be palpable.

Arterial Ulcers.   **Arterial ulcers** are often found on the lower leg, feet, or toes (**Fig. 4–3**). The wound shape is generally irregular with a deep, pale wound base. Exudate is minimal or absent. Diminished circulation delays healing of these wounds. Severe pain is expected with arterial wounds and can be exacerbated with elevation of the extremity. Skin adjacent to these wounds is distinguished by hair loss, is cool to the touch, appears thin and shiny, and displays pallor with elevation.

Pressure Ulcers.   **Pressure ulcers** are most commonly located at sites of anatomic bony prominences, although they can be located over other areas (**Fig. 4–4**). The clinician describes the location and size of the wound. Depth of these wounds is normally documented using the criteria for staging pressure ulcers rendered by the U.S. Department of Health and

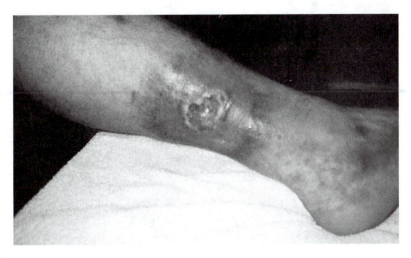

FIGURE 4–2   A venous ulcer located on a medial calf. (*Myers, Betsy, Wound Management: Principles and Practice, 1st Edition, © 2004. Reprinted by permission of Pearson Education, Inc., Upper Saddle River, NJ.*)

Human Services[16] (**Table 4–2**). Once an ulcer has been staged, it is always referred to by its assigned stage, even as the wound heals; for example, a healing stage IV ulcer does not improve to a stage III, stage II, and then a stage I (this is called backstaging). More appropriately, the healing wound is described in terms of changes in its depth, size, or appearance. When healed, it would be documented as a healed stage IV ulcer.

Neuropathic Ulcers.   **Neuropathic ulcers** are most frequently found on the plantar surface of the foot at sites of bony prominence (**Fig. 4–5**). These deep wounds are generally circular in shape. There is often no pain associated with the wound secondary to the sensory neuropathy, and the wounds may easily bleed unless there is associated arterial insufficiency. Skin adjacent to these wounds is regularly healthy but likely will also be affected by sensory deficit.

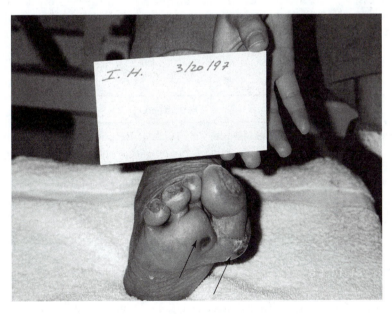

FIGURE 4–3   An arterial ulcer on the plantar surface of a foot. (*Myers, Betsy,* Wound Management: Principles and Practice, *1st Edition, © 2004. Reprinted by permission of Pearson Education, Inc., Upper Saddle River, NJ.*)

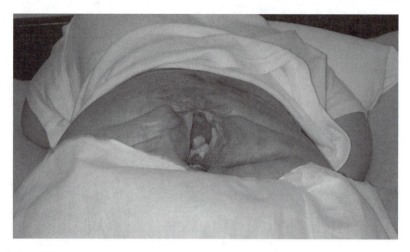

FIGURE 4–4   A stage IV sacral pressure ulcer. (*Myers, Betsy*, Wound Management: Principles and Practice, *1st Edition,* © 2004. *Reprinted by permission of Pearson Education, Inc., Upper Saddle River, NJ.*)

Disease

Although a physician diagnoses and treats primary skin disease, a physical therapist may treat any wound associated with the disease. Etiology, location, size, and depth are used to describe any wound secondary to skin disease. Associated skin is carefully monitored for signs of concern.

Malignant skin diseases (eg, neoplastic skin disease, skin cancer) such as malignant melanoma, squamous cell carcinoma, and basal cell carcinoma do not generally pose wound care challenges. However, the physical therapist must be aware of any such neoplasm because in the presence of any of these diseases, the use of physical agents are contraindicated. Any suspect lesion is a basis for immediate medical referral. Key warning signs of skin cancer include a bump that continually increases in size, a sore that does not heal, new skin growth, and any growth on the skin or growth of a mole that includes changes in size, shape, color, appearance, elevation, or sensation.

TABLE 4–2   *Pressure Ulcer Staging Criteria*

Stage	Definition
I	A stage I pressure ulcer is an observable, pressure-related alteration of intact skin whose indicators as compared to the adjacent or opposite area on the body may include changes in one or more of the following: skin temperature (warmth or coolness), tissue consistency (firm or boggy feel), and/or sensation (pain, itching). The ulcer appears as a defined area of persistent redness in lightly pigmented skin, whereas, in darker tones, the ulcer may appear with persistent red, blue, or purple hues.
II	Partial-thickness skin loss involving epidermis and/or dermis. The ulcer is superficial and presents clinically as an abrasion, a blister, or a shallow crater.
III	Full-thickness skin loss involving damage or necrosis of subcutaneous tissue that may extend down to, but not through, underlying fascia. The ulcer presents clinically as a deep crater with or without undermining of adjacent tissue.
IV	Full-thickness skin loss with extensive destruction, tissue necrosis or damage to muscle, bone, or supporting structures (eg, tendon, joint capsule).

Source: Sussman C and Bates-Jensen BM: *Wound Care.* 2nd ed. Lippincolt, Williams, and Wilkins; 2001:88.

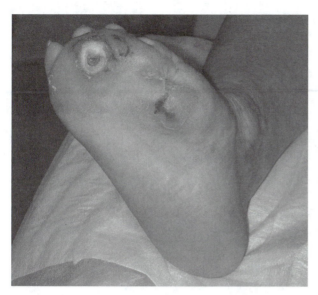

FIGURE 4–5 A Neuropathic ulcer located on the plantar surface of a foot. (*Myers, Betsy,* Wound Management: Principles and Practice, © 2004. *Reprinted by permission of Pearson Education, Inc., Upper Saddle River, NJ.*)

Scar Tissue

As some wounds heal, particularly deep wounds, scar tissue may develop. Scars that remain within the original wound boundaries are referred to as *hypertrophic scars*, whereas those that develop beyond the initial wound boundaries are called *keloid scars*.[15,17,18] The type of scar formation and its location are identified; location of the scar is important because of the implications for impaired mobility secondary to scar contraction as well as the potential impact on cosmetic appearance. The Vancouver Burn Scar Scale based on scar height, pliability, pigmentation, and vascularity provides a method for assessing scars (**Table 4–3**).[19] A higher score on the scale represents more scarring.

PHYSICAL AGENTS IN WOUND MANAGEMENT

Thermal Agents

Ultrasound. Although there are studies that demonstrate effectiveness of ultrasound intervention (US) on wound healing of pressure and venous ulcers,[20–29] the level of significance and the power of the studies do not provide potent evidence for its effectiveness.[30] It appears that any consequence that US has on wounds is likely due to the nonthermal effects of the sound waves, which would suggest that interventions should be in pulsed mode. On the basis of published reports, US might assist in enhancing vascularity during early phases of healing by stimulating angiogenesis.[31,32] Ultrasound may also contribute to increased tensile strength in a healing wound secondary to stimulation of fibroblastic production of collagen early in healing[33] or in the later stages of healing.[34,35] Ultrasound may also have a positive effect on pain associated with wounds; however, no study has demonstrated its efficacy in this regard.

General precautions and contraindications for US can be found in **Chapter 15**. Contraindications of US for wound care include vascular abnormalities or malignancies or precancerous lesions. Precautions with respect to wound care include using US prudently over areas where there is an acute infection or over areas that lack sensation.

Pulsed Diathermy. In using diathermy for wound care, high-frequency (27.12 MHz) radio waves are directed at the wound and associated skin. Diathermy for interventions with wounds is commonly in pulsed mode and known as **pulsed diathermy (PD)**. Depending on the pulse width, the diathermy can produce either nonthermal effects (nonthermal mode PD) or thermal effects (thermal PD).

The evidence for the use of PD in wound care is currently not robust because of the small number of studies published. Nonthermal PD has been studied in interventions with pressure ulcers,[36,37] venous wounds,[38,39] donor sites, and other wounds.[40] These studies generally reported an increase or improvement in wound healing with the use of PD. A suggested mechanism for the potential success of nonthermal PD in improved healing may be an increased vascular perfusion in the area[41] and an increased rate of epithlialization and decreased wound contraction.[42] Thermal PD has not been studied directly for its effects on wound healing in humans, but it is assumed that the increased vascular perfusion that has been demonstrated[43] could benefit wound healing by increasing oxygen tension in the wound.

Standard contraindications and precautions for the use of diathermy can be found in **Chapter 16**. Contraindications that apply more specifically to wound management include avoiding using the devices over areas of neoplasm or on patients with vascular compromise.

TABLE 4–3   *Ratings Used in the Vancouver Scar Scale to Measure Scar Formation*

Pigmentation	Vascularity	Pliability	Height	Score
Normal—color that closely resembles the color over the rest of the body	Normal—color that closely resembles the color over the rest of the body	Normal	Normal—flat	0
Hypopigmentation	Pink	Supple: flexible with minimal resistance	Raised <2 mm	1
Hyperpigmentation	Red	Yielding: giving way to pressure	Raised <5 mm	2
	Purple	Firm: inflexible, not easily moved, resistant to manual pressure	Raised >5 mm	3
		Banding: ropelike tissue that blanches with extension of the scar		4
		Contracture: permanent shortening of scar producing deformity or distortion		5

Note: The higher the score reported, the worse the scar.

Source: Reprinted with permission from T. Sullivan et al., Rating the Burn Scar, *Journal of Burn Care Rehabilitation*, Vol. 11. pp. 256–260. ©1990, Lippincott Williams & Wilkins.

Superficial Heat Modalities.   Although there is clear evidence that most superficial heat modalities enhance vascular perfusion (see **Chapter 13**) and therefore might aid in local wound repair, there are no studies that have investigated the effect of these modalities on wound healing.

Hydrotherapy

In wound management, hydrotherapy may mean the use of a conventional whirlpool or some other means of irrigating a wound; this discussion will focus on the traditional whirlpool. Although there have been studies that have included whirlpool as a component of care, it has not been clear what contribution the whirlpool made to the success of the intervention.[44,45,46] A recent trial comparing the use of moist dressings and whirlpool with the use of moist dressings demonstrated only a greater level of wound healing with the addition of the whirlpool intervention.[47]

When an open wound enters a whirlpool, the wound is exposed to any flora from the other body parts submerged with the wound as well as any conta-minant in the whirlpool; for example, there are published reports that describe infection with *Psuedomonas aeruginosa* after whirlpool intervention.[48,49] This is known as cross contamination and can generally be avoided by meticulous cleansing of the hydrotherapy equipment as well as proper care of the patient in the tub. Reports have demonstrated reasonable wound decontamination with hydrotherapy, particularly when the treated wound is rinsed following removal from the tub.[50] Patients with wounds should not be treated for more than 20 minutes to avoid the risk of superhydration of the skin, which can increase the risk for infection.[48,50]

The turbines or "jets" in the whirlpool are commonly used as a nonselective debridement tool. Either the wounds should not be placed so close to the turbulence that they sustain further damage, or the level of turbulence should be decreased to wound tolerance. Hydration of eschar may make follow-up sharp debridement easier. The Agency for Health Care Research and Quality recommends that whirlpool be used until a wound is clean, at which time it should be discontinued.[51]

General precautions and contraindications for the use of hydrotherapy can be found in **Chapter 26**. Precautions that apply more specifically to wound care include decreasing or not using turbulence with wounds that have a fragile tissue bed or have been recently healed or repaired, and not allowing a patient to remain in the whirlpool for over 20 minutes. Contraindications more relevant to wound care are vascular compromise, incontinence (fecal or urinary), maceration of the skin (superhydration of wound and of normal skin), and moderate to severe edema of an extremity.

Electrotherapy

There may be several reasons that electrotherapeutic intervention contributes to the healing of wounds. One basis may be a unidirectional flow of electrical current in tissues that draws repair cells known as galvanotaxis. **Table 4–4** summarizes the cellular polarity and biologic affects of the cells for each wound healing phase. Further, the skin normally has a negative electrical potential that, when wounding occurs, demonstrates a shift known as the "current of injury." Regenerating tissues show a flow along the current of injury. While an actively healing wound remains moist prior to wound closure, this current of injury is evident.[52] Applying electrical stimulation may initiate or increase healing of a wound because it imitates the usual current of injury associated with the wound.[53]

The effect of electrical current on tissues varies, and any one or a combination of factors may play a role in facilitating wound healing. There is some evidence that blood flow might be enhanced, and therefore oxygen delivery to the healing tissues increased, with the use of electrical stimulation. Kaada demonstrated an increased blood flow in the skin of the web spaces of the hand following application of transcutaneous electrical nerve stimulation (TENS) that may have assisted in the healing of associated wounds.[54] Increased tissue oxygen tension ($tcPO_2$) has been shown,[55,56,57] with this result also reported from galvanic electrical stimulation,[58] monophasic spiked waveform,[59] and high-volt pulsed current (HVPC).[60]

Several studies have demonstrated an antibacterial effect with some applications of electrical stimulation. Positive current through silver electrodes had an inhibitory effect on *Pseudomonas aeruginosa* and *Staphylococcus aureus*.[61,62] Case studies have also reported encouraging results of treating infected wounds with electrical stimulation, including such problems as chronic osteomyelitis, chronic abscess, and spinal thoracic infection.[63,64,65,66] Results were generally noted within 7 days, and a variety of types of electrical stimulation were used.

Managing pain is challenging with many wounds, particularly those of superficial thickness or partial thickness and those wounds extending into deeper

TABLE 4–4   *Cellular polarity and biological effects of the cells for each wound healing phase as it relates to galvanotaxis.*

Phase of Healing	Biological Effects	Cells and Their Polarity	Current/Polarity
Inflammatory	Phagocytosis and Autolysis	Macrophage −	DC (+)[54]
		Neutrophil (−)	DC (+)[55]
		Neutrophil (−)	PC (+)[56]
		Neutrophil (−)	DC (−)[57,58]
		Activated Neutrophil (+)	
Proliferative	Fibroplasia	Fibroblast (+)	PC (−)[59,60]
			DC (−)[61,62,63]
Remodeling	Wound Contraction	Myofibroblast (+)	PC (−)[64]
	Epithelialization	Epidermal (−)	DC (−)[65]
			PC (−/+)[66]
			PC (+)[67]

From Kloth LC: Electrical stimulation for wound healing. In Kloth LC and McCulloch JM (eds.): Wound Healing Alternatives in Management (3rd ed.). FA Davis, Philadelphia, 2002, with permission.

tissues if those tissues are innervated by nociceptors. An abundance of literature describes the beneficial effects of electrical stimulation, especially TENS, in the intervention for pain (see **Chapter 21**). Wound-related pain should respond to similarly directed interventions.

Common precautions and contraindications for electrotherapy interventions can be found in **Chapters 19 through 24.** Precautions that have more direct relevance to wound care include skin irritation under electrodes and pain created by the stimulation. Contraindications include the existence of a malignancy in the area to be treated, an active untreated osteomyelitis in the bone below the wound, or the presence of any electrical implant such as a cardiac pacemaker.

Additional Physical Agents

Ultraviolet Radiation. As described in **Chapter 27**, ultraviolet radiation (UVR) may result in several responses that can contribute to wound healing. These responses to UVR exposure include (1) erythema that may help by increasing local vascularity and capillary permeability, (2) destruction of bacteria that would provide a better healing environment,[67] and (3) exfoliation of epidermal cells. Clinical studies report initially encouraging data to support the use of UVR in healing ulcers, particularly those that have not responded to other interventions.[68,69] One suggested method for application of the UVR is to determine the exposure time (UVB) for a first-degree erythemal dose on the skin adjacent to the wound and to use that as the intervention dose for the wound.[70]

Common precautions and contraindications for UVR are provided in **Chapter 27**. Those contraindications focusing on the wound include serious vascular disease (eg, severe diabetes mellitus) and carcinoma in the wound or surrounding tissue. Photosensitivity, including photosensitivity secondary to medications, must be considered as well when planning the intervention.

Intermittent Pneumatic Compression. Sequential pneumatic compression can be helpful in managing extremity edema. Controlling edema can contribute to the healing of wounds, particularly those secondary to venous disease. Generally, a combination of leg elevation, exercise, and compression therapy are recommended for ongoing management of edema.[71] Intermittent pneumatic compression therapy that is associated with wound care, should also include compression bandages and compression stockings following the intervention to maintain edema reduction.

Familiar precautions and contraindications for the use of intermittent pneumatic compression are discussed in **Chapter 25**. If this physical agent is being considered for use in conjunction with wound management, the presence of cellulitis and active wound infection are additional contraindications.

REVIEW QUESTIONS

1. Identify and describe the three phases of wound healing.

2. Describe the proposed mechanism of how venous insufficiency can lead to wounds.

3. Identify the areas of the body that are most susceptible to pressure ulcers.

4. Identify and describe the staging classification for pressure ulcers.

5. Describe and identify the structures involved in a (a) superficial partial-thickness wound, (b) deep partial-thickness wound, and (c) full-thickness wound.

6. Describe the clinical presentation of an arterial wound.

7. Describe the clinical presentation of a venous stasis wound.

8. Provide a rationale for the use of ultrasound for wound healing.

9. Provide a rationale for the use of electrical stimulation for wound healing.

10. Provide a rationale for the use of external compression for wound healing.

KEY TERMS

inflammatory phase
proliferative phase
remodeling phase
ground substance
superficial wounds

partial-thickness wounds
full-thickness wounds
subcutaneous tissue wounds
scars
total body surface area (TBSA)

venous ulcers
arterial ulcers
pressure ulcers
neuropathic ulcers
pulsed diathermy (PD)

REFERENCES

1. Lehman JF, Masock AJ, Warren CG, Koblanski JN: Effect of therapeutic temperatures on tendon extensibility. *Arch Phys Med Rehabil* 1970; 51:481–87.

2. Warren CG, Lehman JF, Koblanski JN: Heat and stretch procedures: An evaluation using rat tail tendon. *Arch Phys Med Rehabil* 1976; 57:122–26.

3. Browse NL, Burnand KG: The cause of venous ulceration. *Lancet* 1982; 2:243–45.

4. Coleridge Smith PD, Thomas P, Scurr JH, et al: Causes of venous ulceration: A new hypothesis. *BMJ* 1988; 296:1726–27.

5. Reuler JB, Cooney TG: The pressure sore: Pathophysiology and principles of management. *Ann Intern Med* 1981; 94:66–67.

6. Lindon O, Greenway RM, Piazza JM: Pressure distributor on the surface of the human body. *Arch Phys Med Rehabil* 1965; 46:378.

7. Kosiak M: Etiology and pathology of ischemic ulcers. *Arch Phys Med Rehabil* 1981; 62:49–98.

8. *Guide to Physical Therapist Practice.* 2nd ed. *Phys Ther* 2001; 81:S585–S683.

9. Ford-Hutchinson EW, Bray MA, Doig MV, Shipley ME, Smith MJH: Leukotriene B, a potent chemokinetic and aggregating substance released from polymorphonuclear leukocytes. *Nature (Lond)* 1980; 286(5770):264–65.

10. Simpson DM and Ross R: The neutrophilic leukocyte in wound repair: A study with antineutrophil serum. *J Clin Invest* 1972; 51(8):2009–23.

11. Leibovich SJ and Ross R: The role of the macrophage in wound repair: A study with hydrocortisone and antimacrophage serum. *Am J. Pathol* 1975; 78(1):71–100.

12. Fishel RS, Barbul A, Beschorner WE, Wasserkrug HL, Efron G: Lymphocyte participation in wound healing: Morphologic assessment using monoclonal antibodies. *Ann Surg* 1987; 206(1):25–29.

13. Wahl LM and Wahl SM: Lymphokine modulation of connective tissue metabolism. Ann NY Acad Sci 1979; 332:411–22

14. Wahl SM, Wahl LM, McCarthy JB: Lymphocyte-mediated activation of fibroblast proliferation and collagen production. *J Immunol* 1978; 121(3):942–46.

15. Rockwell WB, Cohen IK, Erlich JP: Keloids and hypertrophic scars: A comprehensive report. *Plast Reconstr Surg* 1989; 84(5):827–37.

16. Bergstrom N, Allman RM, Alvarez OM, et al: Treatment of Pressure Ulcers, Clinical Practice Guideline No. 15, Rockville, MD, U.S. Department of Health and Human Services, 1994.

17. Ketchum LD: Hypertrophic scars and keloids. *Clin Plast Surg* 1977; 4(2):301–310.

18. Ketchum LD, Cohen IK, Masters FW: Hypertrophic scars and keloids. *Plast Reconstr Surg* 1974; 53(2):140–54.

19. Sullivan T, et al. Rating the Burn Scar. *J Burn Care Rehabil* 1990; 11:256–60.

20. Paul BJ, Lafratta CW, Dawson RA, Baab E, Bullock F: Use of ultrasound in the treatment of pressure sores in patients with spinal cord injury. *Arch Phys Med Rehabil* 1960; 41:438–40.

21. McDiarmid T, Burns PN, Lewith GT, Machin D: Ultrasound and the treatment of pressure sores. *Physiotherapy* 1985; 71(2):66–70.

22. Nussbaum EL, Biemann I, Mustard B: Comparison of ultrasound/ultraviolet C and laser for

treatment of pressure ulcers in patients with spinal cord injury. *Phys Ther* 1994; 74:812–25.

23. ter Riet G, Kessels AGH, Knipschild P: A randomized clinical trial of ultrasound in the treatment of pressure ulcers. *Phys Ther* 1996; 76:1301–12.

24. Dyson M, Frank C, Suckling J: Stimulation of healing of varicose ulcers by ultrasound. *Ultrasonics* September 1976; 232–36.

25. Peschen M, Weichenthal M, Schopf E, Vanscheidt W: Low-frequency ultrasound treatment of chronic venous leg ulcers in an outpatient therapy. *Acta Dermatol Venereol* 1997; 77(4):311–14.

26. Roche C, West J: A controlled trial investigating the effect of ultrasound on venous ulcers referred from general practitioners. *Physiotherapy* 1984; 70(12):475–77.

27. Lundeberg T, Nordstrom F, Brodda-Jansen G, Ericsson S, Kjartansson J, Samuelson U: Pulsed ultrasound does not improve healing of venous ulcers. *Scand J Rehabil Med* 1990; 22(4):195–97.

28. Callam M, Harper D, Dale J, Ruckley C, Prescott R: A controlled trial of weekly ultrasound therapy in chronic leg ulceration. *Lancet* 1987; 2(8552):204–06.

29. Ericsson S, Lundberg T, Malm M: A placebo-controlled trial of ultrasound therapy in chronic leg ulceration. *Scand J Rehabil Med* 1991; 23(4):211–13.

30. Johannsen F, Gam AN, Karsmark T: Ultrasound therapy in chronic leg ulceration: A meta-analysis. *Wound Repair Regeneration* 1998; 6:121–26.

31. Dyson M: Mechanisms involved in therapeutic ultrasound. *Physiother J Chartered Soc Physiother* 1987; 73(3):8.

32. Dyson M: Role of Ultrasound In Wound Healing. In: McCulloch JM, Kloth LC, Feedar JA, eds. Wound Healing: *Alternatives in Management*, 2nd ed. Philadelphia: Davis; 1995; 3.18–46.

33. Dyson M: Mechanisms involved in therapeutic ultrasound. *Physiother J Chartered Soc Physiother* 1987; 73(3):8.

34. Frieder S, Weisberg J, Flemming B, Stanek A: The therapeutic effects of ultrasound following partial rupture of Achilles tendons in male rats. *J Orthop Sports Phys Ther* 1988; 10:39–46.

35. Jackson BA, Schwane JA, Starcher BC: Effect of ultrasound therapy on the repair of Achilles tendon injuries in rats. *Med Sci Sports Exerc* 1991; 23:171–76.

36. Comorosan S, Vasilco R, Arghiropol M, Paslaru L, Jieanu V, Stelea S: The effect of diapulse therapy on the healing of decubitus ulcer. *Rom J Physiol* 1993; 30:41–45.

37. Seaborne D, Quirion-De Girardi C, Rousseau M, Rivest M, Lambert J: The treatment of pressure sores using pulsed electromagnetic energy (PEME). *Physiother Can* 1994; 48:131–37.

38. Stiller MJ, Pak GH, Shupack JL, Thaler S, Kenny C, Jondreau L: A portable pulsed electromagnetic field (PEPE) device to enhance healing of recalcitrant venous ulcers: A double-blind, placebo-controlled clinical trial. *Br J Dermatol* 1992; 127:145–54.

39. Tood DJ, Heylings DJ, Allen GE, McMillin WP: Treatment of chronic varicose ulcers with pulsed electromagnetic fields. A controlled pilot study. *Ir Jed J* 1991; 84:54–55.

40. Mayrovitz HN, Larsen PB: A preliminary study to evaluate the effect of pulsed radio frequency field treatment of lower-extremity peri-ulcer microcirculation of diabetic patients. *Wounds* 1995; 7:90–93.

41. Mayrovitz HN, and Larsen PB: Effects of pulsed electromagnetic fields on skin microvascular blood perfusion. *Wounds* 1992; 4:197

42. Kelpke S and Feldman D: Alternations in PEME: The effect on wound healing. *Wound Repair Regen* 1994; 2:81.

43. Santoro D, et al: Inductive 27.12 MHz diathermy in arterial peripheral vascular disease. Sixteenth International IEEE/EMBS Conference. *IEEE Press* 1994; 2–3.

44. Gault W, Gatens PF: Use of low-intensity direct current in management of ischemic skin ulcers. *Phys Ther* 1976; 56(3):141–45.

45. Carley PJ, Wainapel S: Electrotherapy of acceleration of wound healing: Low-intensity direct current. *Arch Phys Med Rehabil* 1985; 66:443–46.

46. Shimizu T, Kosaka M, Fujishima K: Human thermoregulatory responses during prolonged walking in water at 25, 30 and 35 degrees C. *Eur J Appl Physiol Occup Physiol* 1998; 78(6):473–78.

47. Burke DT, et al: Effects of hydrotherapy on pressure ulcer healing. *Am J Phys Med Rehabil* 1998; 77(5):394–98.

48. Solomon SL: Host factors in whirlpool-associated *Psuedomonas aeruginosa* skin disease. *Infect control* 1985; 6:402–06.

49. Jacobson JA: Pool-associated *Psuedomonas aeruginosa* dermatitis and other bathing-associated infections. *Infect Control* 1985; 6:398–401.

50. Shankowsky HA, Callioux LS, Tredget EE: North American survey of hydrotherapy in modern burn care. *J Burn Care Rehabil* 1994; 15:143–46.

51. Bergstrom N, Bennett MA, Carlson C, et al: *Treatment of Pressure Ulcers.* Clinical Practice Guideline No.15. Rockville, MD: Agency for Health Care Research and Quality (AHRQ), formerly known as the Agency for Health Care Policy and Research (AHCPR), U.S. Public Health Service (PHS), U.S. Department of Health and Human Services (DHHS); AHRO Publication No. 95-0652; p 52: December 1994: 45–65.

52. Gentzkow G, Miller K: Electrical stimulation for dermal wound healing. *Clin Podiatr Med Surg* 1991; 8:827–41.

53. Gentzkow GD, Pollack SV, Kloth LC, Stubbs HA: Improved healing of pressure ulcers using dermapulse, a new electrical stimulation device. *Wounds* 1991; 3(5):158–70.

54. Kaada B: Vasodilation induced by transcutaneous nerve stimulation in peripheral ischemia (Raynaud's phenomenon and diabetic polyneuropathy). *Eur Heart J* 1982; 3:303–14.

55. Gagnier KA, et al: The effects of electrical stimulation on cutaneous oxygen supply in paraplegics. *Phys Ther* 1988; 68:835.

56. Baker LL: The effect of electrical stimulation on cutaneous oxygen supply. *Rehabil Res Dev Prog Rep* 1988; 176.

57. Baker LL, Chamber R, Merchant L, Park D, Sokolski D, Yoneyama: The effects of electrical stimulation on cutaneous oxygen supply in normal older adults and diabetic patients. *Phys Ther* 1986; 66:749.

58. Peters EJ, Armstrong DG, Wunderlich RP, Bosma J, Stacpoole-Shea S, Lavery LA: The benefit of electrical stimulation to enhance perfusion in persons with diabetes mellitus. *J Foot Ankle Surg* 1998; 37(5):396–400.

59. Dodgen PW, Johnson BW, Baker LL, Chambers RB: The effects of electrical stimulation on cutaneous oxygen supply in diabetic older adults. *Phys Ther* 1987; 67(5):S4.

60. Gilcreast DM, Stotts N, Froelicher ES, Baker LL, Moss KM: Effect of electrical stimulation on foot skin perfusion in persons with or at risk for diabetic foot ulcers. *Wound Rep Reg* 1998; 6(5):434–41.

61. Barranco J, Spadaro J, Berger TJ: In vitro effect of weak direct current on *Staphylococcus aureus.* *Clin Orthop* 1974; 100:250–55.

62. Rowley B, McKenna J, Chase GR: The influence of electrical current on an infecting microorganism in wounds. *Ann NY Acad Sci* 1974; 238:543–51.

63. Thurman BF, Christian EL: Response of a serious circulatory lesion to electrical stimulation. *Phys Ther* 1971; (51)10:137–40.

64. Gault WR, Gatens PF: Use of low-intensity direct current in management of ischemic skin ulcers. *Phys Ther* 1976; 56(3):141–45.

65. Webster DA, Spadaro JA, Becker RO, Kramer S: Silver anode treatment of chronic osteomyelitis. *Clin Orthop Relat Res* 1981; 161:106–14.

66. Fitzgerald GK, Newsome D: Treatment of a large infected thoracic spine wound using high voltage pulsed monophasic current. *Phys Ther* 1993; 73(6):355–60.

67. Conner-Kerr T, Sullivan PK, Gaillard J, Franklin ME, Jones RM: The effects of ultraviolet radiation on antibiotic-resistant bacteria in vitro. *Ostomy Wound Manage* 1998; 44:50–56.

68. Nussbaum E, Biemann I, Mustard B: Comparison of ultrasound/ultraviolet-C and laser for treatment of pressure ulcers in patients with spinal cord injury. *Phys Ther* 1994; 74:812–23.

69. Freytes HA, Fernandez B, Fleming WC: Ultraviolet light in the treatment of indolent ulcers. *South Med J* 1965; 58:223–26.

70. Scott BO: *The Principles and Practice of Electrotherapy and Actinotherapy.* Springfield, IL: Charles C Thomas, 1959; 254–301.

71. Wiersema-Bryant LA, and Kraemer BA: Management of edema. In: Sussman C and Bates-Jensen BM, eds. *Wound Care: A Collaborative Practice Manual for Physical Therapists and Nurses.* 2nd ed. Gaithersburg: Aspen; 2001:235–56.

5

Edema

BERNADETTE HECOX, PT, MA

JOHN P. SANKO, PT, EDD

Chapter Outline

Swelling is a condition in which the amount of fluid within interstitial spaces is greater than normal. Swelling is caused by two different mechanisms. The initial swelling seen immediately following soft tissue injury is the result of vascular damage and hemorrhage, whereas swelling that occurs hours or more after an injury has occurred is the result of edema. **Edema** arises from the disruption of the normal flow of fluid between the capillaries and the interstitial spaces; when more fluid flows into the tissues than is reabsorbed by the capillaries, fluid accumulates in the tissues. The amount of swelling is determined by the degree of fluid exchange imbalance.[1,2,3] This excessive intercellular fluid can be localized to one area of the body, such as a hand or an ankle, or it can be more general, involving an entire extremity or even the entire body. **Effusion** refers specifically to an excess of fluid in a cavity (eg, the pleural space, or excessive synovial fluid in a joint). **Lymph,** the clear fluid that is collected from the tissues throughout the body, flows into the lymphatic vessels and is eventually dumped into the venous blood circulation. Lymph transports protein and other large molecules that cannot be removed directly by absorption into the capillary. **Lymphedema** is the accumulation of interstitial fluid caused by an obstruction in lymph channels that prevents reabsorption of proteins from the interstitium.

Lymphedemia may be classified as primary or secondary. Primary is idiopathic, whereas secondary is acquired. The real incidence of lymphedema is not known because many cases go undiagnosed and untreated.[1,2,3] The major etiology for primary lymphedemia is heredity, whereas the causes of secondary edema include filariasis, metastatic neoplasms, surgery, therapeutic radiation, chemotherapy, infection, venous insufficiency, liposuction, crush injury and other trauma, burns, obesity, and prolonged use of corticosteroids.[3]

When the swelling caused by excess fluid increases pressure on the sensory nerves, it causes pain. When such pressure blocks blood flow to tissues, it can cause necrosis. Excessive fluid, either intra-articular effusion or extra-articular edema, that crowds a joint decreases the range of motion and function of the joint. If edema is allowed to persist, osteoporosis of bone caused by lack of use or infections such as low-grade cellulitis may occur. Edema and slow venous flow predispose the patient to thrombosis or pulmonary embolisms.[4,5] Chronic lymphedema predisposes tissues to bacterial infection.[6] Thus, edema should not be regarded lightly; it should be treated aggressively as soon as possible.

Many physical agents can be useful either for preventing edema or hastening its resolution. However, because some agents have the potential to increase edema, they are contraindicated for some edematous conditions. This chapter provides guidelines for clinicians who must decide whether and how to use physical agents with patients who have edema or have conditions that may cause edema to develop.

ANATOMY OF THE LYMPHATIC SYSTEM

The lymphatic system is composed of lymphatic vessels (superficial, intermediate, deep), lymph fluid, lymph tissues and organs, the right thoracic duct, the right lymphatic duct, and the lymphatic anastomoses.[2] Lymph vessels absorb, collect, and transport lymph throughout the body.[2] The smaller, superficial capillaries empty into the deeper and larger precollection vessels that in turn empty into the deep collectors or **lymphatics.** These are valved vessels with smooth muscle walls that carry lymph centrally to the trunk.[2]

The lymph fluid is a plasmalike substance that normally contains less protein than plasma. Lymph contains water, protein, white blood cells, certain lipids, various microorganisms, and cellular debris.[2]

Lymph tissues and organs are found throughout the body. Lymph tissues include the tonsils and connective tissue nodules found beneath the epitheal linings of the body. Lymph nodes, the thymus, and the spleen are the major lymph organs whose function is to produce and distribute lymphocytes.[2]

PHYSIOLOGIC FACTORS

Approximately 60% of body weight is water.[7,8] The water within the body cells is called *intracellular fluid*, and all that is outside the cells is called *extracellular fluid*. Extracellular fluids include the fluids within the blood vessels, called *plasma*, and the fluids in the interstitial spaces, called *interstitial fluid*. Normally, the interstitial fluid accounts for approximately 16% of an adult's body weight.[9]

Many authorities explain that the content of the interstitial fluid exists in both a "free fluid" and a tissue "gel" state and that, in healthy individuals, most interstitial fluid is in the gel state. Any large concentration in the free fluid state is considered to be edema. Theoretically, the gel serves several purposes. The gel matrix contains negatively charged mucopolysaccharides, which attract and hold positively charged sodium ions (Na⁺). Because sodium is an osmotic substance, its concentration in the gel enhances the passage of water across the capillary membrane, through osmosis, into the gel. The gel also acts as a "filler" holding cells apart and enabling the interstitial fluid to remain relatively immobilized and thus localized. If all the interstitial fluid were free fluid (ie, none was in the gel state), gravity would pull all the fluid to the lower regions of the body. For example, if a person were standing with arms at sides, all the fluid would shift to the distal parts of the arms and legs. Such pooling of interstitial fluid is observed with edema, which is an excess of free fluid.

Because of a pressure gradient between the interstitial space and blood, fluid is constantly being exchanged across the semipermeable capillary membrane between the interstitial space and plasma. A delicate balance between the gradients of the forces drawing fluids in each direction maintains a normal amount of fluid in the interstitium. Guyton[9] stated that the interstitial pressure is normally negative (ie, less than the atmospheric pressure) and that "the *physical* cause of edema is positive pressure in the interstitial spaces." Guyton noted that if edema is prolonged (hours to years), tissues will stretch accordingly, causing the pressure in the spaces to increase and thus leading to still more edema. This possibility underscores the importance of preventing, or hastening the reduction of, edema.

Physical therapists must understand how the delicate balance between the concentrations of fluids in blood and interstitium is maintained, and what may disturb that balance and lead to edema, so a review of the related physiology follows.

In 1896, Starling[10] presented a theory on how fluids are normally transported between blood and interstitium. He postulated that the two-way exchange of fluid between capillaries and interstitium occurs at the capillary membrane because of hydrostatic and osmotic pressure gradients. If all factors were normal, the net effect of the gradients would result in a normal amount of interstitial fluid, thus no edema. This theory is referred to as **Starling's hypothesis of the capillaries.** Witte[10] states that Starling's hypothesis still stands: "although hydrolic and osmotic pressure differ across different barriers, Starling's equation has universal applicability." In the twentieth century, however, new evidence contributed to our current understanding. Figures 5–1, 5–2, and 5–3 illustrate the following brief discussion of the factors that regulate the exchange of fluids between blood and interstitium. Bear in mind that capillaries may be only 0.5 mm long[11] and that the figures are not drawn to scale; they are presented only to clarify the fluid exchange concepts.

Factors Regulating Exchange of Fluids

Hydrostatic Pressure. Hydrostatic pressure always causes fluids moving through a semipermeable membrane to flow from the higher- to the lower-pressure side of the membrane. Plasma pressure is higher than the interstitial fluid pressure at the capillary membrane. In a "model" capillary, the blood plasma pressure approximates 25 mm Hg at the arteriole end of a capillary and 10 mm Hg at the venule end. This pressure within the capillary forces fluids out of the capillary into the interstitium. **Figure 5–1** illustrates the differences at either end.

Interstitial Pressure. As stated earlier, the interstitial pressure is normally negative, averaging approximately −5.3 mm Hg. The negative pressure on the interstitial side of the membrane also favors transport out of the capillary and into the interstitial space. So far, we have shown two forces that cause fluids to flow out of capillaries: (1) the capillary pressure (25 mm Hg at the arteriole end and 10 mm Hg at the venule end), and (2) interstitial pressure, which is negative (−5.3 mm Hg). When the effects of these two forces are combined, a pressure gradient of 30.3 mm Hg at the arteriole end forces fluids out of the capillary (capillary pressure of 25 mm Hg and negative interstitial pressure of −5.3 mm Hg), whereas the pressure gradient at the venule end of the capillary is only 15.3 mm Hg, which forces fluids out (capillary pressure of 10 mm Hg and negative interstitial pressure of −5.3 mm Hg). Thus, the total gradients differ at the two ends—the pressure forcing fluid out of the capillary is 15 mm Hg greater at the arteriole end (see **Fig. 5–1**).

Osmotic Pressure. **Osmotic pressure** is the pressure that causes fluids to pass from areas of lower concentration to areas of higher concentration of an osmotic substance. Both protein and sodium ions are examples of osmotic substances. Most of the osmotic pressure at the capillary membrane is caused by a concentration of plasma protein (primarily albumin). Because protein molecules are large, most are unable to pass from the plasma through the membranes to the interstitium; they accumulate in the capillary at the

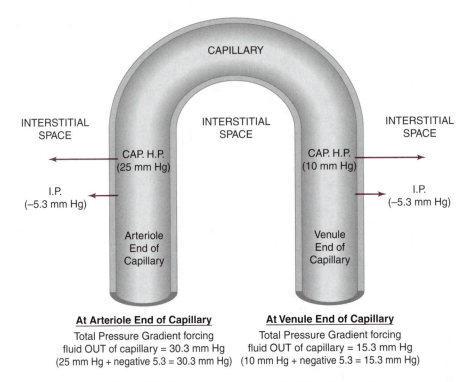

CAPILLARY

INTERSTITIAL
SPACE

INTERSTITIAL
SPACE

INTERSTITIAL
SPACE

CAP. H.P.
(25 mm Hg)

CAP. H.P.
(10 mm Hg)

I.P.
(−5.3 mm Hg)

I.P.
(−5.3 mm Hg)

Arteriole
End of
Capillary

Venule
End of
Capillary

At Arteriole End of Capillary
Total Pressure Gradient forcing
fluid OUT of capillary = 30.3 mm Hg
(25 mm Hg + negative 5.3 = 30.3 mm Hg)

At Venule End of Capillary
Total Pressure Gradient forcing
fluid OUT of capillary = 15.3 mm Hg
(10 mm Hg + negative 5.3 = 15.3 mm Hg)

FIGURE 5–1   Effect of hydrostatic pressure on fluid exchange between a capillary and the interstitial space. The model illustrates the difference in the total pressure gradient forcing fluid *out* of the capillary at its arteriole and venule ends. Although the negative interstitial pressure (IP) is constant, the hydrostatic pressure (CAP H.P.) of the capillary is greater at the arteriole end than at the venule end.

membrane, creating osmotic pressure of approximately 19 mm Hg and drawing fluids into the capillaries. Osmotic pressure resulting from a concentration of protein is called **oncotic pressure (OP)** or **colloid osmotic pressure (COP).** The **plasma colloid osmotic pressure (PCOP)** is augmented approximately 50% by the so-called **Donnan effect,** in which protein molecules, which are negative, attract a large number of positive ions, mainly sodium ions. Because sodium is also an osmotic substance, the concentration of osmotically active sodium molecules increases wherever the proteins accumulate. This increases the total PCOP by 9 mm Hg, making the total PCOP 28 mm Hg, which tends to force fluids into the capillaries.

Although most proteins do not pass through the membrane, a small percentage do pass to the interstitial fluid, creating an opposing osmotic pressure on the interstitial side of the membrane. This pressure is an **interstitial fluid colloid osmotic pressure (IFCOP)** of 6 mm Hg, which tends to draw fluids in

the opposite direction of the PCOP (ie, into the interstitial space). The sum of these osmotic forces (PCOP at −28 mm Hg into capillaries, less IFCOP 6 mm Hg out of capillaries) leaves a net osmotic force of 22 mm Hg, which draws fluids into the capillaries (**Fig. 5–2**).

Direction and Amount of Pressure Gradient. Finally, the direction and amount of the pressure gradient at the arterial and venule ends of the capillaries can be determined. At the arterial end, if the net osmotic pressure forcing fluids into capillaries (22 mm Hg) is subtracted from the net hydrostatic force out (30.3 mm Hg), the remainder is 8.3 mm Hg, which forces fluids out of capillaries (**Fig. 5–3**).

The numbers change, however, at the venule end of the capillary. Here, the net outward force is only 15.3 mm Hg because the capillary hydrostatic pressure at the venule end is only 10 mm Hg. Subtracting the outward force from the net osmotic force drawing fluids into the capillaries (22 mm Hg), the remainder

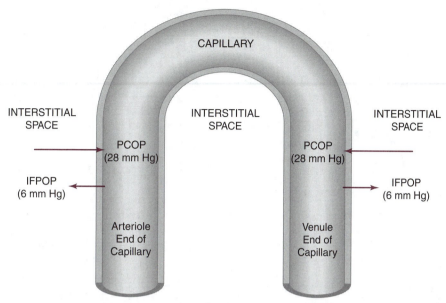

NET Colloid Osmotic Pressure (COP) = 22 mm Hg forcing fluids INTO Capillary
PCOP (28 mm Hg) — IFPOP (6 mm Hg)

FIGURE 5–2   Effect of osmotic forces on fluid exchange between the capillary and the interstitial space. The net colloid osmotic pressure (COP) is the same at both ends of the capillary. PCOP = plasma colloid osmotic pressure, IFCOP = interstitial fluid colloid osmotic pressure.

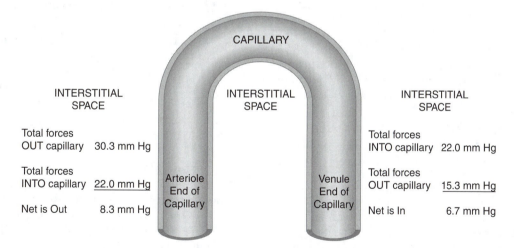

FIGURE 5–3   Difference in net pressure at the arteriole and venule ends of the capillary that effects exchange of fluid between the capillary and the interstitium. Total pressure forcing fluids *out* of the capillary = Cap. hydrostatic pressure and the negative interstitial pressure. Total pressure forcing fluids *into* the capillary = plasma colloid osmotic pressure (PCOP) minus interstitial fluid colloid osmotic pressure (IFCOP). The net pressure at the arteriole end is 8.3 mg Hg, which forces fluids *out* of the capillary. The net pressure at the venule end is 6.7 mm Hg, which forces fluids *into* the capillary. Thus, in this model, the 1.6 mm Hg difference in pressure tends to force fluid *out* of the capillary into the interstitial space.

is 6.7 mm Hg, which draws fluids back into the capillaries. Comparing the net at each end (ie, 8.3 mm Hg out at the arteriole end and 6.7 mm Hg in at the venule end), reveals a difference of 1.6 mm Hg, which tends to force fluids out of the capillaries (see **Fig. 5–3**).

This small, overall resultant effect of forcing fluid out means that a small percentage of fluid will not be reabsorbed into the bloodstream. This interstitial residue is primarily albumin protein. Under normal circumstances, this residue does not cause edema because the proteins will be taken into the lymphatic system (see **Chapter 3).**

Factors That Disrupt Normal Fluid Exchange

The previous discussion showed that the delicate balance that maintains normal volume of interstitial fluid depends on (1) the permeability of the capillary membrane, (2) the hydrostatic pressure of the capillary, (3) negative interstitial pressure, (4) the PCOP, (5) the IFCOP, and (6) an intact lymphatic system. Changes in any of these factors that can disrupt the balance, as we will see.

Capillary Permeability.   The permeability of capillaries appears to increase when vasoactive substances such as histamine or bradykinin are released in the tissues, when tissue temperatures increase, or when the temperatures decrease excessively. The inflammatory process activates vasoactive substances and also increases the temperature of tissues. Capillary permeability may be the factor that causes the edema observed with tissue irritation or with the application of thermal modalities.

Capillary Hydrostatic Pressure.   The hydrostatic pressure of capillaries increases whenever arterial flow to the capillary region increases or when some condition prevents the free return of blood through the veins. Increased arterial flow can occur when metabolic activity is increased (eg, with exercise or increased tissue temperature). Capillary hydrostatic pressure also increases with any pooling of blood in the veins. Pooling occurs when veins are distended (eg, varicose veins) or when systemic problems create an excessive amount of fluids in the body core (eg, renal problems or congestive heart failure). This excessive fluid forces blood to back up in the veins.

Any pressure on veins (eg, fetus pressing on the femoral veins of a pregnant woman) can block the flow. Even straps on leg braces or elastic tops on socks, if narrow and tight, can create strong pressure on leg tissues and block venous return. Standing erect for long periods when one is not using muscle pumps causes pooling in the lower extremities, especially in a hot environment.

Injury to Tissue.   More fluid flows to the interstitium after injury to tissue (eg, burns), because the physical disruption of the capillaries allows more protein to escape to the interstitium. This reduces the gradient between the PCOP and the IFCOPs, thus reducing the osmotic force that draws fluids back into the capillaries. Similarly, any conditions that increase the amount of an osmotic substance (eg, protein or sodium) in the interstitium will destory the balanced osmotic pressure gradient. An example of this is an imbalance in salt-regulatory hormones.

Obstruction in the Lymphatic System.   Finally, obstructions within the lymphatic system prevent the uptake of lymphatic substances. Surgical removal of lymph nodes (eg, during radical mastectomy) or a systemic condition (eg, elephantiasis) can cause lymphedema. **Table 5–1** outlines the common causes of edema and indicates which factor controlling the pressure balance was disturbed.

Although edema ultimately results from disturbances of the delicate balance of capillary membrane pressures, the cause of the disturbances may be many and complex, as illustrated by the shoulder-hand-finger syndrome of the hemiplegic patient. The pain, joint limitations, and swelling that are part of this syndrome interfere with therapeutic exercise and the patient's functional recovery. Impairment of venous and lymphatic circulation and immobilization of the involved extremity—resulting in less muscle-pumping activity—are primarily responsible for these problems. Cailliet[4] pointed out, however, that since the syndrome is seen in patients with and without sympathetic nerve involvement, the motor and sensory deficits of the central nervous system are initially responsible for the syndrome.

The subject of edema can be studied in many ways. This physiologic overview is limited to factors most pertinent for a text about physical agents. More complete information can be found in current physiology texts.[12,13,14]

TABLE 5–1   *Factors Altering Normal Exchange of Fluid at Capillary Membranes*

Physiological Factor Change	Cause	Result
Increased capillary membrane permeability	Inflammatory process Temperature change	Increased flow out of the capillary (edema)
	Release of histamine, kinines, or other vasoactive chemicals	
Increased capillary hydrostatic pressure	Arterial dilatation (increased flow to capillary)	Increased flow out of the capillary (edema)
	Venous obstruction (reduced flow from capillary)	
	Systemic problem: ie, congestive heart failure (blood backflow to capillary)	
	Renal problems causing fluid retention	
Reduced plasma COP*	Reduced plasma protein caused by hypoproteinemia with severe burns or physical disruption of capillaries (eg, trauma)	Reduced flow into the capillary from the interstitium (edema)
Increased interstitial COP*	Increased protein in interstitium	Increased flow out of the capillary (edema)
	Excessive extracellular sodium (eg, imbalance in salt regulating hormones)	
Lymphatic obstructions	Systemic diseases (eg, elephantitis-filariasis)	Lymphedema
	Lymphatic resection (after cancer)	

*COP = colloid osmotic pressure.

CLINICAL ASPECTS

When describing edema, clinicians must consider (1) whether it is acute or chronic, (2) the amount of swelling that has occurred, (3) the consistency of the fluid, and (4) the site and size of the edematous area.

Acute and Chronic Edema

Acute edema, as the term implies, refers to a swelling that has occurred recently and rapidly, for example, the sudden swelling that occurs immediately after an injury such as an ankle sprain. **Chronic** **edema** refers to a swelling that persists for some time, that is, swelling related to a trauma or injury that remains beyond the time expected for normal healing, or a swelling that develops gradually because of systemic problems or other factors that disturb the normal physiologic mechanisms maintaining the balance between the fluids in the capillaries and the interstitial spaces.

Amount of Swelling

The "free fluid" in the interstitium may increase as much as 30% above normal before it is noticeable. But whenever free fluid is increased to the extent that the interstitial fluid pressure changes from negative to positive, marked edema occurs.[9] The extent of edema in a body part can be ranked on a continuum from 1+ (barely detectable) to 4+ (swelling of the area to 1.5 or 2 times its normal size).

Consistency of the Fluid

The consistency of the fluid is the basis for the following classifications of edema: transudate versus exudate and pitting versus nonpitting. **Transudate edema** is the mild edema that is part of the inflammatory process. The fluid, primarily water and dissolved electrolytes, is clear. **Exudate edema** occurs with a more extreme stage of inflammation; it may appear as a milky or puslike fluid because of an increased protein content, primarily leukocytes.[15,16]

Edema is classified as pitting if a depression (pit) appears when the examiner presses a finger into the swollen tissues and the pit remains for a few seconds after the finger is removed, then gradually recedes (**Fig. 5–4**). The fluid moves away from the pressure site, then slowly returns, because the substance was fluid and could move freely. Massive **pitting edema** is seen in cases of extreme neglect in treating the condition.[5]

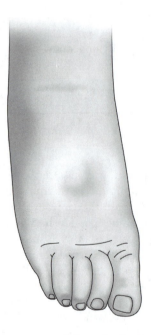

FIGURE 5–4 Severe, bilateral, dependent, pitting edema occurs with some systemic diseases, such as congestive heart failure and hepatic cirrhosis.

Edema is classified as nonpitting if the fluid does not move with the finger pressure (ie, no pitting is observed). This occurs when the interstitial fluid is coagulated or the tissue cells are swollen from disease, trauma, or inadequate nourishment. Longstanding nonpitting edema may progress to a state in which the skin is golden brown in color. This condition is often called **brawny edema.** Eventually, fibrous tissue deposits may form,[17] a condition referred to as **fibrosis edema.**

Site and Size of the Edematous Area

The site of edema must be noted because, if it is near a nerve plexus or major blood vessel, the resultant pressure can block nerve conduction or blood flow and lead to further complications. If it is within a joint, the function of that joint may be decreased. The clinician also needs to note the size of the area because a localized edema that spreads may indicate that the condition is becoming worse. If the edema is generalized (ie, observed throughout the body or in more than one extremity), it may indicate a systemic problem such as heart failure or renal disease.[18] Generalized edema is also called **anasarca** or **dropsy.**

APPLICATION TO PHYSICAL THERAPY

Edema can interfere with any interventions, including mobilization or therapeutic exercise. The pain and discomfort caused by the extra pressure on nerves can precipitate a severe pain cycle. Additional fluid at joints can reduce range of motion, leading to decreased function of those joints. The position of the joint that decreases the fluid pressure is one of flexion; thus, people with edematous joints tend to avoid full extension, which in turn encourages shortening of flexor muscles, tendons, and joints structures. A wisely selected physical modality or combination of modalities and appropriate medication levels may improve and edematous condition before other procedures are initiated. Intervention for edema and lymphedema should begin with the superficial lymphatics.[2] Ignoring the superficial lymphatics may aggravate the situation by slowing the rate of absorption. Heavy pressure and vigorous heating or cooling may cause exacerbation of swelling by overloading the system's ability to absorb the excess fluid.[2]

Physical therapy interventions to prevent or treat edema include the following:

- Application of *mild* superficial heat or cold to reduce pain or spasms.

- Immediate application of cold to prevent or reduce posttrauma swelling. The cold may cause temporary local vasoconstriction and thus decrease the flow of arterial blood to the capillary region and may also reduce inflammatory reactions. This in turn prevents an increase in capillary hydrostatic pressure and in capillary permeability.

- Application of compression bandages or garments to block fluid accumulation in the interstitium.

- Instructions to patients regarding positioning (eg, keep edematous extremities elevated to at least a horizontal position whenever possible and avoid static flexed-joint positions as much as possible). Fluid has less opportunity to accumulate at joints if the joint is in extension or close-pack position.

- Application of external pressure via massage to move the fluids through the vessels. Foldi[19] recommends that massage begin at the "root"—the trunk region just proximal to the swollen extremity—to prevent blockage of fluid as the extremity is massaged. Subsequently, the therapist can massage distally to move fluids back toward the trunk.[19]

- Application of intermittent compression pumps to produce external pressure to vessels that simulates the on-off pressure of muscle contractions.

- Use of ultrasound to deter formation of fibrotic tissue.

- Use of active exercise or electrical stimulation of muscles to increase muscle pumping action and thus encourage venous and lymphatic return of fluids.

The first four modalities may be useful to prevent edema in cases of acute trauma (eg, immediately after a strain or sprain). However, controversy exists regarding the choice of heat or cold.[19,20] (This subject is discussed in **Part 2** of this text.)

Intervention with chronic problems requires an aggressive and a prolonged approach. In such cases, additional modalities such as massage, ultrasound, intermittent positive pressure pumps, electrical stimulation of muscles, or all of these may be recommended.

When generalized edema exists, the therapist must give careful consideration to the use of physical agents. If the condition is extensive, physical agents may be ineffective. With some systemic problems, they may be useful, although incapable of helping the primary problem. For example, if swelling is sufficient to prevent joint movement and thus the functioning of an extremity, even a temporary reduction of the swelling may allow some joint movement and thus some muscle contraction and active movement of the part. This activity, in turn, decreases the edema and improves the function.

The therapist using these modalities in cases of generalized edema must consult with the primary physician because, in some systemic problems (eg, renal problems or congestive heart failure), a modality that reduces edema locally is **contraindicated.** In such cases, the body is attempting to deal with excessive fluid that impinges on heart, lungs, and other organs in the trunk by sending more of the fluid to the extremities, and forcing the fluid back to the body core would be dangerous.

Before applying any physical agents, whether to treat edema or an unrelated problem, the therapist must check the patient's chart, obtain the history, and understand any edema-related physical problems to rule out contraindications. Succeeding chapters address each physical agent and give indications and contraindications for their use. Many are related to how a particular agent may effect edema.

REVIEW QUESTIONS

1. What is the difference between swelling and edema?

2. What are the major causes of primary and secondary lymphedema?

3. Describe how hydrostatic, interstitial, and osmotic pressure affect the fluid balance between the lymphatic system and interstitial space.

4. Which physical therapy interventions would be most appropriate for treating acute edema caused by trauma versus chronic edema caused by lymphatic disruption?

5. How can the use of inappropriate interventions and physical agents increase the severity of swelling and edema?

6. What is pitting edema?

7. What is brawny edema?

8. Describe conditions and situations in which capillary hydrostatic pressure may be abnormally increased and lead to edema.

9. How is acute edema distinguished from chronic edema?

10. Identify the principles of lower-extremity positioning for an individual with ankle and lower-leg edema.

KEY TERMS

edema
effusion
lymph
lymphedema
lymphatics
right lymphatic duct
thoracic duct
starling's hypothesis of the
  capillaries

filtration
reabsorption
hydrostatic pressure
interstitial pressure
osmotic pressure
colloid osmotic pressure
plasma colloid pressure
donnan effect
acute and chronic edema

transudate
exudate
pitting edema
brawny edema
fibrosis edema
anasarca
dropsy

REFERENCES

1. Knight KL: *Cryotherapy in Sport Injury Management.* Champaign, IL: Human Kinetics; 1995.

2. Kelly DG: *A Primer on Lymphedema.* Upper Saddle River, NJ: Prentice Hall; 2000.

3. Goodman CC, Boissonnault WG, Fuller KS: *Pathology: Implications for the Physical Therapist.* Philadelphia: Saunders; 2003.

4. Cailliet R: *The Shoulder in Hemiplegia.* Philadelphia: FA Davis; 1980.

5. Fishman A, Wyngaarden J, Smith L, eds: Heart Failure. In: *Cecil's Textbook of Medicine.* 17th ed. Philadelphia: Saunders; 1985.

6. Staub N, Taylor A, eds: *Edema.* New York: Raven Press; 1984.

7. Carola R, Harley J, Noback C: *Anatomy and Physiology.* New York: McGraw-Hill; 1990.

8. Anthony C, Thiboneau G: Fluid and Electrolyte Balance. In: *Textbook of Anatomy and Physiology.* 11th ed. St. Louis: Mosby; 1983:569.

9. Guyton AC, Hall JE: *Textbook of Medical Physiology.* 10th ed. Philadelphia: Saunders; 2000.

10. Witte CL, ed: The Introduction to Classics in Lymphology. In: *Lymphology.* 1984; 17(4):124.

11. Lockhart R, Hamilton G, Fyfe F: *Anatomy of the Human Body.* Philadelphia: Lippincott; 1965; 580.

12. Boyd W, Sholdon H: *Introduction to the Study of Disease.* 11th ed. Philadelphia: Lea & Febiger; 1992.

13. Berne R, Levy MN: *Cardiovascular Physiology.* 8th ed. St. Louis: Mosby; 2001; Chaps 6 and 7.

14. Guyton AC, Hall JE: *Human Physiology and Mechanism of Disease.* 6th ed. Philadelphia: Saunders; 1997.

15. Baez S, Knobile E, eds: Microcirculation. In: *Ann Rev Physiol.* 1977; 39:391–415.

16. Reed B. Zarrou, Michlovitz S: Inflammation and repair and the use of thermal agents. In: *Thermal Agents in Rehabilitation.* Philadelphia: Davis; 1990; 5–7.

17. Abramson D, Miller D: *Vascular Problems in Musculoskeletal Disorders.* New York: Springer-Verlag; 1981.

18. *Dorland's Illustrated Medical Dictionary.* 27th ed. Philadelphia: Saunders; 1988.

19. Foldi E: Lymphedema. In: Staub N, Taylor A, eds. *Edema.* New York: Raven Press; 1984; 657–77.

20. Marek J, Jezdensky S, Ochonsky P: Effects of local cold and heat therapy in traumatic oedema of the rat hind paw. *Acta Universitatis Palackiane Olomucensis.* 1973; 65–66, 203–226.

6

Pain

JOSEPH WEISBERG, PT, PhD

WILLIAM E. DETURK, PT, PhD

Chapter Outline

Pain is the major complaint of most patients. Finding ways to minimize the devastating effects of pain—psychological,[1] socioeconomic,[2] and physiological[3]—is a major challenge for those who care for people suffering from pain. To deal with the problem effectively, we need to understand that pain is a multidimensional phenomenon: ie, the experience of pain is modulated by a wide range of factors, such as the sensitivity of the particular tissue involved, the person's mental state, the attitudes of the culture toward pain, and the person's previous experience of pain. Patients who suffer from chronic or acute pain are often extremely irritable and depressed. Consequently, the physical therapist must be aware of its psychological as well as neurophysiologic aspects.

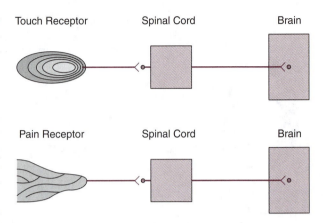

FIGURE 6–1   A diagram representing the concept of the specificity theory of pain.

THEORIES

One of the oldest theories of pain was postulated by Aristotle, who believed that pain was a reaction to excessive stimulation. This stimulation was said to be carried by the blood to the heart, where it was perceived as an unpleasant experience. It should be noted that Aristotle was cognizant of the psychological aspects of pain.[4]

Specificity Theory

Acceptance of the concept that pain is a sensory modality led to the development of neurophysiologic theories of pain. In 1894, Von Frey proposed a doctrine of specific nerve energies—the **specificity theory** of pain. This doctrine implied that each sensory modality was subserved by morphologically specific nerve endings: that is, pain by free nerve endings, light touch by Merkel's corpuscles, flutter (vibration) by Meissner's corpuscles, and pressure touch by pacinian corpuscles. Von Frey's theory grew out of Muller's concept, which stated that the quality of the sensation depended on the properties of the nerve[5] and from the evidence gained by microscopic investigation, especially the identification of specific receptors in the skin. According to Von Frey's theory, pain is a specific sensation that is triggered when specific receptors in the skin are stimulated. This stimulation travels along specific pathways in the spinal cord to reach specific projection areas in the brain, namely, the "pain center," where the stimulus is appreciated (**Fig. 6–1**). The anatomical evidence for this theory was that similar stimulation of a different type of receptor produced different sensations and that a different stimulus to the same type of receptor produced the same sensation. The objections to this theory are many; most obvious is the fact that a wide spectrum of sensations can be transmitted from tissue served by one type of nerve ending. For example, free nerve endings can transmit the sensations of pain, touch, or pressure.

Pattern Theory

The realization that pain and other sensations were not simple stimulus-response phenomena led Goldschneider (1896) to develop the **pattern theory.** This theory suggested that the pattern of stimulation (intensity and frequency) of nerve endings determined whether the brain would interpret the stimuli as pain (**Fig. 6–2**). The theory implied that a group of nerve endings and their associated nerve fibers form a "pain spot." Such spots are the primary areas for initiation of a train of impulses in the pain pathways.[4] The stimulation of these spots results in the perception of pain when the proper "pain centers" in the brain are activated. Actually, the conscious perception of various nuances of pain probably arises from expressions of the stimulation of different combinations of nerve endings and the resulting complex interactions in the "pain centers" in the brain.[6]

In 1943, Livingston expanded on the pattern theory to explain how pain could occur long after an initial injury. Subsequently, Weddell and Sinclair (1947) suggested that the size of the nerve fiber as well as the frequency and intensity of the stimulus were the determinants of the sensation and perception of pain.

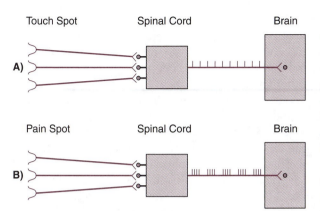

Touch Spot   Spinal Cord   Brain

A)

Pain Spot   Spinal Cord   Brain

B)

FIGURE 6–2 A diagram representing the concept of differentiation between pain and touch according to the pattern theory of pain.

This theory was challenged by the fact that receptor specialization does exist to a great extent.

Both the specificity and the pattern theories were valid to a degree; however, both were criticized for overemphasizing the sensation of pain and underemphasizing the perception of pain.[7] Although the functional role of all known nociceptors and their corresponding afferent fibers has been established, no detectable structural differences of general pain receptors (free nerve endings) explain the functional differences. Moreover, the unimodal nociceptor responds to only one type of noxious stimulus, whereas the polymodal nociceptor may respond equally to mechanical, thermal, or chemical stimuli. In addition, it has been determined that different nerve fibers mediate different sensations. Large myelinated (A-alpha) fibers transmit messages perceived as vibrations, and small myelinated (A-delta) fibers transmit messages perceived as sharp, prickling, dermatomic pain; proprioception; and temperature. The unmyelinated (C) fibers transmit burning sclerodermic pain, a poorly localized deep aching. Pain mediated by A-delta fibers is more severe but of short duration, whereas pain mediated by C-fibers is dull and continuous. Although dull, the effects of this continuous pain accumulate, and it is subjectively viewed as more disabling.

Gate Theory. In 1965, Melzack and Wall proposed the **gate theory** of pain,[8] which they subsequently revised in 1978 (**Fig. 6–3**). They originally postulated that interneurons in the substantia gelatinosa in the dorsal horn of the spinal cord acted as a gate to modulate sensory input. These cells project to second-order

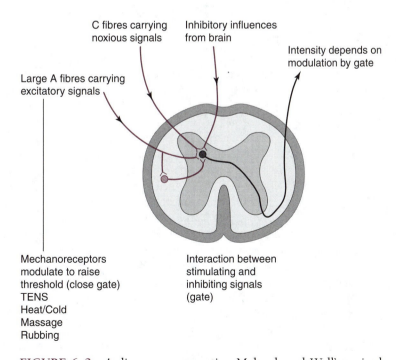

C fibres carrying
noxious signals

Inhibitory influences
from brain

Intensity depends on
modulation by gate

Large A fibres carrying
excitatory signals

Mechanoreceptors
modulate to raise
threshold (close gate)
TENS
Heat/Cold
Massage
Rubbing

Interaction between
stimulating and
inhibiting signals
(gate)

FIGURE 6–3 A diagram representing Melzack and Wall's revised gate theory of pain.

neurons of pain or temperature pathways located in lamina V and called *transmission cells.* Melzack and Wall postulated that this was where modulation of peripheral stimuli occurred through the activity of interneurons. The gate was considered to be related to the different amounts of input from large and small fibers to the system. For example, the input of large A-fibers could be viewed as exciting the inhibitory interneuron in the substantia gelatinosa. This A-fiber input, which reduced the excitation level of the transmission cells, might result in "closing the gate" at that level, thus decreasing the number of ascending nociceptive stimuli. In turn, the small C-fibers could be regarded as stimulators of the excitatory interneurons, thereby tending to "open the gate." The gate could be "opened" or "closed" further by descending excitatory or inhibitory pathways from the brain, thus decreasing or increasing the firing of transmission cells. This original theory was criticized for its simplicity and the fact that it does not explain pain mediated by A-fibers. Nonetheless, it did spark renewed interest in pain control that led to the development of **transcutaneous electrical nerve stimulation (TENS),** which is currently an effective and widely used modality for the relief of chronic and acute pain.

Melzack and Wall revised their theory, incorporating a more complex neural mechanism in the dorsal horn. In this revision, they hypothesized that the control at the gate was the result of the activities of nociceptive and non-nociceptive neurons rather than the activities of large- and small-diameter afferent fibers (see **Fig. 6–3**).[9] The gate theory offered an explanation for a clinical prediction: namely, that direct stimulation of sensory fibers by TENS diminishes the pain. However, the gate control theory remains just a theory. No solid anatomical evidence is available to support the existence of this mechanism.

Endogenous Opiates: Another Theoretical Dimension

The discovery of pain-mediating chemicals produced within the body has added another dimension to the specificity, pattern, and gate theories of pain. These endogenous opioids and their receptors are located within the nociceptive pathways and provide analgesia in much the same way as externally applied electrical stimulation and extrinsic opiates (eg., morphine) reduce pain. Over the past 50 years, our knowledge of analgesic opiates has increased dramat-

ically. Their effects involve a dynamic interplay between pain-transmitting substances, pain-mediating substances, and pain chemoreceptors. Both the central and the peripheral nervous system participate in this interaction.

The *transmission of pain* begins with the release of a peptide called *substance P.* This amino-acid peptide is produced in the spinal ganglia within the dorsal root ganglia. Although synthesized in the cell body, substance P is then transported to the peripheral target area via axonal transport and released by terminal vesicles. Substance P can also be found at the central terminal of the C-fiber in the dorsal horn, and transmits nociceptive information from both somatic and visceral structures. Substance P allows transmission of pain from such tissues as skin, sweat glands, and coronary and cerebral blood vessels, as well as the gastrointestinal tract, the ureters, and the urinary bladder.[10] The close proximity of neurons receiving input from somatic and visceral structures in the dorsal horn, as well as the fact that they may synapse on the same projection neuron, helps to explain the phenomenon of **referred pain:** The release of substance P from primary afferents of the heart can impact on afferents of the upper extremities. For example, it is a common finding that patients complain of left-arm pain when they are experiencing a myocardial infarction.[11]

Although the release of substance P can be blocked by morphine and results in analgesia,[12] other substances within the body may also act to counter nociceptive input from pain fibers. These are the opioids, so-called for their *pain mediating effects* and analgesic properties. Three classes of opioids are currently recognized, each having its own anatomic distribution. These are (1) the enkephalins, (2) the dynorphins, and (3) the beta-endorphins. Each of these substances is associated with its own *pain chemoreceptor binding site* on neurons.

Cell bodies and nerve endings containing **enkephalin** are found in the substantia gelatinosa. In the dorsal horn, enkephalins are released by spinal interneurons. Enkephalins are activated when the perception of pain, or perhaps its anticipation, is transmitted by C-fibers from the periphery and reaches the dorsal horn. This pathway and its neuromediator may be activated when a person picks up a skillet, knowing it to be hot yet needing to remove it from the table before it burns the tablecloth. Enkephalin serves to hyperpolarize the projection neurons such that nociception is blocked at the spinal level.[11]

The substance **dynorphin** is contained in neuronal cell bodies and nerve endings found in the periaquaductal gray matter, rostroventral medulla, and the dorsal horn of the spinal cord.[11] Injection of dynorphin directly into the spinal canal produces dramatic analgesia.[10]

The third class of opioids are the **beta-endorphins.** Unlike the enkephalins and dynorphins, the beta-endorphins are confined to the hypothalamus. The precursor of beta-endorphin is proopiomelanocortin (POMC). The POMC neurons are located in the hypophysis; stress causes beta-endorphin to be released into the bloodstream.[10] Thus there is wide systemic distribution of this powerful analgesic. Removal of the hypophysis disrupts control of stress-induced analgesia (SIA). This is evidence that beta-endorphins may contribute to pain control.[10]

Some nonopiate chemical substances have been associated with producing pain. For example, an imbalance of dopaminergic and serotoninergic substances influences the neurotransmission of pain.[12] Acetylcholine, histamine, bradykinin, prostaglandin, capaicin, and potassium ions have been implicated, and the injection of bradykinin into the viscera actually has produced lasting pain. A good example of pain that is most likely produced by these substances is angina pectoris. During an ischemic attack, bradykinen and prostaglandin are released, probably because of the ischemia in the heart muscle, which causes sensitization of the nociceptor.[13]

Anatomic and Physiologic Aspects

Nociceptive Receptor System

The **nociceptive receptor system** consists of two varieties. The first type is the free nerve ending found mostly in the cornea of the eye, teeth, tendons, and ligaments. The second type is a continuous tridimensional plexus of unmyelinated nerve fibers that weave in all directions throughout the tissue and around blood vessels (except for blood vessels in the central nervous system, CNS).[14] Mechanical distortion, changes in the chemical composition of tissue fluid, or thermal changes may stimulate these receptors. The person suffering from pain elicited by mechanical distortion might describe the pain as pressure pain, stabbing pain, or prickling pain, whereas pain caused by a thermal or chemical agent is usually described as burning pain. When the pain receptors around blood vessels are activated, the pain is usually described as a throbbing pain.

Most nociceptors are innervated by unmyelinated afferent fibers (C-fibers) with small diameters or by finely myelinated (A-delta) fibers. The C-fibers in the skin can be stimulated by mechanical irritation, which is likely to cause a prickling pain (**Table 6–1**).[15]

Certain pain sensations are associated with specific pathologies. Trauma to muscle or nerve cells usually causes a deep, "boring" pain; spasm causes intermittent

TABLE 6–1   *Characteristics of Type A and C Pain Fibers*

Fiber Type	Location	Distribution in a Given Area	Myelinated?	Conduction Velocity	Receptors	Perceived Pain Sensation
A	Skin and mucous membranes	Several spots within 1 sq cm; half as much as C fibers	Yes	Fast: 5–30 m/s	Mechanical, thermal, and chemical	Pricking, localized, sharp, stabbing; short duration, usually of sudden onset
C	Throughout the body except for nervous tissue in the brain	Spotty; twice as much as A fibers	No	Slow: 0.5–2 m/s	Mechanical, thermal, and chemical	Persistent, diffuse, throbbing, burning, itching, aching; often after the initial sharp pain

recurrent pain; cramps cause deep-pressure pain that is initially sharp, then achy; inflammation (myositis, tendinitis) produces a deep ache; and ischemia in the muscle causes deep intermittent pain. Every time a muscle contracts, toxic catabolites are released, then cleared by the circulation. When more catabolites are produced than can be cleared by the circulation (whether because of poor circulation or excessive muscle contraction), they accumulate and irritate the nociceptor, causing pain.[16]

The sympathetic nerves themselves do not mediate sensation. However, because pain-mediating fibers travel with the sympathetic nerves, interruption of the sympathetic nerves (sympathectomy) also cuts these pain fibers, thus obliterating the pain (visceral or neuropathic). Sympathectomy to an extremity may have an additional beneficial effect of decreasing pain by increasing the blood supply to the extremity.[17]

Some pain receptors have high thresholds; others have low thresholds. The stronger the stimulus, and the larger the recruitment of stimulated receptors, the stronger the sensation. Pain threshold is considered by some to differ by age (older people have higher pain tolerance)[18] and between men and women (men have higher thresholds),[19,20] but individuals perceive pain differently. The literature asserts no absolutes on pain thresholds in men and women or by age. Castro de Lopez et al.[21] investigated pain perception between men and women. They found that during assessment of pain perception to venous puncture, there were no differences between men and women. Data did reveal significant variability and suggest that the differences are psychosocial.

Thus an individual's reaction to the stimuli cannot be accurately predicted. For example, the pain threshold of thermal pain receptors is said to be 45°C[8] for some people in whom exposure to a stimulus of 42°C would be perceived as pain, whereas others would find that exposure to a stimulus of 45°C is relatively comfortable.

The action potentials carried by the primary afferent neurons via the A-delta and C-fibers produce neural activity that is conveyed via two basic pathways to the higher centers in the brain. The A-delta and C-fibers terminate in the dorsal horn of the spinal cord where some neural processing occurs. Each pathway transmits somewhat different types of pain sensations.

Lateral Spinothalamic Pathway

The axons of some transmission cells (see **Fig. 6–3**) of the dorsal horn cross over (decussate) and ascend as the **lateral spinothalamic pathway** and terminate in the thalamus. Some collateral fibers of this tract terminate in the brainstem. Other neurons of the thalamus associated with this pathway terminate in the postcentral gyrus (somatosensory cortex) of the cerebral cortex. This pathway transmits information perceived as sharp, discriminative, and relatively localized sensations of pain.

Spinoreticulothalamic Pathway

The axons of other transmission cells ascend in the same tract and terminate in the brainstem (reticular formation) and the midbrain tectum, including the periventricular gray matter. From these regions, neurons have axons that terminate in some thalamic nuclei and in some structures of the limbic system. Axons of neurons of the thalamus project to the structures of the limbic system, basal ganglia, and cerebral cortex. This pathway, known as the **spinoreticulothalamic pathway,** conveys information perceived as diffuse, poorly localized somatic and visceral pain.

TYPES OF PAIN

The three types of pain are acute, chronic, and referred (**Table 6–2**). **Acute pain** may last from seconds to days and is usually a result of potential or actual tissue damage. **Chronic pain** lasts for many months or years, and its mechanism is poorly understood. **Referred pain** is pain that is perceived to be in areas other than where the nociceptors were stimulated (eg, pain in the shoulder that is referred from the gallbladder). At times, this phenomenon may arise because both areas—the area where the pain is perceived and the area where the nociceptors were irritated—are innervated by the same root level, and their afferent fibers all converge in the same area of the spinal cord in close proximity of neurons within the dorsal root ganglia.

In essence, the perception of pain begins with the stimulation of certain receptors. Acute pain is believed to be an alarm that triggers activities to protect the body from noxious stimuli. The actual perception of the sensation occurs in the higher centers of the brain. A good example of this is a person with amputation who feels pain in the absent limb (the phantom limb phenomenon); the pain sensation occurs because the area in the brain associated with the amputated limb is stimulated.

The perception of pain and the reaction to pain are based on a complex of anatomic, physiologic,

TABLE 6–2   *The Characteristics of the Different Types of Pain*

Type of Pain	Onset	Duration	Pain Sensation	Cause	Associated Condition	Medication	Prognosis	Type of Nerve Fiber
Acute	Sudden, recent	Short: seconds–days	Sharp, localized	Tissue damage often easy to localize and diagnose	Usually none	Usually effective	Usually good	A C
Chronic	Slow, gradual	Long: months–years	Dull, diffuse	Prolonged nerve compression or pain spasm cycles poorly understood; often difficult to localize and diagnose	Poor posture, depression, hopelessness, drug abuse	Usually ineffective	Usually poor	Mostly C
Referred*	Dependent on primary cause	Dependent on primary cause	Dependent on primary cause	Irritation in area other than where pain is experienced				

*Referred pain is poorly understood and difficult to diagnose.

chemical, and psychological factors, many of which are still poorly understood. In totality, pain can be defined as an unpleasant sensory and emotional experience that is associated with actual or potential tissue damage or simply the result of an unpleasant emotional state.[22] Because pain is a perceptual experience, it is viewed as a symptom, not a root cause. The clinician must realize that stimulation of pain receptors will not always evoke the experience of pain and that the number of nerve fibers and the frequency of discharge of the fibers carrying the nociceptive impulses will not always be directly related to the intensity of the pain.

ASSESSMENT

Assessing pain is not a simple task. Pain may be present without any objective findings (eg, nonorganic pain). Conversely, healthy normal people may demonstrate objective abnormalities without associated symptoms (eg, an asymptomatic leg-length discrepancy). Measurement of pain is difficult because of the complex interaction of the host of contributory variables previously described. Measurements include a qualitative assessment that describes the nature of the pain and a quantitative assessment that measures the amount or severity of

the pain. Finally, pain assessment includes some indication of the degree of disability that the pain inflicts on the patient.

Nonorganic pain occurs in the absence of standard clinical signs of physical pathology. Although it is tempting to associate nonorganic pain with malingering, this may be unfair. Many other factors contribute to legitimate complaints of pain: the presence of small lesions may go undetected because diagnostic instrumentation lacks sufficient resolution, there may be errors of interpretation, or the patient may demonstrate a heightened psychological awareness. *Waddell's nonorganic physical signs for low back pain* recognizes five variables that distinguish nonorganic from physical pathology. It is an evaluation procedure that is applied to the patient and then scored by the therapist (**Fig. 6–4**).[23] Although the test is specific to low-back pain, it has general application in that it illustrates the need to make the distinction between nonorganic and organic pain because the implications for intervention are different.

Quantitative assessment of pain typically involves the use of pain scales. These may take the form of verbal scales (ie, mild, moderate, severe), or numeric scales (1–10). Visual analog scales (VASs) are also widely used. The VAS consists of a single line, usually 10 cm long, mounted either vertically or horizontally, with anchors at both ends labeled "no pain" and "worst

WADDELL'S NONORGANIC PHYSICAL SIGNS IN LOW BACK PAIN

tenderness: Tenderness not related to a particular skeletal or neuro-muscular structure, may be either superficial or nonanatomic.

> **superficial:** The skin is tender to light pinch over a wide area of lumbar skin not in a distribution associated with a posterior primary ramus.

> **nonanatomic:** Deep tenderness, which is not localized to one structure, is felt over a wide area and often extends to the thoracic spine, sacrum, or pelvis.

simulation test: These tests give the patient the impression that a particular examination is being carried out when in fact it is not.

> **axial loading:** Low back pain is reported when the examiner presses down on the top of the patient's head. Neck pain is common and should not be considered indicative of a nonorganic sign.

> **rotation:** Back pain is reported when the shoulders and pelvis are passively rotated in the same plane as the patient stands relaxed with the feet together. In the presence of root irritation, leg pain may be produced and should not be considered indicative of a nonorganic sign.

distraction tests: A positive physical finding is demonstrated in the routine manner; this finding is then checked while the patient's attention is distracted. A nonorganic component may be present if the finding disappears when the patient is distracted.

> **straight leg raising:** The examiner lifts the patient's foot as when testing the plantar reflex in the sitting position. A nonorganic component may be present if the leg is lifted higher than when tested in the supine position.

regional disturbances: Dysfunction (e.g., sensory or motor) involving a widespread region of body parts in a manner that cannot be explained based on anatomy. Care must be taken to distinguish from multiple nerve root involvement.

> **weakness:** Demonstrated on testing by a partial cogwheel "giving way" of many muscle groups that cannot be explained on a localized neurological basis.

> **sensory:** Include diminished sensation to light touch, pinprick or other neurologic tests fitting a "stocking" rather than a dermatomal pattern.

overreaction: May take the form of disproportionate verbalization, facial expression, muscle tension and tremor, collapsing or sweating. Judgments should be made with caution minimizing the examiner's own emotional reaction.

> **SCORING.** Any individual sign counts as a positive sign for that type; a finding of three or more of the five types is clinically significant.

BASED ON

Waddell, G, et al: Nonorganic physical sign in low-back pain. Spine 5:117, 1980, with permission.

FIGURE 6–4 Waddell's nonorganic physical signs in low back pain. *(Adapted with permission from Rothstein J. et al, The Rehabilitation Specialist's Handbook, 2nd ed. Philadelphia: FA Davis; 1998.)*

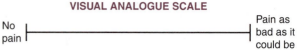

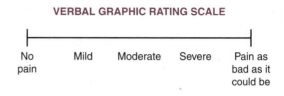

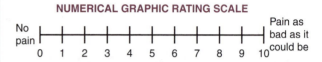

FIGURE 6–5 The Visual Analog Scale and two Graphic Rating Scales of pain intensity. *(Reproduced with permission from Turk & Melzak,* Handbook of Pain Assessment, *p. 140, New York, Guilford Press.)*

simple to explain and easy to administer. It correlates highly with both the verbal and the numeric scales. It possesses ratio scale properties that make it easy to compare measurements obtained from one patient over time or pain measurements from different patients. The main disadvantage of the VAS is its assumption that pain can be described solely on the basis of severity.

The *McGill Pain Questionnaire (MPQ)* provides the *qualitative assessment* dimension lacking in the VAS. Introduced in 1975, this pain inventory recognizes that pain is more than just a sensory experience. Rather, it possesses an unpleasant, affective dimension that adds to the painful sensation a potent combination of past experience, culture, preexisting anxiety, and depression.[12] Imagine a patient with chronic neck pain that resulted from a rear-end collision caused by a burly, bearded driver. This patient may experience a worsening of symptoms whenever interacting with a husky man who wears a beard. The MPQ includes words that reflect these affective feelings, like "horrible" and "vicious."

The MPQ provides a choice of words to describe the sensory, affective, and evaluative properties of the painful experience. The patient is instructed to choose only the words in each category that describe the present pain state. Each word is assigned a rank value. A *pain rating index (PRI)* is obtained by adding

pain ever." The patient is instructed to make a mark on the line that best represents his or her current level of pain. After the scale is administered, the results are quantified as the distance from the bottom of the line to the patient's mark (**Fig. 6–5**).[12] The VAS is up the value of each word. In the example, the patient with neck pain might choose the words "shooting," "vicious," "miserable," and "nagging" to describe the current pain. This yields a total score of 52 (**Fig. 6–6**).[12] The MPQ can be administered in about five minutes; it has been found to be consistent, valid, and reliable.

Many pain centers find that the use of both the VAS and the MPQ provides the quantitative and qualitative data they need to direct intervention. However, information from these scales may not reflect the *degree of patient disability*. This is an important component, particularly given the present emphasis on functional outcomes. The question of disability turns, not on the pain itself, but rather on the degree to which the pain restricts activity. Determination of disability is sometimes not easy; it is task-specific, and it may be compromised by symptom magnification on the part of the patient or by the subjectivity of the examiner.

Functional disability can be assessed by physical examination and by questionnaire. Physical exam may include palpation of target areas designed to illicit pain (eg, myofascial pain, trigger points), and a functional evaluation based on activities of daily living (ADLs) that provoke pain (eg, sitting, bending, lifting). Exercise tests may consist of a series of exercises designed to elicit symptoms. A key factor in these tests is the repetition of certain components randomly placed within the series. The examiner looks for consistency in response to these repeated elements. If reports of pain vary, this may indicate pain of nonorganic origin. For example, the patient with complaints of cervical pain may be given a series of 10 exercises on an isokinetic dynomometer, with measures of force output during each exercise. These exercises provoke reports of pain from the patient, which presumably would reduce force output. Exercises 2, 5, and 8 may be the same, but spaced so that the patient cannot motorically "remember" what force was generated the first time. If force output varies significantly across these three exercises, the patient may be "faking it."

The *Roland and Morris Disability Questionnaire* instrument is a 24-question self-assessment that measures what the patient can and cannot do because of the current level of pain. It is specific to back pain: the stem of each question is followed by ". . . because of my back." However, the questionnaire was derived from an earlier one, the Sickness Impact Profile,[24] that was more general in scope, suggesting that a vari-

ation of the scale could be used for other body parts (**Fig. 6–7**).[25]

MUSCLE SPASM (MUSCLE HOLDING STATE)

Muscle spasm is one cause of pain that is often treated with physical modalities. The literature is unclear about the meaning of the term **muscle spasm.** Even medical dictionaries lack a clear definition of what the term means. For example, *Taber's Medical Dictionary* defines *spasm* as "an involuntary muscular contraction that occurs as a result of some irritant or trauma."[26] If painful, the spasm may be referred to as a cramp. Moreover, the term does not represent a specific pathology or a specific dysfunction. Therefore, the authors suggest that the term *muscle holding state*, which describes the continuous contracted state of muscles, be used.

There are three different types of muscle-holding states: **involuntary muscle holding, voluntary muscle holding,** and **chemical muscle holding.**[27] The interrelationship between the three different types of muscle holding and dysfunction is illustrated in **Figure 6–8**. The pain associated with the spasm is probably caused by stimulation of mechanosensitive or chemosensitive pain receptors or both.[27]

The term *muscle spasm* is often used to describe a pathophysiologic state of muscles. The spasm is a symptom of a pathologic condition, not of the pathology itself. Some authorities combine spasm with the term *cramp*, or *contracture*, or both.[26,28] Others differentiate between the terms simply by stating that the cramp is painful.[26] The EMG recordings of muscle cramps show irregular, high-frequency, high-voltage, profuse bursts of motor unit potential, whereas the EMG recordings of muscle contracture (spasm) show little or no electrical activity in the muscle affected by the contraction.[29] Physiologically, the state of contraction is sustained when there is enough calcium present in the sarcomere to uncover binding sites between the actin and myosin fibers. Therefore, an agent or a condition that promotes release of calcium or inhibits its reaccumulation will cause a muscle to go into spasm.[29]

Spasticity also describes a pathophysiological state of muscles. This term is not interchangeable with the terms *spasm*, *cramp*, and *contracture*. Spasticity is

McGill Pain Questionaire

Patient's Name _____ Date _____ Time _____ am/pm

PRI: S _____ A _____ E _____ M _____ PRI(T) _____ PPI ____
     (1-10)   (11-15)   (16)   (17-20)   (1-20)

1 FLICKERING __ QUIVERING __ PULSING __ THROBBING __ BEATING __ POUNDING __	11 TIRING __ EXHAUSTING __
	12 SICKENING __ SUFFOCATING __
2 JUMPING __ FLASHING __ SHOOTING __	13 FEARFUL __ FRIGHTFUL __ TERRIFYING __
3 PRICKING __ BORING __ DRILLING __ STABBING __ LANCINATING __	14 PUNISHING __ GRUELLING __ CRUEL __ VICIOUS __ KILLING __
4 SHARP __ CUTTING __ LACERATING __	15 WRETCHED __ BLINDING __
5 PINCHING __ PRESSING __ GNAWING __ CRAMPING __ CRUSHING __	16 ANNOYING __ TROUBLESOME __ MISERABLE __ INTENSE __ UNBEARABLE __
6 TUGGING __ PULLING __ WRENCHING __	17 SPREADING __ RADIATING __ PENETRATING __ PIERCING __
7 HOT __ BURNING __ SCALDING __ SEARING __	18 TIGHT __ NUMB __ DRAWING __ SQUEEZING __ TEARING __
8 TINGLING __ ITCHY __ SMARTING __ STINGING __	19 COOL __ COLD __ FREEZING __
9 DULL __ SORE __ HURTING __ ACHING __ HEAVY __	20 NAGGING __ NAUSEATING __ AGONIZING __ DREADFUL __ TORTURING __
10 TENDER __ TAUT __ RASPING __ SPLITTING __	PPI 0 NO PAIN __ 1 MILD __ 2 DISCOMFORTING __ 3 DISTRESSING __ 4 HORRIBLE __ 5 EXCRUCIATING __

BRIEF __ MOMENTARY __ TRANSIENT __	RHYTHMIC __ MOMENTARY __ INTERMITTENT __	CONTINUOUS __ STEADY __ CONSTANT __

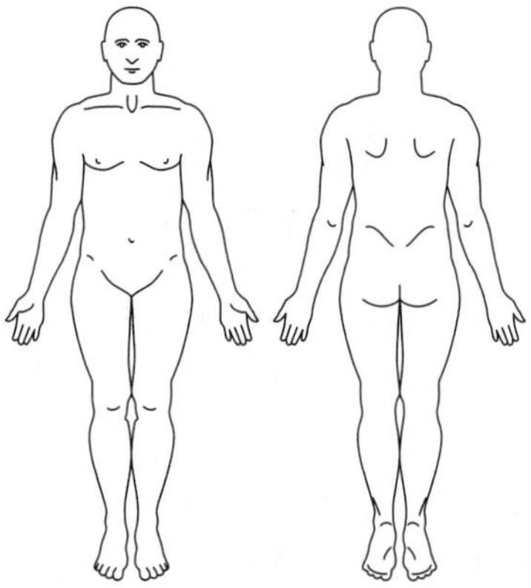

E = EXTERNAL
I = INTERNAL

COMMENTS:

FIGURE 6–6 The McGill Pain Questionnaire. The descriptors fall into four major groups: sensory, 1–10; affective, 11–15; evaluative, 16; and miscellaneous, 17–20. The rank value for each descriptor is based on its position in the word set. The sum of the rank values is the Pain Rating Index (PRI). The Present Pain Intensity (PPI) is based on a scale of 0 to 5. (*Reproduced with permission from Ronald Melzak,* Handbook of Pain Assessment, *140, 1975.*)

**Roland and Morris Disability Questionnaire:
Instrument**

When your back hurts, you may find it difficult to do some of the things you normally do.

This list contains some sentences that people have used to describe themselves when they have back pain. When you read them, you may find that some stand out because they describe you *today*. As you read the list, think of yourself *today*. When you read a sentence that describes you today, put a check beside the number of the sentence. If the sentence does not describe you, then leave the space blank and go on to the next one. Remember, only check the sentence if you are sure that it describes you *today*.

_____ 1. I stay at home most of the time because of my back.

_____ 2. I change position frequently to try and get my back comfortable.

_____ 3. I walk more slowly than usual because of my back.

_____ 4. Because of my back, I am not doing any of the jobs that I usually do around the house.

_____ 5. Because of my back, I use a handrail to get upstairs.

_____ 6. Because of my back, I lie down to rest more often.

_____ 7. Because of my back, I have to hold onto something to get out of an easy chair.

_____ 8. Because of my back, I try to get other people to do things for me.

_____ 9. I get dressed more slowly than usual because of my back.

_____ 10. I only stand up for short periods of time because of my back.

_____ 11. Because of my back, I try not to bend or kneel down.

_____ 12. I find it difficult to get out of a chair because of my back.

_____ 13. My back is painful almost all the time.

_____ 14. I find it difficult to turn over in bed because of my back.

_____ 15. My appetite is not very good because of my back pain.

_____ 16. I have trouble putting on my socks (or stockings) because of the pain in my back.

_____ 17. I only walk short distances because of my back pain.

_____ 18. I sleep less well because of my back.

_____ 19. Because of my back pain, I get dressed with help from someone else.

_____ 20. I sit down for most of the day because of my back.

_____ 21. I avoid heavy jobs around the house because of my back.

_____ 22. Because of my back pain, I am more irritable and bad tempered with people than usual.

_____ 23. Because of my back, I go upstairs more slowly than usual.

_____ 24. I stay in bed most of the time because of my back.

FIGURE 6–7 The Roland and Morris Disability Questionnaire (*Reproduced with permission from Roland M, Morris R. A study of the natural history of back pain, Pt. 1: The development of a reliable and sensitive measure of disability in low back pain. Spine 8: 141, 1983.*)

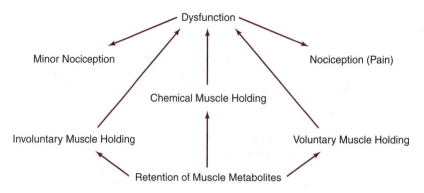

FIGURE 6–8 The interrelationship between the three different types of muscle holding and dysfunction (*Adapted from Paris SV.*)

associated with upper motor neuron lesions; the spastic muscle is hypersensitive to stretching; that is, it will contract strongly even with a small sudden stretch.[30]

An incidental spasm occurs as a result of a noxious stimulus that produces a momentary reaction. The minor derangements of reflex control produced by a muscle spasm may result in a remarkable aberration in the rhythm of body movements. Incidental muscle spasm is also referred to as a protective spasm.[31] Some authors object to the term *protective* primarily because, at times, such a spasm may be destructive, especially if left untreated. For example, a spasm that develops around an infected joint to prevent movement and further deterioration can be viewed as a protective spasm, whereas the severe spasm that may accompany fractures and cause displacement of the bones can be viewed only as a destructive spasm.[31,32]

A muscle spasm also may develop as a response to an abnormality in the physiologic environment of the muscle. For example, a deficiency of muscle phosphorylase or phosphofructokinase or an increase in the concentration of calcium or iodacetate within the myofibril increases the likelihood of a muscle cramp.[29] Consequently, muscle spasm is a dominant response to many pathologic states whether those states are local, systemic, or even psychological.

Muscle spasm is identified primarily by palpation and is characterized by the symptoms of local pain and tenderness, restriction of motion, and, when severe enough, impaired ADLs. Symptoms associated with spasms are part of a vicious cycle. The cycle begins with a specific pathology (trauma or stress) that causes pain, inflammation, dysfunction, muscle spasm, or all of these. The spasm then may cause local ischemia (increasing the concentration of metabolites), which leads to more pain, inflammation, or both, which in turn results in more spasm (**Fig. 6–9**).[32]

Because muscle spasm is a symptom, one must identify the cause and the mechanism by which it developed to treat it effectively. The cause of muscle spasm is not always obvious. The muscle may be susceptible because of its physiologic condition. On the other hand, a spasm can be triggered by irritation of any of the following structures: sensory organ or nerve, motor end plate (the most pain-sensitive site in muscle), motor nerve, or CNS. Whatever the cause of the spasm, one can reasonably assume that, during the early stage, the structure of a muscle in a holding state is essentially the same as that of a contracted muscle.[33]

Although most musculoskeletal spasms are not life-threatening, their impact on quality of life is substantial. Pain associated with spasm is among the most important causes of absenteeism from work.

INTERVENTIONS

Interventions should first be directed at the cause, provided that the cause can be identified. Spasm that is widespread throughout the body might be caused by an abnormal physiologic state, and the intervention might involve medication, a change in diet, or both. Localized spasm is more likely to be induced mechanically, and its intervention might involve correction of a joint dysfunction, improving the patient's posture, or changing the patient's work habits. Psychological stress contributes to overall tension and spasm in specific vulnerable sites and can be treated

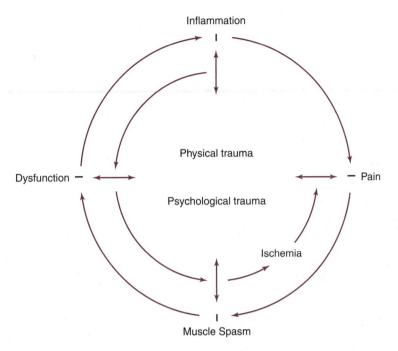

FIGURE 6–9 Pain cycle showing the interrelationship between physical and psychological trauma and signs and symptoms. The outer cycle shows the cause and effect relationship in a clockwise direction. The inner cycle shows other cause and effect relationships in a counterclockwise direction (pain, muscle spasm, ischemia, more pain).

by teaching the patient how to use relaxation techniques and, at times, by suggesting psychotherapy.

In some cases, addressing the cause of spasm may not bring the immediate relief necessary for the patient to function. This problem usually arises either during the acute stage, when the pain is disabling, or when the condition has become chronic and the tissue has already undergone some physiologic changes. Under these conditions, the clinician will have to incorporate specific modalities into the intervention plan that are directed at the spasm itself. Many interventions are available that can effectively reduce muscle spasm and help restore normal length and function of the muscle. Physicians often use local injections, systemic medications, or both to achieve relief. Physical therapists often use massage, exercise, heat, cold, ultrasound, phonophoresis, electrical stimulation, iontophoresis, and biofeedback to reduce pain and promote relaxation. The specific effects of each physical agent are discussed in subsequent chapters.

REVIEW QUESTIONS

1. What are the similarities and differences of the various pain theories?
2. Describe the two neuroanatomical pathways for pain transmission. What types of painful sensations do they each transmit?
3. What are the characteristics for each type of pain?
4. Describe the gate theory of pain. How can you use this information to plan an appropriate intervention for a patient with each type of pain?
5. What are the endogenous opiates, and what is their role in pain control?

KEY TERMS

specificity theory
pattern theory
gate theory
transcutaneous electrical nerve
  stimulation
endogenous opiates
enkephalin

beta-endorphin
dynorphin
lateral spinothalamic pathway
spinorecticulothalamic pathway
acute pain
chronic pain
referred pain

nonorganic pain
quantitative pain assessment
qualitative pain assessment
involuntary muscle holding
voluntary muscle holding
chemical muscle holding

REFERENCES

1. Nolan MF: Pain: The experience and its expression. *Clin Mgt, Phys Ther* 1990; 10(1):22–25.

2. French S: Pain: Some psychological and sociological aspects. *Physiotherapy* 1989; 75:255–60.

3. Bullingham RES: Physiological mechanism in pain. In: Smith G, Covino BG, eds. *Acute Pain.* London, UK: Butterworth; 1985.

4. Luce JM, Thompson RL II, Getto CJ, et al: New concepts of chronic pain and their implication. *Hosp Pract* April 1985:113.

5. De Pace DM: Anatomic and Functional Aspects of Pain: Evaluation and Management with Thermal Agents. In: Michlovitz SL, ed. *Thermal Agents in Rehabilitation*, 3rd ed. Philadelphia: Davis; 1996.

6. Novack C, Demarest R.J.: *The Nervous System: Introduction and Review.* New York: McGraw-Hill; 1986:92.

7. Martin J: Receptor physiology and submodality coding in the somatic sensory system. In: Kandel F, Schwartz J, eds. *Principles of Neural Science.* 2nd ed. New York: Elsevier; 1985:294.

8. Melzack R, Wall PD: Pain mechanism: A new theory. *Science* 1965; 150:971.

9. Wall PD: The gate control theory of pain mechanism: A reexamination and restatement. *Brain* 1978; 101:1.

10. Raj PP: *Pain Medicine: A Comprehensive Review.* St. Louis: Mosby; 1996:21.

11. Kandel ER, Schwartz JH, Jessell TM: *Principles of Neural Science.* 3rd ed. Norwalk, CT: Appleton & Lange; 1991:395.

12. Turk DC, Melzack R: *Handbook of Pain Assessment.* New York: Guilford Press; 1992:19–24, 26–28,139–64.

13. Kantor TG: Physiology and treatment of pain and inflammation. *Am J Med* 1986; 80(suppl 3A):118.

14. Thompson FF: *The Brain: An Introduction to Neuroscience.* New York: Freeman; 1985:141,196.

15. Willis WD, Jr: *The Pain System.* New York: Karger; 1985:264.

16. Kisner C, Colby LA: *Therapeutic Exercise.* 4th ed. Philadelphia: Davis; 2002.

17. Guyton AC: *Basic Neuroscience.* Philadelphia: Saunders; 1987:269.

18. Gagliese L, Katz J: Age differences in postoperative pain are scale dependent: A comparison of measures of pain intensity and quality in younger and older surgical patients. *Pain* 2003; 103:11–20.

19. Koltyn KF, Focht BC, Ancker HM, Pasley J: Experimentally induced pain perception in men and women in the morning and evening. *Int J Neurosci* 1999; 98(1–2):1–11.

20. Chesterton LS, Barlas P, Foster NE, et al: Gender differences in pressure pain threshold in healthy humans. *Pain* 2003; 101,259–66.

21. Lopez de Castro, et al: Do men and women have different perceptions of pain? *Aten Primaria* 2003, Jan; 31(1):18–22.

22. Wyke BD: Neurological aspect of pain therapy: A review of some current concepts. In: Swerdlow M, ed. *The Therapy of Pain.* Philadelphia: Lippincott; 1981:4.

23. Rothstein JM, Roy SH, Wolf SL: *The Rehabilitation Specialist's Handbook*, 2nd ed. Philadelphia: Davis; 1998:204.

24. Bergner M, Bobbitt RA, Carter WB, Gilson B: The Sickness Impact Profile: Development and final revision of a health status measure. *Med Care* 1981; 19:787–805.

25. Roland M, Morris, R: A study of the natural history of back pain, Part I: The development of a reliable and sensitive measure of disability in low back pain. *Spine.* 1983; 8:141.

26. *Taber's Cyclopedic Medical Dictionary.* 18th ed. Philadelphia: Davis; 1997:1791.

27. Paris SV: Institute of Graduate Health Sciences. 1982.

28. O'Donoghue DH: *Treatment of Injuries to Athletes.* 4th ed. Philadelphia, PA: WB Saunders; 1984:86.

29. Kimura J: *Electrodiagnosis in Diseases of Nerve and Muscle,* 3rd ed. New York: Oxford University Press, 2001:836.

30. Carr J, Shepherd R: *Movement Science: Foundations for Physical Therapy in Rehabilitation,* 2nd ed. Gaithersburg, MO: Aspen; 2000.

31. Ritchie AE: Muscle spasm: Its role in the natural order of biological activities. Proceedings of a symposium on skeletal muscle spasm. London: British Medical Association; November 1961:101–105, 111–12.

32. Cailliet R: *Soft Tissue Pain and Disability,* 3rd ed. Philadelphia: FA Davis; 1996.

33. Barer R: Muscle structure in relation to spasm. Proceedings of a symposium on skeletal muscle spasm. London: British Medical Association, November 1961:53.

7

Electromagnetic Spectrum

JOSEPH WEISBERG, PT, PhD
LESLIE SCHONBRUN, MS, PT

Chapter Outline

- QUANTUM THEORY
  - Photon
  - Quantum
  - Frequency
- ELECTROMAGNETIC WAVE THEORY
  - Oscillatory Motion
  - Velocity
  - Wavelength
  - Frequency
- INFLUENCES OF ELECTROMAGNETIC FREQUENCY
  - Level of Energy
  - Depth of Penetration
- REPRESENTATION OF ELECTROMAGNETIC ENERGIES
  - Spectrum
- ELECTROMAGNETIC ENERGY TRANSMISSION
  - Reflection
  - Refraction
  - Absorption
  - Penetration
- DETERMINANTS OF ELECTROMAGNETIC ENERGY TRANSMISSION
  - Target Medium
  - Angle of Application
- ELECTROMAGNETIC ENERGIES
  - Cosmic Rays
  - Gamma Rays
  - X-Rays
  - Ultraviolet
  - Visible Light
  - Cold Laser
  - Infrared
  - Microwave
  - Radar
  - Short Wave Diathermy
  - Long Wave Diathermy
  - Broadcast
  - Electrical Power
- SKIN DETERMINANTS OF ELECTROMAGNETIC ENERGY TRANSMISSION
  - Melanin Content
  - Texture
- LAWS THAT INFLUENCE THE ELECTROMAGNETIC RADIATION DOSAGE
  - Inverse Square Law
  - Cosine Law
  - Bunsen Roscoe Law of Reciprocity

All substances with temperatures above absolute zero (−273° C) emit radiant energy. The emission and transmission of this energy can be explained only by the combined efforts of two theories: (1) the quantum theory, and (2) the electromagnetic wave theory. Radiant energy can be shown to act as a wave by a diffraction grating, but it can also be shown to act as a particle by the photoelectric effect. This apparent contradiction can be explained if radiant energy is thought of as packets (or particles) of energy carried along by propagated waves.

According to the **quantum theory,** the packet of energy is an indivisible unit named the *photon,* which is the smallest entity of radiant energy produced by either electronic or molecular motion of high velocity or by the transformed kinetic energy released from the collision of molecules. The energy (E) content, or *quantum,* of each photon is proportional to the frequency (f) of the photons emitted and is determined by the formula

$$E = H \times f$$

where H is Planck's universal constant and f is the frequency in cycles per second, now commonly called Hertz (Hz). X-rays, for example, are potentially destructive because of their high frequency and photon energy.

According to the **electromagnetic wave theory,** the energy is transmitted by oscillatory motion in the form of electromagnetic waves. The wavelength (λ) and frequency are related by the equation

$$\text{Velocity} = \lambda \times f$$

The shorter the wavelength, the higher the frequency of oscillation. This inverse relationship between frequency and wavelength must be remembered whenever one considers characteristics of different waves. As explained by the quantum theory, the higher the wave frequency, the higher the energy content. The frequency of the wave emitted by the different modalities used in physical therapy determines the depth of penetration. Lower frequencies penetrate more deeply than higher ones. In light of the inverse relationship of frequency and wavelength, this could also be stated as longer wavelengths penetrate more deeply than shorter ones. For example, ultraviolet light is a more superficial agent than infrared light (**Fig. 7–1**) because ultraviolet light has a higher frequency (and therefore a shorter wavelength). In general, all modalities used by physical therapists have low photon energy, and they serve either to increase or decrease the kinetic or thermal energy of body tissues or to induce a photochemical reaction in the absorbing media.

The **electromagnetic spectrum** is a representation of various wave energies arranged in the order of their wavelength, frequency, or both (**Fig. 7–2**). *Wavelength* is defined as the distance from the peak of

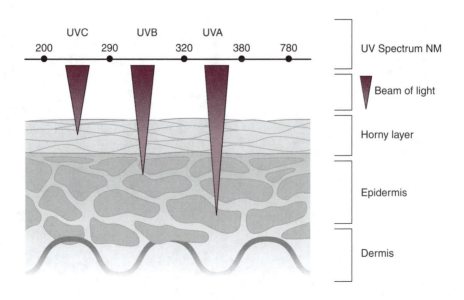

FIGURE 7–1   Depth of penetration of various wavelengths of UV radiation.

0.01nm	0.14nm	12nm	180nm	290nm	320nm	400nm		800nm	1500nm	15,000nm	10cm	1m	3m	30m	30,000m

Cosmic Rays	Gamma Rays	X-rays		UVC	UVB	UVA	Violet Indigo Blue Green Yellow Orange Red	Short or Near	Long or Far	Microwave	Radar	Shortwave		Low Frequency Stimulating Currents
					Ultraviolet		Visible Light	Infrared						

One nanometer (nm) = 10^9 meter (m)
One hertz = one cycle per second

FIGURE 7–2   Electromagnetic Spectrum.

one wave to the identical peak of the next wave and is measured in units ranging from nanometers (10^{-9}m) to meters (**Fig. 7–3**). The frequency is defined as the number of oscillations or cycles per second (Hertz). The spectrum that is commonly used extends from wavelengths of 0.0001 nm or (10^{21}Hz), the cosmic ray, to wavelengths of $.5 \times 10^{15}$nm (60Hz), a long wave of electric power that is in clinical use (see Fig. 7–2).

The wave propagates in a straight line, but it can undergo reflection (**Fig. 7–4**), refraction (**Fig. 7–5**), and absorption by the media that it encounters. The amount of reflection, refraction, and absorption that occurs will depend on the type of media and the angle of the rays in relation to those media. Ideally, any radiated material, including body tissues, should be at right angles to the wave for maximum absorption (**Fig. 7–6**). Different wavelengths have different designations (eg, infrared and ultraviolet), and some waves have specific medical uses. **Table 7–1** displays the wavelength, the frequency of the wave, its designation, and its medical use.

Electromagnetic waves travel through a vacuum at the speed of light, c = (3×10^8m/s). As the density of the medium through which it travels increases, however, the velocity decreases. Sound and ultrasound are not part of the electromagnetic spectrum because they have different physical characteristics; for example, they cannot travel through a vacuum but need an elastic medium for propagation. They differ also in being longitudinal waves, whereas all electromagnetic waves are transverse. These waves are discussed in **Chapter 15**.

Rays of radiant energy such as light can be affected by a medium in four different ways:

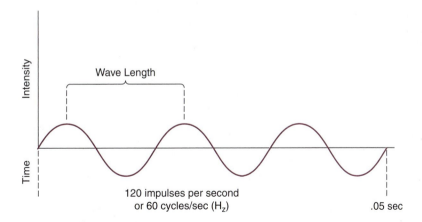

FIGURE 7–3   Wavelength. Wavelength is the distance from the peak of one wave to the identical peak of the next wave. Frequency is the number of oscillations or cycles per second. Here, the frequency is 60 Hz.

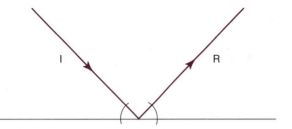

FIGURE 7–4 Reflection (I = rays of incident, R = rays of reflection). The angle-of-incident ray is equal to the angle of the reflected ray.

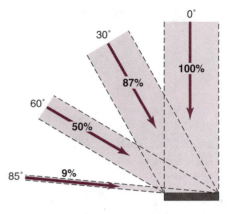

FIGURE 7–6 The cosine of the angle of incidence. The law states that maximum absorption of radiant energy occurs when the source of the energy is at a right angle to the absorbing surface. (*Graph courtesy of International Light, Inc., 1997, www.intl-light.com*)

1. They can be reflected by the medium (eg, a mirror).
2. They can be absorbed by the medium (eg, one with a dark, nonshiny surface).
3. They can be refracted by the medium (eg, a prism, which refracts the sunlight into its different wavelengths, producing a rainbow effect).
4. They can penetrate through the medium (eg, clear glass).

When energy penetrates or transmits through a medium, some of it is absorbed in the process. Therefore, having 100% of emitted energy available at deeper tissues is impossible. Biological tissue exposed to radiant energy will be affected by that energy. According to the **Grotthuss-Draper law,** waves of different wavelengths produce different effects, and the extent of the effect will be determined by the amount of the energy that is absorbed by the tissue.

When radiant energy, such as infrared and ultraviolet, is used in intervention, the skin is invariably exposed and will reflect some of the rays. The amount of reflection will be related to the patient's complex-

ion (amount of melanin in the skin), the texture of the skin (scaly or smooth), and the oiliness or dryness of the skin. The skin will absorb some of the rays, and the energy from those rays will affect the skin. Some rays have a predominantly photochemical effect, whereas others simply increase the skin temperature. Some examples of photochemical effects are skin tanning and erythema.

In addition to the quality of the skin, three laws govern the dosage of radiant energy that the tissue receives: the inverse squares law, the cosine law, and the Bunsen Roscoe law of reciprocity. The **inverse square law** states that the intensity of the wave varies inversely with the square of the distance between the source of the radiant energy and the absorbing tissue because of the divergence of the rays (**Fig. 7–7**). For example, if the distance between the source and the intervention surface decreases from 2 feet to 1 foot, the intensity of the dosage is increased 4 times, as expressed in the following formula:

$$\Delta I = \frac{1}{(\Delta D)^2}$$

where ΔI = change in intensity and ΔD = change in distance (ratio).

In our example the change in distance was $\frac{1}{2}$, making the change in intensity $\Delta I = 1/(\frac{1}{2})^2 = 1/\frac{1}{4} = 4$. To avoid overexposure, the distance must be kept in mind.

The **cosine law** states that maximum absorption of radiant energy occurs when the source is at right an-

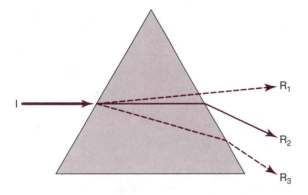

FIGURE 7–5 Refraction through a prism (I = rays of incident, R = rays of refraction).

TABLE 7–1 *The Electromagnetic Spectrum*

Wavelength (range in nm)[*]	Frequency The upper limit (cycle/s, or Hz)	Designation	Medical Use
0.0001–0.01	3.0×10^{21}	Cosmic rays	Not known
0.01–0.14	2.14×10^{18}	Gamma rays	Radium therapy
0.14–120	5.9×10^{15}	X-rays	Diagnosis and treatment
180–280	1.03×10^{15}	Short (far) ultraviolet (UVC)	Diagnosis and treatment
280–315	9.0×10^{14}	Long (near) ultraviolet (UVB)	Diagnosis and treatment
280–400	7.5×10^{14}	Long (near) ultraviolet (UVA)	Diagnosis and treatment
400–800	3.75×10^{14}	Visible light: violet, blue, green	Not fully explored (seasonal depression)
632	4.74×10^{14}	Cold laser	Not fully explored (tissue healing, pain)
800–1500	2.0×10^{14}	Short (near) infrared	Superficial heat
1500–15000	2.0×10^{13}	Long (far) infrared	Superficial heat
$1.5 \times 10^4 - 1 \times 10^9$	$3.0 \ 10^8$	Microwave	Diathermy (deep heat)
$1 \times 10^9 - 3 \times 10^9$	10^8	Radar	Not known
$3 \times 10^9 - 30 \times 10^9$	10^7	Short wave diathermy	Deep heat
$30 \times 10^9 - 300 \times 10^9$	10^6	Long wave diathermy	Deep heat
$300 \times 10^9 - 30 \times 10^{12}$	10^4	Broadcast	Not known
$.5 \times 10^{15}$	60	Electric power	Muscle and nerve stimulation

[*]Millimicron (nm) is equal to 10 angstrom (Å) or 10^{-7} cm.

gles to the absorbing surface. When the source is not at a right angle to the absorbing surface, the angle (θ) formed by the source and the perpendicular to the absorbing surface determines the effect of the energy. The relationship between the angle of the rays and the amount absorbed is expressed by the following formula (Fig. 7–6):

$$\text{Energy absorbed} = \text{Energy available} \times \text{Cos } \theta$$

$$\text{Cos } \theta = \frac{AB}{BC}$$

For example, if ultraviolet light were aimed at the skin at an angle of 30° from perpendicular, using the cosine law, the percent of energy absorption would be 87% (see Fig. 7–6). Now consider the situation of

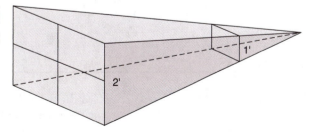

FIGURE 7–7 The law of inverse squares. This law states that because of the diversion of the rays, the intensity of the wave varies inversely with the square of the distance between the source of the radiant energy and the tissue absorbing the rays.

applying ultraviolet light to the thigh of a patient, with the UV generator directly above (and perpendicular to) the top of the thigh. The uppermost area of the thigh would be absorbing 100% of the energy. However, as you assess the upper medial and upper lateral aspects of the thigh, the energy absorption would decline to approximately 87%. Assess the area of the skin that is 60° from the perpendicular both medially and laterally on the thigh, and absorption would decline to 50%.

The **Bunsen Roscoe law of reciprocity** states that the intensity and duration of the dose of radiant energy are inversely proportional:

$$Energy\ (E) = intensity\ (I) \times time\ (T)$$

The practical meaning of this law is that the intensity and duration of the dose can be manipulated even when one wants the amount of energy delivered to the patient to remain constant. This relationship can be shown by rearranging the formula in the following way:

$$I = \frac{E}{T} \text{ or } T = \frac{E}{I}$$

For example, a UV minimal erythema dose (MED) test was previously performed where the optimal amount of energy delivered was determined to be 50 units. This was achieved by an intensity (I) (as determined by the inverse square law and the cosine law) of 25 and an intervention time (T) of 2 min. There, $E = I \times T$; $E = 25\ 2$, or $E = 50$.

For slowly increasing the intervention intensity, various parameters could be changed:

1. The *time* could be increased, with the distance and angle remaining the same. $E = I \times T$; $E = 25 \times 2.2$, or $E = 55$ units.
2. The time could remain at 2 min, with the *distance* decreased (inverse square law) and the angle remaining the same. $E = I \times T$; $E = 30\ s\ 2$, $E = 60$ units.
3. The time and distance could remain as originally set, but the *angle* (cosine law) could be brought closer to perpendicular. $E = I \times T$; $E = 30 \times 2 = 60$ units (different aspect of intensity due to change in angle).

The principles and laws just outlined must be considered when planning interventions using electromagnetic waves (ie, when determining dosage and when positioning equipment) if the interventions are to be both effective and safe.

REVIEW QUESTIONS

1. What is the relationship between the wave frequency and the depth of penetration?
2. What are ways in which radiant energy is affected by a medium?
3. Describe the Grotthuss-Draper law as it relates to radiant energy and biological tissue.
4. What is the significance of the inverse square law as it relates to radiant energy?
5. What is the significance of the cosine law as it relates to radiant energy?
6. Describe the Bunsen Roscoe law of reciprocity for planning therapeutic applications of radiant energy.

KEY TERMS

quantum theory
electromagnetic wave theory
electromagnetic spectrum

Grotthuss-Draper law
inverse square law

cosine law
Bunsen Roscoe law of reciprocity

II

Thermal Agents

Whether using a sunbath to relax aching muscles or splashing cool water on the temples when overheated, people throughout the ages have treated physical complaints and sought relief from discomfort by applying heat or cold to their bodies. Both heat and cold are still widely used physical therapy agents. A physical agent or modality is sometimes the primary aspect of a program of intervention, when it is likely that the physiologic or psychological changes produced can of themselves alleviate an impairment. However, the use of a therapeutic modality or physical agent as the sole intervention does not, in and of itself, constitute physical therapy. Generally, physical agents are used as an adjunct to other physical therapy interventions. For example, before therapeutic exercise, heat or cold may be applied to prepare body tissues or reduce pain, allowing the individual to benefit more fully from the procedures to follow.

In the past, the use of thermal modalities was based on anecdotal evidence—clinical observations that patients exhibited positive reactions following the application of a particular agent. Research has provided us with a scientific understanding of how and why these reactions occur, but additional studies are required if physical therapists and physical therapist assistants are to continue to provide optimal care for their patients and clients. In addition, payers and informed consumers of our services demand evidence-based practice that integrates research with clinical expertise.

With the passive procedures just mentioned, studies have shown that either heat or cold can be beneficial but that the rationales differ for using them. For example, some evidence indicates that collagen tissues become more elongated when heated and that cold, by altering the activity of peripheral nerves, decreases muscle spasm and/or spasticity. Thus, heat might be chosen if scar tissue limits the range of motion, and cold might be chosen if the limitation is the result of muscle splinting or spasm.

Conclusive evidence is lacking regarding some physiologic responses to changes in tissue temperature, and, in some instances, controversy exists concerning the therapeutic benefits. For example, it is generally accepted that heat should be applied before muscle stretching and that warming muscles prior to exercise improves performance; however, research has also shown improved muscle performance after applications of cooling agents (see following chapters). Although studies can be cited for either viewpoint, more research must be conducted regarding clinical implications of thermal modalities on muscle performance and on the prevention of injuries.

To select and apply thermal modalities rationally, the physical therapist must know why and how each modality is employed. Chapter 8 discusses terms commonly used to differentiate the various thermal modalities. Chapters 9, 10, and 11 address basic thermal physics and physiology. Chapter 12 compares the effects of heat versus cold, the therapeutic implications of which aid therapists in choosing specific modalities. Chapters 13 through 16 present specific thermal modalities. Chapter 17 looks at monitoring signs and symptoms and at ambient conditions to consider when applying thermal modalities to patients.

8

Terminology

BERNADETTE HECOX, PT, MA

JOHN P. SANKO, PT, ED.D

Chapter Outline

This chapter defines terms that are often used when discussing thermal modalities that include both heat and cold. Familiarity with these terms and their meanings can help the physical therapist and physical therapy assistant to understand the content of the chapters in this thermal section and to communicate effectively with other health professionals as well.

Categories of Thermal Modalities

Heat Modalities

Heat modalities can be categorized as either superficial or deep. A **superficial heat modality** refers to heat that, when applied at a maximally safe clinical dosage, is capable only of raising the temperature of superficial tissues to a therapeutically significant level (**Fig. 8–1**).[1] Although these modalities may increase the skin temperature by 18°F (10°C), the increase in temperature of tissues 1 cm deep will be less than 6°F (3°C) and that of tissues 2 cm deep about 2°F (1.3°C).[1,2]

Superficial heat can be either moist or dry, depending on the source. If the source is the sun, other sources of infrared radiation, or a modality with little moisture (eg, an electric heating pad or warm dry air), it is called a **dry heat** modality. If the heat source is water, another fluid, moist air, or a modality containing moisture (eg, a hot pack or hydrotherapy), it is called **moist heat.**

The term **deep heat modality** implies that a form of energy other than heat is transmitted through the skin and is absorbed in deeper tissues, where it increases the kinetic action of molecules. Deep heat is capable of heating to 3 cm depth at 40°C.[1] Thus, forms of energy such as electromagnetic energy (diathermy) and acoustic energy (ultrasound), which can be transmitted to deeper tissues, increase the temperature of those tissues. These modalities produce heat as a result of energy conversion (see **Chapter 9**).

Cold Modalities

Because all cold modalities are applied to superficial tissues, they will cool the surface tissue more than the deeper tissues. Cold modalities are categorized

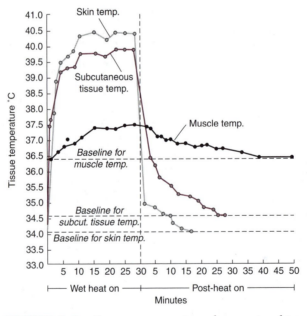

FIGURE 8–1 Curves representing changes in skin, subcutaneous tissue, and muscle temperatures obtained during and after 30 minutes of wet heat topically applied to the forearm. (*Permission from Abramson, PI et al. Changes in blood flow, oxygen uptake and tissue temperatures, produced by the topical application of wet heat. Arch Phys Med Rehab 42:305, 1961, Saunders.*)

according to the specific modality: for example "apply ice" versus "apply a cold pack." The general term used to describe cold modalities is **cryotherapy,** which literally means "cold therapy." Therefore, the terms *deep* and *superficial* are not applicable to cryotherapy.

LOCAL VERSUS GENERAL APPLICATIONS

Local application refers to the application of a thermal modality to only one area of the body: for example, placing a hot-water bottle or ice pack on a painful shoulder. *General application* refers to the application of heat or cold to all or much of the body, as in using a therapeutic pool or staying in a sauna. The terms *local* and *general* refer only to the amount of the body being treated, not to the amount of heat absorbed or given off. Naturally, if heat of the same temperature and duration is used in a general and a local application, the general agent will provide more heat input. However, a brief warm shower, although a general application, may provide less heat input than a heating pad, which is a local agent that is "on" for an extended period of time. The modalities shown in

Fig. 8–2A and B can be clearly described as local or general. However, a modality applied to larger areas of the body (see **Fig. 8–2C**) requires a more specific description.

LOCAL VERSUS SYSTEMIC REACTIONS

A **local reaction** refers to physiologic changes occurring at the site of a **local application,** including localized sweating with heat, pilo erection (goose bumps) with cold, and changes in local metabolic rate, blood flow, and skin condition with both heat and cold. A **systemic reaction** refers to physiologic changes occurring in the various systems of the body following a **general application.** For example, if enough heat is added to or taken from the body (regardless of whether by a prolonged local or general thermal modality), the core temperature may change. The results may include systemic reactions such as generalized sweating or shivering and cardiovascular changes such as increased or decreased pulse rate and blood pressure. With application of a local heat modality, the rate at which the modality is able to increase tissue temperature is an important factor that influences

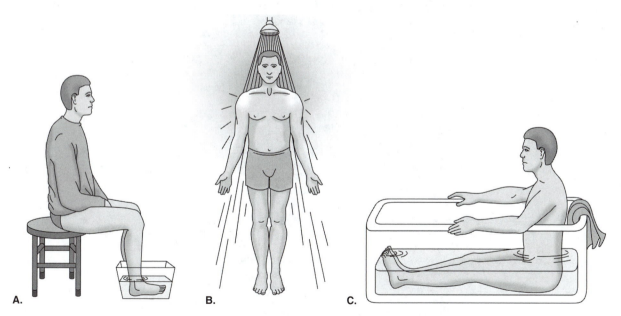

FIGURE 8–2   *Examples of applications of a thermal modality.* The modality is water in this case. (**A**) The immersion of one foot or ankle is a local application. (**B**) A full-body shower is a general application. (**C**) Sitting waist high in water is not considered to be either a local or general application. A more specific description is required.

the degree of local containment of the heat and the duration of the intervention. If the heat input causes the **tissue temperature (TT)** to rise faster than the local vascular system can convect the heat into the general circulation, the result is a greater local heating effect. Conversely, if a modality requires 10 min to increase the TT above 107°F (42°C) and the goal of the therapist is to have a significant **tissue temperature rise (TTR)** lasting 15 min, a 25-min intervention is required. The usual 20-min intervention would not be long enough.[3] These physiologic responses are mentioned here because they affect the dosage given. Such responses will be discussed in more detail in later chapters of this section.

DOSAGE TERMS AND REACTIONS

For safe and effective use, thermal modalities should be applied appropriately. The application will vary with each modality and with each patient's needs.

General dosage terms can be used to describe the effect that the modality has on the patient, whereas **specific dosage** terms describe precise intervention factors.

Heat or cold interventions are often described in the following general terms: mild, moderate, and vigorous. One can say "mild heat may be helpful" or "vigorous heat is indicated." These general terms relate to the degree to which the reactions to the dosage occur, or they describe the desired effect.

Dosage Reactions

Thermal modalities can produce changes in tissue temperature and changes in firing of thermal sensory neurons. Either can result in local or systemic reactions, or both (**Fig. 8–3**).

Changes in Tissue Temperature.   With a mild dose, or dose II, of heat or cold, the desired effect is no

---

QUALITATIVE DOSIMETRY OF SWD THERAPY[a]

DOSE I: NO PERCEPTION OF HEAT
Presumed responses induced: athermal
Recommended application: PSWD with power output <38 W

DOSE II: MILD PERCEPTION OF HEAT
Presumed responses induced: mixed balance of athermal and thermal
Recommended application: PSWD with power output >38 W

DOSE III: COMFORTABLE PERCEPTION OF HEAT
Presumed responses induced: thermal
Recommended application: CSWD with low to medium power output

DOSE IV: MAXIMUM TOLERABLE PERCEPTION OF HEAT
Presumed response induced: thermal
Recommended application : CSWD with medium to high power output

[a]This scale is adapted from Low and Reed's (1990) dosimetric scale. It is strongly recommended that the operator wait approximately 5 min after beginning the application to gather the patient's initial perception of heat to then set the desired therapeutic dosage for the rest of the session, which usually lasts approximately 20 minutes total. At the end of the application, gather the patient's overall perception of heat felt during the entire period of application. Only then can the operator determine which dose level the patient has received during the therapeutic application. This overall perception of heat must be recorded in the patient's chart as the therapeutic dosage (i.e., Dose I, II, III, or IV). Moreover, chart the key dosimetric parameters, such as mean power and other variables, to ensure maximal consistency across repeated applications throughout the treatment schedule.

FIGURE 8–3   Qualitative Dosimetry of SWD Therapy.

more than a slight change in the TT in the area where the modality is applied. Benefits are probably related to the sensation of warmth or coolness. A moderate dose, or dose III, is expected to increase the TT to approximately 102–106°F (39–41°C), with only a slight increase in blood flow. With a vigorous dose, or dose IV, the goal is a TTR to approximately 107–113°F (42–45°C). In this range, one can anticipate maximum beneficial physiologic effects without tissue damage.[10,14] A temperature in deeper tissues of 109–113°F (43–45°C) is required to increase blood flow significantly in those tissues.[3,4]

In general, if the patient's vascular status and thermal sensation is good, it is considered safe to heat tissues up to approximately 113°F (45°C) for 30 min to 50 min, whereas tissue damage occurs at even slightly higher temperatures.[5] However, patients may not tolerate temperatures higher than 109°F (43°C), because at approximately that temperature, an individual begins to perceive pain, signaling the danger of tissue damage at higher temperatures. With prolonged vigorous heating, the patient's core temperature may rise to well above 100°F (37.8°C).[6]

With cold, a TT near freezing may be tolerable for brief periods. However, as the TT falls to 68°F (20°C) or less, the tissues approach a **critical range.** Although tissues are not frozen in the range between 68° and 32°F (20° and 0°C), pain is perceived, neural activity gradually diminishes, and protective vascular adjustments are activated (**Fig. 8–4**).[7] Heating or cooling beyond safe limits may irreparably damage tissues or threaten survival of the individual.[5,8,9,10] **Table 8–1** notes significant physiologic effects that occur at various temperatures.

Changes in Firing of Thermal Sensory Neurons. Thermoreceptors are found in cutaneous tissues throughout the body. Whenever these receptors are subject to any change in temperature, the rate of firing of the thermal sensory neurons changes, and the body responds instantaneously to the sensation of heat or cold. Depending on (1) the size of the area subjected to the temperature change, (2) the temperature gradient between the skin and the applied modality, and (3) the rate of heat exchange, autonomic nervous system responses and behavioral responses, sometimes called **thermal shock reactions,** occur.

If the thermal modality applied is approximately the same temperature as the skin (a mild dose) or if the rate of change in skin temperature is gradual, the responses of the autonomic system are usually those associated with comfort: for example, relaxation and analgesia. With a moderate dose, the therapist can expect a more pronounced sensation of heat or cold and a more stimulating reaction. With a vigorous dose, if

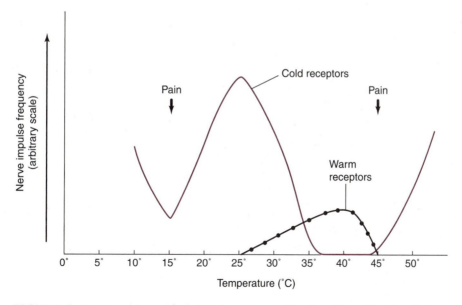

FIGURE 8–4 Responses of thermal receptors in the skin. (*Reprinted from Low, J and Reed, A: Electrotherapy Explained: Principles and Practice. Oxford, Butterworth-Heinemann, 1990, p 177, with permission from Elsevier.*)

TABLE 8–1   *Effects of Various Temperatures on Tissues*

Temperatures	Degrees		Effect
	Fahrenheit	Celsius	
Increased temperature*	109.0	43.0	Pain threshold
	113.0	45.0	Severe pain; safety limit for 30 min of heat application.
	118.0	47.8	Blisters appear in 20 min; tissue necrosis occurs in 1 hr.
	126.0	52.0	Blisters appear in 30 sec; tissue necrosis occurs in 1 min.
	149.0	65.0	Tissue necrosis occurs in 1 sec.
Decreased temperature*†‡§‖	73.4	23.0	Activity of peripheral nerves begins to decline markedly.
	68–32	20–0	Critical range.
	50.0	10.0	Redness and swelling in 1 hr.
	48.2	9.0	Velocity of nerve conduction ceases.
	41.0	5.0	Paralysis of peripheral nerves occurs.
	28.6	-1.9	Marked pain or swelling occurs in 4–7 min.
	28.0	-2.2	Skin freezes.

*Krusen F, ed: *Handbook of Physical Medicine and Rehabilitation.* 2nd ed. Philadelphia, PA: WB Saunders; 1971:261–272.
†Burton A, Edhold O: *Man in a Cold Environment.* London, UK: Edward Arnold; 1955:225, 227, 230.
‡Holdcroft A: *Body Temperature Control.* London, UK: Bailliere-Tindall; 1980:1, 12–26.
§Lehmann J, ed: *Therapeutic Heat and Cold.* 3rd ed. Baltimore, MD: Williams & Wilkins; 1982:65, 128–129, 175, 179, 212–213.
‖Williamson C, Schultz J: Time-temperature relationships in thermal blister formation. *J Invest. Dermatol.* 1949 12(1):41–47.

the temperature gradient and rate of change are sufficient, the result is the "fight or flight" reaction associated with the sympathetic division of the autonomic nervous system and include changes in the activity of the cardiovascular system.[6,7,10,11] For example, if the skin temperature is 84°F (28.9°C) and a person slowly gets into a 90°F (32.2°C) bath or an 80°F (26.7°C) lake, the body will react only slightly to the temperature change—an experience usually perceived as pleasurable. However, everyone is familiar with the strong reactions that occur when one jumps into an extremely hot bath (105°F, 40.6°C) or an extremely cold lake (68°F, 20°C).

Many factors, including age (the very old have lessened ability to thermoregulate), individual sensitivity, past experiences related to thermal sensation, and pathologic conditions, will affect an individual's reactions to thermal shock. Thus, when applying a thermal modality, the therapist must consider the effect of both the temperature gradient and the rate at which the patient experiences the change. For example, when treating a patient in a Hubbard tank, the therapist lowers the patient into the tank slowly to avoid a thermal shock reaction.

Specific Dosages

The following specific factors must be considered for each thermal modality:

- The intensity of the heat or cold per area of the patient to which it is applied: ie, how much and how fast the modality can affect tissues or systems.
- The duration of each intervention.
- The frequency with which the intervention will be made.

Because variations in techniques alter the intensity and therefore the thermal changes, the techniques recommended when applying the modality must be known. If, at a given temperature, one hot pack is applied with only two layers of toweling and another is applied with eight layers, the intensity of heat that the patient receives will obviously be much greater with the former. Recommended dosages for each therapeutic intervention should be guided by evidence-based practice and individualized patient assessment.

The factors that dictate the dosage for each thermal modality differ for several reasons. Each modality is composed of different substances with different thermal qualities, and the means by which each transfers heat to the patient also varies. These factors are discussed in subsequent chapters in this section.

Another important consideration is whether the modality is connected to a constant source of heat production such as a heat lamp or an electric heating pad, which can either maintain or increase its temperature and heat output as long as it is connected to the source of electrical energy. A modality such as a hot pack or a hot-water bottle will not maintain its initial heat output for more than a few minutes, whereas a modality that provides constant heat produces a greater TTR, systemic reaction, or both. The latter modalities pose an inherently greater danger of overheating, both locally and systemically.

Special attention must be paid to the dosages for deep heat modality interventions because the temperature of deeper tissues may be higher than that of superficial tissues. Skin sensation may not indicate the temperature rise in the deeper tissues where the damage may occur because thermal receptors are superficial (approximately 1 cc deep).

To predict the temperature changes in deeper tissues more objectively, the National Council on Radiation and Measurements of the Food and Drug Administration (FDA) has quantified the high-frequency electromagnetic energy absorbed in the tissues per unit of tissue mass through the use of a unit called the **specific absorption rate (SAR),** which is expressed in watts per kilogram (w/kg). The therapeutic range of this absorption extends from approximately 50 w/kg to 170 w/kg, and the rate of TTR corresponds somewhat to the SAR. In vascularized tissues, a low SAR (50 w/kg) will generally cause a TTR of 1.4°F (0.8°C)/min and a high SAR (170 w/kg) will cause a TTR of 4.9°F (2.7°C)/min. As with all thermal modalities, the final TT depends on the duration of the intervention and on physiologic factors, especially the patient's vascular status.[11–13] However, physiologic factors differ for each patient, and because the skin temperature does not indicate the deep TTR, the therapist has no way of determining the exact dosage that each patient should receive.

Although one can use the percentage of power (energy) or the SAR level readout on the high-frequency device as a guide, the dosage for deep heat modalities must ultimately be determined by the patient's report of the sensation of heat being experienced. **Table 8–2** suggests the dosage level, duration, and frequency of interventions to be used when deep heat modalities are used for acute, subacute, or chronic conditions. These suggestions are based on the patient's subjective reporting of the warmth experienced and the SAR dosage factors that produce similar sensations of warmth. These factors include the percentage of power output required to produce a specific SAR that can be predicted to cause a specific rate of TTR.

Finally, the fact that care must be used with all thermal modalities cannot be overemphasized. The specific dosage must be determined according to each patient's physical status and pathology, which can greatly influence the local and systemic reactions that thermal changes may produce. Subsequent chapters discuss recommended dosages for each modality as well as precautions and contraindications based on pathology and physical status.

REVIEW QUESTIONS

1. What are superficial and deep heat modalities? Give examples.

2. What is the difference between a "general application" and a "local application"? Give examples of each.

3. What changes in tissue temperature are desired with

   a. a mild dose?
   b. a moderate dose?
   c. a vigorous dose?

4. If a vigorous heat dosage is recommended, what temperature range may maximize the beneficial effects without damaging tissue?

TABLE 8–2   *Dosage Guide for Deep Heat Treatments*[*†‡]

Condition Being Treated	Treatment			Heat Sensation Reported by Patient	Percentage Output of Energy from the Device	Specific Absorption Rate (SAR) (w/kg)	Rate of Tissue Temperature Rise (°C/min)
	Dosage Level	Duration of Treatment	Frequency of Treatments				
Acute inflammation	1. Lowest	1–3 min	Daily for 1–2 wks	None; dose is just below any sensation of heat	1/4 maximum output	25–50 w/kg	0.4°–0.8°C/min
Subacute resolving	2. Low	3–5 min	Daily for 1–2 wks	Barely felt	1/2 maximum output	50–75 w/kg	0.8°–1.2°C/min
Inflammatory conditions	3. Medium	5–7 min	Daily for 1–2 wks	Distinct but pleasant heat sensation	3/4 maximum output	75–125 w/kg	1.2°–2°C/min
Usual chronic conditions	4. High	5–7 min	Daily or 2 times/wk for 1 wk to 1 mo	Definite heat sensation, well within tolerance	maximum output	125–170 w/kg	2.0°–2.7°C/min

*Kloth L: Lecture delivered at the APTA Combined Section Meeting. Anaheim, CA: February 1986.
†Michlovitz S: *Thermal Agents in Rehabilitation.* Philadelphia, PA: FA Davis; 1986.
‡Therapeutic shortwave and microwave diathermy. *FDA Bulletin* 85–8237. December 1984.

5. What range of tissue temperatures is required to cause a *significant* increase in blood flow to the tissues?

6. What does the term *significant heating* mean?

7. At approximately what temperature do patients begin to perceive pain?

8. What does the term *critical range* mean for colder temperatures? What happens within that range?

9. What is a thermal shock reaction? How can it happen?

10. Compare and contrast a local reaction and a systemic reaction.

KEY TERMS

superficial heat modality
dry heat
moist heat
deep heat modality
cryotherapy
local reaction

local application
systemic reaction
general application
tissue temperature (TT)
tissue temperature rise (TTR)
general dosage

specific dosage
critical range
thermal shock reaction
specific absorption rate (SAR)

REFERENCES

1. Lehmann J, Silverman D, Baum B, Kirk N, Johnston V: Temperature distribution in the human thigh produced by infrared, hot packs and microwave applications. *Arch Phy Med Rehab* 1966; 47(6):291–99.

2. Borrell R, Parker R, Henley E, Masley D, Repinecz M: Comparison of in vivo temperatures produced by hydrotherapy, paraffin wax treatment, and fluidotherapy. *Phys Ther* 1980; 60(10):1273–76.

3. Lehmann J, Warren G, Scham S: Therapeutic heat and cold. *Clin Orthop* 1974; 99:207–45.

4. Sekins K, et al: Local muscle blood flow and temperature responses to 915 mHz (MW) diathermy as simultaneously measured and numerically predicted. *Arch Phy Med Rehab* 1984; 65:1–7.

5. Moritz A, Henrique F: Studies of thermal injury, part II: The relative importance of time and surface temperature in the causation of cutaneous burns. *Am J Pathol* 1947; 23:695–720.

6. Licht S, ed: *Medical Hydrology.* New Haven: E. Licht Pub., 1963; 98–99; 102; 242.

7. Hensel H: *Thermal Sensations and Thermoreceptors in Man.* Springfield: Charles C Thomas, 1982; 6; 36; 91–92; 94.

8. Thorman M: The pathology and management of frostbite. *Clin Manage* 1985; 5:12–15.

9. Dyke P, Thomas PK, Lambert E, Bunge R, eds: *Peripheral Neuropathy.* Philadelphia: Saunders 1984; I:453–76; II:1479–1511, 2303–04.

10. Lehmann JF, DeLateur BJ: Diathermy and Superficial Heat, Laser, and Cold Therapy. In: Kottke F, Lehmann J, eds: *Krusen's Handbook of Physical Medicine and Rehabilitation.* 4th ed. Philadelphia: Saunders, 1990; 283–367.

11. Kloth L: Lecture delivered at APTA Combined Section Meeting, Anaheim, February 1986.

12. Michlovitz S: *Thermal Agents in Rehabilitation.* 3rd ed. Philadelphia: Davis, 1996; 110–12.

13. *Therapeutic Shortwave and Microwave Diathermy.* FDA Bulletin, December 1984; 85.

14. Belanger AY: *Evidence-Based Guide to Therapeutic Physical Agents.* Philadelphia: Lippincott Williams & Wilkins, 2002.

9

Thermal Physics

BERNADETTE HECOX, PT, MA

JOHN P. SANKO, PT EDD

Chapter Outline

To understand the amount of heat or cold that the patient receives and its resulting therapeutic effects, the physical therapist/assistant must be acquainted with basic physical concepts concerning thermal energy and with biophysics, the physical relationship to the body and the physiologic effects produced. Integrating this information helps the clinician determine which thermal effects are therapeutically beneficial or detrimental. This chapter begins that process of integration by discussing the aspects of thermal physics that are relevant to thermal physical agents.

Heat and the First Law of Thermodynamics

Kinetic energy—the movement of molecules or their components (atoms, nuclei, and electrons)—is related to the temperature of a substance. (As the temperature of a substance increases, its molecules move more rapidly.) Thus, kinetic energy, the internal energy of the substance, is **thermal energy.** Movement of the entire molecule is termed *translational*, and movement of the constituents within the molecule can be either *rotational* or *vibrational*. Molecular motion ceases only if the temperature of a substance is absolute zero (ie, it contains no heat or kinetic energy).

Assuming that the sun is the initial source of all energy in our solar system, no molecular motion of any substance occurs without solar energy. As long as a substance has some energy and therefore some random molecular motion, heat is potentially available.

With increased input of energy, kinetic energy increases. This increased molecular motion produces more heat, and the temperature rises. An increase in molecular motion correlates with an increase in the heat of a substance. Therefore, a simple definition of **heat** is molecular motion. However, heat may be better defined as energy in transit from a high-temperature object to a lower-temperature object. An object does not possess "heat"; the appropriate term for the potential energy is an object in *internal energy.* The internal energy may be increased by transferring energy to the object from a higher temperature (hotter) object; this process is properly called *heating.*[1]

The words *hot* and *cold* are relative terms. It can be said that no such thing as cold exists because as long as any molecular motion is present, there is some heat. However, we use the terms for the sake of subjective comparison. If we place a hand previously warmed to 104°F (40°C) in water that is 90°F (32.2°C), the water may feel cold, but if we place a chilled hand is in the same water, the water may feel hot. In each case, the different perception is the result of a different reference point. Thus, cold is not an absolute entity; **cold** is a relative term used to describe an entity that has less heat, or gives the sensation of less heat, than does another entity. However, in everyday situations we call certain temperatures hot or cold for practical purposes. To a snow skier, 50°F (10°C) weather is hot; to a water skier, it is cold. **Table 9–1** indicates how various temperatures of water are generally perceived when a person in a moderate ambient temperature immerses a body part in water.

TABLE 9–1   *Perception of Cold and Hot Temperature of Water for a Body Bath**

°Fahrenheit	Perception	°Celsius
32–55	Extremely cold	1–13
55–65	Cold	13–18
65–80	Cool	18–27
80–92	Tepid	27–33.5
92–96	Neutral	33.5–35.5
96–98	Warm	35.5–36.5
98–104	Hot	36.5–40.0
104–113	Extremely hot	40–46
Maximum tolerance 113–115		Maximum tolerance 45–46

*Adapted from Licht S, ed. *Medical Hydrology.* New Haven, CT: 1963:13, 55, 140, 142, 507.

First Law of Thermodynamics

The **first law of thermodynamics** states that, with the exception of nuclear effects, energy can be neither created nor destroyed, but is transformed from one form to another. Whenever this transformation occurs, some energy is released as heat and is considered to be thermal energy. Any activity of chemical, mechanical, or electromagnetic systems always produces some heat. Through such processes, diathermy and ultrasound modalities convert high-frequency electromagnetic or sound energies to heat (lower-frequency electromagnetic energy) in the tissue, where the original energy is absorbed.[2]

Temperature and Temperature Scales

Temperature is not heat. **Temperature** is a means of measuring or describing heat more specifically than is possible using the relative terms *hot* and *cold*. But even this description is not completely accurate because two substances (eg, water and melted paraffin) at equal temperatures may not necessarily contain equal amounts of heat energy or feel equally hot because of variations in thermal properties specific to each substance. As an example, recall how much colder a tile floor feels on your bare feet than the same-temperature wood floor.

Temperature can be expressed in four different scales. **Table 9–2** compares the four scales, and it

TABLE 9–2   *Four Temperature Scales Noting Specific Temperatures Pertinent to Thermal Modality Treatments*

Rankin[†]	°F		° (Celsius)	Kelvin*
672°	212	Boiling point of water (steam)	100	373°
	194		90	
	176		80	
	149		65	
	131	Melting point of paraffin	55	
	125.6	Approximate melting point of paraffin-oil mixture	52	
	122		50	
	114.8		46	
	111.2		44	
	107.6		42	
	104.0		40	
	100.4		38	
	98.6		37	
	96.8		36	
	95.0		35	
	77.0		25	
	68.0		20	
	59.0		15	
	50.0		10	
	41.0		5	
492°	32.0	Freezing point of water (ice)	0	273°
0°	−460.00	ABSOLUTE ZERO	−273	0°

*Same as Celsius scale (100° between boiling and freezing point of water).
[†]Same scale as Fahrenheit (180° between boiling and freezing point of water).

notes the temperatures that have special meaning to therapists. Clinically, we use both **Fahrenheit (F) and Celsius (C) (centigrade) scales;** therefore, therapists should be able rapidly to convert any information from one scale to the other. One commonly used conversion formula is

$$°F = (9/5°C) + 32 \text{ or } °C = 5/9 (°F - 32)$$

The **Kelvin and Rankin temperature scales** are used for scientific research. The size of a degree is the same for the Celsius and Kelvin (K) scales and for the Fahrenheit and Rankin (R) scales. The difference between the boiling and freezing points of water is 100° in both the C and the K scales, and the difference between these points is 180° (212° − 32°) in both the F and the R scales. Absolute 0° K equals −273.16°C, and absolute 0° R equals −460°F.

HEAT TRANSFER

Heat is always transferred from higher to lower temperature molecules until a state of equilibrium is achieved.[3] This **heat transfer** can occur through radiation, conduction, convection, and conversion. Devices using each of these means of heat transfer are available to clinicians. **Figure 9–1** illustrates four thermal modalities that transfer heat by the different mechanisms: heat lamps, hot packs, ultrasound, and fluidotherapy. The physical therapist can select the modality with the means of heat transfer that is most appropriate for a particular situation.

Radiation

Radiation is the term used to describe the transmission of all energy, including heat through space. All objects can give off (emit) or take on (absorb) thermal energy through the process of radiation. Energy emitted at infrared frequencies (heat) will radiate from a warmer substance and be absorbed by a cooler sub-

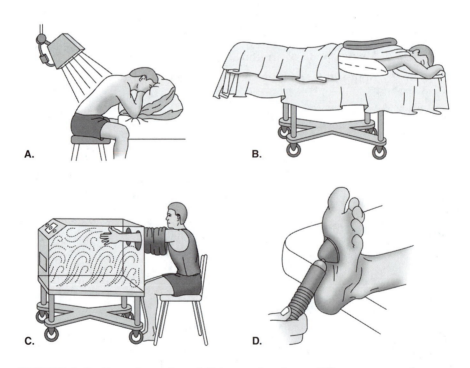

FIGURE 9–1   Four thermal modalities, each using a different means of transferring heat to the patient. (**A**) A heat lamp uses radiation; heat energy is beamed through space to the patient. (**B**) A hot pack uses conduction; a moist heat modality is in contact with the patient. (**C**) Fluidotherapy relies on convection; warm air blows over the patient. (**D**) Ultrasound uses conversion as sound waves create a thermal effect.

stance. The increase in infrared energy causes the molecular motion in the cooler object to increase, thus increasing its thermal energy (heat). Infrared rays are synonymous with heat waves. Therefore, all the physical laws of radiation apply to heat (see **Chapter 7**).

If while you are standing in a room the temperature of your exposed skin is 87°F (30.6°C) and the walls of the room are 65°F (18.3°C), the net flow of energy by radiation will be from your body to the wall. That energy will travel from you to the walls, where it will be absorbed; this transfer will continue until you have cooled and the walls have heated so that temperatures of both are equal. Infrared waves are transmitted through space and thus do not heat the air. However, some waves are absorbed in dust and other substances that may be in the air. Any opaque surface can absorb or reflect infrared rays. Dark or dull objects absorb more rays then they reflect, whereas bright or shiny objects reflect many of the rays that strike them. Materials that are good absorbers are usually good emitters, and good reflectors are poor absorbers. Advertisements for small-area quartz heaters claim that these heaters are "people heaters," not space heaters. This is true, because the infrared rays transmitted through space are absorbed into objects and people, and do not heat the space through which they travel. But it is equally true for the heated-filament units commonly called space heaters. Both types emit infrared rays and thus heat objects rather than the air. The term *space heater* implies that the heater is effective only within a limited space. Both quartz and filament infrared lamps are also used in physical therapy.

Conduction

Conduction is a method of heat transfer from one place to another by successive molecular collisions.[3] Conduction is the only way heat can transfer through an opaque solid. Heat transfer by conduction is a slow process. When two objects of different temperatures touch—for example, when your warm hand touches a cooler object—the more-rapidly moving molecules of the warmer object (your hand) collide with the more-slowly moving molecules of the cooler object. The collision causes the slowly moving molecules to move faster, thus increasing the temperature of that object. Because the warmer object (your hand) gave up some of its energy, its molecules move more slowly after the collision, causing your hand to become cooler.

Paraffin, hot packs, and cold packs use the conduction transfer method. Hot packs and melted paraffin transfer heat directly from the modality to the body.

In the case of a cold pack, however, the rapidly moving, warmer molecules of the body transfer energy to the pack. Consequently, the body cools and the pack becomes warmer.

Convection

Convection is a method of heat transfer between a solid substance and a gas or liquid, in which the heated molecules move from one place to another.[3] This method of heat transfer is more rapid than conduction. Increased input of energy into a system increases the energy of some molecules, which produces more forceful collisions and causes the molecules to travel greater distances after colliding. Thus, as the temperature increases, the space between fluid or gas molecules increases, resulting in a less-dense heated region. A region of lower density is lighter, but it demands more space, replacing the region of higher density. For example, warm air rises and cool air sinks. Circulation of the air or water takes place as the heated, more buoyant gas or fluid rises.

Figure 9–2A and **9–2B** illustrates convection. If the air in a room is initially 50°F (10°C) and a baseboard heater heats the air adjacent to it to 90°F (32.2°C), the warmer air will expand, and the molecules will begin to rise, causing the cooler air nearer the ceiling—because of its greater density—to circulate

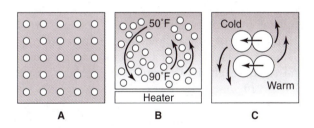

FIGURE 9–2   In this simplified illustration of the convection process, a baseboard heater is used to heat the air in a room. **(A)** All air in the room is the same temperature (50°F): ie, no convection occurs. **(B)** As the heater begins to heat the room, the temperature of the air near the heater increases to 90°F, the warm air expands (becoming less dense) and therefore rises toward the ceiling, which causes the cooler denser air above to circulate toward the floor. **(C)** As the warmer molecules of air rise, they collide with the cooler descending molecules; during this circulation, some heat transfers from the warmer molecules to the cooler ones.

downward to the baseboard, where it will be heated. However, as rising hot-air molecules pass the descending cool-air molecules, they collide (touch). As a result, some heat is conducted (transferred to the cooler molecules). Thus, the "cool" molecules will be warmer than the initial temperature of the air in the room (50°F) as they near the floor (**Fig. 9–2C**).

Nonetheless, as this cooler air, which is now near the floor, is heated, it in turn will rise. The circulatory process will continue until all molecules reach the same temperature. This is analogous to the body's major means of heat transfer between core and surface. As heat is convected in blood flowing through the vascular system, some heat is transferred by conduction to adjacent tissues or blood vessels.

The same principles of convection apply to water. With a temperature gradient, water will circulate without any stirring or agitation until all of it reaches approximately the same temperature. For example, suppose you fill one-third of a whirlpool tank with extremely hot water and then add the same amount of cool water. In a few minutes, all the water will be the same temperature via convection, even without stirring the water. Of course, agitation hastens this circulating process.

Conversion

Conversion is the process whereby nonthermal energy, such as mechanical or electrical energy, is converted to heat energy as it passes through a substance. Rubbing your hands together rapidly to warm them is an example of conversion. Both ultrasound and diathermy increase molecular motion as the sound and electromagnetic waves pass through the tissues. Because the energy generated by these waves is not absorbed at the same rate by different tissues, heating occurs differently in different tissues.[2,4] The power of the energy source determines how vigorously the tissues are heated. (See **Chapter 15, Ultrasound,** and **Chapter 16, Diathermy.**)

THERMAL PROPERTIES OF SUBSTANCES

Many properties of substances depend on and vary with changes in temperature and atmospheric pressure. Such properties include (1) the state of the substance (solid, liquid, or gas), (2) its density and thermal expansion, (3) its specific heat capacity (c),

and (4) its thermal conductivity (k). Because each substance has a unique molecular structure, no specific temperature or pressure affects the properties of all substances in the same way.

State of the Substance

Heat taken in or given up by a substance does not always change its temperature. Some energy is used in the process of changing a substance from one state to another. The heat required to change a substance from a liquid to a solid is called the **heat of fusion,** and the heat required to change a substance from a solid to a gas is called the **heat of vaporization.** Water has a heat of vaporization of 540 cal (more than half a Kcal).

Heat of Fusion.   When water gives up enough heat so that its temperature drops to the freezing point, the next 80 calories per gram of heat (c/g) (336j/g) it gives up will not lower its temperature but will cause the water to solidify and form ice. Conversely, as the solid becomes fluid, its temperature will not rise until all the solid has melted, even though heat is continually being added to the substance. Thus, at approximately the melting point, all substances remain at the same temperature until they have melted completely.

PROBLEM 1

Water can exist in the liquid or solid (ice) state at 32°F (0°C). Why does melting ice remove more heat when applied to the tissues than liquid water at the same temperature?

Answer

Melting ice removes more thermal energy because it is water changing state from a solid to a liquid, which removes an additional 80c/g (336j/g) from the heat source.

The melting and solidifying temperature points of substances vary. Although the exact temperature at which a substance changes from a fluid to a solid depends on the atmospheric pressure, we usually say that water solidifies at 32°F (0°C), whereas melted paraffin solidifies at approximately 131°F (55°C). Adding mineral oil to paraffin lowers the melting point of the mixture, and the exact temperature at which the mixture changes from solid to fluid depends on the amount of mineral oil added. As used clinically, this melting point is approximately 126°F (52°C) (see **Table 9–2**).

Heat of Vaporization.   Water is changed into its gaseous state (steam) at the boiling point. This state requires 540 c/g (2268 j/g). Thus, at 212°F (100°C) the next 540 c/g (2268 j/g) input of heat into the water does not raise the temperature but converts the water into steam.

The same process occurs with vaporization of sweat—an essential mechanism for cooling the body (see **Chapter 8**). Fluids do evaporate below 212°F (100°C), removing significant amounts of heat energy in the process. For example, water left in a dish gradually disappears; the rate of vaporization depends on the humidity of the ambient air. The faster the evaporation of any substance, the more pronounced the cooling effect. Using alcohol, water, or vapor coolant sprays to cool the skin quickly are clinical examples of this phenomenon.

PROBLEM 2

Why will steam at 212°F (100°C) cause a more severe burn than an equal amount of water at the same temperature?

Answer

As in problem 1, this is an example of water changing from one state to another. It requires an additional 540c/g (2268j/g) to convert liquid water into steam. The additional thermal energy of the steam will cause an even greater burn than water of the same temperature.

Density and Thermal Expansion

The **density** of a substance refers to the mass of that substance per unit volume **(Fig. 9–3). Thermal expansion** refers to changes in the density of a substance related to its temperature. How such changes cause heat transfer by convection was discussed earlier.

Nearly all substances expand when their temperatures increase (ie, when the mass per unit volume decreases). Conversely, the density increases when the temperature decreases. The amount of expansion per increase in temperature differs for various substances; the amount has been determined for many substances and accorded a specific coefficient of thermal expansion. This coefficient is used to calculate the effects of changes in density per temperature change.

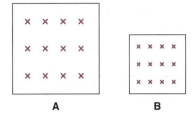

FIGURE 9–3   An example of how the density of a substance changes as its temperature changes. Both parts of the figure represent a substance with a mass of 12 g (each X represents 1 g). (**A**) As the temperature increases, the substance expands: ie, its density (mass per unit volume) decreases. (**B**) As the temperature decreases, the substance contracts: ie, its density increases.

Water is an exception to the rule that density decreases with increases in temperature. Water reaches its greatest density at 39.2°F (4°C). Although it does expand as the temperature increases above that level, it also expands as the temperature drops below that level. Because ice at 0°C is less dense than water at 4°C, it floats slightly above the water level. When the temperature of water in a glass bottle drops to freezing, the bottle may break. The water expands and changes into ice with the decrease in temperature, but the bottle contracts.

The mercury and glass thermometer is a good clinical example of different coefficients of thermal expansion. Mercury passes through a narrow glass tube and rises within the tube when placed in a warmer environment. Both the glass and the mercury expand at the higher temperature; however, mercury, having the higher coefficient of thermal expansion, expands more and therefore rises within the glass tube. Incidentally, when the mercury rises, a design feature holds the mercury in the tube as it cools to allow correct reading.

Of more direct concern to clinicians is an understanding of factors that influence the difference in the quantity of heat contained in various modalities at equal temperatures and in the difference in the rate at which each transfers heat to or from the patient. Among the contributing factors are thermal properties inherent to the substance of that particular modality: ie, the **specific heat capacity** of the substance, which influences the quantity of heat in that modality, and the **thermal conductivity** qualities of the substance, which influence how quickly the substance transfers heat.

Quantity of Heat. Many factors determine the quantity of heat in a specific substance. First, consider the volume. A bathtub one-third full of hot water at any given temperature will not contain as much heat as a tub three-quarters full of water of the same temperature. Thus, if you sit in a tub that is one-third full, your body systems will not be affected as much as if you sat in the three-quarter-full tub for the same length of time. In this example, the substance, water, the temperature of the water, and the time of application are equal, but the volume—the amount of the substance—determines the difference in the quantity of heat available for the body to receive.

Next, consider the same substance, water, at different temperatures and volumes. The temperature of a cup of boiling water may contain less heat than a pail full of warm water. Try pouring the water from each container over a block of ice and observe what happens. Ice melts in the area where the cup of boiling water was poured (a local effect) whereas the remaining block remains much as it was. If the pail of water is poured over the block, the water will melt more of the entire block, thus having a greater effect on the entire object—that is, a more general effect.

Using a clinical example that is relatively analogous, a 20-min local application of heat with a modality such as a towel-wrapped hot pack or hot-water bottle at 140°F (60°C), like the cup of boiling water, it will produce a noticeable local effect but will produce less systemic change than a 20-min Hubbard tank intervention at 104°F (40°C) because the quantity of heat available in the Hubbard tank is much greater.

PROBLEM 3

Which would you expect to cause a greater systemic (cardiovascular and pulmonary) effect: lying up to the neck in Hubbard tank for 20 min at a temperature of 100°F (37.8°C) or sitting in lowboy tank up to the bottom of the rib cage in the same temperature water for the same amount of time? Why?

Answer
The Hubbard tank would cause a greater systemic effect, because more of the body is in contact with the water; therefore, the quantity of heat is greater even though the water temperature is the same. Heart rate and respiratory rate would increase as the body attempts to cool itself.

Variations Among Substances. Two different modalities can be of equal mass and temperature; however, if they are not made of the same substance, one modality may contain a much greater amount of heat than the other. The quantity of heat contained in a substance at any given temperature depends on specific physical properties of that substance. Some substances require more energy input than others to achieve similar increases in molecular motion.

In physics the term *specific heat* is used to represent the amount of heat (energy) input required to increase molecular motion and thus increase the temperature, or the amount of energy released to reduce the motion and thus the temperature of a substance.[3] The joule is the International System Unit (ISU) for thermal, electrical, and mechanical energy. James Prescott Joule, a nineteenth-century English physicist, discovered that if he added a mechanical paddle system to a container of water and began to stir the water, the temperature, a measure of the kinetic energy of molecular motion, increased. After repeating the experiment many times, he observed that it always required the same amount of work to raise the temperature of 1 gram of water by 1 degree celsius. The amount of energy necessary to perform this work became known as a **Joule (J).** The calorie is also a unit of measurement often used to measure heat energy. One **calorie (c)** is equal to 4.18 Joules. Calories are often used when working with water because the specific heat capacity of water (the amount of heat necessary to raise the temperature of 1 gram of water by 1 degree celsius) is 4.18 Joules/gram times the temperature in celsius, which is equal to 1 c/gram times the temperature in celsius. Energy in food is commonly measured in calories as well, but these calories are actually kilocalories and should be represented by an upper-case C (**Calorie**).

The **specific heat** is the amount of heat per unit mass required to raise the temperature by 1°C. The relationship between heat and temperature change is usually expressed in the form shown below where c is the specific heat. The relationship does not apply if a phase change (transition between solid, liquid, or gas states) is encountered, because the heat added or removed during a phase change does not change the temperature.

$$Q = cm \, \Delta T$$

where Q is heat added, c is specific heat, m is mass, and ΔT is change is temperature.

Specific Heat Capacity

The ability of a molecule or its constituents to move depends on the structure of the molecule and differs for every substance. Some substances require more energy input than others to increase the internal random motion; therefore, the quantity of heat energy required to raise the temperature is greater. The specific heat input required to raise the temperature of 1 g of a substance 1°C is designated its specific heat capacity value. The value given to water is 1 and is used as a basis for comparing the specific heat capacities of all other substances. Applying the formula Q = SmT to water, 1c is the quantity (Q) of heat input required to change the temperature of 1g of H_2O, the mass (m), 1°C from 14°C to 15°C. Because the specific heat capacity (S) value for water is 1, the formula can be written as follows:

$$1c = 1 \times 1 \text{ g} \times 1°C \text{ (from 14°C to 15°C)}$$

In British thermal units, quantity = BTU, mass = pounds (lb), and temperature = degrees Fahrenheit. Therefore:

$$1 \text{ BTU} = 1 \times 1 \text{ lb} \times 1°F$$

which is equivalent to 1058.4J or 252c.
Table 9–3 gives the specific heat capacity values of substances that are of interest to physical therapists. Note that paraffin, as used clinically, has a specific heat capacity value of 0.65 compared with that of water (1.0).

To clarify the concept of quantity of heat, use the preceding formula in reverse (SmT = Q) and compare the amount of heat intake required to raise 500 g of water or paraffin 3°C (at no given temperature):

S of water = 1	S of paraffin = 0.65
1 × 500g × 3°C = 1500 c (6300 J)	0.65 500g × 3°C = 975 c (4095 J)

Fewer calories (joules) of heat input are required to raise the temperature of the paraffin. Thus, at any given temperature, paraffin contains less heat than does water.

PROBLEM 4

Equal amounts of paraffin and water are put in two pans of identical size; each pan receives equal amounts of heat from a stove burner. The temperature of both pans was the same at the start, and both were heated for the same amount of time. At the end of a given time, which substance has the greater increase in temperature? Approximately how great is the increase? Which substance has acquired the greatest amount of additional heat?

Answer

The specific heat constant of paraffin is about 1/3 less than that of water (paraffin 0.65, and water 1.0). Thus, per given time, the paraffin temperature will increase about 1/3 more than the water. Both will have had equal amounts of heat (thermal energy) added.

Thermal Conductivity

Some substances conduct heat more readily than others. Thermal conductivity of a particular substance refers to the ability of that substance to conduct heat. Thermal conductivity properties determine the rate at which heat is taken in or given up, by and conducted through, the substance.

Generally, metals are good conductors of heat, stone and sand are moderate heat conductors, and wood is a poor conductor. The following are everyday examples of thermal conductivity. If you are walking barefoot on the beach and the sand is extremely hot, you move to the wooden boardwalk because your feet will not feel as hot; you would avoid walking on any metal that was lying on the beach. Wood does not give up heat as quickly as sand does, but metal gives up heat much faster than either wood or sand.

Similarly, in an extremely cold environment, if you put your hand on a metal versus a wooden doorknob, the metal knob will feel much colder than the wooden one because the metal can more quickly absorb the heat given off by your hand.

The conductivity of many materials has been scientifically determined and given a specific number value for the constant (k). The larger the value of k of a substance, the faster it can transfer heat. **Table 9–3** gives the constant values of thermal conductivity for several substances. The constants given indicate that water is a better conductor than wood

TABLE 9–3   *Constant Values for Specific Heat Capacity and Thermal Conductivity of Nonbiologic and Biologic Substances*[*†]

Substance	Constants	
	Specific Heat Value (S)[‡]	**Thermal Conductivity Value (k)**[§]
Nonbiologic		
Paraffin	0.65	—
Rubber	0.480	0.372
Paraffin and oil	0.45	—
Wood	0.42	0.2
Sand	0.25	93.0
Air	0.24	0.026
Aluminum	0.215	235.0
Plate glass	0.2	2.60
Water	1.0	1.4
Copper	0.0923	401.0
Biologic[॥]		
Skin	0.9	0.898
Muscle	0.895	1.53
Whole blood	0.87	1.31
Average for body	0.86	—
Subcutaneous fat	0.55	0.45
Bone (average)	0.38	2.78

*Lehman J, ed: *Therapeutic Heat and Cold*. 4th ed. Baltimore, MD: Williams & Wilkins; 1990:65, 128–129, 175, 179, 212–213.

[†]Halliday D, Resnick R: *Fundamentals of Physics*. 3rd ed. New York: John Wiley & Sons; 1988.

[‡]Heat required to raise the temperature of a specific substance: $S = Q/mT$ or $Q = SmT$, where S = specific heat value (constant), Q = quantity (c or BTU), m = mass (g or lb), and T = amount of temperature change (°F or °C). Note that S and k are not directly correlated: eg, the k for copper is the highest value given, but the S for copper is lower than that for aluminum.

[§]Speed at which heat transfers through a specific substance: $H = kATG/D$, where H = rate of conduction (c/s), k = value (constant), A = cross-sectional surface area (m²), T = time (s), G = temperature gradient between hot or cold surfaces on opposite sides of the substance $(t_1 - t_2)$ (°C), D = thickness (m).

[॥]The values do not represent in vivo tissues; many are simulated models, animal tissues, or in vitro tissues.

but not as good a conductor as metal, and that paper, cloth, and air are poorer thermal conductors than water. Because they retard the rate of heat transfer, poor heat conductors are considered to be good heat insulators. **Table 9–3** also shows the difference in thermal conductivity values for various body tissues. Bone and tissues such as blood and muscle, which have a high fluid content, are the best heat conductors, whereas fat, a poorer conductor, is

a good insulator. Thus, when applying thermal modalities, the physical therapist must consider the amount of subcutaneous fat of the patient. The fat acts to retard heat transfer, by conduction, to or from the deeper body tissues.

Thermal conductivity principles are constantly applied in daily life. For example, imagine two pans of food are heating on the stove. One pan has a wooden handle, the other a handle of the same metal as the pan. You could comfortably hold the wooden handle but not the metal one. To lift the pan with a metal handle, you would probably use a pot holder made of quilted layers or terry cloth, each with many air spaces. Although air conducts heat slowly, it is not a perfect insulator. Heat will come through eventually, but less heat over time reduces the possibility of burning your hand. For the same reason, fluffy terry-cloth toweling or other materials with air spaces are used to wrap a hot pack: the heat will then conduct to a patient at a slower rate.

Most liquids and all gases are poor conductors of heat. Down jackets, fur coats, and thermal blankets, although lightweight, are good heat insulators because air, a poor conductor, is trapped between the feathers or hairs, or in the spaces of thermal fabrics. The air retards the conduction of heat away from the warm body to the outside colder air. Moist towels will conduct heat more quickly than dry towels because much of the dead air space is replaced by the better-conducting water.

Although good electrical conductors are also good heat conductors, the two uses of the term *conductors* should not be confused. Both are related to the free electrons of the substance. Electrical conductivity depends on the arrangement of electrons in the atoms of a substance: the attraction of negative ions for positive ions, or a flow of energy along the path of free electrons (see **Part 3**). Heat conductivity depends on the arrangement of electrons in a molecule and the way that the electrons react to changes in temperature, not how they react to positive ions or polarity.

PROBLEM 5

You are heating a pan of milk on the stove. You observe that the milk on the surface near the sides of the pan begins to bubble before the milk in the center. Why?

Answer

The thermal conductivity constant (k) is much higher for metal than for milk. Thus, the milk on the sides, adjacent to the pan, absorbed heat conducted up the sides of the pan as well as that conducted through the fluid. Thus the milk on the sides reached a boiling point sooner than the milk in the center.

PROBLEM 6

You use several layers of moist towels rather than dry towels between the patient and a hot pack. Which will feel hotter to the patient, and which is more likely to cause a burn? Why?

Answer

The moist towels will conduct the heat faster because the dead air spaces in the fluffy dry towels is replaced by moisture (water) which conducts heat much better than air.

To differentiate between (1) specific heat capacity, which determines a quantity (how much heat is necessary to raise the temperature of a substance), and (2) thermal conductivity, which determines a rate (how long it takes for heat to conduct through a substance), solve the following problem.

PROBLEM 7

If a patient places a hand in liquid paraffin or water, the temperature of which is 128°F, the hand will instantly feel much hotter in the water. Is this outcome the result of the specific heat properties of the substance, its thermal conductivity, or both?

Answer

As mentioned in problem 4, there is less heat per given temperature in paraffin than in water.

To predict the rate of heat transfer in a given time period, many factors must be considered. This brief overview can only begin to explain the many factors that control the rate of heat conduction through a given substance. The rate (ie, how much heat passes through a specific material in a given time) depends on the cross-sectional area, the temperature gradient between the heated surface (t_1) and cooler surface (t_2) to which the heat will transfer ($G = [t_1 - t_2]$) the thickness of the material, and the thermal conductivity constant for that substance. The greater the area and the temperature gradient, the faster the heat transfer, and the thicker the material, the slower the transfer. Thus, the following equation can be used to determine the rate of heat conductivity through a substance (**Fig. 9–4**) or to predict the rate of heat conduction through body tissues:

$$H = \frac{kATG}{D}$$

where H = heat, k = constant, A = cross-sectional area, T = time, G = temperature gradient between t_1 and t_2, and D = thickness.

In actuality, the thermal conductivity constant (k) of a tissue is not considered as an isolated factor when determining the conductivity properties of the tissue. Instead, the thermal inertia of the tissue is used; that is, the thermal conductivity, the mass, and the specific heat of the tissue are factored into the equation. But no measurements based on constants are ever precise for body tissues in vivo, primarily because they cannot account for individual variations in circulation.[5]

This brief discussion of heat conductivity formulas represents an attempt to explain the many factors that control the actual rate of heat conduction through a mass of a given substance. An understanding of these factors is useful for developing research projects that investigate heat modalities or for determining why there are differences in the results of other researchers.[6]

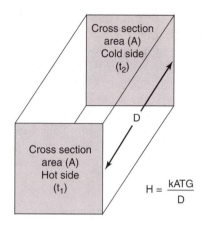

FIGURE 9–4   Determinants of thermal conductivity. (H) = Heat passing through the substance in a given time period (the rate). k = Thermal conductivity constant for given substance. A = Cross-sectional Area of the Substance. T = Given time period. G = Temperature Gradient between hot and cold side surface areas (t1 2 t2). D = Thickness of the substance (the slab).

KEY TERMS

thermal energy	Fahrenheit temperature scale	convection
heat	Celsius (centigrade) temperature scale	conversion
Joule		heat of fusion
calorie	Kelvin temperature scale	heat of vaporization
Calorie	Rankin temperature scale	density
BTU	heat transfer	thermal expansion
first law of thermodynamics	radiation	specific heat
temperature	conduction	thermal conductivity

REVIEW QUESTIONS

1. What is the first law of thermodynamics?
2. Explain how hot and cold are relative terms.
3. Convert the following temperatures from Fahrenheit to Celsius or vice versa:
   a. 52°C
   b. 131°F
   c. 114°F
   d. 37°C
   e. −2.2°C
4. Explain the four methods of heat transfer:
   a. radiation
   b. conduction
   c. convection
   d. conversion

5. Name some substance properties that influence temperature changes within that substance.

6. What is the heat of fusion?

7. What is the heat of vaporization?

8. What is the treatment temperature of the following two items? Why do the treatment temperatures vary?
   a. paraffin
   b. water

9. What is thermal expansion?

10. What three factors determine the quantity of heat required to produce a given change in temperature?

REFERENCES

1. Downloaded from the World Wide Web, December 2003: http://hyperphysics.phy-astr.gsu.edu /hbase/thermo/heat.html#cl.

2. Lehmann J, ed: *Therapeutic Heat and Cold*, 4th ed. Baltimore: Williams & Wilkins; 1990.

3. Serway RA, Faughn JS: *College Physics*, 4th ed. Philadelphia: Saunders; 1995.

4. Williams R: Production and transmission of ultrasound. *Physiotherapy* 1987; 73:113–16.

5. Houdas Y, Ring E: *Human Body Temperature: Its Measurement and Regulation*. New York: Plenum; 1982.

6. Cameron MH, ed: *Physical Agents in Rehabilitation: From Research to Practice*. Philadelphia: Saunders; 1999.

10

Biophysics

BERNADETTE HECOX, PT, MA

JOHN P. SANKO, PT, EDD

Chapter Outline

Human tissues, like all substances, are subject to physical laws. Thus, the topics discussed in **Chapter 9** apply to human tissues but are complicated by factors beyond those considered in inanimate substances. People, because of their thermoregulatory mechanisms, have a special way of dealing with internal and external thermal conditions. Thermoregulation is under neural control, and it integrates adjustments in physiological, psychological, and behavioral mechanisms.

THERMOREGULATION

Human beings and other mammals are warm-blooded (**homeotherms**), which means that they must maintain their internal temperature within a very narrow range in order to survive (**Fig. 10–1**). Unlike cold-blooded animals (poikilotherms), whose survival depends on compensatory behaviors to counter extreme changes in the thermal environment, homeotherms maintain **thermal homeostasis** through a number of complex, integrated physiologic mechanisms

Cold-blooded animals are also known as **ectotherms** because of their dependance on external factors for control of their body temperature. In contrast, warm-blooded animals are classified as **endotherms** because of their ability to maintain thermal homeostasis internally. Humans can tolerate variations in internal temperature of about 7.2°F (4°C) before physical and mental performance become impaired.[1] Consequently, we humans live our lives within a few degrees of death. Body temperature affects numerous biochemical and physical processes necessary to maintain life. Under normal resting conditions, core body temperature is relatively stable and is one of the most frequently assessed vital signs.[2,3] Core temperature, or internal temperature, is the temperature deep within the trunk and is usually measured sublingually, rectally, at the tympanic membrane, in the axilla, or at the lower esophagus near the heart. The best approximation of core temperature is obtained from the esophagus, but this technique is poorly tolerated in unanesthetized individuals. Oral measurement is best tolerated and accurately reflects the temperature of the blood because of the vascularity of the tongue, but this measurement is easily distorted by eating, drinking, and breathing through the mouth. Tympanic thermometers, placed in the ear, are being used consistently because of simplicity of use, rapid response, and minimal distress to the patient. The tympanic thermometer detects thermal infrared radiation from the tympanic membrane in the ear.

It is customary to say that the normal body temperature is 98.6°F (37°C). However, normal body temperature is not that precise or constant. There are normal diurnal fluctuations throughout the course of the day. The lowest temperature, about 97°F (36.1°C), usually occurs between 4:00 A.M. and 6:00 A.M., whereas the maximum temperature of about 98.8°F (37.1°C) generally occurs in the late afternoon. These variations correspond to circadian rhythms (the body's internal clock), sleep, work and activity patterns, food ingestion, body size, age, gender, and physiologic impairment.[4] Travel to different time zones and working different shifts will also alter the patterns of an individual. Patterns in temperature variation are among the first patterns to develop in full-term newborns, beginning about 1 week after birth. The rhythms themselves undergo change until about 5 years of age, when the adult pattern is established.

The ability to regulate body temperature appears to change with age. Infants have difficulty regulating body temperature in both cold and hot environments. This difficulty may be partly due to their higher surface area to mass ratio, which causes them to lose body heat more rapidly in cool environments, and an immature autonomic nervous system and underdeveloped sweat glands that make it more difficult to dissipate heat in warm environments. Preadolescents exhibit lower sweating rates and higher core temperatures than adolescents and adults during physical activity.[5]

Older people may have a cooler core temperature 95°F (35°C).[6,7,8] There is no consensus regarding the effect of aging on thermoregulation during periods

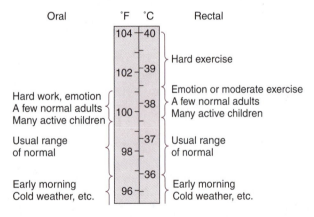

FIGURE 10–1   Estimated range of body temperature in normal people. (*Pandolf RB, Sawkamn MN, Gonzalez RR, eds.* Human performance physiology and environmental medicine at terresterial extreme. *Indianapolis: Benchneris; 1988:106. McGraw-Hill.*)

of physical activity. Some studies have concluded that the elderly exhibit less thermoregulatory control. However, more recent studies that controlled for body size and composition, pathologic conditions, and aerobic fitness level show little or no limitations in the thermoregulatory capacity of older adults.[9] Studies of fit older men and their younger cohorts have demonstrated no difference in their ability to regulate core temperature during heavy exercise. The question then becomes whether the thermoregulatory changes observed in many older adults are a consequence of aging or the changes that often occur concurrently with aging (eg, obesity, cardiovascular and other diseases, and physical inactivity). There is some evidence to suggest that cutaneous circulation becomes less effective in transporting blood from the core to the shell as we age.[10] This may be because of changes in the autonomic nervous system that result in delayed vasodilatation and changes in both sweat rate and sweating threshold. There is also evidence that older adults are less able to sense changes in skin temperature.[11] Thus, the physical therapist must always consider the age of the patient when selecting a therapeutic intervention, including the administration of a physical agent. Finally, a number of commonly prescribed medications may also have a profound effect on a person's ability to regulate body temperature.

The effect of gender on thermoregulation has generated considerable debate. Early studies seemed to indicate that men were better able to manage thermal stress than women. More recent studies that controlled for relative fitness levels and aerobic capacity have shown that women tolerate thermal stress as well as, if not better than, men. Hormonal changes during the menstrual cycle do appear to influence thermoregulation by reducing the cutaneous blood flow and sweat rate near ovulation. Preovulatory females have the same core temperatures as their male counterparts but have an average increase of about 0.72°F (0.4°C) during the follicular and luteal phases of the menstrual cycle.

Diseases such as diabetes may result in autonomic neuropathy, and diabetes will interfere with cutaneous circulation and thermoregulatory control. Spinal-cord injuries within the thoracolumbar column will cause the loss of sympathetic input and severely impair thermoregulation by reducing cutaneous vasoconstriction, shivering, and sweating.

The so-called thermogenic effect of foods increases with fitness levels and varies in proportion to the quantity and type of food ingested. Foods high in protein elicit the greatest thermic effect, followed by carbohydrates and fats. The maximum thermic effect of food is usually seen within 1 hour of ingestion.

Variations in body temperature are sometimes described in relation to the depth of the tissues (**Fig. 10–2**).[8] The temperature of muscles at rest is usually lower than the core temperature, but it increases with exercise as muscle metabolism increases.[10,12] The outside surface of the body can be referred to as the **shell.** If a resting person is nude and the ambient temperature is 86°F (30°C), the shell will be approximately 92°F (33.5°C), assuming low humidity and minimal air flow.[13] Even the shell temperature varies greatly in different areas of the body. For example, skin temperature is higher in the axilla and groin areas, where less heat can escape, than on the back and in areas with poor circulation. The various temperatures on the body surface are well defined in color thermographs. They can also be determined by placing a skin thermometer such as a thermistor on several different areas of the skin.

The temperatures of the tissues beneath the shell also vary greatly. In general, the deeper the tissues, the higher their temperature, especially in the trunk. For convenience, the variations in temperature in relation to depth have been described as **isotherm layers** (ie, areas with similar temperatures).[12] The temperature of each isotherm layer increases so that the deepest isotherm, the center of the body, is represented as the warmest (see **Fig. 10–2**). However, this is not a completely accurate description. The depth at which tissues are equal in temperature (ie, isothermic) varies according to body size and in different areas of the body.[14] Layers outside the shell, such as clothing, are described as outside isotherm layers.

Ideally, the temperature gradient between the shell and the ambient temperature is approximately 7°F (4°C).[1] Disregarding environmental factors such as wind velocity and humidity, when the ambient temperature is about 77°F (25°C) and the shell is about 84°F (29°C), a resting person who is nude feels comfortable. (The temperatures vary, depending on the climate to which the individual is adjusted and on individual differences such as age and sex). However, if the ambient temperature drops to 70°F (21°C), a nude person will begin to feel uncomfortably chilly and begin making behavioral adjustments (eg, putting on clothes or moving around to keep warm. This phenomenon has direct application to therapists. When working with a patient in a room where the temperature is 70°F (21°C), the therapist is comfortable and may forget that a

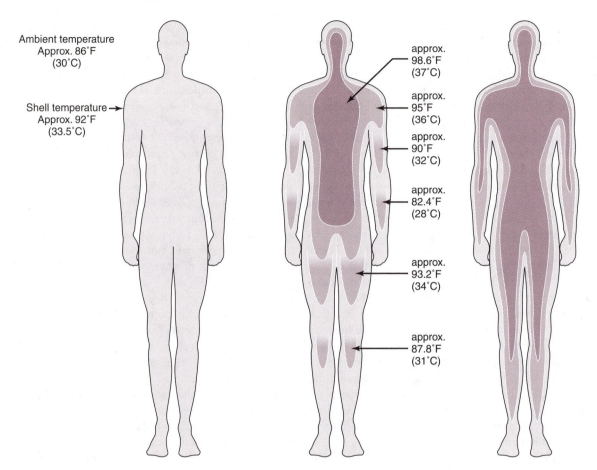

Ambient temperature
Approx. 86˚F
(30˚C)

Shell temperature →
Approx. 92˚F
(33.5˚C)

approx.
98.6˚F
(37˚C)

approx.
95˚F
(36˚C)

approx.
90˚F
(32˚C)

approx.
82.4˚F
(28˚C)

approx.
93.2˚F
(34˚C)

approx.
87.8˚F
(31˚C)

FIGURE 10–2   Schematic illustrations of an average body surface temperature relative to the ambient temperature and to various depths of tissue in various areas of the body. **(A)** Gradient between ambient temperature and the average temperature of a nude resting man's body surface (shell). **(B)** Variations in tissue temperature (shown in °F and °C) relative to depth and area of the body. **(C)** Illustrations of descriptive isotherm layers.

partly nude patient lying quietly on a plinth will be uncomfortable. For this reason, a sheet or blanket—an outside isotherm—should be used to cover the patient.

The behavioral adjustments that people make when the ambient temperature is cold include a preference for warm food and drinks and for food with more calories. The opposite behavioral adjustments occur as ambient temperature increases much above 77°F (25°C); people may have the urge to wear fewer clothes and to select cooler foods and drinks. They will also have the urge either to decrease the amount of physical activity or to perform activities more slowly and with less effort.

Heat Loss

As a by-product of metabolism, heat is constantly being generated within the body. Because metabolism is a continuous process, this heat must be dissipated; otherwise, the body's internal temperature would constantly be increasing. In the ideal environment, the shell is warmer than the environment, and the core is warmer than the shell. Because heat transfer is always in the direction of warmer to cooler, this gradient factor allows the body to release heat and to maintain a constant internal temperature. The heat leaves the body by the same physical means of heat transfer mentioned in

Chapter 9—conduction, convection, and radiation—and through the process of evaporation of moisture (conversion).

Conduction

Some heat will be conducted from the warmer, deeper tissues to the shell. However, as shown by the thermal conductivity constants in **Chapter 9** (**Table 9–3**), tissues differ in their ability to conduct heat. The thermal conductivity of bone and muscle is high relative to that of the skin and fat. Thus, skin and subcutaneous fat act as insulators, retarding the rate of heat conduction through tissues to the surface. Although some heat is conducted through tissues to the surface, this conduction is by no means adequate to prevent a rise in core temperature.

Convection

The primary means of transferring heat from the deeper areas of the body to the shell is internal convection. Heat is first conducted from the deeper tissues into the vascular system circulating through them. The warmed blood flows through the vessels and is convected toward the shell by the peripheral circulatory system. The circulating blood, just like hot water in the heating system of a building, is transported from the source to a cooler area. This convection, bringing the warm blood to the surface, causes the shell temperature to be warmer than the ambient temperature to which the shell is exposed.

Radiation

If the shell is warmer than the ambient temperature, infrared heat waves will radiate from the warmer skin into the cooler environment. The body gives up its heat in the same way the radiator does in a hot-water heating system. Radiation is the primary means by which heat escapes until the ambient temperature rises higher than 86°F (30°C). When the skin and ambient temperatures are equal, usually 95–97°F (35–36°C), there can be no heat lost through radiation.[15] When the ambient temperature is warmer than the shell, net radiation takes place in the opposite direction, and the body, in addition to an inability to rid itself of heat, will gain additional heat from the environment. Similarly, when a superficial heat modality is applied, the direction of heat transfer is reversed, and the body gains heat. In addition to the heat produced through metabolism, will the core temperature

rise with a reversal of heat transfer? Within a limited range of heat application, no, because people have other means of losing heat.

Evaporation

One essential mechanism that enables the body to maintain a constant core temperature is **evaporation of sweat.** In addition to conduction and convection, a large amount of heat can be brought to the body surface in the forms of insensible and sensible sweat. The term **insensible sweat** refers to the constantly occurring diffusion of moisture through the skin. The term **sensible sweat** refers to the moisture brought to the surface by thermally activated eccrine sweat glands. Regulation of sensible sweating is under neurophysiologic control.[15–17] Activation of this sweat mechanism occurs when any increase in core temperature occurs and when the skin temperature rises to approximately 91.4°F (33°C)[18]; these increases can be caused by fever, exercise, or an ambient temperature above 85°F (29°C) (see **Chapter 17**). When local heat is applied, provided that no increase in systemic temperatures has occurred, secretion of sweat is limited to the area where the temperature has increased.

Once sweat is on the body surface, it will evaporate, provided that it is exposed to air and that the moisture content of the air is not too great. This process of evaporation cools the body. When the ambient temperature is greater than the skin temperature and radiation is no longer possible, evaporation is the major means of losing body heat. You may recall that 540 calories per gram (2268 J) is required for vaporization of water to occur (see **Chapter 9**). Similarly, evaporation of sweat uses heat (calories) to cool the shell. When the air is humid, however, sweat cannot evaporate as easily; it either remains on the body surface or drips off—and neither condition assists in cooling the body. It is the process of evaporation that cools and makes the individual feel more comfortable, even when the ambient temperature hovers around 90°F (32.2°C). This effect accounts for the expression "It's not the heat, it's the humidity!" It also explains why it is important to consider both the temperature and the humidity, or "apparent temperature," and to use these apparent temperatures rather than exact temperatures to guide our patients' and our own activities. When the temperature of the air is 80°F (26.7°C) and the humidity is 40%, the apparent temperature is 79°F (26°C), which is usually safe during exercise for people with compromised health. With the same temperature and a humidity of 70%, however, the apparent temperature is 85°F (29.4°C), and exercise could be unsafe (**Fig. 10–3**).

Some evaporation also occurs with respiration. Moisture from the mucous membranes of the respiratory passages can evaporate when passages are open to the environment, but in humans this means of heat loss is far less effective than evaporation of sweat. In an effort to cool off, however, an individual may develop a panting breath pattern when overheated.

Ambient Air Flow (Convection)

Air flow contributes significantly to heat loss. When a breeze allows a flow of air molecules that are cooler than the body surface to pass over the body, heat is given up. First, heat is conducted from the warmer molecules on the body surface to the cooler air molecules, thus cooling the body surface. Then, the heat is convected (ie, carried away) by the moving air molecules. The greater the wind velocity, the greater the cooling effect.

Biophysical Aspects of Heat Loss

Despite the production of heat by metabolism and the heat gained from ambient conditions, a constant internal temperature is maintained by physiologic, physical, and behavioral means that include the following: modifying physical activity (the greater the fitness, the better the thermoregulation), clothing, eating habits, and avoiding environments with extreme temperatures. The body transfers heat from deeper tissues to the surface tissues only minimally by conduction through the tissues and primarily by convection in the bloodstream and by sweating. This heat is then released to the environment by infrared radiation, evaporation of sweat, and respiratory moisture, or by convection via air flow. Ambient temperature, humidity, and wind velocity influence the body's ability to give off heat.

Temperature		Relative Humidity (%)										
°C	°F	100	90	80	70	60	50	40	30	20	10	5
15	59	17.5	17.0	16.5	16.0	15.5	15	14.5	14	13.5	12.9	12.7
18	64	20.2	19.6	19.0	18.4	17.8	17.2	16.6	16.0	15.4	14.8	14.5
20	68	22.2	21.5	20.8	20.1	19.4	18.7	18.0	17.4	16.7	16.0	15.6
22	72	24.2	23.4	22.6	21.9	21.1	20.3	19.5	18.7	18.0	17.2	16.8
25	77	27.5	26.5	25.6	24.7	23.7	22.8	21.9	20.9	20.0	19.1	18.6
28	82	31.0	29.9	28.7	27.6	26.5	25.4	24.3	23.2	22.0	20.9	20.4
30	86	33.5	32.2	31.0	29.7	28.5	27.2	26.0	24.7	23.5	22.2	21.6
32	90	36.1	37.7	33.3	31.9	30.5	29.1	27.7	26.3	24.9	23.5	22.8
35	95	40.4	38.7	37.1	35.4	33.7	32.1	30.4	28.8	27.1	25.4	24.8
38	100	45.1	43.1	41.1	39.2	37.2	35.3	33.3	31.4	29.4	27.4	26.5
40	104	48.4	46.2	44.4	41.9	39.7	37.5	35.3	33.2	31.0	28.8	27.7

Low Risk   Medium Risk   High Risk

FIGURE 10–3   Chart For Calculating Heat Index. (The table above shows how to find the "apparent temperature," that is, how hot various temperature-humidity combinations feel. For example, if the temperature is 95 and the relative humidity is 50 percent, find 95 in the temperature column on the left side, follow that row to the right to the 50 percent humidity column. The apparent temperature is 107. This falls into the "danger" area where outdoor exercise isn't a wise idea. The colors on the chart show the level of danger of various combinations.

PROBLEM 1

If the ambient temperature is 93.2°F (34°C), the humidity is 20%, and little wind is blowing, will the core temperature of a nude individual at rest increase or remain stable? Why?

Answer

The core temperature will remain stable if the patient's sweating mechanism is functioning.

PROBLEM 2

If you place a patient in a Hubbard tank with only his head and shoulders above water for a 20-min intervention and if the temperature of the water is 93.2°F (34°C), would you expect his core temperature to increase or remain stable?

Answer

Assuming that the temperature of the body shell is 84°F (29°C) and the temperature of the water is 93°F (34°C), heat will be conducted into the body. The metabolic process increases because of the input of heat. Little heat is being given off. Core temperature may rise.

PROBLEM 3

The ambient temperature is 95°F, the humidity is 80%, and no wind is blowing. Eighty-year-old Ms. Smith, attempting to stay cool, is rocking in her rocking chair and fanning herself vigorously. Will this activity help? Can you apply this example to a therapeutic situation?

Answer

Although the fan may circulate air, the temperature of the air is dangerously high. The rocking and fanning exercise may increase Ms. Smith's metabolic rate, producing more internal heat and raising her core temperature. Thus, her fanning will probably be more damaging than helpful, although she may gain some relief from the air movement across her face. An electric fan, of course, would be more efficient. Asking Ms. Smith to exercise vigorously in such ambient conditions could be dangerous.

HEAT GAIN

Whenever the ambient temperature is higher than the body temperature, heat is transferred to the body. The body gains heat through the same physical processes by which it loses heat, but the processes occur in the opposite direction. The effects of exposing the entire body to a warmer environment are discussed under **Generalized Heating** in **Chapter 11** and **Ambient Conditions** in **Chapter 17**. The focus in this section is on the effect of applying heat to one area of the body.

When a superficial heat modality is applied to a local area of the body and the body surface is cooler than the modality, as it usually is, the heat will be transferred from the modality to the local area. This transfer occurs by conduction, radiation, convection, or all of these, depending on the modality used.

Once the local body surface is heated, the specific heat capacity and the effective conductivity of those tissues will influence the amount of **tissue temperature rise (TTR)** that will occur. **Effective conductivity** includes both the thermal conductivity properties of the heated tissues described in **Chapter 9** and the vascular supply controlling convection. The heat can then be conducted to adjacent tissues. How much and how fast the TTR occurs in adjacent tissues depends on the thermal properties and the effective conductivity of each type of tissue. Although some heat may conduct to subcutaneous tissues, skin, and fat layers, the surface tissues are not good conductors (see **Chapter 9**, **Table 9–3**).

Surface versus Deep Tissues

Because surface tissues are poor thermal conductors, they will retain much of the heat they receive. Some heat may be transferred to adjacent superficial bone and muscle; however, because these tissues are better thermal conductors, they will retain less heat than do skin and fat. Muscle and bone are also deeper than skin and subcutaneous fat and thus farther from the source of heat. The usual explanation is that any heat conducted into blood in the cutaneous vessels will be transported by convection away from the local area of application. This convection, added to their thermal properties, limits the TTR of superficial muscle and bone. Because the temperature of deeper tissues was originally higher (recall the isotherm layers), it is unlikely that any significant TTR will occur there.

Although straightforward, this explanation is an oversimplification.

Some evidence indicates that as the heated blood travels back toward the heart, some heat will be conducted to adjacent tissues and arterial vessels. However, the deep muscles are not likely to be heated by this process. The cutaneous capillaries and their terminal arterioles and venules pass only through the superficial muscles. Blood flow in deep muscle is independent of cutaneous circulation.[19–21] This anatomic distribution of vessels lends support to studies showing that no change in blood flow in deep muscle occurs when superficial heat is applied and to studies showing that the regulation of blood flow in muscle is related to the oxygen demands of the muscles. Only if the temperature of the deep muscles increases, as when deep heat modalities are applied or during exercise, does the blood flow to those muscles increase.[22,23] **Figure 10–4** illustrates the findings of Lehmann's well-executed study, showing that local superficial heat modalities produce a modest TTR in tissues that are 1 cm deep but that a significant TTR—higher than 107°F (41°C)—occurs only in surface tissues.[24] The figure also demonstrates the effectiveness of vascular convection. The plateau in the TTR appears to be controlled by the blood flow because when the flow is obstructed, the surface tissue temperature increases. Comparing **Fig. 10-4A** and **B**, we see that the peak surface temperature was reached sooner with the hydrocollator pack than with the infrared lamp, whereas the plateau temperature reached with the lamp was slightly higher. Note that the infrared lamp provides a constant source of heat, whereas the hydrocollator pack does not.

The many studies conducted to determine the amount of TTR that can occur in tissues at various depths have produced varying results.[25–32] It is important to compare carefully the methods used and the results obtained in these studies. In some of them, all measurements of temperature or circulatory changes were done with instruments that record surface changes; changes in deeper tissues were theorized but not determined.[31]

Other studies were done in tissues in vitro (taken out of the body) with their vascular supply abolished; the results of these studies cannot be compared with what occurs in normal (in vivo) human tissues. In studies in which no generalized circulatory changes were possible, the tissue temperature could indeed rise significantly. Although much can be learned about physiologic reactions from experiments performed on small animals in vivo, we must remember that the effects of a certain dose of heat that might kill a rat are not directly applicable to humans because the tissue volumes and circulatory capabilities are so different. These studies, however, can be meaningful if a clinician is deciding whether to use heat or cold on tissues with a poor vascular supply.

We must be aware of the ways in which terms are used. For example, the term *deeper tissues* may mean any subcutaneous tissues, tissues deeper than 1 cm, or tissues deep within a particular part of the body. It is possible to raise the temperature as deep as the joints in small body parts such as the fingers or toes with a superficial modality. To heat joints appreciably that are deeper than 1 cm, however, surface tissue would have to be heated to the point of pain or damage. Fortunately, this is not the case with deep-heat modalities. With microwave, shortwave diathermy, or ultrasound, forms of energy other than heat are transmitted to deeper tissues, producing heat where that energy is absorbed.

Factors Determining Temperature Rise

The extent to which a local superficial thermal modality will change the tissue temperature significantly or produce heat gain in the body depends on several factors: (1) the ability of the modality to give heat to the body, (2) the physical properties of the specific tissues, (3) the integrity and response of body systems, and (4) surface area to volume ratios. Fingers heat up with superficial modalities partly because of their large surface area to volume ratios. For deep-heat modalities, the specific absorption rate (SAR) is also a factor (see **Chapter 8**, **Table 8–2**).

Factors Related to the Modality. The ability of the modality to give heat to the body depends on (1) the amount of heat that the modality can provide, (2) its thermal conductivity properties, (3) the temperature gradient between the patient and the modality, and (4) the duration of the application. Many modalities can provide a large amount of heat. For example, a large amount of heated water, an infrared lamp, or a heating pad can maintain a constant output of heat for a prolonged period. The large amounts of heat that these modalities can deliver can cause changes in the body's core temperature, assuming that the vascular system is intact and can convect the heat to the general circulatory system. If the local vascular system is not intact, local tissues can be dangerously overheated

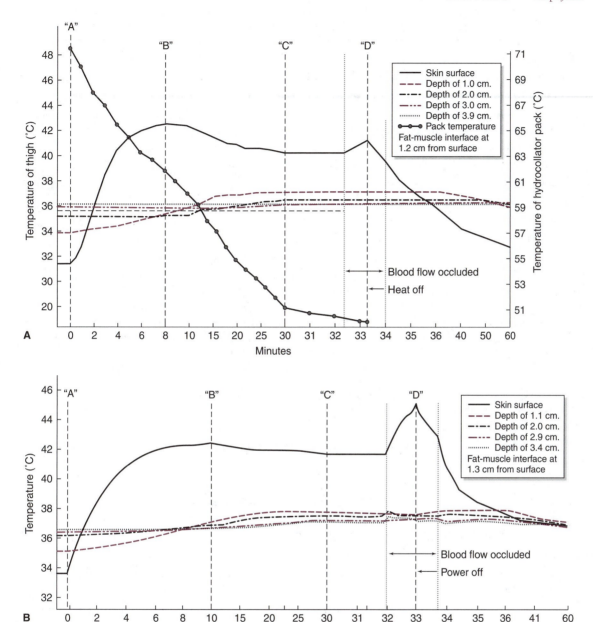

FIGURE 10–4 Comparison of the effects of two superficial heat modalities on surface and deeper tissues. (**A**) Temperatures recorded in the human thigh during application with Hydrocollator hot packs. (**B**) Temperatures recorded in the human thigh during exposure to infrared radiation from a 250 w Mazda lamp (red bulb). (*Reproduced with permission from* Arch Phys Med Rehab *1966; 47:291–299*)

by modalities that provide a constant heat output; thus, such modalities must be carefully monitored. (**Table 10–1** outlines the thermal properties of some commonly used superficial modalities.) Other modalities, such as hot-water bottles and hot packs, provide a limited amount of heat because they are cut off from the source of heating. With these modalities, the amount of heat the body absorbs is limited.

Depending on the thermal conductivity properties and temperature gradient between tissues and the modality, heat can be exchanged quickly or slowly. If the exchange occurs faster than the vascular system is

TABLE 10–1   *Thermal Properties of Common Superficial Heat Modalities*

Hot Pack

- Pack is soaked in and saturated with water that has a relatively high specific heat value (S); thus, much heat is put into the pack to attain a temperature of 145°F or more.
- The pack contains a substance with a lower thermal conductivity constant (k) than water; thus, it conducts heat more slowly—retains heat longer than water alone. Patient's vascular system can normally dissipate the heat readily.
- If a 145°F pack is wrapped in other materials that retard conduction, the temperature reaching the patient is approximately 105°F.
- The hot pack cools down in proportion to the amount of heat given to both the patient and the environment.

Hot Water Bottle

If water is approximately 133°F and the bottle contains approximately 2 quarts of water, compared with water immersion modalities mentioned below, there is relatively little heat contained in the modality. Water is a good conductor, but rubber is an insulator. Thus, the effect on the patient is not the same as direct application of 133°F water. If wrapped in one towel layer, the temperature of the towel may be 122°F. Although the initial rate of heat transfer may be rapid, the initial sensory impression of heat is great, and skin temperature may increase to 110°F, the amount of heat available is limited. Consequently, if the vascular system is normal, there is little additional tissue temperature rise locally.

Immersion

- The quantity of heated fluid is usually larger than the amount of heated substances in the two modalities mentioned above; therefore, it contains more heat/temperature. Actual amount of heat/temperature depends on the specific heat value of the fluid.
- Fluid surrounds the body part; thus, much heat is conducted into the body per temperature of fluid without high intensity per square inch.

Heating Pad

If continuous over time, only an extremely low output can be safely tolerated. If off/on periods are thermostatically controlled and circulation is intact, this modality can give much input to the body, most in general body heating. Only with impaired circulation will it overheat a local area.

Infrared Lamp

- Energy from the lamp radiates to patient and objects. Because of much divergence and reflection of rays, placement of the lamp as well as power output (wattage) determine the intensity.
- A *constant source* of energy output; thus, much heat is available and tissues continue to be heated as long as the lamp is on.

capable of accommodating, the skin temperature may rise quickly. This can occur if a hot pack of 145°F (62.8°C) is placed directly on a patient. If conduction occurs slowly—eg, when several layers of terrycloth are placed between the pack and the patient—the temperature rises gradually over a longer period. Because this method gives the vascular system time for convection, it prevents a dangerous change in temperature. However, a slow rise in an area with good circulation may prevent effective changes in local

temperature or may require intervention for a longer period to be effective. The importance of using the correct amount of insulators and the correct duration of application cannot be overstated.

It should be noted that heat is transferred from a modality in all directions. For example, unless prevented by some insulated covering, a hot pack may radiate heat into the environment rather than conduct it into the patient. If hot pack is wrapped with equal toweling on the side exposed to the environment as on the side adjacent to patient, and if the room temperature is 72°F (22.2°C) and the patient's skin is 84°F (28.9°C), more heat will be transferred to the room than to the patient. Because the temperature gradient is greater on the room side, the rate of transfer is faster. This illustrates the need to cover packs with good insulators such as plastic and terrycloth covers.

Physical Properties of Tissues.   Skin and superficial fat layers are insulators; thus, conduction of heat to deeper tissues is hindered, and applied heat remains in cutaneous tissues. Because bone and muscle are better conductors, any heat reaching these tissues is dissipated more easily than heat from skin and fat. The thermal properties of tissues adjacent to bone and muscle and the circulation in the area determine the rate and amount of heat loss. To a great extent, the vascular system controls thermal changes in tissues, primarily by convection of heat from an area where

the tissue temperature is increased to an area where the tissue temperature is decreased, thus influencing the local effect of a modality (**Table 10–2**).

Integrity and Response of Body Systems.   To prevent tissue damage, the vascular system must function properly. Any vascular problems will prevent normal protective mechanisms. Vascular control is dependent on both sensory and autonomic nervous systems; thus, these systems must also be intact.

Biophysical Aspects of Heat Gain

Whenever the external temperature is higher than the skin temperature, heat is transferred to the body surface by conduction, radiation, convection, or all of these mechanisms. The greater the gradient between the source of heat and the body, the faster the transfer. The TTR of surface and adjacent tissues is determined by the thermal characteristics and vascularity of

TABLE 10–2   *Biophysical Considerations When Heating with Superficial Modalities*

Cutaneous Skin and Fat Layers

- Good heat insulators.
- Retard conduction of heat to or from deeper tissues.
- Much of applied heat is retained in skin or fat layers.
- If the fat layer is less than 1 cm, some of the applied heat conducts to superficial bone or muscle (temperature rise as high as 6°F).
- If the fat layer is thicker than 2 cm (obese), little heat will conduct through skin or/and fat layers.

Local Vascular Vessels

- Heat is conducted to blood in the cutaneous vessels that permeate the area.
- If the circulation in the area is good, heat is convected to the general body and to adjacent tissues and vessels en route.
- If the circulation in the area is poor, more heat is retained in the surface area where applied and the temperature of these tissues will rise. If temperature rises above 113°F (45°C), damage will occur.

Bone

- Bone is a better conductor than overlying skin or fat. Heat in these tissues can conduct to other tissues.
- Little tissue temperature rise (TTR) occurs if the circulation in the area is good, if the bone underlies muscle, or both.
- The TTR at bony prominences may be great enough to cause discomfort.

Superficial Muscle

- Muscle is a relatively good thermal conductor.
- Some TTR is possible but not significant.
- The vascular supply is usually good; thus, heat is convected from the area.

the various tissues. Skin and subcutaneous fat are poor thermal conductors; thus, they retain a large amount of heat and conduct little heat to deeper tissues.

Heat conducted to the cutaneous blood supply will be convected away from the heated area. As this blood travels toward the heart, it may conduct some heat to tissues and adjacent arterial vessels. But neither the heat conducted through surface tissues nor that convected in heated blood through tissues is sufficient to produce a significant TTR beneath the surface, although a slight TTR occurs to about 1 cm below the surface.[33]

Superficial heat modalities will not elevate the temperature of deep muscles or increase the amount of blood flow through them. However, deep-heat modalities are capable of doing both. Superficial heat modalities, such as a full-body hot-water bath or a heat lamp, can transfer enough heat to the body to elevate the core temperature.

Factors that determine the ability of a heat modality to heat body tissues depend on the type of modality, the physical properties of the tissues, and the integrity and responses of the vascular, sensory, and autonomic systems.

Tables **10–1** and **10–2** summarize this discussion as it relates to the thermal effects of superficial heat modalities and their clinical application.

PROBLEM 4

Part 1: Two modalities, A and B, are heating body areas of similar size and contain the same amount of heat, but A has a lower thermal conductivity constant. Which modality will produce less TT change/time? *Part 2:* If the temperature gradient between modality A and the body part being heated is less than the gradient between modality B and the body part, which modality will produce less TT change/time?

Answer

Part 1: A is the answer. *Part 2:* Again, the answer is A. The lower the temperature gradient, the slower the rate of heat exchange. Any TTR is lower because the heat is convected from the area in the vascular system.

REVIEW QUESTIONS

1. What is thermal homeostasis?
2. Explain how each of the following may affect an individual's thermoregulation:
   a. Age
   b. Gender
   c. Body size and composition
   d. Diet
   e. Inactivity
   f. Diabetes
   g. Spinal cord injury
3. What is an isotherm? How does a fan or whirlpool turbine's effectiveness depend on isotherms?
4. What are the four ways that the body can lose heat? Which is most effective? Which is least effective?

5. How does sweating cool the body? How does heat vaporization make sweating a more effective cooling mechanism?
6. Identify the factors that will influence the rise in tissue temperature when using the superficial heating modalities.
7. Which of the body's tissues are most efficient and least efficient in conducting heat?
8. Which superficial heating modality provides a constant source of heat?
9. Explain why exercise is better able to increase muscle blood flow as opposed to a superficial heating modality.
10. An elevation in core temperature is most likely to occur with what type of superficial thermal application?

KEY TERMS

homeotherms
thermal homeostasis
ectotherms
endotherms

shell
isotherm layers
evaporation of sweat
insensible sweat

sensible sweat
tissue temperature rise (TTR)
effective conductivity

REFERENCES

1. Astrand P, Rodahl K: *The Physiology of Work*. New York: Taylor & Francis; 1989.

2. Downy J, Lemons DE: Human Thermoregulation. In: Downey JA, Myers SJ, Gonzalez EG, Lieberman JS: *Physiological Basis of Rehabilitation Medicine*. Boston: Butterworth-Heinemann; 1994.

3. Ivy AC: What is normal or normality? *Q Bull Northwestern Univ Med School* 1994; 18:22–32.

4. Stitt JT: Central Regulation in Body Temperature. In: Gisolfi CV, Lamb DR, Nadel NR. *Perspectives in Exercise Science: Exercise, Heat, and Thermal Regulation*. Carmel, IN: Cooper Publishing Group; 1993.

5. Perlstein PH: Thermoregulation. *Pediatric Annals* 1995; 25:531–37.

6. Collins K: Hypothermic and Thermal Responsiveness in the Elderly. In: Fanger P, Valbjors O, eds. *Danish Building Research Institute*. Copenhagen: 1979; 819–33.

7. Collins K, Dore C, Exton-Smith A, et al: Accidental hypothermia and impaired temperature homeostasis in the elderly. *Br Med J* 1977; 1:353–56.

8. Fox R, Woodward P, Exton-Smith A, et al: Body temperatures in the elderly: A national study of physiological, social, and environmental conditions. *Br Med J* 1973; 1:200–06.

9. McArdle W, Katch F, Katch V: *Exercise Physiology: Energy, Nutrition, and Human Performance*, 3rd ed. Baltimore: Lippincott Williams & Wilkins; 2001.

10. Aschoff J, Wever R: Kern and Schale in Warmehaushalt des Menschen. *Naturwissen-schaften* 1958; 45:477–81.

11. Taylor RA, Allsopp NK, Parkes DG: Preferred room temperature of young vs aged males: The influence of thermal sensation, thermal comfort, and affect. *J Gerontol A Biol Sci Med Sci* 1995; 50(4):M216–21.

12. Houdas Y, Ring E: *Human Body Temperature: Its Measurement and Regulation*. New York: Plenum; 1982.

13. Lehmann J, ed: *Therapeutic Heat and Cold*, 4th ed. Baltimore: Williams & Wilkins; 1990.

14. Folk G Jr: *Textbook of Environmental Physiology*, 2nd ed. Philadelphia: Lea & Febiger; 1974; 44:88–132.

15. Frisancho A: *Human Adaptation: A Functional Interpretation*. St. Louis: Mosby 1979; 44–45.

16. Sloan A: *Man in Extreme Environment*. Springfield, MO: Charles C Thomas; 1979; 9.

17. Slonim NB, ed: *Environmental Physiology*. St. Louis: Mosby; 1974; 94:102–03.

18. Holdcroft A: *Body Temperature Control*. London: Bailliére-Tindall; 1980:1, 12–26.

19. Dentry J-M, Brergelmann G, Rowell L, et al: Skin and muscle components of forearm blood flow in directly heating resting man. *J App Physiol* 1972; 32:506–11.

20. Downey J: Physiological effects of heat and cold. *Phys Ther* 1964; 44:713–17.

21. Weinbaum S, Jiji LM, Lemons D: Theory and experiment for the effect of vascular microstructure on surface tissue heat transfer: part I. Anatomical foundation and model conceptualization. *J Biomech Eng* 1984; 106:321–30; 333–41.

22. Weinbaum S, Jiji LM, Lemons D: Theory and experiment for the effect of vascular microstructure on surface tissue heat transfer: part II. Model formulation and solution. *J Biomech Eng* 1984; 106:331–41.

23. Rowell L: Reflex control of the cutaneous vasculature. *J Invest Dermatol* 1977; 69:154–66.

24. Rowell LB, Shepherd J, Abboud F: Cardiovascular Adjustment to Thermal Stress. In: *Handbook of Physiology*. Bethesda, MD: American Physiological Society. 3: (Sect. 2, pt. 2), 967–1023.

25. Abramson DI, Tuck S, Chu LS, Agustin C: Effects of paraffin bath and hot fomentation on local tissue temperatures. *Arch Phys Med Rehab* 1964; 45:87–94.

26. Borrell PM, Parker R, Henley EJ, Masley D, Repinecz M: Comparison of in vivo temperatures produced by hydrotherapy, paraffin wax treatment, and fluidotherapy. *Phy Ther* 1980; 60:1273–76.

27. Erdman WJ, Stoner EK: Comparative heating effects of moistaire and hydrocollator hot packs. *Arch Phys Med Rehab* 1956; 37:71–74.

28. Hollander JL, Horvath SM: Influence of physical therapy procedures on intra-articular temperature of normal and arthritic subjects. *Am J Med Sci* 1949; 218:543–48.

29. Horvath SM, Hollander JL: Intra-articular temperature as measure of joint reaction. *J Clin Invest* 1949; 28:469–73.

30. Lehmann JF, Silvermann DR, Baum BA, Kirk NL, Johnson VC: Temperature distribution in the human thigh produced by infrared, hot pack, and microwave applications. *Arch Phys Med Rehab* 1966; 47:291–99.

31. Oosterveld FG, Rasker JJ: Effects of local heat and cold treatment of surface and intra-articular temperature of arthritic knees. *Arthritis Rheum Med* 1994; 37:1578–82.

32. Weinberger A, Fadilah R, Lev A, Pinkhas J: Intra-articular temperature measurements after superficial heating. *Scand J Rehab Med* 1989; 21:55–57.

33. Abramson DI: Neural regulation of cutaneous circulation. *Adv Biol Skin* 1972; 12:207–33.

11

Physiologic Responses to Thermal Stimuli

BERNADETTE HECOX, PT, MA

JOHN P. SANKO, PT, PHD EDD

Chapter Outline

Whenever the body gains or loses heat, regardless of cause, physiologic adjustments occur in an effort to preserve homeostasis. This chapter discusses the physiologic responses that are related to (1) the application of heat or cold modalities, (2) the metabolic rate related to physical activity, and (3) ambient conditions. Although the emphasis is on the application of heat or cold, the interrelationship of all three factors must be considered. For example, an intervention program consisting of a heat modality and therapeutic exercise, given in hot weather, may cause physiologic changes that would not occur in cooler weather. Some individuals—the very old or very young, or those who are medically compromised—may be unable to tolerate the combination of effects of a heat modality, hot weather, and therapeutic exercise, although they might be able to tolerate any one factor.

Under what circumstances should the physical therapist or assistant omit the therapeutic exercise or application of the heat modality? When would it be feasible to substitute a cold modality for a heat modality? To answer such questions, therapists and assistants must understand both the local and the systemic physiologic responses resulting from local application or general body exposure to heat or cold. These responses include the effects on specific types of body tissues and on the functions of the body systems. For example, vigorous heat may be indicated for a patient with a chronic ankle-sprain problem because the effect of heat on local tissues and sensory nerves may reduce pain and increase range of motion. However, if the patient also has diabetes and poor circulation, vigorous heat would be contraindicated because the vascular system would be unable to make the adjustments necessary to remove excessive heat or metabolic wastes. In addition, the use of certain medications may alter autonomic and/or nervous system function, making the individual incapable of responding appropriately to the application of heat and cold.

The focus of this chapter is on the physiologic responses to locally applied thermal modalities, although much of the information pertains to all thermal interventions. The effects of full body exposure to heat and cold are discussed further in **Chapter 17**.

MECHANISMS CAUSING RESPONSES TO HEAT AND COLD

The body responds to thermal changes to protect tissues from damage from excessive heat and cold and to maintain a constant core (internal) temperature (thermal homeostasis). Some local responses may be related to the effects that heat or cold have on substances, found naturally in tissues, that modulate microcirculatory blood flow. Such vasoactive substances include the prostaglandins, histamine, bradykinin, and serotonin.[1] In turn, these substances can directly affect the activity of the sweat glands in the skin or the local blood vessels.[2]

In general, however, local and systemic responses are under neural control. Free nerve endings that respond to warm, cold, and thermal pain are situated in the skin and probably in many deep body sites. Other thermal sensors are located in the central nervous system (CNS). Information received from the cutaneous receptors travels through afferent pathways to the hypothalamus and also to the cortex, where conscious awareness of heat and cold sensations occurs (**Fig. 11–1**). Within the hypothalamus are sensor sites that monitor the temperature of the blood flow through the capillaries at the hypothalamus itself.[3]

Although extrahypothalamic deep-body sensors appear to exist, in general the hypothalamus integrates information received from the receptors, then mediates appropriate responses through neural efferent pathways. Some evidence indicates that areas that trigger activities to prevent temperature rise are situated in the anterior hypothalamus, and those that prevent cooling are situated in the posterior hypothalamus. A well-balanced integration of neurotransmitter substances probably mediates these efferent pathways.[4]

Because both local and systemic thermal responses depend on information initiated by receptors, both receptors (especially those in the skin) and their afferent pathways must be intact for appropriate physiologic responses to occur when thermal modalities are applied. In addition, the patient's ability to report excessive heat or cold depends on those receptors. **Figure 11–2** illustrates the frequency of firing of warm, cold, and thermal pain fibers at various temperatures. Note that the frequency of firing, as shown in the figure, approximates the temperatures given in

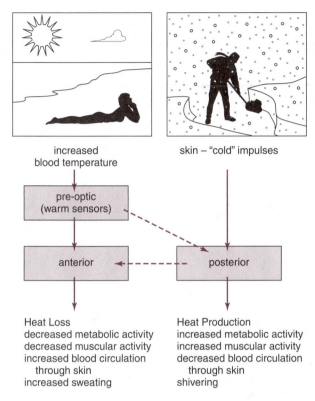

increased
blood temperature

skin – "cold" impulses

pre-optic
(warm sensors)

anterior

posterior

Heat Loss
decreased metabolic activity
decreased muscular activity
increased blood circulation
    through skin
increased sweating

Heat Production
increased metabolic activity
increased muscular activity
decreased blood circulation
    through skin
shivering

FIGURE 11–1 Hypothalamic control of body temperature. The pre-optic area responds to changes in blood temperature by initiating reflexes that prevent overheating. This involves stimulation of the anterior hypothalamus and inhibition of the posterior hypothalamus. The posterior hypothalamus responds only to nerve impulses coming from skin receptors. Cold stimulates these nerves, causing activation of the posterior hypothalamus and reflex mechanisms of heat production. There is also simultaneous inhibition of heat-loss mechanisms of the anterior hypothalamus.

Table 11–1 for perceptions of cold, heat, and thermal pain, and for marked changes in tissue function. For example, the firing of warm fibers decreases and that of heat-pain fibers begins at approximately 109°–113°F (43°–45°C), the temperature above which tissue damage can occur. Similarly, cold fibers decrease and cold-pain fibers increase firing at temperatures below about 59°F (15°C), the temperature at which tissues and physiological functions are endangered.[3]

The responses triggered by the peripheral sensory input are the safety mechanisms that protect against tissue damage. There is a range of about 50°F (10°C) within which one can usually tolerate changes in tissue temperature, but pain is perceived when the temperature rises toward 109°C (43°C) or when it falls below 59°F (15°C). This pain is a warning that tissues are in danger. Depending on the length of time that the temperatures of tissues is beyond the safe range, damage or necrosis can occur (see **Table 8–1**).

To maintain a constant internal temperature, systemic responses occur that are triggered at the thermoregulatory center of the central nervous system (CNS). However, relatively little is known about the central processing of thermal afferents.[5,6] It is thought that various thermoregulatory systems operate from **set points,** which are not necessarily identical for all systems.[7] Set-point temperatures are those that trigger heat dissipation (sweating) or conservation (shivering) mechanisms in the body. These temperatures will change on the basis of skin temperature. **Figures 11–3 and 11–4** display the effect of skin temperature on the set-point temperature control from the hypothalamus. The control of the activities of these systems has been compared with the control of the temperature of a room by a thermostat that acts from a set point. When the temperature of a room rises above the point at which the thermostat is set, the heater switches to off. When the temperature drops below that point, the heater switches to on again. Because the regulation of body temperature appears to occur primarily in the hypothalamic region, we sometimes refer to a "hypothalamic thermostat."

The body strives to maintain an internal temperature of about 98.6°F (37°C) and a mean skin temperature of about 91.4–94°F (33–34.5°C) for men and about 90°–95°F (32.2°–35°C) for women. The information about these temperatures is integrated at the hypothalamus.[6] When either the skin or the internal temperature changes or the relative difference between the two temperatures varies, the thermoregulatory centers trigger appropriate responses to reestablish the set-point temperatures.

Although the set point theory is useful to explain how humans maintain thermal homeostasis, it is open to criticism and leaves many questions unanswered. For example, experiments have shown that thermoregulatory responses are elicited by changing the temperature of the spinal cord, although the hypothalamic temperature remains constant. However, changes as small as 0.36°F (0.2°C) in the temperature of blood passing near the hypothalamus can cause systemic responses proportional to the temperature change, that act to restore homeostasis.[8]

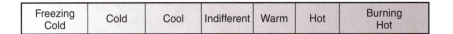

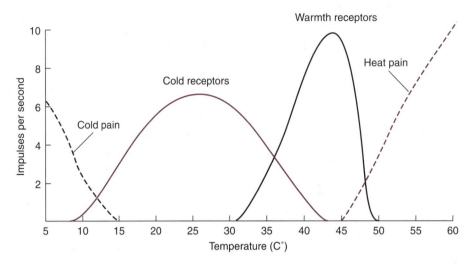

FIGURE 11–2   Frequencies of discharge of (1) cold-pain receptors, (2) cold receptors, (3) warmth receptors, and (4) heat-pain receptors. Note that the frequencies of firing shown in this figure approximate the temperatures at which pain
related to hot and cold are perceived as shown in Table 7–1. (*Adapted with permission from* Human Physiology and Mechanisms of Disease. A Guyton. 6th ed. 1981)
1881, WB Saunders. Drawn from original data collected in separate experiments by
Zotterman, Hensel, and Kenshalo.)

IMMEDIATE RESPONSES

When either a heat or cold agent is applied to the skin,
specific reactions relative to the temperature gradient
between the modality and the skin may occur before
any appreciable change occurs in tissue temperature.
Figure 11–5 illustrates these responses. The immediate reactions caused by the thermal sensory experience
of either hot or cold may be similar. However, other
responses to heat differ from those to cold because
they are appropriate for preventing tissue injury from
opposite problems—either excessive heating or cooling. Thus, this discussion of immediate responses proceeds as follows: (1) thermal sensory reactions to hot
and cold, (2) other responses to tissue temperature
rise, and (3) other responses to tissue cooling.

Responses to
Thermal Sensory Experiences

Sometimes called *thermal shock reactions*, reactions to
thermal sensory experiences occur whenever the
skin comes in contact with something that is hotter or
colder than it is.[9] The specific response depends on the
size of the surface area and the temperature gradient
between the skin and the modality. More precisely, the
reaction depends on the temperature change at the site
of the cutaneous thermal receptors.[5] **Figure 11–2** indicates that the frequency of firing of thermal neurons is
stable at any given temperature (a static response).
However, with a change in temperature at the receptor
sites, the rate of firing changes (a dynamic response).
Depending on the amount and rate of temperature
change, the frequency of neuron firing at first overshoots, then settles at the predictable frequency for any
given temperature. These responses will differ according to the area experiencing the thermal change: the
smaller the area, the less the response. The individual's
perception of and attitude toward such changes in thermal sensation also influences the reaction.

An initial sensation of mild heat or coolness may
produce an analgesic effect in the area of application.
Mild warmth or coolness applied to a local area can
reduce local pain and/or muscle spasms and promote
general relaxation.[10] If the temperature of a modality
is such that the individual experiences a greater sensation of hot or cold, other reactions occur. A moderate
temperature change may serve as a general stimulant

TABLE 11–1   *Summary of Physiologic Responses to Applied Heat and Their Clinical Significance*

Physiologic Response	Effects	Clinical Significance
	Mild: analgesic/sedative.	Decreases pain spasms, and aids relaxation.
Thermal sensory experience (thermal shock).	Moderate: autonomic responses. Severe: fight or flight responses.	Invigorating general stimulant. Pain and fear.
Changes in skin color.	Observable sign is erythema.	Usually increases blood flow.
Increased metabolic rate.	Increased healing and waste production.	Increases heat production and tissue temperature.
Increased blood flow.	Increase bleeding.	Increase healing (increases nutrients to and waste removal from the area).
Reflex response.	Increased cutaneous blood flow in areas of body other than where heat applied.	Effect is transitory.
Increased capillary permeability.	Increase (or decrease) interstitial fluid.	Increased (or decreased) edema.
Increased sweating.	Increased cooling.	Decreases fluid/salt balance in body.
Fluctuations in cardio-vascular (CV) activity.	Changes in heart rate/blood pressure.	Stresses CV system and/or can cause fainting if excessive.
Increased respiration.	Little value in maintaining thermal homeostasis.	Indicates heat distress.
Decreased joint stiffness.*	Increase speed and freedom of joint movement.	Increases agility.
Increased extensibility of nonelastic tissues.*	Assist in elongating or stretching tendons, scar.	Increases range of movement of any body segment.
Increased peripheral nerve conduction velocity and motor nerve activity.*		Increases speed and motor function.

* Indicates responses that are discussed in Chapter 12.

that produces an arousing, invigorating effect.[11] For example, a hot or cold shower often helps us get going in the morning. However, if the temperature change is perceived as too hot or too cold, we may experience pain or fear. Fight-or-flight responses of eye dilation and changes in facial and skin color, increased blood pressure, and increased pulse may be observed. If the temperature of the modality is within the therapeutic range, these reactions subside quickly as we adapt to the temperature change, that is, as the rate of neuron firing stabilizes.

Other Responses to Heat

Local sweating and erythema also increase in immediate response to the local application of heat. Although the erythemal response is observed, the reasons for it are not clearly established; it may be related to a spinal reflex. It also has been theorized that because sensory axons have many branches, the excitation of hot, cold, or noxious afferent neurons may result in action potentials that travel back to the area of stimulation through another branch of the same sensory axon, causing release of a vasodilatory substance—possibly a hormone, histamine, or acetylcholine. These substances produce a local capillary dilation, thus erythema. Because this is an event that is separate from any action potentials reaching the spinal cord, it has been termed *axon reflex.*[12,13] **Figure 11–6** illustrates this axon activity. However, it is important to note that current researchers consider an axon reflex improbable.

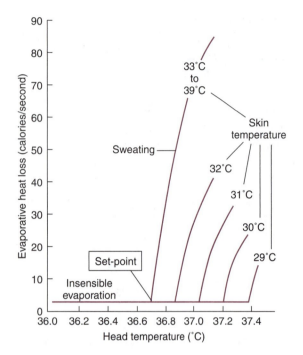

FIGURE 11–3 Effect of changes in the internal head temperature on the rate of evaporative heat loss from the body. Note also that the skin temperature determines the set-point level at which sweating begins.

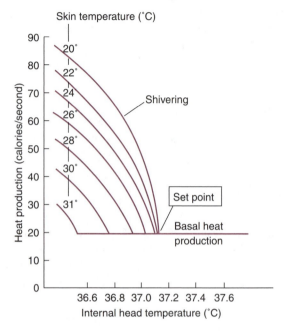

FIGURE 11–4 Effect of changes in the internal head temperature on the rate of heat production by the body. Note also that the skin temperature determines the set-point level at which shivering begins.

Temperature increases may act directly on smooth muscles of blood vessels and on the sweat glands. Immediate local sweating has been shown to release bradykinin, which in turn causes erythema.[1] Bradykinin is formed as the enzyme kallikrein interacts with alpha$_2$-globulin and forms kallidin, which is eventually converted to bradykinin from the action of various tissue enzymes.[3] The observed erythema occurs as a result of bradykinin's actions of increasing arteriolar vasodilatation and capillary permeability.

Other Responses to Cold

In addition to the thermal shock reactions, other immediate responses to cold include local vasoconstriction, with blanching of the skin, and local piloerection. Some investigators believe that the cold inhibits the release of histamine and thus blanching occurs.[14,15] Others explain the vasoconstriction as being part of the initial reaction of the body to maintain core temperature—an autonomic neural response acting to prevent that part of the body from giving up heat to the colder environment. Whatever the cause, vasoconstriction restricts the rate of blood flow. It thus decreases the amount of

warm blood arriving at the site of the cold application and enhances the ability of applied cold to lower the local tissue temperature.[11]

In animals, piloerection, also an autonomic neural response, causes body hair to stand up. This increases air space between hairs, producing insulation that prevents body heat from escaping. Goose bumps in humans are a remnant of this response, but because we have little hair, the response is ineffective.

Therapeutic Implications

The correlation among the afferent inputs resulting from firing of cutaneous thermal receptors, the sensory perception, and the thermoregulatory responses is based primarily on information derived from animal studies.[5] The immediate responses occurring with the application of a thermal modality may be caused by the direct effect of temperature change on the activity of sweat glands, vessels, nerves, or mediator substances in the treated area; from central control of information from skin receptors; by the conscious recognition of a noticeable temperature gradient between skin and the thermal agent; or by any combination of these factors.

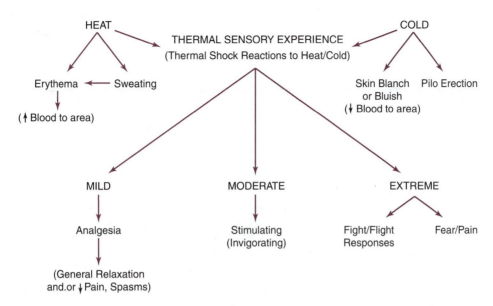

FIGURE 11–5   Immediate responses to the local application of heat and cold.

Many beneficial results attributed to the use of thermal modalities (eg, decreased pain, general relaxation, or both) may be the result of effects of the perceived sensations. However, other benefits are the result of physiologic responses caused by the actual changes in tissue temperature, as the next section will show.

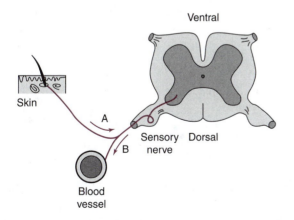

FIGURE 11–6   An axon reflex. (**A**) A cutaneous sensory receptor is stimulated, which sends impulses along the axon toward the spinal cord. (**B**) Theoretically, the impulses could then travel on another branch of the axon back to a capillary, where it could release vasodilatory substances.

RESPONSES TO A RISE IN TISSUE TEMPERATURE

A series of physiologic changes occur whenever tissue temperature rises. This chapter discusses these changes step-by-step as they relate to localized tissue temperature rise (TTR). **Figure 11–7** indicates that an applied heat initially increases the tissue temperature. Vertical and horizontal arrows indicate reactions produced as a result of TTR.

The viscosity of blood is temperature-related. As the temperature increases, the viscosity decreases, and the blood becomes more fluid. Increase in local tissue temperature also causes an increase in local sweating.[16]

As indicated by the two-way arrows in **Figure 11–7**, a feedback system exists between an increase in tissue temperature and metabolic rate. Metabolism is an ongoing cellular activity, and its rate is related to the tissue temperature. The metabolic process speeds up as the temperature increases and slows down as the temperature decreases. As a general estimate, for every 10°C rise in body tissue temperature, the metabolic rate may increase twofold or threefold, depending on the type of tissues.[17] This change in metabolic rate per 10°C is referred to as the **Q_{10} Ratio.** Centuries ago, van't Hoff presented information relating tissue temperature to metabolic rate that was the basis for future investigations in this area. Consequently, the terms **van't Hoff's law** or **van't Hoff effect** are

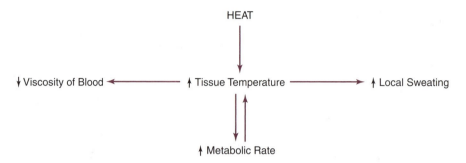

FIGURE 11–7   Physiologic responses to an increase in tissue temperature. The rise in tissue temperature leads to decreased blood viscosity, increased local sweating, and increased metabolic rate. Because metabolism produces heat, an increased metabolic rate, in turn, increases the tissue temperature, which then increases the metabolic rate and so on in a cyclic pattern.

sometimes used when referring to the relationship between tissue temperature and metabolic rate.[18]

The metabolic activity itself—the oxygen consumption and chemical interactions that synthesize body proteins—produces heat as well as an accumulation of acids and other metabolic wastes as by-products. When metabolic activity increases, both heat production and waste accumulation increase. The feedback system operates so that TTR increases the metabolic rate, which increases heat production, producing further TTR. The metabolic wastes are cleared through sweat, urine, and blood, so that a normal pH balance is maintained.

Metabolic Responses

Figure 11–8 indicates two interrelated reactions that are produced with the increase in metabolic rate. The diagonal arrow indicates an increase in phagocytosis. The normal inflammatory process for healing tissues involves activity of the leukocytes and phagocytes of white blood cells. An increase in metabolic rate will increase this activity, which in turn may hasten the healing process and the restoration of damaged tissues. (See the discussions about inflammation in **Chapters 2 and 15**.)

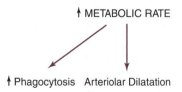

FIGURE 11–8   Effects of an increase in the metabolic rate in relation to a rise in tissue temperature.

The vertical arrow indicates the beginning of vascular changes—arteriolar dilatation. As the metabolic rate increases, the activity of the vascular system, acting through its neuronal and hormonal controls, also increases. Arteriolar dilatation increases blood flow at the heated site. This increased flow is essential to provide the white blood cells for the stepped-up leukocytic and phagocytic activity and the nutrients needed to meet the increased demands of the metabolic process. Because the metabolic process uses O_2 and increases production of CO_2, acids, and other by-products, the tissues must have a constant and sufficient flow of arterial blood to bring oxygenated blood to the heated area. A sufficient venous flow is also needed to remove the metabolic wastes and retard increases in tissue temperature, because heat is convected away from the site through the venous flow. The fact that stepping up the metabolic rate increases phagocytic activity and local circulation explains why the application of local heat is indicated to hasten the healing of damaged tissues and the clearing of interstitial exudates resulting from inflammation, hemorrhage (hematomas), or edema. The erythema observed, which continues as long as the tissues are heated, is an indication that this process is occurring.

In addition to localized healing effects, the application of a superficial heat before exercise often enables an individual to move more easily. Some people mistakenly believe that this improvement occurs because they have "warmed up their muscles" and consequently have increased muscle metabolic rate and blood flow. A deep-heat modality could possibly increase the metabolic rate and blood flow in muscle in a local area, but as Rowell[19] emphasized, even the most intense heating of skin does not increase blood flow to underlying muscle.[20–22] In general, exercise physiologists believe that a "warm-up"—increasing the general metabolic rate and blood flow in muscles in preparation for strenuous activity—should be attained through activity rather than a passive heat application. Nonetheless, local modalities, either superficial or deep, are used before the active warm-up for both therapeutic and athletic exercise, and they do appear to enhance movement. The benefits are likely the result of some other effects of heating, such as analgesic (possibly through pain gating mechanisms) or relaxation effects, but not the increase in general muscle metabolism.

Precautions Related to Increased Tissue Temperature and Metabolic Rate

When tissues are heated within the therapeutic range, the accumulated by-product (metabolic acids) can escape with body fluids to maintain homeostasis. By-product includes an increase in uric acids excreted in urine and lactic acids excreted in sweat. Thus, vascular, renal, and sweat balance mechanisms all come into play. If any of these mechanisms is compromised, the pH balance may be upset, and unfavorable reactions may occur. Therefore, vigorous heat modalities should be used with caution in patients with Addison's disease or metabolic problems, or in any deconditioned individuals whose systems cannot meet the required demands (eg, an individual with advanced diabetes mellitus).

When the tissue temperature rises above 113°F (45°C), tissue damage can occur. If the metabolic rate increases beyond its capacity to function, enzymes are denatured, and proteins are destroyed. Above this temperature, the rate of chemical activity decreases.

Vascular Responses

As stated earlier, the viscosity of blood decreases and arteriolar dilation occurs as blood temperature increases, causing increased flow to the capillaries. **Figure 11–9** shows the vascular responses that then occur in the capillary region. The increased blood flow to the capillary beds increases the capillary pressure, perhaps increasing the number of patent (open) channels and the permeability of the capillary membranes (see **Chapters 3 and 5**).

Further research is needed to investigate the exact mechanisms that increased blood flow may have for promoting tissue healing and for decreasing pain and muscle spasms. Increased blood flow has been speculated to increase the nutrients and cells involved in the healing process (for tissue healing) and clearing of inflammatory by-products (for relief of pain and muscle spasms). Conversely, increase in blood flow may cause bleeding to increase or to resume at injured tissue sites or to lead to hemorrhage in patients with conditions such as ulcers or hemophilia.

The precise means by which substances are transported between the blood and interstitium, including the causes and effects of increased capillary pressure and permeability, are still being investigated. It may be that an increase in capillary permeability permits more wastes and fluids to be reabsorbed into the bloodstream from the extracellular space, thus enhancing tissue healing and clearing of exudates, including long-standing edema. Conversely, an increase in permeability allows more fluids to flow from the bloodstream to the extracellular space, thus encouraging the formation of edema.

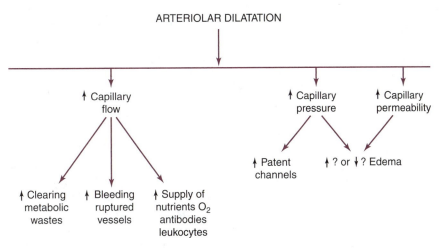

FIGURE 11–9   Vascular responses resulting from a rise in tissue temperature.

On the basis of these responses, heat interventions may at times be beneficial and at other times may increase problems; therefore, they should not be used indiscriminately. With patients whose conditions suggest the possibility of edema or bleeding, only mild heat, if any, is advised. To prevent edema, the body parts to be heated should be elevated to encourage flow of fluid away from the area and toward the heart. When bleeding or edema is anticipated (eg, after an acute injury), heat is contraindicated for at least 24 to 72 hours; rest, ice, compression, and elevation (RICE) are chosen instead.

Finally, the integrity of the vessels must be considered. It is important for vasodilatation to occur so that more arterial blood can flow to the tissues to meet increased metabolic demands. In conditions such as arteriosclerosis, arterial wall compliance is compromised, thus limiting dilatation. If local heat is applied and the increased demand for blood cannot be met, tissue damage, ischemia, or necrosis may occur. Other vascular considerations include local vascular shunting and reflex heating.

Local Vascular Shunting.   Some researchers have hypothesized that when overheating endangers the superficial tissues, the branching of the peripheral system that usually supplies blood to the muscles or other tissues underlying the heated tissue may constrict, shunting blood flow to the cutaneous area in need.[23] This shunting occurs at the expense of temporary deprivation of blood to the underlying tissues. If this is the case, superficial heat modalities not only would be ineffective in enhancing blood flow to deep muscles but also would be decreasing such flow. However, because the circulation to deeper muscles is independent of that to cutaneous tissues, this hypothesis cannot be supported (see **Chapter 3**).

Application of even vigorous superficial heat may have no effect on blood flow to deep muscles, and a superficial heat modality cannot be expected to cause a significant TTR of any tissues at a depth greater than 1 cm.

Reflex Heating.   The term **reflex heating** refers to a technique of applying heat to one area of the body that results in an increase in cutaneous circulation and other reactions in another area. Because the effect occurs almost immediately (ie, before systemic changes have the opportunity to be an influencing factor), it is called reflex heating. This technique also is termed *consensual heating, remote heating,* or—since the studies

by Landis and Gibbons first called attention to the phenomenon—the *Landis-Gibbons reflex.*[24]

Many studies have reported that heat applied to one body part, either by local modalities or by immersion in hot water, results in increased cutaneous circulation, sweating, and hyperemia in other parts of the body.[10,25,26] These include reactions on (1) the leg or arm opposite to the one heated, (2) the ipsilateral upper extremity when the lower extremity is heated, and (3) the lower extremity when heat is applied to the back or abdomen.

A reflex heating technique may be useful for patients with circulatory problems such as diabetes or peripheral vascular diseases, especially if dermatologic conditions such as stasis ulcers are present. These patients could benefit from increased blood flow to their extremities, but they cannot tolerate a great increase in tissue temperature in those extremities. Heating an extremity when the circulation cannot meet its metabolic needs or cannot dissipate the added heat may cause tissue damage. In such cases, heating another part of the body may reflexively increase the cutaneous blood flow to the involved extremity. An extremity with poor circulation that initially appeared blanched and cool will appear pinker, and the skin temperature will increase. This response, however, lasts only for a brief period.[27]

Bisgard and Nye[28] reported that visceral changes occur beneath the area where superficial heat is applied. These visceral changes include a decrease in gastrointestinal activity, relaxation of gut muscles, and a decrease in peristalsis. Thus, a time-honored household remedy, placing heat on the abdomen to decrease stomach or menstrual cramps, is verified.[28]

Whether superficial or deep-heat modalities are more effective in producing remote changes needs more investigation. One unpublished study showed that a hot pack applied to the back for 20 minutes produces significantly greater changes in the skin temperature of the foot than does a 10-min ultrasound intervention to the same area.[29] There is no evidence that deep circulation improves with any remote techniques.

Systemic Responses

Recall that, when the temperature of the blood near the site of thermal integration in the hypothalamus rises or when the normal difference between skin and core temperature changes, the CNS activates body-heat-loss mechanisms to maintain thermal homeostasis. These are not local responses but reactions that affect the entire body. General vasomotor and **sudomotor** (sweat control) **systems** respond to bring heat to the body surface to be released by radiation and evaporation. These systemic reactions will occur regardless of the cause of the rise in the circulating blood temperature. General heating from ambient conditions, physical exercise, general heat modalities, such as whirlpools and Hubbard tanks, or even a local heat modality can provoke systemic reactions if their intensity and duration is sufficient to increase the temperature of the blood in the peripheral system.

Cardiovascular Responses.   With any increase in general body temperature, the responses are (1) generalized vasodilation of cutaneous vessels to allow more heat to reach the surface; (2) a drop in peripheral blood pressure caused by vasodilatation and decreased blood viscosity, which could cause a temporary decrease in peripheral blood flow until the body responds to the drop in pressure; and (3) by increasing heart rate. The increased heart rate occurs to maintain the cardiac output that would naturally be decreased as the stroke volume is reduced by the drop in peripheral blood pressure. The clinical signs that occur with increased core temperature (eg, a fever) signify these changes: the skin will be warm and have a pink flushed color, and the pulse rate will be increased.

However, the body's regulators may overshoot their mark slightly when adjusting to different temperatures in a manner that resembles a room thermostat, as explained earlier. A slight temperature rise above or a drop below the set point is needed to stimulate the reactions of regulators. As the heart rate increases, it overshoots slightly, resulting in an increase in blood pressure. The heart rate then drops. This decrease in heart rate may cause a drop in blood pressure to below its set point; thus, the heart rate will increase again. These temporary fluctuations during adjustments to temperature changes are normal, but eventually the blood pressure can be expected to stabilize with a slightly higher heart rate, which maintains the increase in peripheral blood flow. **Figure 11–10** summarizes these reactions.

It is interesting to observe these fluctuations occurring in normal adults. If we monitored several young, healthy adults sitting waist deep in a hot tub in which the water is 105°F, each person might have rises and drops in both pulse and blood pressure. However, the duration and amount of fluctuation would differ for each person, as would the recovery time.

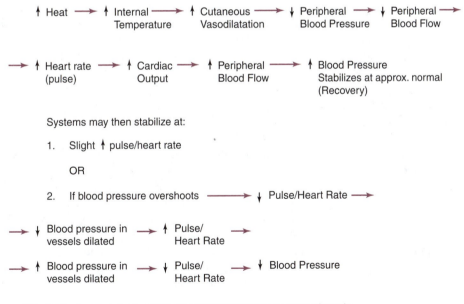

FIGURE 11–10   Cardiovascular responses when applied heat is sufficient to increase the internal (core) temperature. (*Based on data in J Hales*: Thermal Physiology. *New York: Raven Press; 1984.*)

Systemic vascular responses may produce therapeutic effects. The increase in cutaneous blood flow may, in addition to cooling the body, bring additional nutrients to the skin. But unwanted effects such as increased bleeding may also occur. A drop in blood pressure resulting in less blood flow to the brain may cause fainting. It is not uncommon for debilitated people to faint as a result of systemic responses to a rise in temperature. Patients in moderately heated hydrotherapy pools or those receiving prolonged heat from a constant output source such as infrared or diathermy must be monitored carefully.

Systemic Vascular Shunting. Shunting to protect tissues in a localized area from excessive changes in temperature was discussed in **Chapter 3**. Systemic shunting occurs when the internal temperature is high. In an effort to cool the body, blood may be shunted from deep circulatory systems, such as the renal system, to the peripheral system.[30] Thus, more blood reaches the surface to give off heat to the environment. Of course, only a temporary reduction of blood flow from these systems can be tolerated without serious damage to those organs because they, too, need their blood supply.

Sudomotor Responses. Central thermoregulators also control the sudomotor systems. Sensible sweat resulting from activation of eccrine sweat glands begins when the skin temperature rises above approximately 91.4°F and when there is virtually any rise in core temperature above normal. Some eccrine sweat glands, primarily those located in the palms of the hands and soles of the feet, react to emotional stress, but most of the eccrine glands throughout the body are thermoregulators. These sweat glands, controlled by the autonomic nervous system, may be activated by adrenal activity or by epinephrine, norepinephrine, or both circulating in the bloodstream.[3] As mentioned in **Chapter 10**, insensible water loss through the skin is an ongoing activity that preserves thermal homeostasis. All sweat acts to prevent an increase in body temperature as follows: (1) the heat is brought to the surface in the fluid; (2) if exposed to the air, the fluid may then evaporate, using calories of heat to vaporize the sweat and thus cool the surface; (3) and heat may transfer from sweat molecules on the body surface to adjacent cooler air molecules and then be removed by air flow (ie, convection).

Normally, the salt concentration in sweat is low, as little as 5 mEq/L, and most salt intake is reabsorbed by the body. However, unless a person is acclimatized, the salt concentration in sweat will increase as sweating increases. With profuse sweating, the salt concentration may be as high as 60 mEq/L, and the body supply may become greatly diminished. Problems related to excessive salt loss are discussed in **Chapter 17**. Sweat contains potassium ions, urea, and lactate, and with profuse sweating, the lactate concentration in sweat also increases. Thus, the excess lactate, produced by the increase in metabolism, escapes and helps to maintain homeostasis. **Fig. 11–11** summarizes this process. The concentration of other ions also will increase with increased sweating, but not markedly so.[3]

Respiratory Responses. The warm air given off by breathing rids the body of some heat. This expired air is saturated with moisture. Evaporation of the moisture in this air and from the moist mucous membrane of the respiratory passages contributes to the body's cooling. When a person is resting in a neutral environment, as much as a third of the evaporative heat loss is through the respiratory tract. Panting is an effective means of heat loss in many animals, but not in humans, although humans do maintain this mechanism. If a person is extremely hot, a panting exhalation that is a response to metabolic acidosis may be observed. This is a signal that heat or exercise interventions should be terminated. Vigorous, prolonged heat is not advised for any cardiopulmonary patients.

Renal Responses. Some heat, but not a significant amount, is lost during urination. Of greater significance is the increase in the phosphate and hydrogen ion concentration in the urine that occurs and, when excreted, serves to rid the body of the increase in these metabolic by-products.[31] Thus, to prevent acidosis, patients with renal disease or urine retention problems should not receive prolonged or frequent heat interventions, which would increase the internal temperature.

↑ Heat ⟶ ↑ Metabolism ⟶ ↑ Lactic Acid in Tissues ⟶ ↑ Sweat ⟶

↑ Lactic Acid in Sweat ⟶ Assists in maintaining pH balance

FIGURE 11–11   Sudomotor responses to generalized heating when applied heat increases the internal (core) temperature.

Therapeutic Implications

Table 11–1 summarizes the physiologic responses to local heat gain. The responses include both local and systemic initial neurophysiologic responses to the sensation of hot or cold and changes resulting from a rise in tissue temperature, core temperature, or both. The TTR causes an increase in the metabolic rates, which in turn produces changes in arteriolar blood flow and capillary activities. Under certain circumstances, these reactions may have therapeutically beneficial effects; in other circumstances, the effects may be detrimental. Local application of superficial heat may cause physiologic changes in other areas of the body, such as a temporary increase in cutaneous blood flow or a decrease in deep smooth-muscle activity. Recall that this procedure is termed reflex, remote, or consensual heating. Blood also may be shunted from other channels to the cutaneous vessels if damage from externally applied heat occurs and from other circulatory systems as a response to an excessive rise in core temperature. However, blood flow in deep muscles acts independently of cutaneous circulation. Local heating, either superficial or deep, may enhance the movement of individual joints, but it is not an appropriate warm-up for strenuous exercise. Such general warm-ups should involve active, not passive, heating of the body.

Thermoregulatory sites in the body integrate information from skin and deep receptors. Whenever these sites receive information that the internal temperature has risen above normal, systemic changes occur to preserve thermal homeostasis. Depending on the severity of the heat, cardiovascular, sudomotor, respiratory, and renal systems may react to prevent a rise in internal temperature. Any person with systemic problems or indications that any of these systems cannot adapt may not tolerate vigorous heat. Therefore, dosage and the severity of the pathological state must always be considered when applying heat.

RESPONSES TO A DECREASE IN TISSUE TEMPERATURE

When cold is applied locally to the body surface, we might expect reactions to be the opposite of those occurring with heat, but this is not always the case. In general, the metabolic responses are the opposite, but the vascular responses are not.

As with heat, the ability of a cold modality to affect local and systemic changes depends on (1) the temperature of the cold, (2) the skin-modality temperature gradient, (3) the duration of application, (4) the vascular supply to the area, (5) the thermal conductivity and thickness of each tissue layer, and (6) the surface area/volume ratio of the area treated. A modality cooled to 59°F (15°C) may initially draw heat from the body, although not as rapidly as a colder modality; and as the skin temperature decreases and the modality becomes warmer, there will be no significant gradient between them. Various forms of cold packs represent this type of modality. Ice slush pots, ice water, or other modalities remaining just about 32°F (0°C) can be more effective in cooling superficial tissues because the skin modality temperature gradient is greater, and the temperature remains near freezing until the ice melts.[32] However, the danger of cold-related tissue damage is also greater.[33] When supercooling modalities are used (ie, modalities below freezing), there may be more marked cooling effects, but there also will be more danger of damaging tissues.[34] (See **Table 11–2** for critical cold temperatures.)

TABLE 11–2   *Classification of Cold Injuries*[*]

Classification	Type of Damage
First-degree damage	Tissues appear red, inflamed, with perhaps a mild edema.
Second-degree damage	Marked edema, blisters, or both.
Third-degree damage (frostbite)	Necrosis and a blue-gray skin color are probably the result of the formation of ice crystals in tissues.
	These crystals can damage blood vessels and cause dehydration in interstitial spaces.
Fourth-degree damage (severe frostbite)	Gangrene and neurological complications.

[*]Modification of Hardy's classification, from J Lehmann[18] and B Washburn.[56]

The immediate responses to cold were discussed earlier in this chapter. These immediate responses are related to the thermal sensory experience (thermal shock) caused by the increase in the frequency of the firing of cold sensory receptors. The amount of increase in the frequency of firing is related to the temperature gradient between the skin and the modality. In addition to these responses that are related to the sensation of cold are those related to the lowered tissue temperature.

Initial Vascular and Metabolic Responses

Figure 11–12 summarizes the initial responses that can occur in tissues cooled by cryotherapy modalities. As the tissue temperature decreases, both local blood flow and metabolic rate decrease. The local cutaneous vessels constrict, increasing resistance in the vessels proximal to the capillaries and causing the fall in capillary perfusion (blood flow).[9] The viscosity of the blood increases slightly as the tissue temperature begins to drop, and it increases markedly if the tissue temperature falls below 80°F (27°C).[35,36] These temperature-related changes in blood flow can reduce bleeding or hemorrhage. The reduced flow of warmer blood to the cooled area enhances the effect of a cold modality. The slower rate of flow of cooled blood away from the local area back toward the core serves to prolong the local cooling effect[37] and to prevent a decrease in core temperature as well. This initial vasoconstriction response is only transitory, lasting approximately 10 to 30 min.

However, this decrease in incoming arterial blood results in less oxygen and other nutrients being brought to the cooled area. The decrease in venous flow from the area results in increased retention of metabolic wastes and CO_2. The increased content of CO_2 in the blood accounts for the blue color of cooled skin,[3] although skin receiving ice is initially redder than normal because of changes in the hemoglobin/O_2 dissociation curve. As tissue temperature reaches a critically low level (50°F or 10°C), there will be a **cold-induced vasodilation (CIVD).** This is a protective mechanism to reward the cooled area and is believed to be mediated by the release of histamine.

Evidence suggests that the retardation of wound healing that occurs when tissues are cooled may be related to the hypoxia caused by this decrease in blood flow.[38] Because metabolic rate is temperature dependent, it too will decrease at the site of the cooled tissues, as will the heat produced as a metabolic byproduct. With a decreased metabolic rate, there is less demand for O_2 and other nutrients and less production of, or need to rid the area of, metabolic wastes. But this slower metabolic rate may contribute to the retardation of the healing process, as the inflammatory process (ie, the action of leukocytes and phagocytes) is decreased. Lundgren et al[39] showed that the wounds of animals placed in a cooler environment took longer to heal than did the wounds of animals placed in a warmer environment. These investigators suggested that the retardation in healing

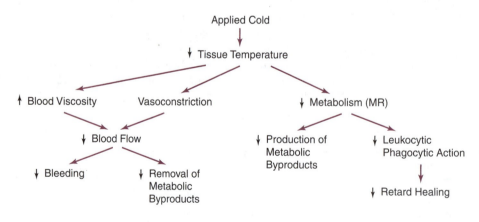

FIGURE 11–12 Initial physiologic responses when applied cold lowers the tissue temperature.

might be caused by the decrease in nutrients at the wound area related to the decrease in blood flow, but it was more likely that the decreased metabolic rate caused the slower healing. Such evidence suggests that cold should not be applied after the acute or subacute phases of injury, when bleeding has stopped and swelling subsided.

It is commonly accepted that cooling tissues for 10 to 30 min periods prevents or diminishes formation of posttraumatic edema in the acute phase. However, some studies have shown that cold may actually increase rather than decrease edema or that, even if diminished during application, edema may increase as tissues rewarm.[40-42]

Schmidt et al[42] studied the effects of heat and cold on the edema resulting from artificially induced inflammation in rats and found that the effects of cold on swelling varied with the type of chemical mediator used to cause the inflammation. Like posttraumatic edema, inflammation induced by mediators such as histamine and serotonin could be inhibited significantly during the acute stage (as long as 24 hours), but other forms of inflammation, particularly those mediated by prostaglandins, could be aggravated by cold.[42]

A more recent study compared the effects of heat, cold, and contrast baths on posttraumatic edema.[43] This study used common clinical duration parameters: 20 min for the heat or cold modalities and, for the contrast baths, immersion for 3 min in hot water alternating with 1 min in cold water with alternations continuing for 20 min. On day 3 the edema treated with cold had decreased slightly, whereas it had increased with the other two modalities. But on days 4 and 5, the edema increased with all three modalities, although the increase with cold was significantly less than with the other two modalities.

The preceding studies exemplify the importance of clinicians' not only keeping abreast of the literature but also carefully considering its direct implications. Findings of studies in which the duration of cold applications ranged from 1 hour to days may not be directly applicable to a 10 to 30 min clinical intervention. However, studies such as the one by Schmidt et al[42] may have direct significance. Schmidt's findings suggest that all rheumatic conditions should not be treated the same way because the chemical mediators of the swelling related to various rheumatic conditions may not be similar.

Intensity as well as duration influences the effect of applied cold. In their experiments, Schmidt et al[42]

used deep-frozen gel packs for 1 hour. They suggested that extremely brief applications of cold (eg, ice massage) cannot suppress any inflammation as effectively as longer-duration cold applications. Other investigators reported an immediate increase in edema when a cold compress soaked in cold water at 53.3°F (12°C) was applied.[41] This suggests an immediate response of increased inflammation.

The conflicting results of various studies may be attributed to the differences in the duration and temperature of the modality used in the investigations. The results of cryotherapy also may depend on these factors. The intensity of the cold per duration should be considered carefully for each condition and for each patient intervention. Individual patients react differently.

Responses of Peripheral Nerves

Both motor and sensory peripheral nerves are affected by cooling. Cold fibers fire minimally at temperatures as high as 109°F (43°C). The rate of firing peaks at about 77°F (25°C), gradually decreasing and ceasing at approximately 47°F (8.5°C). Cold-pain fibers begin firing at approximately 59°F (15°C), and the rate increases as their temperature lowers to approximately 40°F (4.7°C). Thus, between 59°F and 47°F (15°C and 8.5°C), the sensation of cold diminishes as cold-pain increases.[43] **Figure 11–2** illustrates the firing temperature of the thermal neurons.

As the temperature lowers, the firing of all pain and tactile neurons gradually decreases. At a temperature near freezing, all sensory neuron activity ceases. Based on these neural changes, the sensations felt as tissues become colder may first be cold, then painfully cold, then less cold and more painful, which is sometimes perceived as warmth or burning. Eventually, numbness and anesthesia occur.[6,44] During ice massage, patients often report sensory changes in this sequence. The motor nerves also are affected by cold. Both the excitation and the nerve conduction velocity of these neurons decrease relative to the temperature. Obviously, this response has an effect on motor performance.

Responses of Deeper Tissues

It is generally agreed that a superficial cold modality can affect the temperature of tissues to a greater depth than can a superficial heat modality.[11] There are several reasons for this. First, the temperature gradient between the modality and the skin is greater.

Recall that heat always transfers from the hotter to the cooler substance and that the rate of transfer depends on the temperature gradient. If a superficial heat modality at 110°F (43.3°C), about as hot as can be tolerated, is applied to skin that is 85°F (29.4°C), there is a 25°F (13.9°C) temperature gradient. But if a cold modality at 45°F (7.2°C) is applied, there is a 40°F (22.2°C) temperature gradient. Thus, the rate of heat transfer *from* the body surface to the cold modality is much more rapid than is the rate *to* the body from the heat modality.

Second, cold is not convected from the area as rapidly, since there is not an initial vasodilation to send warm blood to the cool area. Recall that because heat modalities increase superficial circulation, much of the heat is quickly convected from the site, deterring conductive transfer to the deeper tissues, and only superficial tissues are heated significantly. But with a cold modality, the vasoconstriction deterring *convective* heat transfer to the cooled site prolongs the surface cooling and allows more time for heat from deeper tissues to *conduct* toward the cooled surface. Thus, the increased temperature gradient—increasing the rate of heat transfer and decreasing the rate of blood flow—increases the ability of cold to change the temperature of deep tissues more than heat.

Other factors that influence the depth at which tissue cooling is effective include the thickness of the subcutaneous fat layer and the vascular status in the area. Because fat is a heat insulator, heat transfer from the deeper tissues by conduction is related to the thickness of the subcutaneous fat layer. Studies have shown that with application of ice, muscles at a maximum depth of 2 cm will cool approximately 3.4°F (2°C) in 10 min if the subject's fat layer is less than 1 cm thick. But if the subject has more than 2 cm of subcutaneous fat, tissues even 1 cm deep are scarcely cooled at all in 10 min; more than 30 min are required to achieve a temperature change similar to those obtained in subjects with less than a 1 cm thick fat layer in 10 min.[45] However, after deep tissues are cooled, because fat is a thermal insulator, the fat layer and any vasoconstriction caused by cold help prolong the time that tissues remain cool. Consequently, we can assume that if a modality with a temperature of 50°F (10°C) (a less intense cold with less gradient than ice) is applied for 15 to 20 min, it is unlikely to cool deeper tissues significantly. The relief obtained when cold at approximately 50°F (10°C) is applied for purposes such as relief of deep muscle spasms may be related to effects other than the change in the temperature of those muscles.

Vascular factors also influence the depth at which cooling occurs. Some heat conducted from arterial vessels to tissues along the route to the cooled site and to adjacent outgoing venous blood via countercurrent heat exchange (see **Chapter 3** and a later section of this chapter) lowers the temperature of blood arriving at the cooled site. Consequently, incoming blood is less able to warm the tissues. In areas with a poor blood supply, the effect of cooling is enhanced even more, perhaps dangerously, because less blood flows to the area. Pugh et al[45] theorized that constriction of superficial vessels may shunt incoming blood to deeper branches, thus supplying underlying tissues with an increased volume of warmer blood and retarding the cooling of these deeper tissues.[46] This theory, if true, discourages the use of cold to prevent bleeding of deeper tissues but makes cold beneficial for nourishing them; however, this kind of reciprocity in blood flow is questionable. The theory may, in part, be based on misinterpretation of published reports.[22,47]

Reports conflict about the amount of temperature change per depth and per duration of application of cold modalities. They also conflict about the length of time that tissues remained cool after intervention. One investigation found that tissues 2 cm deep were cooled in 5 min but that cooling was minimal thereafter.[48] Another study[49] reported that tissues 2 cm deep were cooled 4.1°C (approximately 7.3°F) in 5 min. Continuing the ice massage for 10 min longer cooled the deep tissues an additional 1.1°C, but the skin temperature reached maximum cooling in the first 5 min. This study also found that when a similar ice massage was applied to calf muscles and posterior thigh muscles, the temperature changes at the same depth were different from calf to thigh.[49]

Investigators using supercooling at 20°F (−7°C) for 20 min were able to cool deep muscles much more. Although they found considerable variation among subjects, regarding the time required both for cooling and for fluctuations in temperature that occurred over time, they reported an important finding: supercooling *decreased the spasticity* in all of their subjects who had multiple sclerosis.[35]

On the basis of the findings just described, it appears that ice can reduce the temperature of tissues 2 cm deep about 7°F (4°C) in 5 min with little or no further decrease in the next 5 min. A supercool modality applied for a longer duration, 20 min, can cool deeper muscles markedly. But similar applications do not achieve similar results in all subjects or in different muscle tissues.

Secondary Vascular Responses

If the duration of application or exposure to intense cold is prolonged, tissue damage can occur. Fortunately, unless the cold is excessive, when the local tissue temperature drops significantly, secondary responses occur that act to prevent damage. After 15 to 30 min, depending on the vascular status of the area, blood flow to the endangered tissues increases.[50]

Current theories suggest that the vessels are no longer constricted because neuronal transmission controlling vasoconstriction has diminished or ceased below a critical temperature and because arterioventricular (A–V) shunts open.[15] (See **Chapter 3** for a description of these shunts.)

Figure 11–13 illustrates the A–V shunt mechanism, as reported in a famous study by Lewis in 1930.[50,51] In this study, a finger was immersed in crushed ice. As expected, with time the skin temperature decreased and the finger looked blue, indicating that the vessels had constricted and the amount of blood flowing through the capillaries had decreased. After the temperature had dropped to approximately 2.5–4°C (36–39°F), the temperature began to increase, and the normal pink/red skin color returned. Because there was no flow through local capillary beds, this warming of tis-

sues was attributed to the opening of the shunts. When the tissue temperature rose above 4–10°C (39–50°F), depending on the subject, the temperature again began to decrease, and the blue color of the skin returned, indicating that the shunts had closed down. The alternating of skin temperature and color continued for up to 2 or 3 hours, gradually diminishing over time. This alternation in blood flow is referred to as the *hunting reaction* or *Lewis's hunting phenomenon*. Although the underlying mechanisms are unknown, severe cold may affect the interaction of adrenergic neuroeffectors in the cutaneous vessels.[15] The actual tissue temperature and time required for these shunts to open and close are highly variable, depending to some degree on the acclimatization of the individual. Snow skiers and others who have spent much time outdoors in extremely cold weather are familiar with the changes that occur in color of the skin on cheeks and fingers. Blue cheeks and fingers indicate vasoconstriction and closed shunts. Then, after a few minutes, although still exposed to the cold, the cheeks and fingers turn red, indicating that the shunts are open. These alternations in skin color continue throughout the period of exposure, provided that the exposure time is not prolonged. Depending on the individual, after 1 to 3 hours of exposure to extreme cold, this shunting mechanism will cease to function, and tissue damage may occur.[52–54]

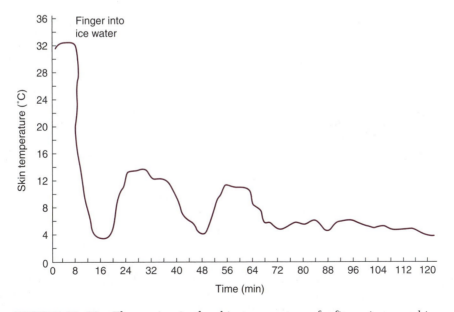

FIGURE 11–13 Fluctuation in the skin temperature of a finger immersed in crushed ice for a prolonged period. (*Modified from Lewis, T., ed., Observations upon the reaction of the human skin to cold. In:* Heart. London: Shaw; 1929/31; 15:177–208.)

Systemic Responses

Systemic responses, which act to maintain the body's constant internal temperature, are based on integration of information received from the superficial cold receptors (free nerve endings) and centrally located thermoreceptors and on the temperature of the blood in the general circulation. Responses are activated when the temperature of blood passing the central sites of integration (primarily the hypothalamus) falls below normal. Theoretically, the responses that occur depend on the amount of temperature change from an original set point. To conserve body heat, there will be generalized cutaneous vasoconstriction. To increase internal temperature, three mechanisms commence: nonshivering thermogenesis, unconscious tension of muscles, and shivering. Nonshivering thermogenesis refers to the production of internal heat by sympathetically controlled, cold-induced chemical reactions that increase the rate of cell metabolism. This means of heat production is not related to shivering.[6,12,55] Although several sites in the body contribute to nonshivering thermogenesis, its effectiveness appears to be related to brown fat content, which is more prevalent in animals and in infants than in adult humans. Thus it may be a more

important factor in the thermoregulation of infants than of adults. Shivering is a tremorlike continuation of brief muscle contractions throughout the body, an exhausting form of exercise. This exercise, which increases the metabolic rate and the production of heat, is a metabolic response to preserve homeostasis.

Sufficient exposure to cold can cause a decrease in the temperature of the blood in the general circulation, resulting in a lower core temperature and systemic responses. But because of the exchange of heat by conduction between vessels and the tissues through which they pass and, to a lesser extent, from arteries to their adjacent veins through the process of **countercurrent exchange (CCE),** the temperature of the cutaneous venous blood is warmed before returning to the general circulation. Although it appears that the heat exchange occurs predominantly between the vessels and the tissues, the CCE theory is used, for purposes of simplification, to explain how internal temperature is preserved.[56] **Figure 11–14** is a theoretical example of how, disregarding all other heat exchange procedures, CCE acts to preserve core temperature. **Figure 11–14A** indicates how markedly venous blood could cool, and consequently lower core temperature, if CCE did not exist. The blood at approximately core temper-

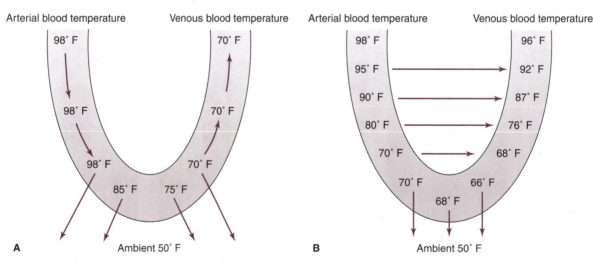

FIGURE 11–14   Schematic illustration of heat convection through the vascular system from deep in the body to the skin and return (ambient temperature, 50°F). (**A**) Hypothetical blood temperatures without countercurrent exchange. At an ambient temperature of 50°F, if the blood flowing to the skin remained at approximately core temperature, there would be a temperature gradient of approximately 40°F that would encourage rapid heat transfer from the blood. The blood returning to deeper circulation would be considerably cooler. If a large area of the body was exposed to this condition, a considerable drop in core temperature could occur. (**B**) Hypothetical blood temperatures with countercurrent exchange. Arteriole blood gradually gives heat to the returning venous blood, which results in a lower gradient between the blood and ambient temperatures and a gradual increase in the temperature of the returning venous blood.

ature would travel from the deeper body to the skin. In a cold environment, a considerable temperature gradient would exist between the temperature of the blood and the environment. Consequently, as blood reached the surface, it would rapidly give up its heat to the environment. The venous blood returning to the general circulation would be considerably cooler than under normal ambient conditions and cause the internal temperature to drop below normal.

Figure 11–14B illustrates the CCE. Proceeding distally toward the periphery, the temperature of the arterial blood gradually lowers, having given off heat to the parallel, returning venous blood. By the time the blood reaches the body surface, the blood temperature has dropped somewhat. With this lower-temperature blood in surface tissues and capillaries, the gradient between the body surface and the cooler environment is decreased. This, in turn, decreases radiation and the rate of heat transfer to the environment. Of course, some heat is given off to the cooler environment, so the venous blood is cooler than its adjacent arterial blood; however, it gains heat as it moves toward the heart until an equilibrium with arterial temperature is reached.[56] Although less than formerly presumed in humans, this mechanism, even when an individual is exposed to great temperature changes, helps the core temperature to remain constant. The heat exchange occurring between vessels and adjacent tissues and between tissues and the environment is similar.

Sometimes the goal of cold interventions is to lower core temperature (eg, if a patient has a dangerously high fever). Generally, when physical therapists intervene, the goal is to *lower local tissue temperature without lowering core temperature.* DonTigny and Sheldon[57] suggested that when cold is applied to one part of the body, application of heat to another part of the body will prevent a drop in core temperature that might initiate undesirable shivering, tensing of muscles, or both.

Tissue Damage

As with heat modalities, tissue damage may occur with cold modalities, depending on the duration or intensity of the exposure as well as on the sensory and vascular condition of the area being cooled. With prolonged cooling, even if the temperature is not low enough to freeze tissues, injuries can occur.[33] Chilblains, a mild injury, causes redness, swelling, tenderness, and itching. It occurs primarily in fingers and toes, and is most commonly seen in people with peripheral vascular deficiencies such as Raynaud's disease and syringomyelia.[58]

Tissue damage resulting from cold can be divided into stages according to severity and is related to both the temperature (at or near freezing) and to the duration of exposure. The reader is referred to articles by Thorman[59] for a good overview and to Meryman[60] for a more comprehensive discussion of cold injuries. **Table 11–2** categorizes cold injuries according to their severity (ie, the depth of tissue damage.[18,61]

Although we usually associate cold injuries with prolonged exposure to ambient cold conditions, the possibility does exist of injury occurring with intervention: it is not unusual to be treating patients with peripheral vascular deficiencies, with whom any intense cold should be avoided; or to be treating some conditions such as spasticity by applying ice wraps for up to an hour in an effort to cool deep tissues. The authors know of a group of physical therapy students who were piercing each others' ears. Knowing that ice could anesthetize, some of the students sandwiched their ear lobes between two ice cubes long enough to cause first-degree damage.

In the past, it was believed that the best emergency intervention for frostbite was slow rewarming. However, experience has shown that rapid rewarming is more successful in preventing permanent tissue damage. Thorman[59] has suggested immersing the part in a whirlpool bath at 104–110°F (40–43.3°C).

Other adverse reactions can occur with cold. Many people are hypersensitive, and the neurochemical activity caused by cold can result in severe local or systemic reactions, or both. Patients with certain systemic diseases are especially prone to hypersensitive reactions. Related specific precautions and contraindications are given in **Chapter 14**.

Therapeutic Implications

When cold modalities are applied to the body, local and systemic physiologic changes can occur. The physiologic effects of cold can be categorized as those resulting from (1) changes in the firing of cold sensory receptors, (2) a decrease in tissue temperature—initial responses lasting about 10 to 30 min followed by secondary responses, and (3) a decrease in internal body temperature. The amount of physiologic change is related to dosage (ie, the temperature gradient between the body surface and the modality); the intensity of the cold, which is generally measured by the temperature of the modality; the duration of application; and the size of body surface area to which it is applied.

Each of these effects has therapeutic implications. On the basis of the skin-modality temperature gradient, the firing frequency of sensory neurons will be altered. These changes in thermal sensory experience may result in general relaxation, a "hyperstimulating analgesic" (counterirritant) effect, or general arousal invigorating effects. As cold decreases nerve temperature, there will be a decrease in **nerve conduction velocity (NCV).** The reduction in NCV is proposed to decrease pain transmission and decrease muscle spindle firing, which will reduce muscle spasm. Local vasoconstriction and piloerection also may occur; the latter has no therapeutic value. As the tissue temperature falls, the viscosity of blood increases, and initially, superficial vessels constrict for as long as 30 min. The initial vasoconstriction causes a fall in capillary perfusion at the cooled area, thus decreasing bleeding and, probably, the formation of edema. After the initial period, cutaneous blood flow increases, which tends to increase the tissue temperature. This increase in cutaneous circulation may be caused by the opening of A–V shunts, by dilatation of the constricted vessels, or both. The latter occurs because cold has inhibited the function of the neurotransmitters that affected constriction. If this secondary response is not desired (eg, after an acute injury), cold application should be limited to 10 to 30 min.

As the tissue temperature declines, the metabolic rate also decreases, resulting in a decrease in the inflammatory process. This may decrease the production of edema, retard the healing process, or both; however, the effect of cold on edema needs further investigation. As the temperature decreases, a decrease in the firing of sensory neurons may cause numbness and anesthesia. Eventually, all sensory and motor activity ceases.

If the application of intense cold, or even moderate cold, is prolonged, or if intense cold is applied to much of the body, the core temperature may fall. Countercurrent exchange and the transfer of heat from adjacent tissues to the circulating blood help prevent applied cold from decreasing the core temperature, and the accompanying shivering or other heat-producing mechanisms act to increase internal temperature. A heat modality applied proximal to the cold also may help prevent a decrease in core temperature.

Superficial cold modalities can affect tissue temperature to a greater depth than superficial heat modalities can, and the temperature change is more prolonged. The effects of cold on deeper tissues are not yet completely understood. The vascular supply, the amount of subcutaneous fat, and the intensity and duration of application are all factors to be considered. Cold can reduce spasticity. This effect can be attributed to a cold-induced decrease in the activity of various neurons or contractile elements of the muscles. **Table 11–3** outlines physiologic effects and therapeutic implications.

Application of cold may cause tissue damage, the severity of which depends on the intensity and duration of the application. At present the recommended intervention is rapid rewarming. Cold well above freezing can cause tissue inflammation and damage. Therapists also must be aware that cryotherapy can cause adverse reactions in patients who are hypersensitive to cold and that certain systemic diseases increase an individual's hypersensitivity. Such conditions, with precautions and contraindications, are discussed in **Chapter 14.**

REVIEW QUESTIONS

1. What does thermal homeostasis mean?
2. In general, what controls local and systemic responses to thermal modalities?
3. What part of the brain appears to regulate body temperature?
4. Why should thermal modalities be avoided if a patient's heat receptors are not intact? Give two reasons.
5. At what temperature range do heat-pain fibers begin firing?
6. Below what temperature do cold-pain fibers begin firing?
7. What damage can be caused by high tissue temperatures? By low tissue temperatures?
8. Explain the set point theory of the thermoregulatory system.
9. What internal temperature does the body strive to maintain?
10. What mean skin temperature does the body strive to maintain for
    a. men?
    b. women?
11. In addition to thermal shock, what are the other two immediate reactions to local application of
    a. heat?
    b. cold?
12. How does an increase in local tissue temperature affect
    a. blood viscosity?

TABLE 11–3   *Summary of Physiological Responses to Applied Cold and Their Clinical Significance.*

Physiologic Response	Effect	Clinical Significance
Thermal sensory experience (thermal shock).	Mild: analgesic/sedative.	Decreases pain and spasms and promotes relaxation.
	Moderate: autonomic responses.	Invigorating general stimulant.
	Severe: fight or flight responses.	Pain and fear.
Initial superficial vasoconstriction.	Decreased superficial bleeding.	May not alter or may increase deep blood flow.
Secondary vasofluctuations.	Blood flow varies accordingly.	Protects tissues from cold injury.
Observable change in skin color.	Initial: blanching.	Decreases superficial blood flow.
	Secondary: redness.	Increases superficial blood flow.
Increased blood viscosity.	Decreased blood flow.	Retards bleeding/hemorrhage.
Decreased metabolism.	Decreased inflammation; may decrease edema.	May retard healing.
Rapid muscular contractions (shivering).	Increased metabolic rate.	Mechanism to maintain thermal homeostasis.
Piloerection—contraction of muscles of skin hair.	Skin hair rises to an erect position (goose bumps).	Ineffectual mechanism for maintaining thermal homeostasis.
Decreased extensibility of nonelastic tissue.*	Decreased ability to elongate tissues eg tendons and joint capsules.	Decreased range of motion and increased probability of rupturing soft tissue fibers.
Decreased peripheral nerve activity.*	Decreased firing and conduction of motor and sensory nerves.	May decrease spasticity.
Possible decreased temperature of joint tissues and fluids.*	Increased joint stiffness. Decreased activity of fluid enzymes.	Decreased speed of joint motion. May decrease destruction in degenative joint disease (eg Rheumatoid arthritis).

* Indicates responses that are discussed in Chapter 10.

   b. local sweating?
   c. the metabolic rate?

13. Define the Q_{10} ratio, or the van't Hoff effect.

14. An increase in metabolic rate also increases phagocytosis. What is the effect of this phagocytosis?

15. An increase in metabolic rate also increases arteriolar dilatation. What is the effect of this increased dilatation?

16. How long does the initial vasoconstriction response last during the application of a cold modality?

17. What are the negative effects of vasoconstriction?

18. How are motor nerves affected by cold?

19. Why can superficial cold modalities change the temperature of deep tissues more than heat modalities can change them?

20. How can fat affect the effectiveness of a cold modality?

21. How can poor vascular status affect the effectiveness of a cold modality?

22. Approximately how long does ice take to cool the temperature of tissues that are 2 cm deep?

23. Approximately how long do supercooling modalities take to cool the temperature of tissues that are 2 cm deep? Is this constant?

24. What happens approximately 15 to 30 min after the tissue temperature drops significantly? Why?

KEY TERMS

set points
thermal sensory experiences
Q_{10} ratio

van't Hoff's law
van't Hoff's effect
reflex heating

Sudomotor systems
cold-induced vasodilation (CIVD)
countercurrent exchange (CCE)

REFERENCES

1. Fox R, Hilton S: Bradykinin formation in human skin in heat vasodilatation. *J Physiol (Br)* 1958; 142:219–32.

2. Baez S. Microcirculation. *Ann Rev Physiol* 1977; 39:391–415.

3. Guyton AC, Hall JC: *Textbook of Medical Physiology*, 10th ed. Philadelphia: Saunders; 2000.

4. Ogawa T: Regional differences in sweating activity. In: Hales J, ed. *Thermal Physiology*. New York: Raven; 1984:229–34.

5. Hensel H: *Thermoreception and Temperature Regulation*. New York: Academic Press; 1981:199.

6. Hensel H: *Thermal Sensations and Thermoreceptors in Man*. Springfield, MO: Charles C Thomas; 1982:6, 36, 91–92, 94.

7. Mekjavic IB, Sundberg CJ, Linnaisson D: Core temperature "null zone." *J App Physiol* 1991; 71:1289.

8. Downey J: Physiological effects of heat and cold. *Phys Ther* 1974; 44:714.

9. Licht S, ed: *Medical Hydrology*. New Haven: Elizabeth Licht; 1963:98–99, 102.

10. Kottke F, Lehmanns, eds: *Krusen's Handbook of Physical Medicine and Rehabilitation*, 4th ed. Philadelphia: Saunders; 1990:261–72.

11. Hartviksen K: Ice therapy in spasticity. *Acta Neurol Scand* 1962; 38 (suppl 3):79–84.

12. Guyton A: *Function of the Human Body*, 3rd ed. Philadelphia: Saunders; 1969:311–12.

13. Pieriau Fr-K, Mizutani M, Taylor D: Do dichotomizing afferent nerve fibers transmit the axon reflex? In: Hales J, ed. *Thermal Physiology*. New York: Raven Press; 1984:17–20.

14. Berne R, Levy M: *Cardiovascular Physiology*, 7th ed. St. Louis: Mosby; 1997.

15. Vanhoutte P, Leusen I, eds: *Vasodilatation*. New York: Raven Press: 1981:263–71.

16. Holdcroft A: Body *Temperature Control*. London: Bailliére-Tindall; 1980:12–26.

17. Brooks G; Fahey T: *Exercise Physiology*. New York: Wiley; 1984:20.

18. Lehmann J, ed: *Therapeutic Heat and Cold*, 4th ed. Baltimore: Williams & Wilkins; 1990.

19. Rowell L: Reflex control of the cutaneous vasculature. *Invest Dermatol* 1977; 69:154–66.

20. Astrand P, Rodahl K: *Textbook of Work Physiology*. New York: McGraw-Hill; 1977:563.

21. Berger R: *Applied Exercise Physiology*. Philadelphia: Lea & Febiger; 1982:199–201.

22. Morehouse L, Miller A: *Physiology of Exercise*, 7th ed. St Louis: Mosby; 1976:236–38.

23. Davies C, Young K: Effect of temperature on contractile properties and muscle power of tricep surae in humans. *J App Physiol* 1983; 55(1):191–95.

24. Gibbons J, Landis E: Vasodilatation in the lower extremities in response to immersing the forearm in warm water. *J Clin Invest* 1932; 11:1019.

25. Bennett R, Hines EA, Krusen F: Effect of SWD on the cutaneous temperature of the feet. *Am Heart J* 1941; 21:490.

26. Lota M: Optimal exposure time for development of acclimatization to heat. *Fed Proc* 1965; 22:704.

27. Downey J, Darling R: *Physiological Basis of Rehabilitation Medicine*. Philadelphia: Saunders; 1971.

28. Bisgard J, Nye D: Influence of hot and cold application upon gastric and intestinal motor activity. *Surg Gyn Obstet* 1940; 71:172–80.

29. Schulman L: A Comparative Study of the Effects of Ultrasound vs. Hot Packs on Increasing Cutaneous Blood Flow to the Lower Extremities Utilizing the Reflex Heating Technique. New York: Columbia University; 1983. Master's thesis.

30. Henrikien O, Bulow J, Kristensen J, et al: Local tissue temperature: An important factor for regulation of blood flow in peripheral tissues during

indirectly induced hyperthermia. In: Hales J, ed. *Thermal Physiology*. New York: Raven Press; 1984:255–58.

31. Halperin ML, Goldstein MB: *Fluid, Electrolyte, and Acid-Base Physiology*, 2nd ed. Philadelphia: Saunders; 1994.

32. McMaster W, Liddle S, Waugh T: Laboratory evaluation of various cold therapy modalities. *Am J Sports Med* 1978; 6:291–94.

33. Burton A, Edholm O: *Man in a Cold Environment*. London: Edward Arnold; 1955:225–30.

34. Mai J, Pedersen E, Arlien-Sobory P: Changes in afferent discharge during cooling. In: Koni P, ed. *Biomechanics-VA*. Baltimore: University Park Press; 1976:171–75.

35. Popovic V, Popovic P: *Hypothermia in Biology and in Medicine*. New York: Grune & Stratton; 1974:66.

36. Rand P, LaCombe E, Hamilton E, et al: Viscosity of normal human blood under normothermic and hypothermic conditions. *J Applied Physiol* 1964; 19(1):117–22.

37. Michlovitz S. *Thermal Agents in Rehabilitation*, 3rd ed. Philadelphia: Davis; 1996.

38. Lundgren C, Muren A, Zederfeldt B: Effect of cold-vasoconstriction on wound healing in the rabbit. *Acta Chir Scand* 1959; 118(1):1–4.

39. Lundgren C, Muren A, Zederfeldt B: Effect of cold-vasoconstriction on wound healing in the rabbit. *Acta Chir Scand* 1959; 118(1): 1.

40. Marek J, Jezdensky J, Ochononsky P: Effects of local cold and heat therapy of traumatic oedema of the rat hind paw. *Acta Univ Palack Olomucensis* 1973; 65–66:203–266.

41. Matson F, Questa K, Matson A: The effect of local cooling on postfracture swelling. *Clin Orthop Rel Res* 1975; 109:201–06.

42. Schmidt K, Ott V, Rocher F, et al: Heat, cold and inflammation. *Zeit Rheumatol* 1979; 38:391–404.

43. Cote D, Prentice W Jr, Hooker D, et al: Comparison of three treatment procedures for minimizing ankle sprain swelling. *Phys Ther* 1988; 68:1072–1076.

44. Fox P: Local cooling in man. *Br Med Bull* 1961; 17(1):14–18.

45. Pugh L, Edholm O, Fox R, et al: A physiological study of channel swimming. *Clin Sci* 1960; 19:257–73.

46. Coles D, Cooper K: Hyperaemia following arterial occlusion of exercise in the warm and cold human forearm. *J Physiol Br* 1959; 145:241–50.

47. Abdel-Sayed W, Abbourd R, Cavelo M: Effect of local cooling responsiveness of muscular and cutaneous arteries and veins. *Am J Physiol* 1970; 219:1773–78.

48. Lowdon B, Moore R: Determinants and nature of intramuscular temperature changes during cold therapy. *Am J Phys Med* 1975; 54:223–33.

49. Waylonis G: The physiologic effects of ice massage. *Arch Phys Med Rehabil* 1967; 48(1):37–42.

50. Lewis T, ed: Observations upon the reaction of the human skin to cold. In: *Heart*. London: Shaw; 1929/31; 15:177–208.

51. Frisancho A: *Human Adaptation: A Functional Interpretation*. St. Louis: Mosby; 1979:44–45.

52. Clark R, Hellon R: Vascular reactions of the human forearm to cold. *Clin Sci* 1958; 17:165–79.

53. Fox R, Wyatt H: Cold-induced vasodilation in various areas of the body surface in man. *J Physiol* 1962; 162(1):289–97.

54. Keating WR: The effect of general chilling on the vasodilation response to cold. *J Physiol* 1957; 139(3):497–507.

55. Stanier MW, Mownt LE, Bligh J: *Energy Balance and Temperature Regulation*. Cambridge, UK: Cambridge University Press; 1984:292.

56. Slonim NB, ed: *Environmental Physiology*. St. Louis: Mosby; 1974:94.

57. DonTigny R, Sheldon K: Simultaneous use of heat and cold in treatment of muscle spasms. *Arch Phys Med Rehabil* 1962; 43:235–37.

58. Wyngaarden J, Smith L Jr, eds: *Cecil's Textbook of Medicine*, 17th ed. Philadelphia: Saunders; 1985:358, 2229, 2304–06.

59. Thorman M. The pathology and management of frostbite. *Clin Management*. 1985; 5:12–15.

60. Meryman H: Tissue freezing and cold injury. *Physiol Rev* 1957; 37:233–51.

61. Washburn B: Frostbite. *N Eng J Med* 1962; 2:266, 974.

12

Clinical Effects of Thermal Modalities

BERNADETTE HECOX, PT, MA

JOHN P. SANKO, PT EdD

Chapter Outline

Decisions regarding which thermal modality to use for specific intervention programs should be based on an understanding of which modalities can improve the condition of the involved tissues or systems most effectively. For example, the functional problem—the limited range of motion of a joint—may be caused by several conditions, including edema, soft-tissue contractures, muscle tension, pain/spasms, peripheral nerve damage, and spasticity or other conditions involving the central nervous system (CNS). Some conditions respond to superficial heating while others respond better to deep heating and still others respond better to cold. Therefore, the therapist must determine the best modality for the patient and not simply apply their favorite modality.

For some conditions, the relative values of heat and cold are supported by consistent findings in scientific studies. For others, studies are either lacking, or the reported results are inconsistent. If the rationale for choosing a specific modality is based on objective findings, we can assume that the results obtained will be relatively predictable. For example, at the site of a wound, the blood flow will predictably increase if heated and will decrease if cooled. When objective findings are lacking, clinical judgments must be based on the information available, which may be theoretical or arising from subjective clinical observations or the patient's report of benefits. To help the physical therapist make intelligent selections and uses of thermal modalities, this chapter summarizes the information that is currently available regarding some frequently treated pathologic conditions.

Effects on Soft Tissue

Nonelastic Tissues

If limited range of motion or nerve compression is the result of shortened collagen tissues, the value of heat is well documented.[1-5] A study comparing the effects of a sustained load on rat tendons at room temperature, 78.8°F (26°C), and at 113°F (45°C) showed that at the higher temperature, the **extensibility** of the collagen tissues was increased.[6] Nonelastic fibrous tissues, joint capsules, and/or scar tissue as well as tendons will yield to a prolonged stretch when heated, but similar results are not obtained if the stretch is applied after the tissues have been cooled.

Warren and colleagues[7,8] demonstrated that although a prolonged low-load stretching procedure produced some **residual elongations** of tissues at 98.6°F (37°C), better results and less damage occurred when tissues were heated before beginning the stretch. These investigators recommended the use of the highest possible therapeutic temperature with low-force load and the maintenance of the stretch for a few minutes after the heat is removed to achieve the greatest lengthening of collagenous tissues. They attributed the elongation of the tissue to organizational changes in the collagen fibers and to changes occurring in the viscoelastic properties of the tissues. If the involved tissues (eg, ligaments and capsules) are deeper than 1 cm, only deep-heat modalities can increase their temperature sufficiently. Ice packs are sometimes applied immediately after the heat is removed to help stabilize the elongation just achieved, but evidence for this procedure is limited.[9]

Contractile Muscle Fibers

Wessling and associates[10] showed that the effect of a passive stretch procedure for increasing range of ankle dorsi flexion was enhanced when heat (ultrasound) was applied to the tricep surae muscle before and during the procedure. They focused the ultrasound more on the belly than on the tendon portion of the muscle, and that suggested that the heat contributed to the overall increase in joint range by increasing the plasticity of the muscle belly rather than by altering the viscoelastic properties of the tendons.

When muscles remain in a shortened position for a prolonged period, the number of contractile units (sarcomeres) in the muscle fiber decreases. This factor may influence the reduced range of joint motion. Although prolonged stretch may increase the number of sarcomeres, evidence is lacking that direct application of thermal modalities enhances changes in the sarcomeres.

Muscle Spasms with Pain

Both heat and cold have been shown to be effective for reducing pain and for relaxing muscle tension and spasms. Fountain, Gersten, and Sengir[11] compared the effects of ultrasound, hot packs, and infrared radiation on the relief of pain and spasms in subjects with spasms of the neck and on subjects who were polio patients with tight, painful hamstrings, and found that all three modalities produced subjective relief. They also found that the three modalities reduced the spasms, as determined by a significant reduction in the amount of force required to initiate movement. The maximum decrease in spasms was apparent 10 to 15 min after termination of intervention. Both of the superficial modalities were significantly more effective than ultrasound for the subject with neck spasms, whereas hot packs were significantly more effective than the other two modalities for the subjects with tight hamstrings. These investigators suggested that the intense sensory stimulation provided by hot packs might play a significant role in the greater relaxation that was apparent. However, before concluding that hot packs are best, the clinician must note the following dosage factors.

Hot packs were changed every 5 min for a 20-min period. For neck spasms, the ultrasound (1 MHz frequency at either 0.95 w/cm^2 or 1.5 w/cm^2) was applied to painful tendon sites of both the upper and the middle trapezius, using a continuously moving head for a total of 5 min. A 1000-w infrared lamp was positioned 16 inches from the skin surface. This study was published in 1960.

One might assume that all three modalities, if applied using methods and dosages similar to those used by Fountain and colleagues, would produce similar subjective and objective benefits. But one hot pack left on a patient for 20 min—a procedure commonly practiced in clinics—may not demonstrate the same results. If ultrasound had been applied to the upper and middle trapezius muscles for 5 min each, more closely approximating a clinically recommended area per time (5 sq in for 3 to 5 min), the results might have been more effective.

Prentice[12] investigated the value of combining ice packs or hot packs with either static or proprioceptive neuromuscular facilitation stretching techniques to determine which combination would decrease spasms best (ie, elicit the greatest muscle relaxation) as determined by a decrease in **electromyographic (EMG) activity.** Each modality was applied for 20 min. All experimental groups as well as a control group displayed some decrease in EMG activity. However, the group treated with ice packs and static stretch was the only one that differed significantly from the control group. Consider that the temperature gradient between an ice pack and skin is great; a less intense form of cold might not produce the same results.

EFFECTS ON JOINTS

Joint Stiffness

Thermal modalities can affect the freedom with which a joint moves. In general, joint freedom refers to the amount of time and force required to move through a given range. Heat enhances this freedom (less force and time are required), whereas cold increases stiffness.[1,13–15]

Wright and Johns[16,17] showed that when skin is heated to 113°F (45°C), the underlying joint moves about 20% more freely than when the skin temperature is 91.4°F (33°C). When the skin is cooled to 64.4°F (18°C), the stiffness increases 10 to 20%. They believed that the stiffness is caused by tension in the periarticular structure rather than by the changes in the viscous properties of the joint.

Backlund and Tiselius[18] also showed that stiffness increases with cold and decreases with heat. However, they found that marked changes occurred with cold when hands were placed in water at 50°F (10°C) for 10 min—whereas the changes occurring with heat were slight when hands were placed in water at 109.4°F (43°C) for 10 min. Note that the study using the more intense heat increased the joint freedom more effectively, whereas the one using intense cold increased stiffness more.

Wright,[19] in his review of research on joint stiffness, reported that Ingpen and Kendall found that "wax baths" caused fingers to move faster. This supports the use of paraffin baths for reducing joint stiffness. Wright also reported that studies on the knee joint showed increased stiffness when the knee was immersed in "ice water" (50°F, 10°C) compared with 91.4°F (33°C) conditions. Of interest in that Wright reported that, although shortwave diathermy reduced stiffness about 20%, the effect was transient; it disappeared about 10 min after intervention. Although the testing methods and specific findings of these studies differ, all indicate that heat is the preferred modality for decreasing joint stiffness.

Intra-Articular Structures and Fluid

In general, the application of heat tends to increase the temperature within a joint, and cold tends to decrease the temperature. However, Hollander and Hovath[20] found that when hot or cold packs were applied to knee joints, a temporary, paradoxical phenomenon occurred. Hot packs increased the temperature of the skin but reduced the temperature of the underlying joint, whereas cold packs increased the temperature of the joint. They attributed this phenomenon to a reflex reaction in which the circulation in the joint opposed the circulation at the surface. However, with other heat modalities, the intra-articular temperature increased. Some increase was observed with infrared radiation, more was observed with paraffin wraps, and the most was observed with deep heat.

Although either heat or cold can be used to relieve symptoms, which in turn permits an increase in joint range of motion, and heat is preferred to gain freedom of joint movement, the therapeutic value of applying heat modalities to joints affected by rheumatoid arthritis has been questioned. Evidence indicates that increasing the temperature of synovial fluid may increase the proteolytic enzyme activity and thus the destruction in a rheumatoid joint.[21,22] Because metabolic activity is temperature-related and enzyme activity decreases as temperature declines, presumably the destructive enzyme activity that occurs in joints will also decrease. At present, no studies have conclusively verified this assumption. However, this assumption, plus the fact that some patients are relieved of symptoms when cold is applied, suggests the positive effects of cold. Nonetheless, the use of heat also should be considered.

Both the heat modality being used and the location of the joint must be taken into account. Only ultrasound or a diathermy such as a 915-MHz microwave (not commonly found in clinics) can be expected to raise the temperature significantly in deep-seated joints. However, the temperature of wrist or finger joints could be elevated with even superficial heat.[23] Of interest is a study by Mainardi,[24] in which one hand of a patient with rheumatoid arthritis was placed in an electric mitten heated to 104°F (40°C) and the other hand acted as a control. The study failed to show that daily heating had any effect on progression of the disease. Lehman and DeLateur[25] pointed out that some investigators[22,26,27] did not study temperatures higher than 105.8°F (41°C) and that at temperatures between 102.2–105.8°F (39–41°C), the rate of enzyme activity *decreased*. Lehmann[28] suggested that bringing the temperature of a joint into the range of 105.8–113°F (41–45°C) may in fact inactivate destructive collagenase, as at higher temperatures the protein component is denatured. Obviously, the final answer concerning the effects of heat versus cold on intra-articular structures is not yet in. However, Lehmann[28] suggested

that, because arthritic joints may be stiff and have contractures that require stretching, the use of heat may be appropriate but should be used cautiously. This is especially true with a modality such as ultrasound, because it is most likely to heat joint fluids.

NEURONAL ACTIVITY

Peripheral Nerves: Sensory and Motor Firing

The activity of peripheral nerves varies with changes in temperature. As shown in **Chapter 11**, **Figure 11–1**, the firing rate of the receptors of warm fibers peaks at approximately 109°F (43°C) and declines rapidly at higher temperatures. Heat-pain fibers begin firing at a temperature of 113°F (45°C), which is only slightly higher than the temperature at which the firing of warm fibers peaks, and their rate of firing increases as the temperature increases.

Cold-pain fibers begin firing at a temperature only slightly lower than the one at which the firing of warm fibers peaks. The temperature at which the firing rate of cold fibers peaks is approximately 77°F (25°C), and their firing stops at approximately 46.4°F (8°C). The firing of cold-pain fibers begins at approximately 59°F (15°C), and the rate increases until the temperature reaches 40°F (4.7°C). Thus, firing of the warm and the cold fibers overlaps with their respective pain fibers, with the firing rate of the pain fibers increasing as the temperatures reach those at which the tissues are endangered.

Impulses conveyed by thermal fibers are fed into the CNS, where they are integrated with information from the internal environment. Cutaneous receptors set up mechanisms to protect local tissues and preserve thermal homeostasis. The face has a large number of clusters of thermal receptors, cold spots, and hot spots; the forehead is especially sensitive to cold.[29,30] Thus, there is a valid rationale for the common practice of placing cool compresses on the forehead to reduce the physiologic effects of, and relieve the discomfort caused by, excessive heating.

Temperature affects the activity of all peripheral nerves, both sensory and motor.[31] De Jong et al[32,33] found that when a neuron is stimulated electrically, the threshold for the firing of an action potential increases as the temperature decreases below 73.4°F (23°C), that is, the current intensity (amperage) required to evoke an action potential increases. However, above that temperature, the threshold for firing remained constant. This study suggests the value of cooling tissues if a decrease in neuronal activity is desired. Tissues are often heated before intervention with electrical stimulation so that less voltage is required to excite the neurons. This procedure is not done specifically to lower the threshold for firing of action potentials; it is done because the increase in sweat and blood at the heated tissue site (usually skin) lowers the electrical impedance of the tissue.

Nerve Conduction Velocity

The **conduction velocity** of both sensory and motor nerves increases and their conduction latency decreases when the temperature is increased. These neuron conduction parameters are discussed in **Part 3**. The rate of change in nerve conduction velocity is approximately 2 m/s per degree centrigrade change in temperature. However, investigators do not agree about the exact rate of change, probably because of variations in testing procedures.[34] In the temperature ranges studied by de Jesus et al[35] for each 1°C change in temperature, the conduction velocity of motor nerves changed 2.4 m/s, and the conduction velocity of sensory nerves changed 2.0 m/s. Studies also have shown that cold receptor neurons conduct faster than warm receptor neurons and that humans react faster to cold than to warm stimuli.[36,37] These results support the use of cold over heat as a neurofaciliatory technique.

Nerve conduction velocity is related to the diameter of the fibers. However, the decrease in velocity relative to cooling does not appear to be based solely on fiber size. Douglas and Malcolm[38] studied the effects of localized cooling on retarding the activities of cat nerve fibers of various sizes. They found that the small myelinated A fibers, both motor and sensory, required less lowering of the temperature to retard their activity than did large myelinated A fibers. Furthermore, the small nonmyelinated C fibers were least susceptible; they required the greatest lowering of temperature to block conduction.

On the basis of these findings, Till[39] suggested cooling toward 32°F (0°C) if the primary goal is to reduce pain traveling via C fibers. If the goal is to decrease pain or spasms in conjunction with muscle reeducation, however, cold must be less intense to avoid slowing the conduction of motor nerves, the myelinated A fibers. Till regarded modalities at 53.6–59°F (12–15°C) as ideal.

Evidence pertaining to cat nerve fibers cannot be applied directly to humans. Some studies of human nerve fibers have found that changes in nerve conduction velocity per temperature change are the same for all fibers regardless of size.[35]

Brown[40] attributed the alterations in neural activity to changes in "sodium channels: kinetics"—the lower the temperature, the slower the opening of the sodium channels of the membrane. Brown believed that this accounted for the slower rise time and prolonged duration of an action potential that is known to occur with decreases in temperature. Brown also suggested that the slower conduction velocities resulted from depolarization taking longer to occur at the next Node of Ranvier.

Cold decreases pain. Theories suggest that the increased stimulation required to activate the pain fibers, the reduced velocity along the pathways, or both diminish the pain. As the temperature continues to decrease, electrical activity decreases, and numbness or anesthesia is produced, which in turn may reduce pain. All nerve conduction velocity ceases at approximately 48°F (9°C).[41]

Application of either heat or cold reduces both tension- and pain-related muscle spasms and CNS-related spasticity.[42–44] Both superficial and deep heat (hot packs and inductance diathermy), each applied for 20 min on trigger point areas, have been shown to be effective in relieving pain.[45]

Central Nervous System

Many investigators have studied the effects of temperature on neuromuscular activity, attempting to determine why the changes in muscle tone occur.[43,46–48] For example, Mense[43] studied muscle spindle activity and found that with warming, the rate of firing of primary ending (I-A) fibers increased (as did Golgi tendon organs, I-B fibers) but that the firing of spindle secondary ending (II) fibers decreased. More recent neurologic theories and evidence suggest that although fusimotor activity (output from the central nervous system) accompanies skeletal muscle activity, excessive fusimotor activity may not be involved in either spasticity or Parkinson rigidity.[49] If this is true, other factors, rather than changes in muscle spindle activity, may be altering spasticity when heat is applied. In spite of ample clinical evidence and countless anecdotal reports indicating that both heat and cold reduce spasms and spasticity, conclusive explanations of the reason why this occurs are not yet available.

Although both heat and cold can reduce **spasticity,** the effects of heat last for only a brief period, whereas the effects of cold have been shown to last from a few minutes to as many as 90 min. Lehmann and DeLateur[25] suggested that the decreased blood flow in cooled tissues permits the effects of cold to last longer.

When treating spasticity, Scholz and Campbell's[50] advice is worth considering. "A therapist cannot assume that a particular technique will be effective by virtue of the fact that it has worked with similar patients. . . . Clinical research under controlled therapeutic conditions, in concert with modern neurodiagnostic techniques for lesion characterization is needed to document: (1) effectiveness of specific techniques, (2) variations in responses under different parametric conditions, and (3) variation in response in different pathological conditions."

Muscle Performance

When the temperature of muscles increases, the speed of movement increases.[43] When a muscle is cooled, a twitch response is prolonged; thus, a decreased rate of action potential firing is required to produce a tetanic contraction. This muscle reaction is consistent with findings regarding changes in action potential responses—slow rise time and prolonged duration—when peripheral nerve fibers are cooled. Studies relating muscle strength and performance to temperature have seldom been duplicated, and the results are so inconsistent that few conclusions can be reached. For these reasons, none of these studies are cited here. Reviews and summaries of many of the investigations are available.[2,51] It may be that with ordinary intervention dosages and clinical conditions, one modality is not consistently more effective than the others in affecting muscle strength, or it may be an oversimplification to relate a motor activity to muscle temperature alone.

Of interest is the work done by Asmussen et al,[52] who compared the height of a jump starting from a squat when the muscle temperature was 89.6°F (32°C) versus 98.6°F (37°C). They found that the jump was higher at the higher muscle temperature. However, when the upward jump was preceded by a downward jump from an elevated level (0.4m), the upward jump was higher at the cooler muscle temperature. These findings suggest that other factors interact with muscle temperature to affect muscle function.

Effects on Visceral Tissues

Application of thermal modalities on the surface of the abdomen appears to have a paradoxical effect on visceral tissues. Evidence indicates that a superficial heat applied on the abdomen reduces blood flow to the mucous membranes of the stomach and intestines, and decreases gastric acidity. Such heat also decreases exaggerated peristaltic actions (stomach cramps), whereas an ice pack aggravates peristalsis.[53]

The effects of a sitz bath also have been studied (see **Part 4**). A significant decrease in internal anal pressure occurred when subjects were immersed in water at 104°F (40°C).[54] But when the temperature was cooler or cold, this decrease did not occur. Because this change in pressure appears to reduce pain, immersion in hot water is recommended for hemorrhoidal disease or fissures and after childbirth or anorectal surgery.[54]

Abnormal Tissues: Hematomas and Malignant Tumors

Local deep-heat modalities are known to modify abnormal deep structures. The time required to resolve hematomas can be reduced significantly when a deep-heat modality is applied daily.[55] Deep heating, alone or in conjunction with radiation, has been used in therapy for malignant tumors. The intervention is highly specialized, requiring the temperature of the tumor to be raised to an extremely high level without damaging normal adjacent tissues.[25]

SUMMARY

This chapter is designed to help the clinician select appropriate thermal modalities for interventions. For some conditions, strong evidence has been presented to support the selection of certain modalities. For other conditions, especially neurologically related problems, investigations continue because the results

TABLE 12–1   *Guidelines for Selecting Heat and Cold for Clinical Problems*

Clinical Problem	Responses Desired or Expected	Is Heat Recommended?	Is Cold Recommended?
Pain	Analgesia by hyper-stimulation (counterirritant).	Yes.	Yes.
	Anesthesia.	No.	Yes.
Muscle spasms	Reduction of pain by clearing metabolites.	Yes.	No.
Upper motor neuron spasticity	Affects motor nerves (mechanism is not clearly established).	Yes. May decrease spasticity for a brief period.	Yes. May decrease spasticity for up to 90 min, but neurological "rebound" may follow.
Bleeding, hemorrhage	Retardation of blood flow to affected area (vasoconstriction).	No. May increase flow.	Yes. May decrease flow for initial period (15–30 min), but flow may increase after initial period or when cold is removed.
Edema	No clear evidence of effectiveness of either heat or cold.	May increase acute edema. May decrease chronic edema.	May decrease formation of acute edema, but edema may increase if treatment is prolonged.
Wound healing	Increased blood flow and metabolism at wound site.	Yes. Hastens healing.	No. Retards healing.
Frostbite	Hastened healing, as indicated by clinical observation.	Yes.	No. See Chap. 14.
Orthostatic hypotension	Vascular reaction.	No. May enhance the problem.	Yes. See Chap. 17.
Joint stiffness	Increased mobility of periarticular structures.	Yes.	No.
Inability to perform *skilled* movements	Increased neuron firing and nerve conduction velocity. Increased mobility of tissues.	Yes.	No.
Arthritic joints osteoarthritis and nonacute rheumatoid	Decreased pain and joint stiffness.	Yes.	Yes. May reduce pain.
	Increased mobility and function.	Yes.	No. Will increase joint stiffness.
Acute rheumatoid arthritis	Reduced enzyme activity of joint fluid. Decrease pain.	Superficial heat, yes. Mild or moderate heat will not increase enzyme activity significantly. Deep heat, no. May increase enzyme activity.	Yes. May reduce enzyme activity.
Shortness of soft tissues	Increased extensibilty of nonelastic tissues.	Yes.	No.
Any need for general stimulation or relaxation	Response of stimulation or relaxation due to mild or moderate sensory stimulation.	Yes.	Yes.
CNS Problems	Increased firing and NCV of sensory neurons to neuro-logically facilitate movement.	Yes. Less than cold.	Yes.

of various studies do not agree. Thus, the choice of modality for these conditions must be based on clinical evidence and observation.

Heat is definitely the thermal modality of choice for lengthening collagen tissues and reducing joint stiffness. However, for intervention with joints affected by rheumatoid arthritis, only superficial heat is advised, and controversy exists regarding the possibility that heating joint fluids may cause further destruction of the joints. Some evidence indicates that heat reduces stomach cramps and internal anal pressure and that cold has the opposite effect.

Both heat and cold may reduce spasms and pain. The fact that the results of comparative studies conflict may be caused by differences in the methods used, including the intensity of the heat or cold. Although both heat and cold appear to reduce spasticity, cold seems to be more effective and for a longer period. Cold is also recommended for neuromuscular facilitation.

With regard to muscle function, cold is more effective for producing tetanic (ie, holding) muscle contractions, whereas heat is more effective for increasing speed of movement. The effectiveness of heat versus cold on muscle strength requires further investigation. **Table 12–1** summarizes the clinical effects of thermal modalities as they relate to information gathered from scientific investigations, empirical observations, or clinical experience.

REVIEW QUESTIONS

1. Which interventions, heat or cold, have been well documented as the best interventions for
   a. limited range of motion caused by shortened collagen tissues?
   b. joint stiffness caused by osteoarthritis?
   c. joint stiffness caused by rheumatoid arthritis?

2. Why has the therapeutic value of applying heat modalities to joints affected by rheumatoid arthritis been questioned?

3. Why is placing a cool compress on the forehead often effective in reducing the effects of a fever?

4. Why do humans react more quickly to cold than to warm stimuli?

5. In what way are the conduction velocities of sensory and motor nerves changed by
   a. an increase in temperature?
   b. a decrease in temperature?

6. Is heating or cooling suggested if the desired effect is to reduce the sensation of pain traveling along small nonmyelinated C fibers? What temperature is recommended?

7. Is heating or cooling suggested if the desired effect is to reduce pain or spasms in conjunction with muscle reeducation? What temperature is recommended?

8. At approximately what temperature does nerve conduction velocity cease?

9. Compare the effects of heat and cold when treating spasticity. Which effects last longer? Why?

10. What is the effect of increased temperature on the speed of muscle movement?

11. What is the effect of reduced temperature on the speed of muscle movement?

12. How are stomach cramps affected by
    a. superficial heat?
    b. superficial cold?

13. For what conditions can a hot sitz bath be helpful? Why?

14. How can treatments with deep heat modalities affect hematomas?

KEY TERMS

extensibility
residual elongations

electromyographic (EMG) activity
conduction velocity

spasticity

REFERENCES

1. Bromley J, Unsworth A, Haslock I: Changes in stiffness following short- and long-term application of standard physiotherapeutic techniques. *Br J Rheumatol* 1994; 33:555–61.

2. Kaurenen K, Vanharanta H: Effects of hot and cold packs on motor performance on normal hands. *Physiotherapy* 1997; 83:340–44.

3. Lentell G, Hetherington T, Eagan J, Morgan M: The use of thermal agents to influence the effectiveness of a low-load prolonged stretch. *J Orthop Sports Phys Ther* 1992; 16:200–07.

4. Taylor BF, Waring OA, Brashear TA: The effects of therapeutic application of heat or cold followed by static stretch on hamstring muscle length. *J Orthop Sports Phys Ther* 1995; 21:283–86.

5. Hardy M, Woodall W: Therapeutic effects of heat, cold, and stretch on connective tissue. *J Hand Ther* 1998; 11 (4–5):148–56.

6. Lehmann J, Masock A, Warren C, et al: Effect of therapeutic temperatures on tendon extensibility. *Arch Phys Med Rehabil* 1970; 51:481–87.

7. Warren C, Lehmann J, Koblanski J: Elongation of rat tail tendon: Effect of load and temperature. *Arch Phys Med Rehabil* 1971; 52:465–74; 484.

8. Warren C, Lehmann J, Koblanski J: Heat and stretch procedures: An evaluation using rat tail tendon. *Arch Phys Med Rehabil* 1976; 57(3):122–26.

9. Sapega A, Quedenfeld T, Moyer R, et al: Biophysical factors in range-of-motion exercise. *Physican Sports Med* 1981; 9(12):57–65.

10. Wessling K, DeVane D, Hylton C: Effects of static stretch versus static stretch and ultrasound combined on tricep surae muscle extensibility in healthy women. *Phys Ther* 1987; 67:674–79.

11. Fountain F, Gersten J, Sengir O: Decrease in muscle spasm produced by ultrasound, hot packs, and infrared radiation. *Arch Phys Med Rehabil* 1960; 41(7):293–98.

12. Prentice W Jr: An electromyographic analysis of the effectiveness of heat or cold and stretching for inducing relaxation in injured muscle. *J Ortho Sports Phys Ther* 1982; 3(3):133–40.

13. Ayling J, Marks R: Efficacy of paraffin wax baths for rheumatoid arthritic hands. *Physiotherapy* 2000; 86:190–201.

14. Weinberger A, Fadilah R, Lev A, Pinkhas J: Intra-articular temperature measurements after superficial heating. *Scand J Rehab Med* 1989; 21:55–57.

15. Yung P, Unsworth A, Haslock I: Measurement of stiffness in the metarapophalangeal joint: The effects of physiotherapy. *Clin Phys Physiol Meas* 1986; 7:147–56.

16. Wright V, Johns R: Physical factors concerned with the stiffness of normal and diseased joints. *Johns Hopkins Hosp Bull* 1960; 106:229.

17. Johns R, Wright V: Relative importance of various tissues in joint stiffness. *J Appl Physiol* 1962; 17:824–28.

18. Backlund L, Tiselius P: Objective measurements of joint stiffness in rheumatoid arthritis. *Acta Rheum Scand* 1967; 13:275–88.

19. Wright V: Stiffness: A review of its measurements and physiological importance. *Physiotherapy* 1973; 59(4):107–111.

20. Hollander JL, Horvath M: The influence of physical therapy procedures on the intra-articular temperature of normal and arthritic subjects. *Am J Med Sci* 1949; 218:543–48.

21. Febel A, Fast A: Deep heating of joints: A reconsideration. *Arch Phys Med Rehabil* 1976; 57:513–14.

22. Harris E Jr, McCroskery P: The influence of temperature and fibril stability on degradation of cartilage collagen by rheumatoid synovial collagenase. *N Engl J Med* 1974; 290(1):1–6.

23. Borrell R, Parker R, Henley E: Comparison of in vivo temperatures produced by hydrotherapy, paraffin wax treatment, and fluidotherapy. *Phys Ther* 1980; 60:1273–76.

24. Mainardi C, Walter J, Spiegel P: Rheumatoid arthritis: Failure of daily heat therapy to affect its progressions. *Arch Phys Med Rehabil* 1979; 60:393–99.

25. Lehmann J, DeLateur B: Therapeutic Heat. In: *Therapeutic heat and cold*, 4th ed. Baltimore: Williams & Wilkins; 1990. Chap. 9.

26. Kottke F, Stillwell G, Lehmann J, eds: *Krusen's Handbook of Physical Medicine and Rehabilitation.* Philadelphia: Saunders; 1982; 275–350.

27. Castor C, Yaron M: Connective tissue activation: VIII. The effects of temperature studies in vitro. *Arch Phys Med Rehabil* 1976; 57:5–9.

28. Lehmann J: Letter to the Editor. *Arch Phys Med Rehabil* 1977; 58:232–33.

29. Clark R, Edholm O: *Man and His Thermal Environment.* London: Edward Arnold; 1985; 155:136–155.

30. Noback C, Demarest B: *The Human Nervous System.* New York: McGraw-Hill; 1981:87–88.

31. Holdcroft A: *Body Temperature Control.* London: Bailliére-Tindall; 1980:1,12–26.

32. DeJong R, Hershey W, Wagman I: Nerve conduction velocity during hypothermia in man. *Anesthesiology* 1966; 27:805–810.

33. Tremblay F, Estephan L, Legendre M, Sulpher S: Influence of local cooling on proprioceptive acuity in the quadriceps muscle. *J Athl Train* 2001; 36:119–23.

34. Currier D, Kramer J: Sensory nerve conduction: Heating effects of ultrasound and infrared. *Physiother Can* 1982; 34:241–46.

35. De Jesus P, Housmanowa-Petrusewicz I, Barchi R: The effect of cold on nerve conduction of human slow and fast nerve fibers. *Neurology* 1973; 23:1182–89.

36. Fruhstorfer H, Guth H, Pfaff U: Thermal reaction-time as a function of stimulation site. *Pflug Arch* 1972; 335:49.

37. Zotterman Y, ed: *Sensory Function of the Skin: Primates.* Oxford, UK: Pergamon, 1976; 331–53.

38. Douglas W, Malcolm J: The effects of localized cooling in conduction in cat nerves. *J Physiol (Br)* 1955; 130(1):53–71.

39. Till D: Cold therapy. *Physiotherapy* 1969; 55:461–66.

40. Brown W: *The Physiological and Technical Basis of Electromyography.* Boston: Butterworth; 1984; 26–27, 385–88.

41. Clark R, Edholm O: *Man and His Thermal Environment.* London: Edward Arnold; 1985.

42. Bishop B: Spasticity: Its physiology and management: IV. Current and projected treatment procedures for spasticity. *Phys Ther* 1977; 57:396–401.

43. Mense S: Effects of temperature on the discharges of muscle spindles and tendon organs. *Pflug Arch Eur J Physiol* 1978; 374(suppl):159–66.

44. Petajan J, Watts N: Effects of cooling on the triceps surae reflex. *Am J Phys Med* 1962; 41:240–51.

45. McCray R, Patton N: Pain relief at trigger points: A comparison of moist heat and shortwave diathermy. *J Ortho Sports Phys Ther* 1984; 5:175–78.

46. Hartviksen K: Ice therapy in spasticity. *Acta Neurol Scand* 1962; 38 (suppl 3):79–84.

47. Knutsson E: Topical cryotherapy in spasticity. *Scand J Rehabil Med* 1970; 2:159.

48. Miglietta O: Action of cold on spasticity. *Am J Phys Med* 1973; 52:198–205.

49. Burke D: Critical examination of the case for or against fusimotor involvement in disorders of muscle tone. In: Desmedt J, ed. *Motor Control Mechanisms: Health and Disease, Advances in Neurology.* New York: Raven Press; 1983; 39:133–50.

50. Scholz J, Campbell S: Muscle spindles and the regulation of movement. *Phys Ther* 1980; 60:1416–24.

51. Cutlaw K, Arnold B, Perrin D: Effect of cold treatment on concentric and eccentric force-velocity relationship of the quadriceps. *J Ath Train* 1995; 30(2):S31.

52. Asmussen E, Bonde-Peterson F, Jorgensen K: Mechano-elastic properties of human muscles at different temperatures. *Acta Physiol Scand* 1976; 96:83–93.

53. Bisgard J, Nye D: Influence of hot and cold application upon gastric and intestinal motor activity. *Surg Gynecol Obstet* 1940; 71:172–80.

54. Dodi G, Bogoni F, Infantino A: Hot and cold in anal pain? *Dis Colon Rect* 1986; 29:248–51.

55. Lehmann J, Dundore D, Esselman P: Microwave diathermy: Effects on experimental muscle hematoma resolution. *Arch Phys Med Rehabil* 1983; 64(3):127–29.

13

Superficial Thermotherapy

BERNADETTE HECOX, PT, MA

JOHN P. SANKO, PT, EdD

Chapter Outline

The previous chapters discussed the physics, biophysics, and physiologic effects of heat as well as evidence supporting or refuting the value of the available methods of heating. This chapter briefly reviews the physiologic effects of local heating. It sets forth the general indications and contraindications that are common to all superficial heating modalities, before presenting each individual modality with its specific effects, indications, contraindications, and intervention procedures.

PHYSIOLOGIC EFFECTS OF SUPERFICIAL HEATING

Any addition of heat to the body may trigger certain physiologic responses. For example, local application of superficial thermotherapy in the form of hot packs, paraffin, and infrared radiation can lead to many beneficial local physical changes and may or may not affect systemic factors such as the core (internal) temperature.

Some physiologic responses to heat include increases in tissue temperature, in local metabolism, and in blood flow. In addition, heat causes both analgesia and sedation (relaxation), which are helpful in chronic conditions. Local heating also leads to increased nerve conduction velocity.[1] **Figure 13–1** summarizes some of the physiological and therapeutic effects of local heating.

Heat has been used throughout history to soothe aches and pains. Many people enjoy sitting in the sun more for the heat and relaxation benefits they receive than for its tanning effects. Most households have a heating pad in a closet for use at some future time. Both the sun and the heating pad are forms of **superficial heat,** that is, they heat the surface of the body or the underlying tissue to a depth of a few millimeters. Any transfer of heat that takes place is a result of radiation, conduction, or convection.[1]

The decrease in muscle spasm and the decrease in pain resulting from local heating are closely interrelated. Sometimes a patient guards a painful affected part and thereby increases muscle tension in that area. If this cycle can be broken by local heating, then the part can be treated easily with massage, exercise, or other modalities. Local heating also may help reduce skin resistance, thus making this modality desirable to use before other modalities such as electrical stimulation are applied.

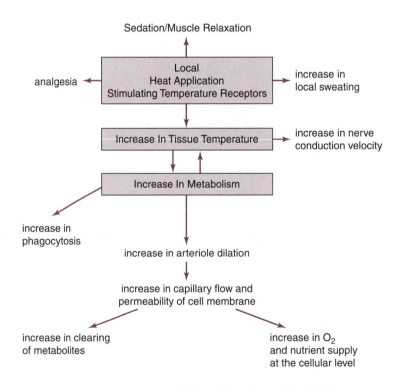

FIGURE 13–1   Summary of the physiological and therapeutic effects of local superficial heating.

Heat is not recommended during the first 24 to 36 hours after an injury if a hemorrhage and swelling is present, but it can be used subsequently to hasten healing, alleviate local edema, and aid in resorption of a hematoma. Once the subacute stage is present, heat is no longer considered contraindicated. To prevent the further accumulation of edema or help reduce the amount of local, chronic edema present, an extremity receiving heat should be elevated to a level above the heart, if possible. As was mentioned in earlier chapters, vigorous heating should not be used if a patient has severe edema caused by renal or cardiac failure or has severely impaired circulation (and therefore an impaired thermoregulatory system).

ALL SUPERFICIAL HEAT MODALITIES
General Indications

Box 13–1 lists common clinical uses and their rationale for superficial thermotherapy. Remember, however, that superficial heating affects only superficial tissue—that the effects on deeper tissues such as muscle are minimal or nonexistent.[2] Moist heat is preferred by most individuals, although no studies have been published that support this statement. Moist heat should provide a better conduction medium; Abramson[3] did find that dry heat will produce a greater increase in skin temperature compared with moist heat but that moist heat produces a deeper heating effect. Although direct heating effects are primarily superficial, research has shown that blood-flow increases occur deeper after application of 30 min of topical heat. Results after applying a heating pad to the trapezious muscle showed vascularity increased 27%, 77%, and 104% with temperatures of 38°, 40°, and 42°F respectively when compared with preintervention baseline measurements. Depth of vascularity changes occurred up to approximately 3 cm below the surface of the skin.[4]

If vigorous or prolonged, superficial heating can cause systemic changes. Heat should be only used when the conditions being treated are in the subacute or chronic stage. Superficial heat modalities are indicated:

General Contraindications

The contraindications and their rationale listed in **Box 13–2** are relative to the intensity of the heat: vigorous heat will cause greater reactions than mild heat.

Postintervention Procedures.   Take care in removing the modality from the patient. Check the patient's skin immediately. Mottling, red and white patches that often occur, can indicate that the superficial dermis has been pushed to its limit with respect to heat control. If there is mottling, a temporary paralysis of the nerves to the arterioles may occur, resulting in vasodilation that could take a number of hours to

Box 13–1 *Clinical Uses of Superficial Heat*

Clinical Use	Rationale
Prior to active exercise.	Increase superficial soft tissue extensibility.
Prior to passive stretching and joint mobilization.[5]	Increase superficial soft tissue extensibility and decrease joint viscosity.
Prior to traction and soft tissue mobilization.	Increase superficial soft tissue extensibility and decrease joint viscosity.
To help reduce pain and muscle spasms.	Increase pain threshold.
	Promote relaxation.
	Increase local blood flow.
Following acute inflammation to promote tissue healing.	Increase tissue metabolism.
	Increase oxygen delivery.
	Increase local blood flow.
Prior to electrical stimulation.	Decrease skin impedance.

Box 13–2 *Contraindications for Superficial Heat Applications*

Contraindications	Rationale
Over tissue during acute inflammation.	Increase secondary hypoxia.
	Promote increased edema.
	Increase bleeding by decreasing blood viscosity.
Over an area with suspected thrombophlebitis.	Promotion of vasodilation and increased blood flow may dislodge thrombus.
Over tissue devitalized by radiation or X-ray therapy.	Tissue unable to tolerate extreme temperature changes.
Over tissue with poor circulation.	Inability to shunt cool blood and deliver oxygen to heated area with increased metabolism.
Over tissue with anesthesia or dysesthesia.	Decreased ability to report overheating.
For individuals with impaired mentation.	Decreased ability to report overheating.
For individuals with fever.	Avoid adding further heat with increased systemic temperature.
Skin or lymphatic cancer (safety in the presence of cancer has not been determined).	Increase in tissue metabolism.

resolve. With repeated intense interventions, erythema ab Igna, skin pigmentation, may occur from overexposure to any infrared energy source. If a patient has been applying modalities at home, it is important to have inspected the skin prior to application of a modality in a clinical setting. Any adverse response to an intervention should be immediately and clearly documented.

USE OF SPECIFIC MODALITIES

The most common superficial heat modalities include hot packs (chemical-silica gel), paraffin, Fluidotherapy®, and water immersion. Paraffin and Fluidotherapy® are considered by most clinicians to be superficial heating modalities. However, when applied to the hands or feet, these two interventions can produce significant temperature increases to muscle and joint capsules beneath the area of application.[2] These general procedures should be followed before any superficial heat modality is applied:

1. Remove any heavy clothing that may induce generalized sweating or temperature rise plus all clothing from the area to be treated.
2. Explain the purpose of the intervention to patients, and tell them what to expect—especially the type of heat sensation that they will experience.
3. Prepare patients by positioning and draping them properly for the intervention.
4. Inspect the area to be treated to note any blemishes, discolorations, open wounds, or indicators of circulatory problems.
5. Make certain that the patient can respond normally to changes in temperature.

Hot Packs

Chemical hot packs, a frequently used superficial heat modality, transmit moist heat to body tissues by conduction. The patient experiences a sensation of pleasant warmth.

Duration. The usual duration of intervention is 20 to 30 min.

Equipment. **Hot packs,** also known as *hydrocollator packs*, consist of silica gel in a canvas cover that has many stitched divisions so that the pack can be placed over body parts with different contours. The packs are immersed in water in a stainless steel tank containing water that is between 165 and 175°F (73.9–79.4°C). Water temperature in the tank should be checked at least weekly and documented in a procedure manual. New packs should be left in the tank for at least 24 hours to absorb as much moisture as possible and achieve the desired temperature. Between interventions, the packs should be left in the tank for at least 20 to 30 min. Many clinics have a rotation system for the packs so that therapists know which ones are the hottest.

Hot packs come in many different sizes and shapes. Those most commonly used are the standard or low back packs and the cervical packs (**Fig. 13–2**). Hot pack covers and terry cloth towels are also needed (**Fig. 13–3**).

Technique of Application.   The hot pack method of heating is not a constant source of heat (unlike a heating pad). The temperature of a hot pack drops quickly once the pack is removed from the tank.[6] Therefore, the more quickly the pack is covered and placed on the patient, the warmer it will be during the intervention.

The following procedures are implemented when using a hot pack:

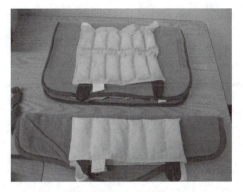

FIGURE 13–3   Hot packs and turkish towel covers.

1. If a patient must lie on top of a hot pack, although it is preferable to avoid doing this, extra toweling must be used between the patient and the pack. Because the pressure and weight of the body or body part will increase the contact with the heat source, less heat can dissipate to the environment, and more heat will conduct to the body, which increases the danger of burns and can elevate the core temperature. Also, pressure from the weight of the body may compromise cutaneous circulation, making it less able to dissipate the elevated tissue temperature.

2. Remove the hot pack from the tank with metal or wooden tongs, allow the excess water to drip off, and place it immediately in a terry cloth cover or towel. At least 6 to 12 layers of toweling or the equivalent should be placed between the hot pack and the patient. A hot pack cover (envelope), when new and fluffy, is equivalent to about three layers of toweling (five layers if the envelope contains a sponge insert). So that the cover does not require laundering after each use, at least one extra layer of toweling must be placed between the pack and the patient's skin. Additional toweling can be added to achieve the required number of layers. More or less toweling may be necessary, depending on the patient's physical condition and heat tolerance, the fluffiness of the cover and the towels, and the actual temperature of the hot pack.

3. Place the pack on the appropriate body area, and secure it firmly to prevent it from slipping off the area. Hot pack covers are equipped with velcro straps for this purpose.

4. Cover the pack with a rubber sheet or plastic (eg, materials such as those used for incontinent

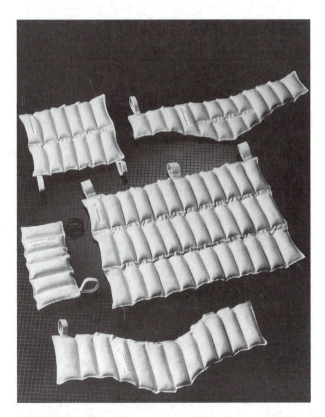

FIGURE 13–2   This photograph shows a variety of hot packs shaped to conform to specific parts of the body. In the top row are the standard "low back" and "cervical" styles. (Reproduced with permission from GE Miller, Inc., Yonkers, NY.)

patients) to prevent loss of heat to the surrounding environment. (Some envelopes have a plastic top layer.) The patient should then be properly draped with a sheet to prevent a chill if the air in the room is cool.

5. Always explain to the patient that he or she should feel a "comfortable warmth." In addition, provide a method of calling should the patient experience any discomfort. It is always necessary to explain to a patient that if the therapist is not immediately available and the pack feels too uncomfortably hot, the patient can remove the hot pack.

6. The skin should be inspected after 5 min to ensure that no extremely hot red areas or burns have developed. The therapist should continually check with the patient to make certain that no severe discomfort is felt.

7. It is advisable to have timers in each intervention room so that the duration of intervention can be monitored.

Postintervention Procedures.   After the intervention is completed, the therapist must do the following:

1. Dry and inspect the patient's skin.

2. Replace the drape sheet or clothes to avoid the patient's becoming chilled.

3. Replace the pack in the tank, following the rotation procedure.

4. Hang the covers and toweling to dry.

5. Put the towel layer that was next to the patient's skin in the laundry hamper.

Indications.   Hot packs are often used before or in conjunction with other techniques to achieve relaxation and sedation, or used when moist rather than dry heat is more comfortable for a patient. If the hot pack is an adjunct to subsequent techniques (modalities or exercise), remember to begin those interventions as soon as possible after the pack is removed so that the treated area does not cool down.

Contraindications.   When a patient has a local infection that could be exacerbated by moist heat, a hot pack should not be used. Furthermore, some dermatologic conditions may respond adversely to heat and moisture; therefore, the use of hot packs should be avoided in their presence. Further contraindications include use of heat

- over an area susceptible to hemorrhage;
- over a malignant area;
- over pelvic, abdominal, or low back area of a pregnant woman;
- on skin that must be visually monitored;
- over insensitive skin; and
- on a patient when direct pressure must be avoided.

Precautions.   Although a hot pack is not a source of constant heat, do *not* let the patient fall asleep on it. Make certain that the patient is aware of the true heat of the pack and will speak up if more toweling is required. Frequent (every 5 to 10 min) inspection of the area being treated is important during the first application burns must be avoided. Some patients cannot tolerate the weight of a hot pack. In such a case, another superficial heat modality should be used.

Keep in mind that hot packs heat only the superficial structures significantly. However, a study by Lehmann et al[6] did show a slight rise in TT at a depth of 1 cm and even a slight rise at a depth of 2 cm.

Home Uses

Thermotherapy is a modality that many individuals can independently apply at home. At-home modalities could include hot showers, foot or hand basins, microwaveable gel packs, single-use chemical heat wraps, and hot-water bottles. Providing patients with general safety precautions would allow safe application of moist heat at home. Patients must be informed about appropriate preparation of the modality, method of application, duration, frequency, and signs or symptoms of potential injury.

ThermaCare® and electric moist heating pads are also readily available. ThermaCare® HeatWraps are single-use devices with contents that react with oxygen when unwrapped. It takes 30 min of exposure for the wrap to reach its therapeutic temperature of 40°C (104°F), and it continues to stay warm for 8 hours. Electric heating pads are available with safety switches that allow the heating pad to increase in temperature only while the control is held in the on position. This feature will help prevent undue overheating if someone falls asleep with the unit turned on. Both devices are available in various sizes to accommodate different body segments.

Paraffin

Paraffin is another superficial heating method used to treat chronic joint disorders. This modality also transfers heat by conduction. Initially, the patient will experience a hot, but not painful sensation of heat, but the sensation will be one of pleasant warmth after about 3 to 5 min.

Duration. The intervention usually lasts 15 to 20 min. Because the paraffin solution is in the fluid state, its use is especially practical when treating distal joints that are difficult to heat evenly.

Equipment. A mixture of paraffin wax and mineral oil in a ratio of about 6 to 1 or 7 to 1 is melted in a tank.[7] The oil helps lower the melting point of the paraffin and make's it easily removable after intervention. The tank contains a built-in heating unit thermostat that should maintain the temperature at about 126–135°F (52.2–57.2°C) for upper extremities and 113–126°F (45–52°C) for lower extremities.[8,9] The temperature of the paraffin must be checked with a thermometer immersed in the solution before each intervention. Some tanks have thermometers that remain permanently inside (**Fig. 13–4**). The tanks currently used in

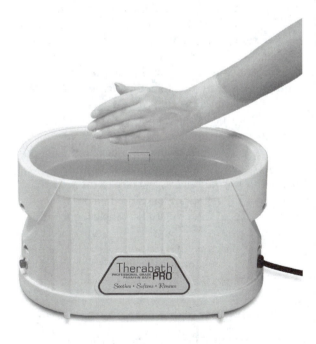

FIGURE 13–4 Paraffin bath application to the hand and wrist. (*Reproduced with permission from WR Medical Electronics Co., Stillwater, MN.*)

beauty salons are similar to those used in clinics but are set at lower temperatures, and the premixed paraffin mixtures used must contain more oils to lower the melting point. Insulated wrapping material (eg, plastic bags, aluminum foil, toweling, or commercially available paraffin) must be available and near the tank.

Techniques of Application. Because the skin temperature of the part being treated is lower than the temperature of the paraffin in the tank, a solid layer of paraffin forms on the skin when the part is immersed in the tank. This layer insulates the part, and the air trapped between each additional layer of paraffin also acts as an insulator. Therefore, the patient should be instructed not to move the part to avoid cracking the insulating layers. Even if the part remains in the tank, as is prescribed in one method, it will have the beneficial effects of the paraffin.

Before intervention the patient's skin should be checked for discolorations associated with circulatory problems, for open wounds or infections, and for a lack of thermal sensory integrity. If any of these conditions are present, the patient should *not* be treated with paraffin. If a wound is minor, it should be protected with gauze and a nonpermeable material such as a plastic strip. The part to be treated should be washed and dried before the intervention because the tank is used by many people. All rings and jewelry should be removed. The patient should be instructed that he or she should experience a "comfortable warmth" and that if the heat is intolerable, he or she should inform the clinician immediately.

Note that care must be taken to check the temperature of the paraffin *before* each use. It is best to leave a thermometer in the tank for accurate, satisfactory readings. If the thermostat is not checked, the patient could be severely burned by paraffin that is too hot. Thermometers that can be held and dipped into the tank for temperature readings are available.

Paraffin can be applied by three different methods: (1) the glove technique, (2) the dip-immersion technique, and (3) the brush technique. The most commonly used method is the glove technique, which involves dipping the relaxed body part (eg, the hand) into the tank several times. The fingers of the hand should be slightly abducted, if possible, to allow the fluid to surround them. Before the part is dipped into the paraffin, however, the patient must be instructed not to move or crack the layers of the paraffin glove or to touch the metal bottom or sides of the tank because they will feel hot. (Remember, metal is an excellent conductor of heat.) After the part is dipped into the paraffin, it is immediately removed, and the paraffin solidifies. This dipping is then repeated 8 to 10 times so that a glove of paraffin layers forms. The part should not be held out of the tank for more than a few seconds between dips to minimize heat dissipation. After the final dip, the treated part is immediately placed in a loose-fitting plastic bag, wax paper, plastic wrap, or aluminum foil, then wrapped in a mitt or several layers of towels to help maintain the heat. To increase the duration of the heat, the wrapped hand or foot may be placed between two small hot packs wrapped in the appropriate amount of toweling. Finally, the patient rests for 15 to 20 min with the treated part in a comfortable position with the extremity elevated above the heart.

In the second method, the dip-immersion technique, following the procedure, the part is immersed into the tank and allowed to remain there for about 15 minutes. With this method, much more heat is transferred to the body.

With the third method, the brush technique, an angular or difficult-to-reach part such as the elbow is painted with multiple layers of paraffin, wrapped as described in the glove technique and covered with towels for about 20 min.

Postintervention Procedures. With all three methods, the wax should be removed over the tank or a protective covering so that wax does not get on furniture or floors. Ask the patient to move the part so that the wax cracks, and then peel it off as if removing a glove or stocking. Encourage the patient to exercise the part immediately while it is still warm. Wipe the part to remove excess oil and perspiration, or use the oil to massage the part.

The three techniques just described heat only superficial tissues; however, one method described in the literature[9] claimed to achieve heating of deeper tissues (the joint capsule) without having a detrimental effect on superficial tissues. This method involved a seven-dip immersion method lasting for 30 min. The hand was then removed and wrapped in plastic and toweling for an additional 30 min.

Advantages. Because of its fluid nature, paraffin can heat areas that are difficult to reach because of bony prominences or uneven contours (eg, the hand). The paraffin-oil mixture softens the skin and prepares the part for massage or other modalities. The immersion technique of paraffin evenly heats the part being treated and therefore is useful for treating arthritic joints of the hands or feet. Paraffin is indicated for the patient with pain because of its soothing, comfortable heating properties.

Disadvantages. Paraffin interventions with open wounds are contraindicated because the wound and the tank can become contaminated. For other contraindications, see all of those listed in the previous section. The literature generally supports the use of paraffin with patients who have rheumatoid arthritis,[10] although some caution that joint temperatures could rise sufficiently to cause injury.

Some joints of the body are not accessible for immersion techniques. Although the brush method can be used, other heating methods may be more advantageous and easier to apply. Paraffin can be a messy procedure if the wax is not removed directly over the tank or protective covering.

Home Use. Paraffin units are now commonly available in drug or department stores, are safe, and are relatively inexpensive. They are useful for patients with chronic pain who cannot come often to the clinic or have been discharged from the physical therapy department.

The paraffin mixture is heated until it reaches a temperature of about 125°F (51.7°C); a candy thermometer can be used to measure the temperature. Then the mixture is removed from the heat source. If no thermometer is available, the wax should be cooled until a thin white coating appears on top. Dip the hand as described earlier.

Studies on the value of paraffin interventions are relatively limited in number.[2] Studies on the temperature of skin and underlying tissues following a 20-min intervention would help substantiate the value of this method of intervention that is used so often by physical therapists. An in vivo study comparing paraffin intervention with Fluidotherapy® and hydrotherapy found that paraffin intervention raised the temperature of the small joint capsule of the hand 13.5°F (7.5°C) at a depth of about 0.5 cm below the skin.[2]

Fluidotherapy®

Another form of superficial heating available to physical therapists is **Fluidotherapy®**, a piece of equipment that can be used as an alternative to paraffin or hydrotherapy in some instances, or when dry heat is desirable. This modality transfers heat by convection.

Fluidotherapy® has been in existence since the 1970s, but the construction of the unit has changed slightly over the years. Extremely small solid particles are heated and suspended by circulating air, thus producing an effect similar to circulating warm liquid. The thermal conductivity and specific heat of the particles and air allow the temperature of the unit to be higher than that of water used therapeutically; that is, the patient can safely tolerate a higher temperature. The feeling produced by the unit resembles that produced by placing a hand in a small enclosed box with heated, air-blown particles.

Minimal research has been published comparing this modality with other forms of superficial heat. Clinicians are encouraged to assist in the validation of this modality.

Duration.   The duration of intervention is recommended to be between 15 and 20 min.

Equipment.   The machine stands 3 feet high (**Fig. 13–5**) and contains a heating element, an air com-

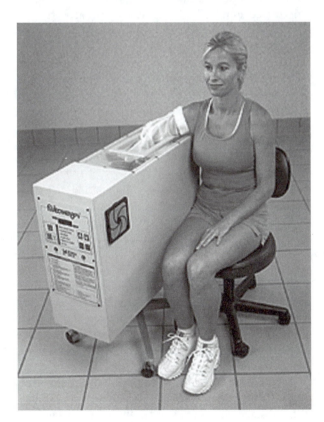

FIGURE 13–5 Fluidotherapy application to the hand, wrist, and forearm. (*Courtesy of Chattanooga Group, Hixson, TN.*)

pressor, tiny silicon or corncob particles in an enclosed see-through container into which the limb is inserted, a timer, a temperature gauge, and a mesh sleeve. The sleeve can be closed snugly around the proximal portion of the arm or leg, thus preventing the circulating particles from blowing into the room. There are usually four openings for the insertion of a limb: two on the top of the unit, which are best for a hand, and two on the side for hand or foot. In addition to this unit for limbs, larger units are available to accommodate the lower back and thigh areas. All the information that follows refers to the smaller units.

Technique of Application.   As is the case for other superficial heat modalities, before initiating the following procedures, the therapist or therapy assistant must inspect the body part for skin integrity, good circulation, and sensitivity to heat. The patient should be instructed that he or she should experience a "comfortable warmth" and should notify the clinician if the heat becomes intolerable. Application is as follows:

1. Wash and dry the part to be treated because other patients will be using the same container.

2. Remove all jewelry from the part being treated.

3. Check the part for open wounds. The manufacturer recommends that if an open wound is present, the body part should be placed in a plastic bag or large rubber glove so that no particles enter the wound.

4. Insert the body part into the sleeve, and close the sleeve snugly around the more proximal portion of the limb so that particles do not come out once the blower is turned on.

5. Set the thermostat at the desired temperature (usually between 115°F and 123°F (46.1–50.6°C), depending on the patient's tolerance.

6. Turn the timer on (usually for 15 to 20 min).

7. Instruct the patient about ways to exercise or stretch (or help the patient perform these activities) during the intervention if these activities are appropriate for the condition being treated. If a patient's hand is being treated through the side opening, the therapist can insert his or her hands through the top openings to help the patient exercise. The therapist also can watch what is going on.

Postintervention Procedure.   When the intervention is finished, loosen the sleeve. Before removing the limb from the unit, help the patient remove all the particles from the limb so that the intervention area remains clean and few particles are lost from the tank. Then, inspect the limb once again, and continue with other interventions as necessary.

Advantages.   The remarkable aspect of Fluidotherapy® intervention is that the circulating, air-blown, warmed particles give the patient the feeling of lightness and surrounding warmth provided by a whirlpool bath. In addition, because the limb is free to move, active exercise is possible. As mentioned, the therapist or assistant can insert his or her hand or hands through a separate access sleeve to perform passive range of motion or stretching procedures to the part being treated or to assist the patient in exercise.

A limb can be inserted in the unit and positioned in the horizontal plane, thus minimizing the effects of gravity; remember, the dependent position can lead to edema. Because this is a dry-heat method, the patient can tolerate a higher temperature than in a hydrotherapy intervention. Like paraffin or water, the circulating particles can surround uneven, bony parts. Finally, because the unit does not require a water source, it can be placed anywhere in the physical therapy department.

Disadvantages.   The limb units are too small to accommodate more than a distal limb; thus, they cannot be used to treat a back, hip, or shoulder. The larger units have a nylon cloth on which a patient can lie if the lower back or thigh is treated. Open wounds cannot be treated unless they are protected. Furthermore, wounds cannot be debrided (unhealthy tissue removed) as in the whirlpool.

As is the case with other superficial heat interventions, more studies must be done to validate the effects of this modality on the tissues being treated. Studies performed by Henley[11] indicated that Fluidotherapy® intervention did, in fact, increase the temperature, blood flow, and metabolic rate in the treated area. In another study, Valenza et al[12] found that a maximum increase in the temperature (measured with a thermistor) of the medial capsule of the first metatarsophalangeal joint occurred at the temperature provided by Fluidotherapy® (115–123°F; 46.1–50.6°C) compared with a 102°F (38.9°C) hydrotherapy intervention and a 126°F (52.2°C) paraffin (glove) intervention, all of which were performed for 20 min.

An in vivo study by Borrell et al[3] compared the glove method of paraffin intervention (126°F;

52.2°C) with hydrotherapy (102°F; 38.9°C) and Fluidotherapy® (118°F; 47.8°C). Fluidotherapy® appeared to raise the temperature of the small joint capsule the most; however, this study has been criticized for not using the optimal methods for the paraffin intervention or hydrotherapy. (We would have recommended higher temperatures for the hydrotherapy and the immersion technique for the paraffin intervention.)

Alcorn et al,[13] described a study using Fluidotherapy® and exercise for patients in crisis from sickle cell anemia. The authors reported that the results were positive: the intervention reduced the length of the patients' hospital stays and need for analgesics.

Infrared Radiation

Infrared radiation is an extremely useful modality for providing superficial heat. The physical laws governing radiated energy are discussed in **Chapter 7**, which contains a graphic representation of various waves of electromagnetic energy in ascending order of wavelength (see **Fig. 7–2**). Infrared rays are a portion of the electromagnetic spectrum and are just beyond the red portion of visible light. As discussed in **Chapter 7**, the depth of penetration to which electromagnetic energy is absorbed depends on the wavelength.

When a material is heated, it gives off electromagnetic rays in the infrared ranges (the result of electrons vibrating in their orbits). The range of infrared rays for heating superficial tissue is divided into **near infrared** (800–1500 nanometers) and **far infrared** (1500–150,000 nanometers).

Certain principles must be understood before a discussion of the clinical uses of infrared energy can proceed. When rays strike the skin or travel from one tissue to another, they can either be absorbed or be reflected (turned back) toward the source. The proportion of rays reflected depends on the angle at which they strike the surface, the type of surface they encounter, and the actual wavelength of the rays. According to the cosine law (**see Chapter 7**), optimal absorption will occur when the rays strike perpendicularly (at a right angle to a surface). Even then, however, some rays may be reflected.

According to the inverse squares law, the intensity of rays from a source varies inversely with the square of the distance from the source. Because equal energy is dispersed over a larger area, the intensity per area is diminished. Similarly, the patient will receive four times as much heat per area from an infrared lamp at a distance of 2 feet than at a distance of 4 feet, providing that the rays reach the patient at a 90° angle (obeying the cosine law).

Duration.   Interventions last about 20 min for maximum heating. However, the time depends on the intensity desired and the distance of the lamp from the body part. The distance should be increased if the skin turns more than a rosy pink or if the patient complains of too much heat.

Equipment.   Two types of therapeutic infrared instruments are available: luminous and nonluminous. The **luminous infrared instrument** produces mainly near infrared rays, and the **nonluminous infrared instrument** produces mainly far infrared rays. As determined by their specific wavelengths, the near rays penetrate to subcutaneous tissue, whereas the far rays are absorbed primarily by the superficial epidermis.[14]

Luminous (near) rays are produced by an incandescent tungsten and carbon filament encased in a quartz tube (similar to a lightbulb). Nonluminous (far) rays are often produced by a metal spiral coil around a nonconducting material such as porcelain. As electricity flows through the coil, it encounters resistance, thus producing heat. Most machines used in clinics radiate electromagnetic energy in the near, far, and visible light ranges of the spectrum. Even the nonluminous lamps give off a minimal glow, indicating the presence of some visible light.

Both luminous and nonluminous machines have a reflecting hood designed to reflect the rays downward, thus evenly radiating the area directly under the lamp (**Fig. 13–6**). This method of reflection minimizes the focal points of heat, thus minimizing the possibility of spot burns (areas of concentrated heat energy). Coverings must be available to protect eyes, hair, and the skin areas not to be treated.

Techniques of Application.   Again, before initiating the following procedures, the therapist or assistant must inspect the part for skin integrity, good circulation, and sensitivity to heat. The patient should be instructed that he or she should experience a "comfortable warmth" and should notify the clinician if the heat becomes intolerable. Then the following steps should be followed:

1. The therapist should allow a few minutes for the nonluminous instrument to warm up before beginning the intervention. The luminous lamp can be used immediately.

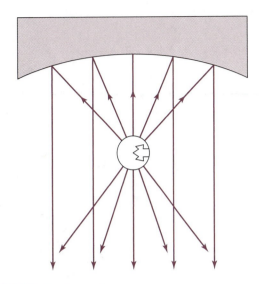

FIGURE 13–6   A diagrammatic representation of a reflecting hood on an infrared lamp showing that energy is radiated most evenly to the area of the body directly beneath the lamp.

2. The patient is placed in a relaxed, comfortable position with the body part to be treated properly exposed and devoid of all creams, ointments, and the like.

3. Position the lamp between 18 and 36 inches from the part being treated (luminous unit, 18–24 inches; nonluminous unit, 29–36 inches). Depending on the patient's tolerance to heat, condition (ie, the competency of the patient's vascular system), and the specifications of the particular piece of equipment, the distance between the part and the machine can be increased. Do not change the height of the lamp while it is above the patient because the lamp itself may fall on the patient while bolts or other parts are loosened. Make certain that the lamp is aligned with the body part being treated to avoid reflection and to allow as much absorption of rays as possible (**Fig. 13–7**).

4. All jewelry in the area must be removed or, if not removable, covered with reflecting tape to avoid burns. If an area near the face is being treated, covering the eyes with cotton balls, gauze, or goggles may be advisable. Cover hair (it can dry out) and all of the body other than the intervention area with reflecting material such as white sheets or pillowcases.

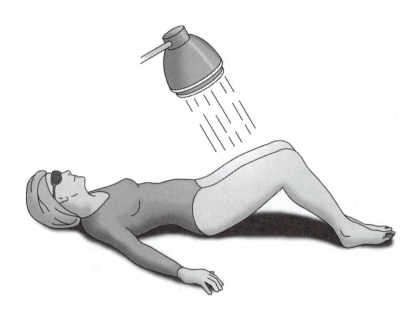

FIGURE 13–7   An infrared lamp aligned parallel with the body part being treated so that direct rays are at a 90° angle for maximum absorption.

5. During intervention, the therapist should periodically check the patient's skin and wipe off perspiration so that spot burns do not develop. Some therapists place a single layer of thin toweling over the part being treated to absorb perspiration; however, the skin must still be checked for redness.

Special Techniques.   If the therapist wants to use a moist heat intervention, but hot packs or whirlpools are unavailable or cannot be tolerated, a turkish towel that has been moistened and wrung out can be used in conjunction with infrared therapy. The towel should be placed over the part to be treated.

When prolonged mild heat is indicated and the heat cannot be applied directly to the skin—for example, in cases of drying out pressure sores (decubitus ulcers) or trying to increase circulation in that area—infrared radiation can be used at a greatly reduced intensity. For example, a 150-w lamp at a distance of 40 inches for 30 min.

Precaution.   If the patient lacks sensation in the treated area, burns can occur. As was noted earlier, if mottling is already present in the area, it signals that the superficial dermal heat control mechanism is being pushed to its maximum. (Refer to the general contraindications for superficial heat presented earlier.)

Advantages.   Infrared intervention may be used to treat a larger body part, such as the lumbar and thoracic area of the back, that cannot always be covered completely by a hot pack. Patients who cannot tolerate the direct contact or weight of another modality such as a hot pack or ultrasound may feel comfortable during an infrared intervention. Because the heat from infrared lamps is so soothing and gentle, patients who are extremely tense may become more relaxed and ready for additional interventions.

Disadvantages.   The use of any heating modality on open wounds requires caution since exposed subcutaneous tissues are less tolerant of heating. Infrared radiation dries the skin more than other thermal modalities, and therefore its application over open wounds is questionable since wounds heal better in a moist environment. In addition, burns may occur when an irregular or a bony body part such as the shoulder is treated if the machine is too close or if the intervention time is not closely monitored. Thus, patients must be watched closely to ensure that the skin is not becoming too red. Finally, some patients may find dry heat to be agitating or irritating.

Although infrared is a superficial heat source, Kramer[15] compared the heating effects of continuous ultrasound and infrared radiation with placebo and found that both the conduction velocity of the ulnar nerve (distal humeral segment) and the temperature of the subcutaneous tissue increased with both modalities.

When deciding on which superficial thermal modality to use, the advantages and disadvantages of each should be considered. **Box 13–3** summarizes the advantages and disadvantages of the different superficial thermal modalities.

REVIEW QUESTIONS

1. If a patient has an open cut on the hand that requires intervention for arthritis, which superficial heat modality would you select? Why?

2. Should heat be used on an acute injury?

3. Identify the contraindications for the use of local heating.

4. How long is the usual intervention time for the following modalities?
   a. hot packs
   b. paraffin
   c. Fluidotherapy®
   d. infrared radiation

Box 13–3 *Advantages and Disadvantages of the Superficial Thermal Modalities*

Modality	Advantages	Disadvantages
Hot packs	Are safe as they cool during treatment.	Weight of packs may be uncomfortable.
	Have good access to trunk and proximal limbs.	Treatment area is not visible. There is risk of infection with open wounds.
Paraffin	Is good for distal extremities and joint contours.	Cannot use with presence of open wounds and skin lesions.
	Softens and soothes skin.	Treatments may be messy.
	Has effective elevation of tissue temperature in the hands.	
Fluidotherapy®	Patient can exercise during intervention.	Is difficult to use on proximal extremities and trunk.
	Is good for distal extremities and joint contours.	Treatment area is not visible.
	Has increased mechanical stimulation.	
	Has good temperature control.	
Infrared	Is good for treating large areas.	Is difficult to treat localized area.
	No pressure exerted on treatment area.	Excessive heating with changes in patient position.
	Treatment area is visible.	Excessive drying associated with infrared radiation.

5. When placing a hot pack on a patient, approximately how many layers of toweling should be used in addition to the hot pack cover?

6. On what part of the body other than the neck might you use a cervical hot pack? Explain.

7. What sanitary precautions need to be taken with hot packs? With paraffin?

8. Why should the therapist check the skin and wipe off the patient's perspiration during infrared interventions?

9. Should infrared radiation ever be used to treat decubitus ulcers? Why?

10. To what level does each of the following infrared interventions penetrate?
    a. luminous rays
    b. nonluminous rays

KEY TERMS

superfical heat
hot packs
Fluidotherapy®

near infrared
far infrared

luminous infrared instrument
nonluminous infrared instrument

REFERENCES

1. Lehmann JF, ed: *Therapeutic Heat and Cold*, 4th ed. Baltimore: Williams & Wilkins; 1990.

2. Borrell RM, Parker R, Henley RJ, et al: Comparison of in vivo temperature produced by hydrotherapy, paraffin wax treatment, and Fluidotherapy. *Phys Ther* 1980; 60:1273–76.

3. Abramson DI: Comparison of wet and dry heat in raising temperature of tissue. *Arch Phy Med Rehab* 1967; 48:654.

4. Erasala GN, Rubin JM, Tuthill TA, et al: The effect of topical heat treatment on trapezius muscle blood flow using power Doppler untrasound. *Phys Ther* 2001; 81(5):A5.

5. Lehmann JF, Massock AJ, Warren CG, et al: Effect of therapeutic temperature on tendon extensibility. *Arch Phys Med Rehabil* 1970; 51:481–87.

6. Lehmann JF, Silverman DR, Baum BA, et al: Temperature distribution in the human thigh produced by infrared, hot pack, and microwave applications. *Arch Phys Med Rehabil* 1966; 47:291–99.

7. Krusen FH, ed: *Krusen's Handbook of Physical Medicine and Rehabilitation*. Philadelphia: Saunders; 1982.

8. Griffin JE, Karselis TC: *Physical Agents for Physical Therapists*, 3rd ed. Springfield, MO: Charles C Thomas; chap 5, 1988; 212.

9. Abramson DL, Tuck SI, Chu LSW, et al: Effects of paraffin bath and hot fomentations on local tissue temperature. *Arch Phys Med Rehabil* 1964; 45:87–94.

10. Belanger AY: *Evidence-Based Guide to Therapeutic Physical Agents*. Philadelphia: Lippincott Williams & Wilkins, 2002.

11. Henley EJ: Engineering and medicine—Fluidotherapy. *Chemtech* 1982; 215–20.

12. Valenza J, Rossi C, Parker R, et al: A clinical study of a new heat modality—Fluidotherapy. *J Am Podiat Assoc* 1979; 69:440–42.

13. Alcorn R, Bowser R, Henley E, et al: Fluidotherapy and exercise in the management of sickle cell anemia: A clinical report. *J Am Phys Ther Assoc* 1984; 64:1520–22.

14. Kitchen S, Bazin S, eds: *Clayton's Electrotherapy*, 10th ed. Philadelphia: Saunders; 1981.

15. Kramer JP: Ultrasound: Evaluation of its mechanical and thermal effects. *Arch Phys Med Rehabil* 1984; 65:223–27.

14

Cryotherapy

BERNADETTE HECOX, PT, MA
JOHN P. SANKO, PT, EdD

Chapter Outline

Cryotherapy, or cold therapy, has been used in medicine over the centuries. The Greek word *cryos* means "cold." The physical and physiologic effects of cooling localized tissues or generalized body cooling have already been detailed in **Chapters 8 through 11.** This chapter introduces the reader to the clinical aspects of cryotherapy as used in physical therapy. Physical therapists and assistants frequently use cold in the intervention for various orthopedic, neurologic, and other disorders.

COMMON CONSIDERATIONS

Tissue temperature can be reduced by (1) applying a low-temperature solid—ice, liquid, or slush—directly to the skin (heat transfer by conduction); (2) immersing a body part in cold or ice water (heat transfer by conduction and convection); (3) blowing a volatile liquid (eg, Spray & Stretch®) on the part being treated (heat transfer by evaporation); and (4) blowing cold air on a part being treated (heat transfer by convection), a method not used often in physical therapy. Because heat always travels from hot to cold, the tissues are cooled because they transfer their heat to the cold modality. The cold does not transfer to the body.

Cryotherapy in its various forms is recognized as an important intervention because it can reduce pain and spasms,[1–6] thereby breaking the cycle of pain, spasms, and ischemia.[7] It can also decrease the inflammatory process, bleeding and hemorrhage, and possibly traumatic edema. Application of a cold modality can also diminish the effects of central and peripheral nerve disorders. Spasticity, such as that caused by a stroke or spinal cord lesion, can be diminished for brief periods,[8] and motor responses in patients can be facilitated by using specific techniques—for example, the quick icing technique described by Rood.[9] Some patients may experience a "rebound phenomenon" with increased spasticity from 30 min to 2 hours after removal of the cold modality.[10] **Box 14–1** lists common clinical uses and rationale for cryotherapy.

Prior to the application of a cold modality, the clinician and patient need to be familiar with cryotherapy contraindications. **Box 14–2** lists contraindications and their rationale when considering the use of cryotherapy.

Numerous methods of intervention with cold are available, including ice massage, chemical cold packs, ice towels, ice packs, vapocoolant sprays, quick icing, cold combined with compression, and cold immersion (baths). Before applying any form of cryotherapy, the physical therapist or assistant should do the following:

1. Inspect the patient's skin to determine whether any rashes or discolorations are present.
2. Test a small area of skin (not on the part to be treated) to determine whether the patient is hypersensitive to cold.
3. Perform a sensory test in the intervention area to assess the patient's ability to perceive hot and cold stimuli.
4. Verify that the circulatory status of the body part is good.

Box 14–1 *Clinical Uses of Cryotherapy*

Clinical Use	Rationale
Following deep friction massage, joint mobilization, and strenuous exercise	Minimize acute inflammation associated with therapeutic intervention
Reduction of edema and bleeding	Decrease tissue metabolism to reduce secondary hypoxia and increase blood viscosity
Reduction of pain and muscle spasm	Decrease neural input and nerve conduction velocity in pain and muscle spindle afferents
Reduction of spasticity	Decrease neural input and nerve conduction velocity in muscle spindle afferents
Immediate intervention for small acute burns	Reduce pain and subsequent blistering
Increasing tolerance for graded exercise (cryokinetics)	Elevate pain threshold by decreasing neural input and nerve conduction velocity

Box 14–2 *Contraindications for Cryotherapy*

Contraindication	Rationale
Severe hypertension and unstable cardiac conditions	Extensive vasoconstriction occurs with generalized applications.
Poor peripheral circulation	Inability to shunt warm blood to treatment area may lead to tissue damage.
Cold hypersensitivity (cold uticaria, Raynaud's phenomena)	Cold may trigger allergic reactions and exacerbation of symptoms associated with certain diseases.
Over open wounds	Loss of superfical insulation. Hypothermia decreases metabolism and may impede tissue healing.
Over ansesthetic skin	Decrease the ability to report excessive cooling.
For individuals with impaired mentation	Decrease the ability to report excessive cooling.
Over regenerating peripheral nerves	Reduction in tensile strength of new neural tissue.

5. Make certain that the patient has not had frostbite in the area to be treated.

6. Make certain that the patient has never previously experienced an exacerbation of spasticity when cold was used.

7. See that the patient is positioned comfortably and draped well to avoid chilliness during the intervention.

Forms of Intervention

Ice Massage

Ice massage, the stroking of ice on a body part, is generally used to anesthetize the skin. Longer exposure is required to lower intramuscular temperature. When performing an ice massage, the therapist must take into account the size and the amount of fat of the area being treated[11] (see **Chapter 11**).

Equipment. Ice massage can be performed in three ways. The therapist can use (1) ice that has been frozen in an insulated cup, (2) a "lollipop," a small cylindrical container with a tongue depressor frozen in the middle, or (3) an ice cube wrapped in paper towels or a washcloth. In the first two techniques, the container helps form a smooth, rounded surface. With the ice cube, however, the therapist must round the end of the cube so that the patient does not feel a sharp edge. In all three techniques, the therapist's hand is protected from the cold either by the insulation of the cup, by holding the tongue depressor, or by the paper towels or washcloth (**Fig. 14–1**). Extra towels should be available to absorb water dripping from the melting ice.

Technique. The therapist describes for the patient the most likely sensations felt during an ice massage: first cold, then burning, then aching, and finally numbness. In addition, the therapist informs the patient that the part being treated may become pale and eventually red. Color changes are the result of the hunting reaction described in **Chapter 11**. If the normal responses mentioned before are not explained properly, the patient may want to end the intervention because of discomfort or fear.

The ice should be applied in smooth circular, rhythmical strokes over the intervention area, reducing the size of the circles as the massage proceeds. Because water from the melting ice can be uncomfortable for the patient, it is wiped up with extra towels. The therapist avoids bumping into bony prominences because this too can be uncomfortable.

Duration. To anesthetize an area, the intervention should last from about 3 to 10 min or more, depending on the size of the area being treated. For example, the lateral aspect of the ankle might be treated for only 3 min, whereas 10 min might be required to treat the hamstrings. Of course, the intervention time may vary, depending on the patient. Note that

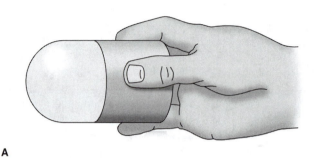

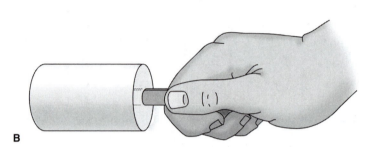

FIGURE 14–1   Ice massage modalities. Ice is frozen in a cylindrical container. (**A**) Ice frozen in a paper cup. The top half of the cup is cut away so the ice will come in contact with the patient. The therapist holds the lower part of the cup while stroking the ice over the part to be treated. (**B**) The "lollipop" technique. A tongue depressor is frozen in the center of the container, the ice is then removed from the container, and the therapist uses the tongue depressor as a handle.

ice massage should stop when the patient reports numbness.

Advantages.   Because ice massage easily and rapidly anesthetizes the skin, a painful technique such as deep friction massage can be performed without causing discomfort to the patient. Ice is colder than the chemical cold packs that will be discussed next. Small areas near bony prominences can be treated easily without directly affecting the surrounding skin and underlying tissues. Finally, ice in some form is usually readily available.

Disadvantages.   The disadvantages are few, except for the drips of cold water that can cause the patient discomfort. The therapist's hands must be protected

from the cold by the insulation of the cup, the paper towels, or the tongue depressor. Because the ice may cause frostbite, the therapist must always check the color of the patient's skin. If the skin turns blue, ice should be removed immediately.

Chemical Cold Packs

Three types of **chemical cold packs** are available. The clinical type of cold pack has a durable plastic cover around a silica gel (similar to a hot pack) and is stored in a refrigerator tank. The second type is similar to but smaller than the clinical cold pack; these can be purchased in most pharmacies and can be stored in the freezer of a home refrigerator. The third type must be activated by breaking an inner seal that mixes the chemicals within. This type must be disposed of after one use because the ice pack will warm up once the chemical reaction has taken place; these cold packs are usually readily available at health spas or gymnastic and other sports events for immediate emergency use. This section focuses on the chemical cold packs available in most clinics: for example, **Hydrocollator®** **cold packs** or **Col-Pack® cold packs**.

Equipment.   Chemical cold packs are stored in a refrigeration tank resembling the one used for chemical hot packs. A thermostat maintains the temperature at about 10–15°F (–12.2 to –9.4°C). The cold packs should remain in the tank at least 24 hours before the first use and at least 30 min between subsequent uses. The chemical cold packs, like hot packs, are available in different sizes and shapes. The most common are those for the cervical and low-back areas (**Fig. 14–2**).

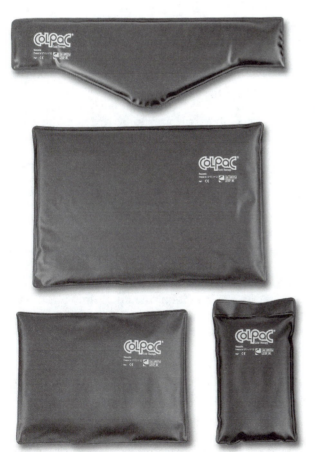

FIGURE 14–2 Variety of clinical gel cold packs. (*Courtesy of Chattanooga Group, Hixson, TN.*)

Technique.   The chemical cold pack should not be placed directly on the patient's skin, not only to ensure hygiene but also to prevent irritation. Many therapists advocate using a wet, well-wrung-out towel or cloth (cold or warm, depending on the patient's tolerance of cold). The wet towel hastens the cooling of the part being treated because the moisture increases the rate of thermal conductivity. Some therapists choose to use a dry towel or pillowcase to enhance the patient's comfort; the cooling effect is slower and permits the patient to adjust gradually to the cold temperature. The pack should be insulated by covering it with a towel or rubber mat to prevent its being warmed by the ambient air. The patient is draped with a sheet or light blanket to prevent chilling. The therapist checks the skin after 5 min to make sure that it is not bluish; if it is, the pack should be removed immediately.

Duration.   The cold pack should be kept on the part for 10 to 15 min. Duration of intervention depends on the amount of subcutaneous fat and the desired depth of cooling. After 15 min the temperature of the pack will have increased substantially.

Advantages.   Chemical cold packs are found in almost all physical therapy facilities and, as mentioned earlier, come in different shapes and sizes to fit the contours of many different body parts. These packs are reusable. Once it has been determined that the patient can tolerate a cold pack, the therapist can leave the patient and work with another patient when necessary. Chemical cold packs can be used immediately after injuries such as sprains or fractures.

Disadvantages.   The cold offered by some chemical cold packs may be less intense than that provided by an ice massage or ice pack. Chemical cold packs must be kept in the refrigeration unit at least 30 min before reusing, whereas ice can be used immediately. In addition, the chemical cold packs are more sensitive than homemade crushed ice packs and tend to break.

Ice Towels

Ice towels are towels containing ice shavings. They can be used if chemical cold packs and their refrigeration units are not readily available.

Equipment.   Terry cloth towels and a container of ice water with ice shavings are the only necessary equipment. The ice shavings are caught in the nap of the towel, allowing a substantial cooling effect.

Technique.   A terry cloth towel should be thoroughly soaked in the water and ice-shaving mixture. The towel is then wrung out and applied to the part being treated. Because the ice shavings melt quickly, the procedure is repeated every few minutes to achieve the greatest cooling possible.

Duration.   As with cold packs, the intervention time should be about 10 to 15 min.

Advantages.   The equipment required is available almost anywhere. No special refrigeration unit is required, although some type of freezer to make ice or ice shavings must be available.

Disadvantages.   The main disadvantage of ice towels is that the therapist must keep changing the towels because they warm rapidly. In addition, because ice water can wet the floor, it must be cleaned up so that no one slips or falls.

Ice Packs

Equipment.   **Ice packs** are simply plastic bags filled with ice cubes or crushed ice. As this definition implies, all that is required is a heavy plastic bag filled with ice or crushed ice. The crushed ice is preferable because the bag will be more easily molded to the part being treated. Towels also must be available.

Technique.   The bag should be filled with ice or ice shavings and be sealed well to prevent melting ice from leaking on the patient or the floor. The technique is the same as that for chemical cold packs. It is usually preferable to place a warm, damp towel between the plastic bag and the patient's skin, mainly for comfort. As is the case for all other interventions, the patient should be placed in a comfortable position and draped well if the ambient air is cold.

Duration.   The ice pack should remain in place from 5 to 15 min, depending on the amount of fat in the treated area and the depth of cold penetration desired, as well as whether there is a towel between the pack and the skin. When striving to cool deeper muscles in some cases of spasticity, the time can be extended to 20 to 40 min (see **Chapter 9**).[12]

Advantages.   The ice pack is useful because it can be molded around the part being treated, and it usually allows the subcutaneous areas to get much colder than does a chemical cold pack.

Disadvantages.   The plastic bag can leak, making it uncomfortable for the patient and dangerous for people in the area if the floor becomes wet. Furthermore, the therapist must continually check the patient's skin because ice can cause frostbite.

Cryo-Cuff®

Cryo-Cuff® is a system for applying cold compression to various areas of the body. Cuffs are available for the shoulder, knee, foot and ankle, and thigh and calf (**Fig. 14–3A, B**). Cryo/Temp®, which is the coldest form of cryotherapy available, is discussed in **Chapter 26**.

Equipment.   The system includes the cuff, cooler, and tube.

Technique.   The cuff is applied to the appropriate area of the body and attached to a tube connected to the cooler. The cooler is filled with ice and water, and is positioned above the area to be treated. The water fills the cuff, and the hydrostatic pressure provides a compressive force to the intervention area. The hydrostatic force is determined by the elevation of the cooler. Every inch above the intervention area produces a pressure of 1.8 mm Hg. When the water in the cuff becomes warm, the cooler is lowered until the cuff is drained, then it is raised again in order to refill the cuff with colder water.

Duration.   The desired length of intervention is dependent on the condition, the intervention goal, and the individual's tolerance. An ice- and water-filled cooler can provide cold water for 6 to 8 hours.

Advantages.   The Cryo-Cuff® allows the therapist to apply cold and compression simultaneously. Because the system is closed, there is no melting ice or dripping water.

Disadvantages.   Special cuffs are needed for various parts of the body. Only one individual per cooler can be treated. Also, they are more expensive than other cooling choices.

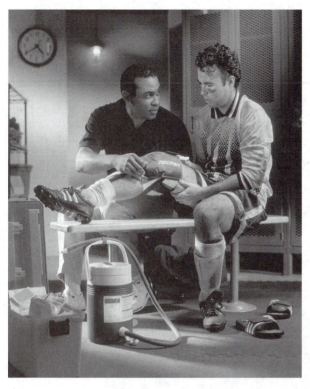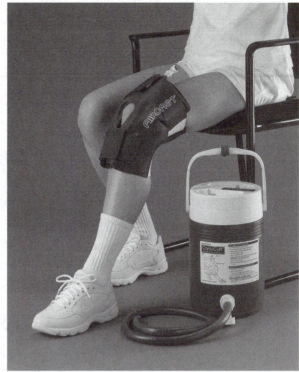

FIGURE 14–3   Cryotherapy may be provided by the Cryo/Cuff®. Simplicity of design and ease of operation permit its use for the ER, post-op, training room, or home. (*Courtesy of Aircast Incorporated, Summit, NJ.*)

Vapocoolant Spray

Vapocoolant spray is a method of cooling the skin by the evaporation of a substance sprayed on the skin. Travell[12] used Kraus's method of spraying ethyl chloride on a sprained joint of the middle finger of a young patient and found that the joint was less painful after the spraying and that the normal range of motion was restored quickly. Travell developed the "stretch and spray" technique for treating trigger points. (Trigger points are discussed in **Chapter 6**.) Theoretically, through cooling and desensitization the pain cycle can be broken. However, some authors believe that counterirritation is the means by which the pain is alleviated[13,14] (ie, stimulation of cold or touch can diminish transmission of pain signals).

Equipment.   Two vapocoolant sprays are available: ethyl chloride and Spray & Stretch®. Today, ethyl chloride is used less frequently because it is highly flammable when heated and may cause general anesthesia in patients who inhale large amounts. Ethyl chloride places pressure (as does any aerosol spray) on its container when at room temperature and can explode if dropped. In clinical physical therapy, the use of Spray & Stretch® has replaced ethyl chloride. When sprayed from an inverted bottle, the liquid begins evaporating. It continues to evaporate upon contact with the skin, thus cooling the skin for a brief period. Spray & Stretch® is a fluorocarbon. Although fluorocarbons were banned in 1990 because of their potentially harmful effects to the earth's ozone layer, Gebauer, the maker of Spray & Stretch®, was granted a medical exemption from this ban, and Spray & Stretch® continues to be available.

Technique.   The area to be treated is exposed, and the other parts should be covered for warmth and comfort. The patient is draped and positioned so that the eyes are protected. The bottle of Spray & Stretch® must be held in an inverted position to ensure flow of the liquid. According to Travell,[12] the liquid should be sprayed at a 30° angle, 18 inches away from the skin, moving at a rate of 4 inches per second (**Fig. 14–4**).

Travell[12] advises beginning at the origin of pain and continuing out over the area of referred pain, spraying the entire length of the muscle once it is in a stretch position. The muscle is stretched passively before and during spraying. This pattern of spraying is repeated a couple of times. Note that the speed of spraying depends on the patient's condition and response to the technique.

Duration.   Spraying should not exceed 6 seconds, so that frosting of the skin can be avoided. Should frosting occur, a quick, light massage to the area will help defrost it.

Advantages.   Vapocoolant spray offers a quick reaction for immediate reduction of pain. It has also been cited in the intervention of

- joint sprains to relieve pain and swelling and possibly lead to early restoration of motion,[12]
- thermal burns to decrease pain, erythema, and blistering (especially in first-degree burns),[15] and
- painful areas in acute myocardial infarction to replace some pain medications.[16]

Travell[12] advises placing a hot pack briefly over the area after intervention with stretch and spray to avoid subsequent muscle soreness.

Disadvantages.   The therapist must be careful not to spray the patient's eyes; the patient must be draped carefully to protect the face when treating the anterior

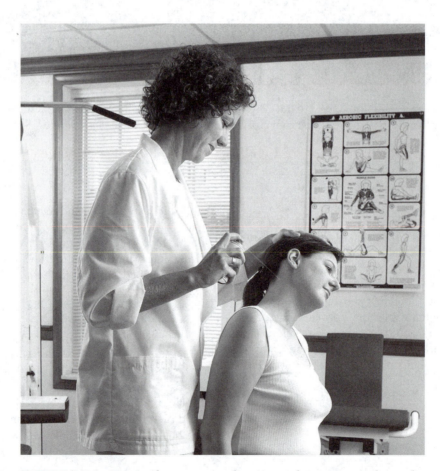

FIGURE 14–4   Vapocoolant spray application to the paracervical muscles (care by the clinician should be taken to protect the patient's face). (*Reproduced with permission from the Gebauer Company, Cleveland, OH.*)

cervical musculature, for example. Frosting of the skin needs to be avoided because it can lead to ulceration. When using ethyl chloride, the therapist must take extreme care not to drop the bottle because it could explode. Finally, the spray cools only a limited area, and the propellent is destructive to the environment.

Quick Icing

Quick icing involves the use of 3 to 5 swipes of ice along an area to be facilitated. Although this special technique of facilitating muscle contractions is used primarily in patients with central nervous system (CNS) disorders, it can certainly be used on patients with peripheral nerve injuries. This technique should be used with care over any area of inadequate sensation.

Equipment.   An ice cube held in a paper towel or gauze (see the section Ice Massage) plus towels to absorb water are the only equipment necessary.

Technique.   According to Margaret Rood,[9] who developed this technique, quick swipes with an ice cube over the belly of the involved muscle must be performed 3 to 5 times to produce the desired effect, which might occur immediately or from 27 to 42 min after application.

Advantages.   A motor response may be seen—in a hemiplegic patient, for example—once the patient is past the flaccid stage. The technique is not uncomfortable or dangerous.

Disadvantages.   A response may not be seen immediately, a possibility that can be frustrating for both the patient and the therapist.

RICE Therapy

In the acute stages of trauma, such as a sprain, strain, or fracture, cryotherapy can be combined with compression and elevation of the involved part to reduce or prevent pain, bleeding, and swelling. Cold packs, ice towels, or ice packs may be used. The technique is known by the acronym **RICE therapy** because it includes the following:

Rest (removing weight-bearing pressure and temporarily immobilizing the part).

Ice (or another cold modality).

Compression (usually with an ace bandage or an air splint).

Elevation of the involved limb as much as possible for the first 24 to 48 hours.

If Cryo/Temp is used (see **Chapter 26**), because it is a modality combining cold and compression, the therapist must take great care to avoid pressure sufficient to increase bleeding or inflammation in an already painful, sensitive area. Intervention should be limited to about 20 min and can be repeated after about 30 min to 1 hour.

When deciding which cold modality to use, the advantages and disadvantages of each should be considered. **Box 14–3** summarizes the advantages and disadvantages of the different forms of cryotherapy

SPECIAL CONSIDERATIONS

The application of cold can lead to reduced speed of muscle contraction because of slower nerve conduction velocity. In addition, increased viscosity of joints, tendons, and ligaments may decrease the patient's ability to perform quick movements. Therefore, asking a patient to perform rapid exercises immediately after a cold application could be counterproductive (see **Chapter 12**).[17] The application of cold before exercise remains a controversial issue. Cold reduces the ability of collagen tissues to elongate. If the tissue is anesthetized, stretching procedures may tear muscle, tendon, or joint fibers. Therefore, if stretching is prescribed, it must be done with great care and ease.

Some people are extremely sensitive to cold and may experience a rapid rise in blood pressure as a result of a cold application. Others may develop severe itching and erythema. Still others may suffer from Raynaud's phenomenon, leading to sudden spasm of the small arteries of the feet, hands, and fingers, which can become extremely painful; there may be a change in color to pale, then blue, followed by red. Before treating a patient with ice, the therapist must test a small area of the patient's body to note the response. Patients who lack sensation to temperature must be monitored very carefully. To avoid reactions (eg, frostbite or edema), ice packs used in intervention for pain and acute injuries should be applied intermittently (ie, after a 15 to 20 min intervention, remove

Box 14–3 *Advantages and Disadvantages for Cold Modalities*

Modality	Advantages	Disadvantages
Ice massage	Quick cooling	Decreased tolerance for some patients
	Treatment area being visible	Difficult to treat large areas
	Cost and availability	
	Effective treatment of small and irregular areas	
	Effective "numbing" to target tissue	
Commercial cold packs	Good contour to treatment area	Weight of packs
	Available in many shapes and sizes	Need for refrigeration to recool
	Allows treatment of large areas	Treatment area not visible
	Packs being reusable	
	Good patient tolerance	
Ice packs	Cost and availability	Decreased tolerance for some patients
	Potential for more effective subcutaneous cooling	
Vapocoolant spray	Quick "numbing" effect	Some sprays containing flammable chemicals that can harm the environment and are toxic if inhaled, ingested, or exposed to the eyes
	Allows stretching without decreasing soft tissue extensibility	The numbing effects tends to be very short term and degree of cooling limited when compared with other cold modalities
Cryo-Cuff®	Allows for simultaneous compression and cooling (complete RICE with immobilization and elevation)	Requires more equipment with modest expense
	Various sleeve shapes for good contour of knee, ankle, shoulder, and foot	

for the same length of time and then reapply) (see **Chapter 11**).

As with heat modalities, problems and/or injuries may occur with the improper use of cryotherapy. It is imperative that any individual being considered for cryotherapy be thoroughly evaluated in order to rule out any contraindications or precautions. In an individual with intact sensation and normal cutaneous circulation, it is very unlikely that the short-term (1 hour or less) application of an ice pack would result in an injury.[18] As the ice melts, it absorbs a significant amount of heat energy, but the temperature will remain at 32°F (0°C) (the heat of fusion). Chemical cold packs have lower freezing points and reach temperatures below 32°F (0°C) and thus warrant special considerations. **Table 14–1** summarizes adverse effects of cold.

Nerve palsy has, on rare occasions, resulted following the application of cryotherapy. The exact mechanism is still under study. It is unclear whether the cold itself, the compression on the nerve from wrapping the injured part, or a combination of both is responsi-

TABLE 14–1   *Adverse Effects of Cold*

Adverse Effect	Description
Thermal discomfort	Intolerable pain associated with cold application
Cold urticaria	Allergic skin reaction with elevated patches that are discolored in comparison with surrounding tissue
Chilblain	Erythema, itching, and burning in fingers and toes related to vascular constriction
Frostbite	Local tissue damage marked by erythema, blistering, persistent edema, and/or gangrene
Hypothermia	Core temperature significantly lower than 94.6°F (37°C)
Exacerbation of systemic disease symptoms	Asthma, angina pectoris, rheumatoid arthritis, Raynaud's syndrome, etc.

ble. When applying ice and compression for an acute injury in an area such as the elbow (ulnar nerve) or distal knee (peroneal nerve), the clinician should monitor the patient for signs of sensory or motor loss and remove the cold source and compression if they appear.

In patients with cold hypersensitivity, other modalities should be used to accomplish intervention objectives without causing the patient undue discomfort or the aggravation of vasospastic disorders such as Raynaud's syndrome.

As is the case with many other physical agents used in physical therapy, more experimental work must be done with cold modalities to validate what clinicians see empirically.

REVIEW QUESTIONS

1. A 25-year-old runner has just sprained an ankle in a marathon. What type of cold application would you select if you could choose any of the cold modalities described in this chapter? Explain your answer.

2. A 40-year-old woman comes to you with a spasm in her left posterior cervical musculature. You know that cold is a good choice because it reduces pain and spasm. What would you do before choosing a cold modality? Why would you do this?

3. A patient with chronic spasm of the upper trapezius muscles is no longer covered by insurance. Yet you believe that cold, in addition to gentle stretching, is the best way to rid her of her spasm and pain. You have written out a home exercise program for her. What type of cold would you tell her to use at home? Why?

4. A patient comes to the physical therapy area with a severely swollen lower extremity on which there appears to be a diabetic ulcer. Would you use the Cryo-Cuff®? Why?

5. One of your patients has had a stroke, and now his left bicep brachii are spastic. What could you do for this patient in addition to or before therapeutic exercise?

6. Name two contraindications to ice massage on the foot or hand.

7. How does Vapocoolant Spray cool the skin?

8. What are the suggested intervention durations for ice massage, chemical cold packs, and ice packs?

9. Identify the warning signs of frostbite during a skin inspection.

10. Provide a rationale for using cryotherapy prior to and after deep friction massage.

KEY TERMS

cryotherapy
ice massage
chemical cold packs
Hydrocollator® cold packs

Col-Pack® cold packs
ice towels
ice packs
Cryo-Cuff®

vapocoolant spray
quick icing
RICE therapy

REFERENCES

1. Lehmann JF, ed: *Therapeutic Heat and Cold*, 3rd ed. Baltimore: Williams & Wilkins; 1982.

2. McMaster WC: Cryotherapy. *Physician Sports Med* 1982; 10(11):113–19.

3. Fox RH: Local cooling in man. *Br Med Bull* 1961; 17(1):14–18.

4. Goodgold J, Eberstein A: *Electrodiagnosis of Neuromuscular Disorders*, 3rd ed. Baltimore: Williams & Wilkins; 1983.

5. Swensen C, Sward L, Karlsson J: Cryotherapy in sports medicine. *Scand J Med Sci Sports* 1996; 6:193–200.

6. McDowell J, McFarland E, Nalli B: Use of cryotherapy for orthopedic patients. *Orthop Nurs* 1994; 13:21–30.

7. McMaster N, Liddle S, Waugh T: Laboratory evaluation of various cold modalities. *Am J Sports Med* 1978; 6:291–94.

8. DonTigny RL, Sheldon K: Simultaneous use of heat and cold in treatment of muscle spasm. *Arch Phys Med Rehabil* 1962; 43:235–37.

9. Weisberg J: Influence of icing and brushing on the achilles tendon reflex in human subjects. *Physiother (Can)* 1976; 28(1):21–23.

10. Price R, Lehmann JF, Boswell-Bessette S, et al: Influence of cryotherapy on spasticity at the human ankle. *Arch Phys Med Rehab* 1993; 74:300–04.

11. Lowdon BJ, Moore RJ: Determinants and nature of intramuscular temperature changes during cold therapy. *J Phys Med* 1975; 54:223–33.

12. Travell J, Simons D: *Myofascial Pain and Dysfunction: The Trigger Point Manual.* Baltimore: Williams & Wilkins; 1983.

13. Melzack R, Jeans M, Stratford J, et al: Ice massage and transcutaneous electrical stimulation: Comparison of treatment for low back pain. *Pain* 1980; 9:209–17.

14. Simons D, Travell J: Myofascial trigger points: A possible explanation. *Pain* 1981; 10:106–09.

15. Travell J, Koprowska I, Hirsch BB, et al: Effect of ethyl chloride spray on thermal burns. *Pharmacol Exp Ther* 1951; 101:36.

16. Rinzler SH, Stein I, Bakst H, et al: Blocking effect of ethyl chloride spray of cardiac pain induced by ergonovine. *Proc Soc Bio and Med* 1954; 85:329–33.

17. Chatfield PO: Hypothermia and its effects on sensory and peripheral motor systems. *Ann NY Acad Sci* 1959; 80:445–48.

18. Knight KL: *Cryotherapy in Sport Injury Management.* Champaign, IL: Human Kinetics; 1995.

15

Ultrasound

RONALD W. SWEITZER, PT, MS

Chapter Outline

Ultrasound, a form of acoustic energy, is often used by physical therapists because of its deep-heating and pain-relieving effects. In 1980, Stewart et al[1] estimated that 15 million ultrasound interventions are given each year in hospital settings alone. In 1988, Robinson[2] estimated that 64% of the physical therapists in the northeastern United States use ultrasound at least once a day. Turner[3] surveyed 230 physiotherapists in England and determined that the therapeutic techniques used in high frequency were exercise therapy, passive mobilization, and ultrasound; his replication study in Australia found a similarly high frequency of ultrasound use.[4] In 1998, Roebroeck et al[5] reported that 23% of the 17,201 patients treated in the Netherlands primary health care system from 1989 to 1992 received at least one ultrasound intervention during their care. Linsay et al[6] found that ultrasound ranked second after hop packs in a survey of 208 Canadian physical therapists. A present-day study of ultrasound application related to managed care and insurance reimbursement/denial would be useful.

The frequent use of this modality is probably related to its large number of indications, few contraindications or detrimental effects, relative ease of application, and clinically reported success. The large number of indications has come into question, however, because of lack of controlled, double-blind studies. The purpose of this chapter is to educate the reader not only in the basic physics and physiologic effects of ultrasound but also in specific techniques and clinical applications of this modality. A thorough understanding of ultrasound as a physical agent is necessary to ensure safe and optimally effective interventions.

Sound waves are mechanical pressure waves that are described in terms of their frequency. Audible sound has an approximate frequency range of 20 to 20,000 cycles per second (cps or Hertz).[7] Ultrasound waves have frequencies greater than 20,000 Hz. The most common frequency used in therapeutic ultrasound is 1 MHz (1 million Hertz), although in recent years 2 MHz and 3 MHz have become available for clinical use by the physical therapist. There are many other frequencies and parameters of ultrasound, being used for therapeutic intervention by physicians, that are outside the realm of physical therapy. Ultrasound units with a low frequency (1 MHz) are more effective in treating deep tissues, whereas units with a higher frequency (3 MHz) are more effective in treating superficial tissues. It should now be the standard for clinics to have multiple frequencies available for adequate intervention in the range of clinical conditions being referred for physical therapy. Throughout this discussion, the term **ultrasound** refers to therapeutic ultrasound of the type used by physical therapist unless stated otherwise. These units should not be confused with diagnostic units or other ultrasonic tools used in medicine and dentistry, as described by ter Haar.[8]

INSTRUMENTATION AND BIOPHYSICS

A description of the way ultrasound is produced gives an introduction to the physical characteristics of ultrasonic energy. The ultrasound generator uses common house current (ie, 60 Hz at 110 volts) as a power source. The conversion of this electrical energy to ultrasonic energy occurs as follows: (1) a transformer boosts the voltage from 110 to as much as 300 volts, (2) an oscillating circuit converts the incoming frequency to the desired higher frequency, (3) the modified electrical energy is transmitted through a coaxial cable to the transducer, and (4) the transducer converts the high-frequency electrical energy to ultrasonic energy.

Transducers

Ultrasound is delivered to the patient through the sound head, or applicator. In most units, the applicator consists of a metal faceplate with a piezoelectric crystal cemented to it. The crystal is a transducer, a device that converts one form of energy into another—in this case, from electrical to ultrasonic energy. This conversion occurs through a reverse piezoelectric effect. A **piezoelectric effect** is the phenomenon of developing an electric charge on certain crystals by applying mechanical pressure to them. The reverse piezoelectric effect is the production of mechanical energy released by imposing electric charges across a crystal. When a direct current (DC) voltage is applied across a crystal, the crystal is deformed in one direction; it will remain deformed as long as the current continues in that direction. The degree of deformation is proportional to the amount of voltage applied across the crystal. When alternating current (AC) is applied, as in the generation of ultrasound, the crystal deformation changes direction as the current changes direction, the crystal becoming thicker during one-half of the AC cycle and thinner during the other half of the cycle. The reverse piezoelectric effect allows the production of mechanical vibrations by the crystal. These oscillations produce pressure waves that are known as ultrasound waves (**Fig. 15–1**).

Today synthetic ceramic crystals of lead zirconate, titanate, or barium titanate are generally used because of their lower cost and lower voltage requirements. Quartz crystals, which require 2000–3000 volts for activation, were used originally because of their natural piezoelectric properties.

Characteristics of Ultrasound Waves

The frequency of ultrasound waves is predetermined by the frequency of the modified current delivered to the soundhead from the oscillating circuit. A natural relationship exists between the frequency and the velocity, as defined by the formula

$$V = \gamma f$$

where V is velocity, f is frequency, and γ is wavelength. Once the frequency of the energy waves is established, the energy is propagated throughout a medium at that frequency. The velocity of sound waves (1) is related to the physical properties of the medium through which it travels and (2) changes as the densities of tissue change. Acoustic energy travels best through a solid medium and cannot be transmitted through a vacuum. The average velocities for sound waves through different media include the following: 3360 m/sec in bone, 1500 m/sec in water and soft tissues, and 330 m/sec in air at sea level.[9]

Ultrasound travels poorly through air. Air transmits the vibratory energy from the transducer so poorly that the excessive nondispersed mechanical energy may cause physical damage to the crystal or to the seal around it if the ultrasound is directed into the air rather than into body tissue or another medium. To prevent this problem from occurring, a coupling medium is needed between the transducer and the skin. The couplant, usually a gel or water, replaces the air that lies on the skin and in the pores. The couplant also acts as a surface lubricant to allow the applicator to glide easily.

The primary mode of propagation of ultrasound in soft tissues is the **longitudinal (compression) wave.** This type of wave produces a movement of molecules in the same direction as the flow of energy; therefore, the activated molecules will flow parallel to each other and to the flow of energy. The analogy of a piston moving forward and backward may help to illustrate the concept of a piezoelectric crystal expanding and contracting to produce a longitudinal wave. Imagine a piston at one end of a closed tube containing a fluid medium. If the piston is at rest, the fluid density should be uniform throughout the tube. The piston now moves forward, causing compression of adjacent molecules, which increases the density in this area. The molecules are pushed forward, exerting compressive forces on the molecules lying in their paths. Now, withdrawing the piston to its starting point removes the compressive force and produces a decreased density or rarefaction of molecules in the immediate area. The cycle is repeated, and another wave of compression and rarefaction occurs (**Fig. 15–2**).

The waves are propagated in the medium until the energy is absorbed. Consider the ultrasound crystal to be like a piston oscillating back and forth 1 million times per second. When it is in contact with a patient,

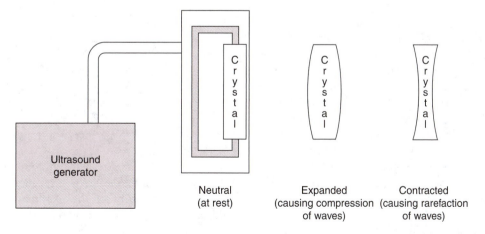

FIGURE 15–1   The production of ultrasound waves.

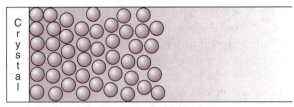

(Equal molecular density)
AT REST

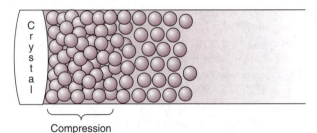

Compression
(Molecules next to crystal are compressed)
COMPRESSION PHASE

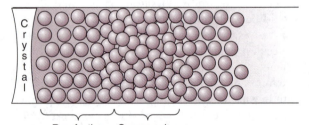

Rarefaction   Compression
(Molecules next to crystal less dense,
compressed molecules move forward)
RAREFACTION PHASE

FIGURE 15–2 The compression and rarefaction phases of the longitudinal wave. The cycles repeat as the piezoelectric crystal continues to expand and contract.

compression and rarefaction of the molecules of the body occur. This molecular flow that occurs parallel to the direction of wave propagation can be referred to as *microstreaming of molecules*. We can create a similar, but visible, streaming effect by holding the ultrasound applicator just below the surface of water in a basin. Direct the ultrasound waves parallel to the surface, and gradually increase the intensity. Notice a streaming and rippling effect, which increases as the intensity is raised. Ultrasound is transmitted in a straight line, as if in a cylinder, when it first leaves the transducer. This area of the ultrasound beam closest to the transducer is referred to as the *near field*, or **Fresnel zone.** As the energy travels farther from the

transducer, the waves begin to diverge. This point of divergence is the start of the *far field*, or **Fraunhofer zone (Fig. 15–3).**

Another type of ultrasound wave that may occur in the body is the **shear (transverse) wave,** which causes particle oscillation perpendicular to the direction of the wave propagation. Shear waves are produced by the frictional forces of molecules contacting other molecules as they pass. Production of shear waves can occur effectively only in solid media. It is the solid state of a substance rather than its chemical composition that allows propagation of shear waves. Ice can conduct shear waves, whereas water cannot. Solids have strong three-dimensional intramolecular bonding, which allows transverse forces to be transmitted. Williams[10] gave the following example: If you hold a steel bar at one end and twist it, the other end will also twist. If you put your hand into a cylinder of water and try to twist the water, no twisting will occur at the opposite end of the column. Liquids, with their weaker intramolecular bonds, are ineffective transmitters of shear waves. The shear wave does not transmit ultrasonic energy or produce significant heating in the soft tissue of the body.[11] In the body, the shear wave has a role in heating bone, particularly when striking the bone from an oblique angle of incidence.[12]

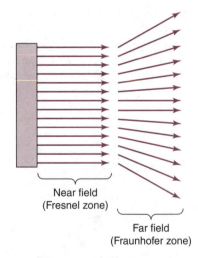

Near field
(Fresnel zone)

Far field
(Fraunhofer zone)

FIGURE 15–3 The Fresnel and Fraunhofer zones. When ultrasound first leaves the transducer, it is transmitted in a straight line in the area known as the near field (Fresnel zone). As the energy travels farther from the transducer, the waves begin to diverge in the area known as the far field (Fraunhofer zone).

Biophysical Characteristics

Ultrasound has some of the same characteristics as radiant energy. It can be transmitted, absorbed, reflected, and refracted. The type of tissue that the energy affects and the angle of incidence of the energy will determine the nature of each characteristic. Ultrasound is transmitted most effectively through a homogeneous medium. A highly homogeneous and dense medium such as steel will transmit ultrasonic energy in a relatively straight pathway at a high velocity. A less homogeneous, lower-density medium such as water will allow less transmission at a lower velocity. Transmissiveness is directly related to depth of penetration. If an adequate power supply is available, a highly transmissive medium will allow for a deep penetration. The effective depth of penetration for therapeutic ultrasound is generally considered to be from 3 to 5 cm.[13,14]

Frequency.   Depth of penetration is inversely related to the frequency of the ultrasonic energy. The lower the frequency, the deeper the penetration. As the frequency increases, more attenuation occurs, and consequently less energy is available for penetration to the deeper tissues. Griffin and Karselis[11] reported that 90 KHz ultrasound penetrated soft tissue as far as 1 MHz. They found a penetration of 10 cm versus 5 cm, respectively. Conversely, 6 MHz ultrasound will not penetrate beyond the depth of the skin.[15] The 1 MHz frequency of the commercially available ultrasound generators allows adequate depth of penetration to treat most soft-tissue problems without posing the potential risks associated with the greater penetrating abilities and cavitational potential of the lower-frequency generators. The dangers of cavitation will be discussed later. Three-MHz ultrasound units are also available to the clinician; however, because of the greater attenuation, energy is absorbed more superficially. Refer to the section on thermal response for a comparison of heating at different depths with different frequencies.

Attenuation.   **Attenuation** refers to the combination of absorption and scattering of ultrasonic energy as it passes through a medium. **Scattering** refers to the production of spherical waves that radiate the reflected ultrasound in all directions. As ultrasonic energy strikes a tiny reflecting surface such as a cell nucleus, which is smaller than the wavelength of the incident energy, scattering occurs. In fact, scattering occurs in all living tissues because of the nonhomoge-neous composition of different cellular structures. Tiny blood vessels or cell nuclei are examples of scattering structures within living tissue. Attenuation coefficients have been determined for various substances. Two substances may have similar attenuation coefficients but may possess different proportions of absorption and scattering. Attenuation coefficients increase as the frequency of the ultrasound increases; therefore, as the frequency of ultrasound increases, absorption and scattering occur at a higher rate, resulting in less energy being available for penetration to the deeper tissues.

Depth of penetration is also inversely related to the coefficient of absorption of the medium. If energy is absorbed, it is no longer available for penetration. According to Piersol et al,[16] the tissue with the highest protein content demonstrates the highest absorption of ultrasonic energy. These authors have listed several body tissues according to their absorption coefficients. Wells[17] compiled a similar list of absorption coefficients showing that tissues with a high collagen content demonstrate the highest absorption. Both sources list the following tissues in order from highest to lowest in their ability to absorb ultrasound: bone, peripheral nerve, skeletal muscle, fat, blood, and water. Frizzell and Dunn[18] added cartilage and tendon to the list between bone and skeletal muscle. The clinical significance of this information is that ultrasound will be transmitted relatively well through water and fat with little absorption of the energy. For heating to occur, the ultrasound must be absorbed. A more detailed discussion of heating will follow.

Reflection and Refraction

Reflection and refraction occur when ultrasound is transmitted from a material of one density to material of another density. The angle of reflection equals the angle of incidence. If a wave has a 60° angle of incidence from the left, it will be reflected at a 60° angle to the right. If the angle of incidence is perpendicular to the surface, reflection will occur directly toward the source (**Fig. 15–4**).

If the ultrasound source is stationary, energy waves can be cyclically transmitted and reflected to and from the source. When energy waves overlap and are in phase, summation of the energy occurs. If overlapping ultrasonic energy waves reach equilibrium, they become standing waves. Standing waves are potentially hazardous to biological tissues because high concentrations of energy are produced when multiple waves are in phase.

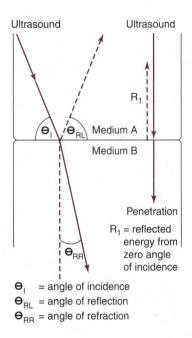

Θ_I = angle of incidence
Θ_{RL} = angle of reflection
Θ_{RR} = angle of refraction

FIGURE 15–4 Reflection and refraction of sound waves.

Refraction, the deflection of energy waves, depends on the changes in velocity and wavelength that occur when ultrasound passes from one medium to another. When ultrasound is transmitted from a high-density medium to a lower-density medium, the velocity and wavelength decrease while the angle of refraction becomes less than the angle of incidence (see **Fig. 15–4**). In the body, reflection, refraction, and attenuation occur largely at tissue interfaces. These interfaces include (1) fat to muscle, (2) muscle to fascia, (3) tendon to periosteum, and (4) ligament to periosteum. The proportion of reflection to refraction depends on the acoustic impedance of the material or tissue on each side of the interface. Acoustic impedance (z) is the product of the density (p) of a material and the velocity (v) of the sound waves in it. Thus,

$$Z = pv$$

For a more detailed description of acoustic impedance, see Williams.[10]

Thermal Responses

Ultrasound has been used by physical therapists primarily for its deep-heating effects. For heating of tissues to occur, the energy must be absorbed. The absorption of the high-frequency vibrational energy results in the production of heat. Transmission, reflection, and refraction are *means by which the ultrasonic energy is distributed* to the various tissues in different patterns; they should not be confused with heat production. However, if standing waves are produced because of reflection at an interface (eg, between bone and ligament), a greater energy concentration is available for absorption by the tissue between the transducer and the reflecting surface. Not all reflections result in standing waves. If a tissue has a high concentration of ultrasound energy and a relatively high absorption coefficient, it has the potential to produce a strong thermal response. This is the case at the myofascial or tenoperiosteal interfaces. Fat, on the other hand, is a homogeneous tissue with a low absorption coefficient; therefore, it transmits ultrasound effectively without being heated significantly. This low heat-producing ability in fat is considered an advantage in choosing ultrasound rather than the electromagnetic diathermy to heat deep tissues.

The tissue with the highest absorption coefficient will not necessarily be the hottest. Although thermal energy can be produced in the tissue, the following factors also contribute to the total tissue temperature rise (TTR): (1) the rate at which energy is applied, (2) the length of time the energy is applied, (3) the thermal conductivity of the tissue, and (4) the rate of perfusion of blood to the tissue.

The first consideration, the rate at which energy is applied, is controlled by the *intensity adjustment* and *the mode of application* of the ultrasound. If the intensity of ultrasound is too low, the energy required to produce a significant TTR will be inadequate. If the energy is applied at an extremely high intensity, the local thermal response may be so great and sudden that pain from overheating will occur before heat can be conducted away from the local area to produce a more general TTR.

Lehmann et al[19] demonstrated this result in a study of human thighs exposed to ultrasound. His results indicated that, for ultrasound to heat the soft tissue adjacent to the bone effectively, the energy level must be (1) kept low enough to allow the energy to heat the bone and soft tissue to a safe, pain-free level, (2) kept high enough to allow adequate depth of penetration, and (3) applied long enough to allow for conduction of the heat away from the bone into the surrounding tissue. While this conductive heating is occurring, a long application time will also be available for more energy absorption and thus conversive heating directly into the soft tissues. If the energy is applied too quickly, heat production will be so rapid that the thermal nociocepters of the body will be stimulated. The patient's painful response will require a withdrawal of the ultrasound before a general TTR in the surrounding soft tissue can be produced.

The third consideration is thermal conductivity. For example, bone has a higher thermal conductivity than surrounding tissues. With its high absorption coefficient, bone does not become proportionately hotter than the muscle or tendon lying next to it. As the energy is absorbed, the heat produced is quickly dissipated throughout the bone to the cooler, nonsonated areas. Another reason that excessive bone temperatures are not observed is that about 20% to 30% of the incident energy striking bone is reflected into the surrounding tissue.[20] This reflected energy is available to be absorbed by the soft tissue rather than the bone.

The fourth consideration is the rate of blood perfusion in the tissues. If a local body tissue with an impaired circulation is heated, it may not be able to dissipate the excess heat. Therefore, the risk of thermal injury to the tissue is higher than it would be if the circulation were normal. For example, a healthy muscle belly will be less likely to suffer thermal injury than would a poorly vascularized tendon. The vascularity of tissue must be considered when determining the dosage level for ultrasound.

Recent studies can be used to reinforce the preceding principles. Draper et al[21] sonated human triceps surae muscles with both 1 MHz and 3 MHz ultrasound at .5, 1, 1.5, and 2 w/sq cm for 10 min. They evaluated temperature changes every 30 sec at depths of 2.5 cm and 5 cm for the 1 MHz group and 0.8 and 1.6 cm for the 3 MHz group. They discovered greater rates of temperature rise at the higher intensities and higher overall temperatures as time progressed. Also, the rate of rise for the 3 MHz group was as much as four times that of the 1 MHz group. The subjects also reported feelings of warmth on the skin. This finding demonstrates the greater superficial absorption rate of the higher-frequency ultrasound. Kimura et al[22] treated a tissue preparation with 1 MHz continuous ultrasound at 2 w/sq cm for 5 min and confirmed that greater the time of sonation, the higher the temperature. They also applied the ultrasound at angles 60, 70, 80, and 90 degrees. The greatest increases in temperature occurred at the 80° and 90° angles as predicted. They did all their trials with two different brands of ultrasound units that were calibrated prior to the study. The results were parallel but to different degrees. This finding demonstrates the need to be familiar with the intensity characteristics of the equipment being utilized.

These studies used small intervention areas of 1 or 2 times the effective radiating area (ERA) of the transducer, which allows a concentration of the energy to maximize the thermal response. The temperature changes were not necessarily linear and were less predictable in the first minute or two of application. This outcome may be a result of blood flow and thermal conductivity in the body. We do know that these conditions are dynamic and may also be effected by pathology.

Nonthermal Responses

Suggested nonthermal effects of ultrasound include (1) micromassage, (2) increased membrane permeability, (3) arteriolar vasoconstriction or dilatation, and (4) cavitation. Nonthermal effects, sometimes described as mechanical effects, are changes that are not related to heat production. Remember that the absorption of energy is on a continuum. A nonthermal response occurs as energy absorption does not cause a detectable increase in tissue temperature.

Micromassage.   The term **micromassage** refers to the microscopic movement, or oscillations, of the body fluids and tissues as a result of exposure to ultrasound. The term was used as early as 1942 to describe the action of ultrasound.[23] The other nonthermal effects of ultrasound are probably produced as a result of this micromassage to the body tissues.

Increased Membrane Permeability.   *Acoustic streaming* has been described as a mechanism that induces changes in diffusion rates and **membrane permeability**.[13] Ultrasound causes a stirring effect in the fluid near a biological membrane. This agitation of the ions increases the ionic concentration gradient, thereby accelerating the diffusion rate. These mechanical effects were similarly documented by analyzing membrane potentials that were altered by exposure to ultrasound.[24]

Lota and Darling[24] demonstrated that the membrane permeability of erythrocytes to potassium increased because of mechanical rather than thermal effects. Dyson et al[25] suggested that streaming might be an important mechanism in tissue regeneration because of its effect on weak secondary bonds in the tissue. They hypothesized that the making and breaking of these bonds, which are important to the enzyme activity necessary for tissue repair, are enhanced by the types of stresses placed on them during streaming. So far, the scientific documentation for this theory is inadequate.

Further evidence supports changes in membrane permeability during exposure to ultrasound. Coble and Dunn[26] observed changes in frog skin that suggested changes in membrane permeability. Mortimer and colleagues, in a series of experimental studies,[27,28,29] confirmed changes in membrane transport by documenting changes in the action potential of cardiac muscle and increased oxygen transport through frog skin and silastic membranes. In the last study, the changes occurred in the absence of a temperature rise or transient cavitation. This finding further confirms the nonthermal effect of ultrasound on membrane transport.

Arteriolar Vasoconstriction or Dilation.   The nonthermal effect of arteriolar vasoconstriction or vasodilation is not clear. Hogan et al[30] used pulsed ultrasound at supraclinical intensities of 5–10 W/sq cm with a stationary technique to demonstrate vasoconstriction of the smallest arterioles of rat cremaster muscle. They later used pulsed ultrasound at a clinical intensity to demonstrate arteriolar vasodilation and increased opening of capillary beds in chronically ischemic muscles.[31] These results were obtained in the absence of thermal responses. The mechanism that produced the preceding reaction is unknown. (Results from these reports may encourage clinicians to use nonthermal ultrasound in the clinical intensity range.) However, much more research is needed before any conclusions can be reached.

Cavitation.   **Cavitation,** the most widely known of the nonthermal responses, refers to the formation and collapse of gas- or vapor-filled cavities in liquids.[32] It occurs within the biologic system when small gas pockets (bubbles) are subjected to the compression and rarefaction cycles of ultrasound. As the bubble grows to a stable size characteristic of the resonant frequency, it pulsates in the sound field and is considered to be a stable cavity. This stage is not destructive but, with further sonation, induced microstreaming may produce increased cellular stress and disruption.

As the bubble or cavity grows larger, the tissue membrane becomes thinner and more fragile. If a compression wave causes a collapse of the cavity, transient cavitation has occurred. Transient cavitation causes spotty cell destruction and tissue damage. It should be noted that cavitation occurs much more readily in vitro than in vivo (ie, transient cavitation will occur at therapeutic intensities in a suspension of cells in a laboratory but not in intact tissues).[33] Cavitational thresholds are much more attainable when using low-frequency ultrasound. For example, at a frequency of 10 KHz, cavitation may occur in vitro at 0.1–1 W/sq cm; at a frequency of 1 MHz, however, 100 W/sq cm may be required to produce the same level of cavitation. Most research states that transient cavitation will not occur in the body using a 1 MHz frequency at therapeutic intensities, with a moving sound head technique, of less than 3 W/sq cm.[10]

Williams[10] agreed that transient cavitation has not been convincingly demonstrated in vivo at therapeutic intensities and frequencies. However, he cautioned that stable cavitation has been documented within the therapeutic range. Nonacoustic factors, such as muscular exercise and muscular contraction induced by electrical stimulation, enhance the formation of gas bubbles. Williams implied that it may be more hazardous to apply the combination intervention of ultrasound with electrical stimulation than to apply each intervention individually. Therefore, to justify the use of electrical stimulation with ultrasound, further research is needed to show that the combination intervention is more effective than the individual techniques.

CLINICAL USES

Ultrasound, as we have noted, is used clinically to treat a variety of conditions. For clarity, the effect of ultrasound on inflammation, pain, edema, tissue healing, circulation, and extensibility of collagen tissue are discussed separately. However, the goal, when possible, should be to restore tissue function rather than to treat symptoms alone. The following descriptions of potential biophysical effects of therapeutic ultrasound are derived from many studies done in laboratory settings. One must not assume that the in vivo effects are the same as in vitro. The body possesses many dynamic mechanisms to adapt to external stresses imposed on it. Many of these mechanism will not occur in a cell preparation. Baker et al[34] performed a very thorough analysis of many of the studies that follow and assert that there is inadequate evidence to assume that the following therapeutic effects of ultrasound may actually occur in the clinical setting. We will see how ultrasound usage has been justified to this point.

Inflammation

Following an injury, the body tries to repair itself. The first stage of this process is acute inflammation. The area of damage becomes walled off, and the flow of fluid into the extracellular space eventually ceases. The tissue remains swollen because the excessive extracellular fluid and waste products have not been reabsorbed by the body. Next, the body begins to lay down collagen tissue in order to strengthen the weakened area. However, if the acute inflammation becomes excessive, uncontrolled edema can lead to tissue damage and scarring. Frequently, the collagen tissue, commonly called scar tissue, is distributed in a manner that impairs the normal function of the tissue.[23] The end result for the patient is a chronic condition resulting from periodic microtearing and further scarring. Ultrasound is widely used to treat conditions related to the effect of inflammation on tissue. With its dual effect, thermal and nonthermal, ultrasound may prevent the development of chronic conditions. Obviously, ultrasound should not be used at an intensity that would produce a temperature rise in the acute inflammatory process. However, the clinician can consider the use of ultrasound at extremely low intensities or in the pulsed mode during the acute phase of inflammation. The nonthermal micromassage and alteration of tissue permeability may be beneficial to enhance reabsorption of interstitial fluid. Enhanced reabsorption from ultrasound was demonstrated by Reid et al[35] in their intervention of experimentally produced hematoma in rabbit's ear.

Pain

The concept of pain remains elusive and has been described differently by many authors (see **Chapter 6**). Wyke[36] described pain as "an abnormal emotional state that is aroused by unusual patterns of activity in specific afferent systems." This emotional situation is created by activation of a nociceptive afferent system. However, many factors are involved in interpreting a patient's report of pain. Although it is important to relieve a patient's pain to allow for increased func-

tion, one must not assume that because pain is absent, healing has occurred. The pain may be temporarily masked.

Numerous clinical studies describe the effectiveness of ultrasound in relieving the pain of bursitis, tendonitis, osteoarthritis, and other musculoskeletal conditions. In addition to considering the direct effect of ultrasound on an injured tissue, the physical therapist examines the effect of ultrasound on nerves to understand the mechanisms of pain that may be related to ultrasonic therapy. Pain relief is often associated with an increase in temperature. Ultrasound was shown to raise pain thresholds in human subjects similar to the level produced by raising tissue temperature by other means.[37]

Szumski[38] summarized the effects of ultrasound on nervous tissue as follows: (1) it selectively heats peripheral nerves, (2) it may alter or block impulse conduction, (3) it may increase membrane permeability, and (4) it may increase tissue metabolism. He pointed out that any of these mechanisms may occur from heating and may effect pain relief. Pain impulses are transmitted by small-diameter axons. Anderson et al[39] established that B and C type fibers are more sensitive to ultrasound than is the A type. Perhaps this selective absorption by smaller fibers allows for decreases in pain transmission (see **Chapter 6**).

Some authors addressing the effect of ultrasound on the conduction velocities of motor and sensory nerves have suggested a relationship between changes in nerve conduction velocities and pain. This relationship may not be explained by the thermal effects of ultrasound alone. Some initial studies of **motor nerve conduction velocities (MNCV)** showed that when certain intensities of ultrasound were applied over peripheral nerves, a reduction in nerve conduction velocity occurred, whereas an increase in MNCV occurred at other intensities. Zankel[40] found no significant reduction of ulnar MNCV at 1 W/sq cm applied for 5 min to the flexor forearm but did find a significant decrease in MNCV after 10 min or by applying 2 W/sq cm for 5 min. Farmer[41] found a decrease in MNCV when the intensity range was 1–2 W/sq cm, but found an increase in MNCV when 3 W/sq cm was applied to the ulnar nerve. These results cannot be explained but indicate that there is more than just a thermal effect on nerve. Although the preceding authors did not report changes in tissue temperature, one would expect an increase at the intensities of 1–2 W/sq cm.[42] Why the preceding differences occurred is not understood.

Studies performed on sensory nerves are more supportive of a parallel relationship between increased temperature and increased **sensory nerve conduction velocity (SNCV)**.[43] This finding has been supported by several studies on SNCV. Currier et al[44] exposed the lateral cutaneous branch of the radial nerves of 5 men to 1.5 W/sq cm for 5 min and found that the speed of conduction increased as the subcutaneous temperature increased. Similarly, Halle et al[45] demonstrated an increase in conduction of superficial radial nerve associated with an increase in subcutaneous temperature. Consentino et al[46] attempted to clarify the previous findings with a study on the sensory fibers of the median nerve. However, they were unable to show any significant difference between the control group and the experimental groups, which received ultrasound at 0.5, 1, or 1.5 W/sq cm for 10 min.

The previous studies were done on normal nerve. Hong[47] found decreased amplitude of the compound motor action potentials and increased proximal latencies in patients with painful polyneuropathies treated for 2 min with 1 MHz continuous ultrasound at 1 and 1.5 W/sq cm. He found no changes at 0.5 W/sq cm in the same group and no changes in the normal and nonpainful patient groups. He did not note whether the patients reported relief of symptoms during the intervention.

The studies reported here demonstrate that changes in nerve conduction velocity do occur. They are not as predictable as we would like, and they have not been done with 3 MHz ultrasound. One can only hypothesize that these changes, whether through thermal or nonthermal mechanisms, may be responsible for the reduction in pain reported by many patients after receiving ultrasound.

Edema

Subacute inflammatory edema can be treated by the physical therapist in the following ways: (1) compression, (2) massage, (3) ice, (4) electrical stimulation, (5) heat, and (6) ultrasound for its thermal and nonthermal effects. Middlemast and Chattergee[48] reported better reduction of swelling, tenderness, and pain in soft-tissue lesions by using ultrasound rather than other forms of heat such as shortwave diathermy, infrared radiation, and paraffin baths.

Ultrasound may stimulate the production of joint fluid when applied at high intensity. White et al[49] applied 1 MHz continuous ultrasound at the maximal tolerable dose (1 to 1.8 W/sq cm) for 10 min to the wrists of normal subjects. An average increase of 52.8% wrist joint fluid was produced in 3 of the 6 subjects as determined by MRI.

Tissue Healing

The scientific literature is perhaps the most abundant in the area of tissue healing. Although most clinicians have never treated an open wound with ultrasound, it is valuable to review the physiologic effects that have been stimulated by therapeutic ultrasound. Research has been performed on experimental tissue preparations, animal, and human subjects. The review of literature is often contradictory because of the many different and often changing parameters. The clinical section that follows will sort through this information and give it a more practical application.

Ultrasound has been found to enhance tissue repair in both subcutaneous injuries and open wounds. Vanharant et al[50] had limited success in producing a long-term rise in glycosaminoglycan (GAG) metabolism in normal adult rabbit knees after 5 days of intervention with ultrasound through water at 1 W/sq cm for 5 min. Glycosaminoglycan is a product of connective tissue cells and can be used as an indicator of metabolic activity. Concentrations in articular cartilage, menisci, and collateral ligaments were unaltered one day after the last intervention. The only significant finding—an increase in radioactivity in the medial collateral ligament in the treated knees—reflects increased metabolic activity. These authors evaluated the response in normal rather than pathologic tissue.

Stratton et al[51] discovered an increase in the number of tissue repair cells (macrophages, lymphocytes, fibroblasts, endothelial cells, and myoblasts) in sonated rat thighs. Collagen, required for tissue strengthening, also was increased in the sonated group. The significant number of healing cells was present only in the group sonated with continuous ultrasound at 1.5 W/sq cm. Lower intensities and pulsed ultrasound were ineffective. Young and Dyson[52] used lower intensities of 0.1 W/sq cm at 0.75 MHz and 3 MHz to increase the responsiveness of macrophages in vitro. They also used 0.1 W/sq cm at 0.75 MHz and 3 MHz to increase granulation tissue and fibroblasts in the first 5 days after experimentally produced full-thickness lesions in rat skin. They suggested that ultrasound is useful in accelerating the inflammatory and early proliferative stages of repair.[53] Using the same parameters, they stimulated new blood-vessel formation in the flank skin of adult rats.[54] Byl et al[55] were able to increase the breaking strength of incisional wounds in pig skin with 1 MHz ultrasound in the continuous mode at 1.5 W/sq cm and in the pulsed mode (20% duty cycle) at 0.5 W/sq cm for 5 min. However, only the low-intensity pulsed ultrasound group had increased collagen deposition after 5 and 10 days. Byl et al[56] also found low-intensity ultrasound to increase tensile strength, increase collagen deposition, and decrease wound size in the first week of experimentally induced wounds in Yucatan pigs. Pulsed ultrasound at 0.1 W/sq cm for 5 min a day was shown to have a positive effect on the proliferative phase of experimental rat wounds.[57] This study found the same effect for wounds treated with electrical stimulation but found electrical stimulation to be superior to ultrasound at the maturation phase.

Open wounds may benefit from intervention with ultrasound. In 1960, Paul et al[58] reported clinical success in completely healing 13 of 23 pressure sores and significantly improving five others. Since then, various controlled studies have documented the effectiveness of ultrasound in wound repair. Shamberger[59] summarized several studies demonstrating that tissue healing increased after intervention with ultrasound as compared with a control group. Some studies measured wound size; others measured tensile strength or fibroblast proliferation. Dyson and colleagues,[25,60] using 3 MHz ultrasound, documented increased tissue regeneration in rabbit ears and in chronic varicose ulcers in humans. They theoretically attributed the increased rate of healing to ultrasound-induced protein synthesis and perhaps to the vibrational micromassaging effect, which may reduce edema and thus facilitate repair. In a clinical report, Ferguson and Noel[61] described the use of pulsed ultrasound, 0.5 W/sq cm at 1 MHz for 3 min, in the intervention of episiotomy wounds on the first and second postoperative days. They claimed that hematomas were resolved more quickly and that patients reported a soothing effect on the pain. Peschen et al[62] used 30 KHz ultrasound successfully in a placebo-controlled, single-blind clinical study on venous leg ulcers. However, this is not a frequency presently available to the clinician. Research is also being conducted using low frequency for phonophoresis (discussed in a later section of this chapter).

Not all studies have confirmed accelerated healing as a result of ultrasound exposure. Eriksson et al[63] found no significant difference in the proportion of area of healed chronic leg ulcers between an experimental group and a placebo group. They used 1 MHz ultrasound at 1 W/sq cm by direct contact for 10 min. Compared with the results of the Vanharanto et al[50] underwater technique, the effective intensity was higher, and the exposure time was longer in the Eriksson et al study. The Eriksson study also was done on chronic human ulcers rather than on fresh animal lesions. Lundeberg et al[64] were unsuccessful in using 1 MHz pulsed ultrasound (11% duty cycle) at 0.5 W/sq cm for 10 min to improve the healing rate of venous ulcers at 4, 8, and 12 weeks. Pressure ulcers were not successfully treated with 3.28 MHz pulsed ultrasound (20% duty cycle) at 0.1 W/sq cm for 4 to 7.5 minutes for 5 times a week for 12 weeks.[65] Ultrasound at 3 MHz in both continuous mode at 0.3 W/sq cm and pulsed mode (20% duty cycle) at 0.25 W/sq cm delivered 5 days a week for 6 weeks was found to be ineffective in healing experimentally induced burns in Fischer rats.[66]

Enwemeka's research[67] supports the use of ultrasound to promote tendon healing. He emphasized that all correct parameters of application must be addressed for successful results. In 1989, he treated rabbit Achilles tendons in deionized water with 1 MHz continuous ultrasound at 1 W/sq cm for 5 min with a moving sound head technique. The ultrasound was applied daily for the first 9 postoperative days. The results showed an increase in overall tensile strength of the tendons because of increased cross-sectional area in the sonated tendons. In 1990, Enwemeka et al[68] repeated these studies using 0.5 W/sq cm of continuous ultrasound instead of 1 W/sq cm and produced greater increases in tensile strength and capacity for energy absorption after sonation. Da Cunha et al[69] found increased healing rates in Achilles tendons of Wistar rats at 14 days post tenotomy using 0.5 W/sq cm of pulsed 1 MHz ultrasound. They found decreased healing when using the continuous mode. These studies support the rationale for low-intensity ultrasound in acute stages of healing. Jackson et al[70] also found increased breaking strength and collagen synthesis in rat Achilles tendons in the first 5–9 days of intervention with ultrasound. They treated puncture wounds and used 1.5 W/sq cm of continuous ultrasound with a stationary sound head technique under water for 4 min. Although these authors obtained favorable results, a stationary technique should not be used in the clinic. Gan et al[71] increased range of motion and advanced scar maturation, and they decreased the inflammatory infiltrate on surgically lacerated chicken tendon. They found the ultrasound application to be most effective when applied early (starting day 7 postoperatively) versus later (starting day 42 postoperatively). Gum et al[72] stimulated regeneration of rabbit Achilles tendon with combined ultrasound and laser photostimulation; however, the results were not as dramatic as ultrasound intervention alone. This finding implies a counteracting effect of the two modalities applied together in early tissue healing.

Karnes and Burton[73] treated contraction-induced muscle injuries in rats for 7 days using continuous 1 MHz ultrasound at 0.5 W/sq cm underwater before finding an increased force production ability compared with the nontreated limbs.

The studies on tendon healing just described emphasize the effectiveness of clinical doses of ultrasound for tendon repair immediately after the injury. Prolonged use of ultrasound may be of no value, or even harmful. Turner et al[74] found a significant difference between treated and untreated tendons after 5 weeks of intervention given 3 times a week. Roberts et al[75] demonstrated reduced strength and healing in surgically repaired tendon after intervention with pulsed ultrasound of 0.8 W/sq cm at 1.1 MHz after 5 min per day for 6 weeks.

Circulation

Ultrasound-induced heating has been shown to increase local circulation by both direct and reflex means. In 1953, Bickford and Duff[76] reported an increase in blood flow after ultrasound at intensities high enough to heat tissue. This finding was supported by other investigators.[77,78,79] Abramson et al[80] demonstrated increased blood flow 26 min after the termination of experimental ultrasound interventions. Lota[81] demonstrated not only that as tissue temperature increases so does blood flow but also that a reflex vasodilation may be initiated by the application of ultrasound. He sonated the sympathetic lumbar ganglia in human subjects to produce an increase in superficial circulation to the big toe.

Not all studies have confirmed increase in blood flow following the application of ultrasound.[82,83] Fabrizio et al[84] compiled a summary table of twelve previous investigations of blood flow following ultrasound. Various techniques of assessment, mode of ultrasound, frequencies, and time of application were compared. In general, if ultrasound was applied

for 5 min or less, at intensities below 2 W/sq cm, increases in blood flow were not demonstrated. There are other factors, such as size of the irradiated area, stationary versus moving sound head technique, continuous versus pulsed mode, and animal versus human subjects. Fabrizio produced increased blood flow velocity in the popliteal artery of human subjects after treating their triceps surae with 1 MHz ultrasound for 5, 10, and 15 min at intensities of 1 and 1.5 W/sq cm. Those treated with 3 MHz ultrasound at 1 and 1.2 W/sq cm showed no increase in blood flow velocity.

Extensibility of Collagen Tissue

Collagen tissue is an effective absorber of ultrasonic energy. Ligaments, joint capsules, and tendons (all high in collagen composition) are common sites of pathology for which ultrasound is indicated. These structures often lie deeper than the effective heating range of the diathermy and superficial heating modalities. Ultrasound may be the only clinical modality that can produce a TTR in these deeper structures, which are heated effectively because of their close proximity to bone and their high absorption coefficients. Lehmann et al[85] demonstrated the effectiveness of a stroking technique of continuous ultrasound at 1.5 W/sq cm for 5 min in heating intra-articular menisci and joint capsules in the knees of hogs. Lehmann et al[86] also studied the effect of heating on the extensibility of rat tail tendon. They found that the greatest increase in tendon length occurred when heat and sustained stretch were simultaneously applied and the stretch was maintained during the cooldown period. This experimental model provides a rationale for using ultrasound and stretching for tight joints.

Ultrasound can be applied locally to the sites of small fibrous lesions to produce relaxation of the scar tissue. Griffin and Karselis[14] reported the relaxation of polypeptide bonds after the application of ultrasound. Relaxation of collagen tissue bonds would allow increased extensibility of the scar, which in turn would permit normal function of the joint, tendon, or muscle and subsequent pain reduction. While administering the ultrasound, the therapist also can stretch the tissue, which will further break up the scar.

Knight et al[87] demonstrated the usefulness of continuous 1 MHz ultrasound at an intensity of 1.5 W/sq cm for 7 min on the plantar flexors of human subjects prior to static stretch to display the greatest increase in ankle range of motion. They compared this group to a control group and to others simply performing active exercise or exercise with superficial heat.

Ward et al[88] were unsuccessful in their use of ultrasound to increase range of motion in eight joints of burn patients. They used 1 MHz at 1 W/sq cm for 10 min. This intensity may have been inadequate to obtain the heating necessary for tissue elongation. The authors were not specific in their description of patient positioning or the size of the area sonated. This type of detail will be discussed in a later section because of its extreme importance to the success of many therapeutic procedures we use.

Phonophoresis

Phonophoresis is the use of ultrasound to enhance the transdermal absorption of medications into body tissues. Hydrocortisone, dexamethasone, and lidocaine are medications commonly administered by phonophoresis.[89] The skin, particularly the stratum corneum, is normally resistant to the passage of chemical substances through it. Ultrasound, as described in the thermal and nonthermal response sections of this chapter, alters membrane permeability and therefore enhances the absorption of medications in its path. Utrasound's thermal effect on tissue is believed to be an important mechanism in determining the effectiveness of phonophoresis. Heat increases circulation to the area and dilates hair follicles and sweat glands to allow diffusion through the skin. Kassan et al[90] describe these mechanisms and a review of literature showing the benefits of both phonophoresis and iontophoresis in enhancing drug penetration through the stratum corneum.

Williams[10] described the phonophoretic effect as a synergistic interaction of ultrasound and drugs. He documented the positive effects of phonophoresis with viricidal ointments, such as increased tissue regeneration in rabbit corneal ulcers following penicillin phonophoresis. The synergistic effect was also demonstrated by the increased clinical effectiveness of sonating soft tissue after injection of anti-inflammatory or analgesic medications. After the physician injected the drug into the inflamed periarticular structure, the physical therapist applied an ultrasound intervention over the same area. The ultrasound was assumed to have distributed the drug through the inflamed tissue and enhanced its absorption.[91,92] Ultrasound also has increased penetration and absorption of topical medications into deeper tissues.[88,93] Griffin and colleagues[94,95] reported that phonophoresis was effective in driving hydrocortisone through the skin of pigs by measuring the cortisol levels in muscle and nerve. Griffin et al.[96] later studied the effectiveness of hydrocortisone phonophoresis in patients with periarticular conditions. Sixty-eight percent of the subjects treated with phonophoresis showed significantly improved range of motion and decreased pain compared with only 28% who improved with ultrasound and a placebo instead of hydrocortisone.

Kleinkort and Wood[97] demonstrated the superiority of a 10% hydrocortisone preparation over a 1% mixture in the intervention of 285 patients with a variety of inflammatory conditions. Effective clinical results have been achieved using intensities in a mid to high range of 1–2 W/sq cm.[93,94,98] However, phonophoresis of low intensity and long duration proved to be more effective in driving cortisol into pig muscle and nerve in a study involving only 10 subjects.[99] In contradiction to the preceding studies, Bare et al[100] were unable to produce hydrocortisone penetration through the epidermis using 1 MHz continuous ultrasound at 1 W/sq cm for 5 min. Their blood analysis was done within 30 min of the intervention. They unfortunately did not repeat the blood work at later time intervals, which may have yielded a positive result. The stratum corneum acts as a chemical reservoir that may release medication slowly over time. Benson et al[101] also failed to demonstrate enhanced absorption of benzydamine by phonophoresis. Additional studies are needed to document the most efficient mode of application for this noninvasive alternative to injection of medication into painful and inflamed structures.

The choice of conductive media used for phonophoresis must be seriously considered. In a survey of directors of California physical therapy practices that use phonophoresis, 81% used 10% hydrocortisone, and 19% used 1% hydrocortisone cream. Ninety percent of them used a preparation in a thick white cream or a thick white cream mixed with ultrasound gel. Cameron and Monroe[102] compared this preparation and many others to degassed water and discovered 0 transmissiveness through a 5 mm layer of cream and 7% transmissiveness for a mixture of hydrocortisone and ultrasound gel. They found the following products to be highly transmissive: Lidex® gel, fluocinonide 0.05%a, Thera-gesic®

cream, methyl salicylate 15%b, Betamethasone 0.05%c in US geld.

Although 5 mm is a very thick layer as compared with the amount of cream used in an intervention, the authors felt that thickness was needed to be precise consistently in their evaluation of transmissiveness.[103]

Chemical enhancers are also being evaluated for their ability to increase transdermal drug delivery. Johnson et al[104] found 50% ethol alcohol (EtOH) saturated with linoleic acid (LA/EtOH) to be the most effective chemical enhancer of the six chemicals tested for increasing the corticosterone flux. They found the permeability of human cadaver skin to corticosterone to be increased significantly when therapeutic continuous ultrasound of 1 MHz at 1.4 W/sq cm was applied to all of the chemical enhancers. The most dramatic increase was 14 times greater with LA/EtOH. They explain that ultrasound and linoleic acid are both bilayer disordering agents with a synergistic action when used together. They also found permeability enhancement to occur with ultrasound and LA/EtOH when used with dexamethasone, estradiol, lidocaine, and testosterone. This information should be shared with pharmacists who are formulating phonophoresis drug preparations.

Technique. The technique for phonophoresis is similar to a routine ultrasound intervention except that the medication is placed on the skin immediately over the target structure. The clinician can enhance the effectiveness of the intervention by following recommended procedures. Byl[105] made the following suggestions after a very thorough literature review: (1) the medication and its transmission medium should transmit ultrasound; (2) the skin should be prepared by heating, moistening, or shaving; (3) the patient should be positioned to maximize circulation to the part being treated; (4) a moisture barrier should be applied after the intervention; (5) an intensity of 1.5 W/sq cm should be used for its combination of thermal and nonthermal effects; and (6) use lower intensities (0.5 W/sq cm) when treating open wounds and acute conditions. These suggestions seem appropriate on the basis of current knowledge. In number (6) one might also recommend the use of pulsed ultrasound so as to reduce the overall amount of ultrasonic energy and thermal effect. This use may reduce the effectiveness, as demonstrated by Asano et al[106] in rats. The greatest transdermal absorption of indomethacin was observed in the pulsed ultrasound group with the longest on time (1:2 vs. 1:4 or 1:9). They also noted increased absorption as the intensity increased and the time increased to 15 min. However, if the intensity went too high (1.5 to 2.0 W/sq cm stationary technique), tissue damage occurred. Most of the studies were done with 1 Mhz continuous ultrasound, but two studies investigating the phonophoresis of methyl nicotinate with 3 Mhz continuous ultrasound on human subjects demonstrated enhanced absorption.[107,108]

Warning. Physical therapists or assistants must be aware of indications, contraindications, and adverse reactions for any medication that they are delivering even if it has been prescribed by a physician. This includes systemic as well as local reactions. Franklin et al[109] used 1 MHz continuous ultrasound at 1.5 W/sq cm for 8 min every other day for 2 weeks on human shoulders to determine that there was no systemic effect on adrenal function as assessed by 24-hour cortisol levels. More studies of this type are needed to evaluate the amount of systemic absorption that may occur with the various medications driven by phonophoresis.

Low-Frequency Ultrasound for Phonophoresis. Recently there have been numerous scientific investigations into the use of low-frequency ultrasound to enhance transdermal delivery of medications. Mitragotri et al[110] showed that low-frequency ultrasound dramatically increased skin permeability to numerous chemicals compared with the higher frequencies generally used by physical therapists. They also found that the amount of transdermal delivery increased as the intensity of the ultrasound increased. In a prior study they demonstrated the ability to deliver insulin, interferon gamma, and erythropoetin across human skin.[111] Ueda et al[112] found 150 KHz ultrasound to increase the diffusivity across the aqueous region in the stratum corneum of rat skin for the polar compound antipyrine. This also occurred through a nonthermal mechanism. Singer et al,[113] in an attempt to establish the safety parameters for low-frequency ultrasound, used 20 KHz (0.02 MHz) ultrasound at a 60% duty cycle at various intensities on dog skin with a stationary technique and found that only low intensities did not produce tissue damage. Further studies may lead to the development of a low-frequency ultrasound unit designed to administer phonophoresis efficiently and safely.

INDICATIONS, CONTRAINDICATIONS, AND PRECAUTIONS

Indications

Ultrasound is indicated for the intervention **of many musculoskeletal, neuromuscular, and integumentary conditions.** Box 15–1 lists the most common clinical uses for ultrasound, and the text provides additional clinical applications that are sited in the clinical and research literature. Many of these conditions have already been discussed in this text. Additional information is supplied for some conditions for which the intervention may not be obvious. Although many references are listed here, they are often from poorly controlled studies. Therefore, the therapeutic efficacy for the use of ultrasound is often inconclusive.[114,115,116,117,118,119,120,121] Robertson and Baker[122] systematically reviewed 35 randomized controlled trials in which people with pain and musculoskeletal problems were treated. They eliminated 25 articles that did not meet the acceptable inclusion criteria that they had established. Eight of the remaining articles showed ultrasound to be no more effective than the placebo intervention, and the remaining two articles showed ultrasound to be beneficial. Draper[123] is not ready to rule out the effectiveness of ultrasound

after review of the literature. He feels that the choice of clinical parameters such as effective radiating area (ERA), size of intervention area, and intervention time are factors that need to be more closely evaluated for ultrasound to be used effectively. Parameters for therapeutic dosage will be discussed in a following section.

Arthritis. The pain of chronic osteoarthritis and rheumatoid arthritis may be relieved by ultrasound, probably because of its deep-heating ability.[124] Casimiro et al[125] conducted a comprehensive search of the literature for treating rheumatoid arthritis and concluded that ultrasound to the palmer and dorsal surface of the hand significantly increases grip strength. Experimental animal studies are showing beneficial effects in both early stage and later stage repair of chemically induced arthritis.[126,127]

Carpal Tunnel Syndrome. Significant relief of pain, increase in motor-nerve conduction velocities, and decrease in motor distal latencies were documented by treating the wrists with 1 MHz pulsed (20% duty cycle) ultrasound for 15-min sessions. Interventions were given 5 days a week for the first 2 weeks followed by 2 sessions per week for the next 5 weeks. These results lasted at least until the follow-up testing 6 months later.[128]

Box 15–1 *Clinical Indications and Rationale for Therapeutic Ultrasound*

Clinical Use	Rationale
Tightness in soft tissue (ie, joint restrictions, adaptive muscle shortening, scar tissue)	Elevate tissue temperature to increase soft tissue extensibility during stretching.
Subacute and chronic inflammation (ie, bursitis, tendonitis)	Increase blood flow and cellular activity to assist in the inflammatory and healing phases following trauma.
	Use of anti-inflammatory topical medications during phonophoresis.
Musculoskeletal pain and associated muscle spasm	Increase blood flow to wash out inflammatory chemicals associated with pain and muscle spasm.
Bone fractures	Stimulate callus formation with nonthermal effects of ultrasound (very low intensity in a pulsed mode).
Wound healing	Increase activity in those cells involved in the inflammatory and proliferative phases of healing (very low intensity in a pulsed mode).

Contracture: Joint Capsules or Adhesive Scars. Tightness and scarring of periarticular structures have a variety of causes. Adhesive scars result from excessive proliferation of collagen, which may occur secondary to a laceration, incision, or burn, or may occur insidiously. Success in treating Dupuytren's contracture has been documented. Increased softening of the fibrous tissue has been accomplished with ultrasound.[129,130] In other conditions of fibrous hypertrophy, pain is a factor. Ultrasound has been reported to be effective in relieving pain, reducing curvature of the penis, and altering the consistency of the fibrous plaque in Peyronie's disease.[131,132,133]

Periarticular Conditions. The symptoms of bursitis, tendonitis, and ligamentous sprains may be relieved by ultrasound because of its thermal, and possibly nonthermal, effects.[134,135] Calcific tendonitis is frequently treated with ultrasound. Ebenbichler[136] used radiograph to document the complete resolution on one subject and a considerable decrease in size on two other subjects after being treated according to the following protocol for 30 sessions. One MHz pulsed ultrasound (25% duty cycle) at 2 W/sq cm for 10 min was administered 1 to 2 times a day, 4 to 5 times a week, for 4 to 8 weeks. This treatment sounds impressive, but the author warns that it is common for calcifications to resolve spontaneously.

Muscular Problems. The symptoms and decreased function of strains, spasm, fibrosis, myositis, and hematoma may be relieved by ultrasound.[137]

Neuromas. The pain of neuromas may be relieved by ultrasound because of its effects on nervous tissue. Griffin[14] stated that pain relief might be a result of relaxation of excessively proliferated connective tissue.

Sympathetic Nervous System Disorders. The reflex dystrophies, such as causalgia and Sudek's atrophy, can be treated by paravertebral sonation of the involved segments or underwater over the segment of hyperpathia.[138]

Plantar Warts. Several authors reported success with the elimination of pain, or the wart itself, after exposure to ultrasound.[139,140,141] Vaughn, in particular, reported excellent results with the direct-contact technique at a mean intensity of 0.69 W/sq cm for 15 min. These findings are from clinical reports rather than from controlled studies, however.

Open Wounds. Refer to the discussion earlier in this chapter about pressure sores and tissue repair studies. Ultrasound can be administered to open wounds with a water immersion technique or with a direct contact technique using a sterile couplant.

Chronic Systematic Peripheral Arterial Disease. Griffin and Karselis[14] advocated sonation directly over vessels affected by vasospasm or sonation of the sympathetic nervous system. Warning: If signs of thrombophlebitis are present, direct sonation is contraindicated.[10]

Temporomandibular Joint Pain. Shin and Choi[142] demonstated the pain-relieving effect of indomethacin phonophoresis for TMJ pain in a double-blind, placebo-controlled clinical trial. They successfully used 1 MHz continuous ultrasound at 0.8–1.5 W/sq cm for 15 min. They began interventions at 1.5 W/sq cm and lowered the intensity if the subject felt anything but a mild warm.

Contraindications

There are relatively few contraindications for therapeutic ultrasound. Ultrasound will be contraindicated for any condition for which a TTR is contraindicated for the use of ultrasound in a manner that will produce a thermal response. Refer to the list of contraindications to therapeutic heat in **Chapter 13 and those listed in Box 15–2.** The rationale and research literature related to these contraindications are further reviewed in this chapter.

Cardiac Pacemakers. If a pacemaker or its surrounding tissue is exposed to the ultrasound field, it may malfunction. Note that the use of ultrasound is not excluded for a distal part of the patient's body, where the sound field will not affect the pacemaker.[143]

Pregnancy. The effects of therapeutic ultrasound on the fetus are not known. Therefore, if pregnancy is suspected, avoid sonating the abdomen, pelvis, and lumbar-sacral areas. Diagnostic ultrasound is not included in this contraindication.

Tumors. Whether a tumor is malignant or benign, sonation of the tumor is probably best avoided because the heat and mechanical energy may increase the rate of tumor growth or cause metastasis. Three MHz continuous ultrasound at 1 W/sq cm for 5 min, administered 10 times in a 2-week period over murine

Box 15–2 *Therapeutic Ultrasound Contraindications*

Near a pacemaker

Near the uterus in a pregnant woman

Near a malignant or benign tumor

Near a suspected thrombophlebitis

Near an area with infection

Over areas with active bleeding or susceptible to hemorrhage

Over growing epiphyseal plates (skeletally immature individuals)

Over areas that have recently been exposed to radiation and radioactive isotopes

Over the cervical ganglia, stellate ganglia, or heart (especially for those individuals with cardiac disease)

Over the vertebral bodies (especially for those individuals with laminectomy)

Over the eyes, ears, and genitalia

Over joint replacement and superficial metal implants

---

tumors in mice, increased the size and weight of the tumors. In this study there was no increase in metastatic lymph nodes.[144] In a subsequent study, lower-intensity continuous (0.75 W/sq cm) ultrasound was compared with energy-matched pulsed ultrasound (20% duty cycle). The same amount of energy was applied but at a different rate for a different amount of time. The results were smaller tumors than had previously been seen with high-intensity ultrasound but no difference in the energy-matched ultrasound groups. All tumors in groups treated with ultrasound were larger than the control-group tumors.[145] (Note: Ultrasound at different parameters is being used medically for the destruction of tumor cells.[146,147,148,149,150] It has also been used successfully to produce regression of psoriatic lesions, which are caused by benign hyperproliferative disease.[151]

Thrombophlebitis.   The mechanical energy may disrupt a clot, resulting in the formation of an embolus that may travel to the brain, heart, or lungs.[139]

Infected Areas.   Ultrasound may promote the spread of infection.

Areas with a Tendency to Hemorrhage.   Increased blood flow and capillary permeability produced by ultrasound may encourage bleeding.

Epiphyses of Growing Bone.   Ultrasound has been shown to cause bone-growth disturbances in experimental situations.[152] Therapeutic ultrasound has been shown to have an effect on endochondral ossification in the developing metatarsal long-bone rudiments of fetal mice.[153] Although 1 MHz, low-intensity (0.1 to 0.77 W/sq cm SATP), pulsed ultrasound at a 20% duty cycle produced increases in longitudinal growth, continuous ultrasound at 0.1–0.5 W/sq cm had either no effect or possible decrease in growth. Therefore, clinicians must continue to use caution in the application of ultrasound over unclosed epiphyseal plates.

Deep X-ray, Radiation, or Radioactive Isotopes.   There may be an interaction effect a low-intensity ultrasound and ionizing radiation on surface tumor cells. Six months should pass after termination of radiation intervention before ultrasound begins. Routine diagnostic X-rays are not included in this contraindication.

Cardiac Disease.   Ultrasound over the cervical ganglia, stellate ganglia, or heart area may stimulate a coronary reflex that could be hazardous to a person with cardiac disease.

Over the Eyes.   Ultrasound in this area may have a cavitational effect because of the fluid medium.[12]

Over the Spinal Cord in Areas with Inadequate Protection.   In cases of laminectomy or other conditions that reduce the normal bony and muscular protection of the spinal cord, ultrasound may cause cavitation or overheating of the spinal fluid.[12]

Precautions

Unhealed Fracture Sites. Although many manufactures state that the use of ultrasound over unhealed fractures is contraindicated, it is the intensity and mode that determine whether there is a detrimental or beneficial effect of ultrasound on fracture healing. There is evidence that continuous ultrasound at mid to high intensities produces deleterious effects on healing bone.[154,155,156] There are more indications that therapeutic ultrasound may be effective in the stimulation of bone formation.[157,158,159] Low intensity appears to be the key to appropriate use. The stimulatory effects are from nonthermal mechanisms rather than from heating. Therapeutic ultrasound was found significantly to stimulate the synthesis of both collagenous and noncollagenous bone matrix proteins.[152] The 3 MHz ultrasound was pulsed with a 20% duty cycle and delivered at 0.1 w/cm for 2 to 5 min. Ultrasound at 1 to 2 W/sq cm inhibited synthesis of both proteins. Pilla et al[160] found that low-intensity ultrasound stimulated fracture repair in fibular osteotomies in rabbits. They used 1.5 MHz ultrasound delivered in 200 microsecond bursts at a burst frequency of 1 KHz and an intensity of about 30 mW/sq cm (SATA) for 20 min from postoperative Day 1 to Day 28.

The clinician must determine whether using low-intensity, pulsed ultrasound over a fracture site will produce a therapeutic effect on the target tissue. If the purpose is to heat the surrounding soft tissue, low intensity would be ineffective.

Primary Repair of Tendon or Ligament. This category may include a partial tendon rupture in the early stages. Look back to the section on Tissue Healing.

Osteoporosis. Use ultrasound with caution over osteoporotic bones until research is available to rule out a detrimental effect on the already demineralized bone.

Plastic Implants. High-density plastics used for joint replacements have high coefficients of absorption of ultrasonic energy. Theoretically, this factor would pose a potential risk. Although the risk has not been documented in any controlled studies or clinical reports, direct sonation over plastic implants should be avoided until it can be proved to be safe.[13]

Metal Implants. Lehman et al[161] investigated the acoustical properties of various metals used for surgical implants and found that a large amount of ultrasonic energy was reflected at the tissue-metal interface, thus creating standing waves of increased intensity in front of the metal. In addition, little penetration of sound occurred through the metal. Other studies using animal or human tissues have shown that no appreciable temperature rise occurred in the metal implant and that the soft tissues surrounding the isolated metal implant were actually heated less than if the bone had been present.[162,163] The most probable explanation is related to the high thermal conductivity of metal, which is able to transmit the heat generated at the metal-tissue interface away from the sonated area more quickly than the heat can be produced.

Metal plates and screws are commonly used for the internal fixation of fractures. Does ultrasound have detrimental nonthermal effects on the strength of internal fixation? Skoubo-Kristenson and Sommer[164] implanted metal plates fastened by three cortical screws into the femora or humor of dogs. After 2 weeks, half of the dogs were treated with low intensity (0.5 W/sq cm) ultrasound, and the other half were treated with high intensity (3 W/sq cm) ultrasound for 5 min a day for 14 days. The authors found no significant difference in the torque used to insert the screws with the torque needed to remove the screws in the sonated and control groups. Thus, they supported the notion that internal fixation does not contraindicate the use of ultrasound therapy.

THERAPEUTIC DOSAGE AND MODE

Physical therapists must understand the quantification of ultrasonic energy for several reasons: (1) to ensure selection of the safe and appropriate intensity for a patient's condition, (2) to apply a consistent dosage from intervention to intervention, and (3) to keep accurate clinical records so that more reliable and meaningful descriptive information can be obtained about the clinical success and failure of ultrasound techniques. To be meaningful, these considerations require regular calibration of the ultrasound unit. The many inconsistencies in reports of clinical trial may be related to lack of calibration and accurate documentation of dosages and techniques. Even with calibration, the dosage that the patient receives at similar meter readings varies among ultrasound units. The therapist must be aware that many ultrasound units currently in service are inaccurate. Stewart et al[165] tested 56 different units and found that 20% of them emitted at least 20% more energy than the power meter indicated. Fyfe and Parnell[166] further confirmed the inaccuracy of power output and effective radiation surface. Only 5 to 18 transducers tested met the required +/−15% of power expected according to the manufacturers' data. Although these studies were done on machines that may not be in use today, similar findings of inaccuracy were discovered in the 1980s[167,168] on the types of ultrasound units that may still be in use in some clinics. Recently, Arthro et al[169] found that 39% of the 83 ultrasound units they tested were outside the +/−20% standard for at least 1 of the 4 intensity settings tested. Three machines produced no output at any of the settings tested. Pye and Milford[170] found 69% of the 85 ultrasound units they tested in Scotland to have power outputs that differed by more than 30% of the expected values. The ultrasound units designed in the 1990s have built-in feedback mechanisms designed to control accuracy and warn the clinician if contact with the patient is inadequate. Even new ultrasound equipment must be checked regularly. A quick check by the clinician can be performed to determine whether energy is being emitted from the sound head. Face the sound head toward the ceiling, and wrap a piece of tape around it. Fill with water the cylinder that you have created, and slowly increase the intensity of ultrasound (**Fig. 15–5**). You should initially see tiny ripples in the water, and as the intensity is increased, the water should become more turbulent. This procedure shows only that there is output proportional to the intensity setting but does not quantify it. It can also be used as a demonstration for patients who seem doubtful that energy is really being emitted.

A more accurate method to test the average power output from an ultrasound unit is using a device that adheres to the Radiation Force Balance principle. These devices vary in sensitivity and price, but provide accurate information on power output (**Fig. 15–6**).

Power

Power, measured in watts, is the amount of acoustic energy in the radiating beam per unit of time. The power value is the only indicator of the total amount of ultrasonic energy that a patient receives. If a therapist treated a patient one day with an intensity of 1.5 W/sq cm with a 10 sq cm transducer, the patient would receive 15 watts of energy. If, on a subsequent day, the therapist treated the patient at 1.5 W/sq cm using an ultrasound unit with a 7 sq cm transducer, assuming the treated area to be the same, the patient would receive only 10.5 watts of energy (1.5 W/sq cm × 7 sq cm), which may indicate a less-effective second intervention. This example demonstrates the need to record both power and intensity in the patient's

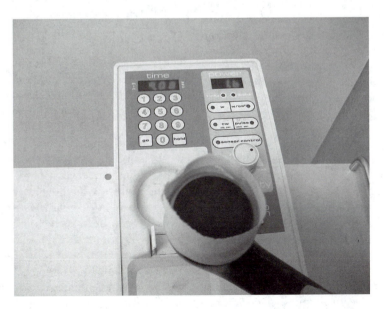

FIGURE 15–5   Ultrasound unit showing water cylinder.

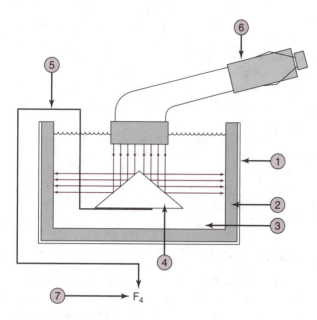

FIGURE 15–6   Schematic illustrating ultrasound test based on the radiation force balance principle.

record. The term **time average power** is sometimes used with pulsed ultrasound generators to represent the total watts applied to the patient during an intervention.

Intensity

Intensity (I) is the term used most frequently when discussing ultrasound dosage. The more accurate term is **spatial average intensity,** which is the acoustic power (W) divided by the effective radiating area (ERA) (sq cm) of the transducer. In medical ultrasonics, the units are watts per square centimeter (W/sq cm). If 15 watts of acoustic energy is radiated from a crystal, the area of which is 10 square centimeters, the intensity is 1.5 W/sq cm, or

$$I = W/\text{sq cm}$$

Intensity represents the strength of the acoustic energy at the point of application. The effective radiating area is not necessarily the same size as the metal face of the sound head, but rather the size of the radiating surface of the crystal within. The ERA should be stated in the specification list of each ultrasound generator.

Continuous- versus Pulsed-Wave Mode. **Continuous-wave ultrasound,** as the name implies, is acoustic energy transmitted without interruption from the time

the transducer is energized until the intensity control is returned to zero. **Pulsed-wave ultrasound** is acoustic energy with brief cyclical breaks in transmission throughout its application. These breaks in transmission reduce the overall amount of energy available to the patient for a given time interval compared with ultrasound at the same peak intensity. If 1 W/sq cm of pulsed ultrasound is applied for 1 min, the patient receives less energy than if continuous ultrasound is applied at 1 W/sq cm for 1 min. How much less energy depends on the ratio of on-time to off-time (duty cycle).

Many clinicians use the rationale that pulsed ultrasound produces only nonthermal effects because of the interruptions in transmission of energy. It would be more accurate to say that less heating occurs with pulsed ultrasound than with continuous ultrasound at similar peak intensities. It should be noted that similar thermal effects can be obtained if the same time-average intensities are used. The clinician can use extremely low intensities of continuous ultrasound to minimize its thermal effects. Perhaps the mode of ultrasound is less important than the average intensities and power used. However, if the nonthermal effects of ultrasound are required when treating deeper structures, it may be more advantageous to choose the pulsed mode at a low duty cycle (20%) and a high spatial average intensity. This method would provide enough energy to be available for absorption at the target tissue. Of course, the proper frequency is also required so that the most energy will be available for absorption at the depth of the target tissue.

Duty Cycle

When pulsed ultrasound is used, the duty cycle must be considered to determine the overall amount of energy that the patient receives. **Duty cycle** is a percentage or ratio of the pulse duration (on-time of the pulse) to the pulse period (the sum of the on-time and off-time of the pulse during each cycle). **Figure 15–7** shows two different pulse modulations being applied at the same spatial average intensities. The raised rectangles represent the flow of energy, the on-time; the return to baseline begins the rest period, the off-time.

In **Figure 15–7**, which modulation is providing the most ultrasound to the patient? How much more energy is modulation B providing than modulation A during the same time period? Modulation B is providing twice as much energy as modulation A, although only half as much as if it were continuous ultrasound at the same spatial average intensity. Note that in

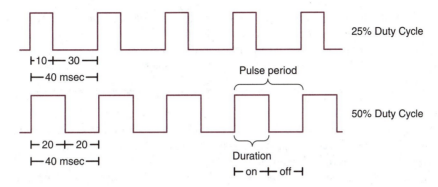

FIGURE 15-7 Pulse modulation of ultrasound energy. Modulation B provides twice as much energy as modulation A because its on-time is twice as long.

both A and B in **Figure 15-7**, the complete cycles are 40 milliseconds in duration. Pulsed ultrasound intensities should be stated as both spatial average and temporal (time) average intensities. The **temporal average intensity** is the average intensity of ultrasound emitted throughout the pulse period. Find it by multiplying the duty cycle as a percent by the pulse average intensity on the meter. If the pulse average intensity (the maximum intensity during the on cycle) is 1 W/sq cm and the duty cycle is 20% the temporal average intensity would be 0.2 W/sq cm. If the duty cycle were 80%, the temporal average intensity would be 0.8 W/sq cm.

Beam Nonuniformity Ratio

The **spatial average intensity** represents the intensity averaged over the area of the beam of energy. This implies that the ultrasonic energy is not distributed evenly throughout the beam. In some areas within the beam, the intensity is much higher than it is in the adjacent areas. The **beam nonuniformity ratio (BNR)** is a numerical value that represents the ratio of the peak intensity (ie, the highest intensity in the ultrasound field) to the spatial average intensity indicated on the ultrasound meter.[171]

Figure 15-8 represents the variation in intensity at different points in the cross section of a near ultrasonic field. The spatial average intensity is the average of the shaded area under the curve. In this example, the BNR is 6 to 1, and the peak intensity is 12 W/sq cm in a field of spatial average intensity of 2.0 W/sq cm. Therefore, if a patient is treated with an intensity of 2.0 W/sq cm, as indicated by the ultrasound meter, the beam may create a hot spot with an intensity of 12 W/sq cm if the sound head remains stationary.

The BNR should be considered when purchasing an ultrasound unit. Examine the specifications and an ultrasonic beam diagram showing the relatively even energy distribution with low BNR.

Irradiation Time and Surface Area

In addition to power, intensity, and duty cycle, the total amount of time that the patient is treated must be noted. Logically, if a patient receives 10 W of ultrasound for 2 min, twice as much energy has been administered than if the patient had received 10 W for only 1 min.

The other major consideration when determining dosage is the size of the surface being treated. Assuming the same total watts and time, the larger the area sonated, the smaller the amount of energy available per unit of tissue. Consider this example: A physical

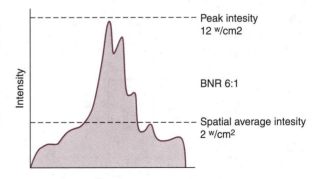

FIGURE 15-8 The variation in intensity at different points in the cross section of near ultrasonic field. The beam nonuniformity ratio (BNR) is 12:2, or 6:1, the ratio between the peak intensity and the spatial average intensity. If kept stationary, the sound head will create a hot spot of 12 watts per square centimeter.

therapist treats the right lumbar paravertebral muscles of a patient at 2 W/sq cm for 5 min. The effective radiating area of the transducer is 10 sq cm. Thus, the therapist administers a total of 20 W at 2 W/sq cm for 5 min to the 50 sq cm area. On the other hand, if the therapist decides to include more of the musculature and doubles the length and width of the sonated area, the surface area quadruples (**Fig. 15–9**). In other words, the exposure time of each section of tissue is reduced to one-fourth the amount of energy that would be received if only the smaller area were treated.

In this example, only 10 sq cm of each section can be sonated at any time. During the course of a 5-min intervention, each portion of tissue can receive only 1 min of ultrasonic energy if the intervention area is 50 sq cm. If the 5-min intervention is distributed over an intervention area of 200 sq cm, each section of tissue receives only 15 sec, or one-fourth the previous amount of ultrasound. In this example, one would not expect a significant TTR or other therapeutic effect in the larger area of intervention because the exposure time per unit area of tissue would be inadequate. This subject will be discussed in more detail in the intervention protocol section.

METHODS OF APPLICATION

Three techniques of applying ultrasound are available (1) direct contact, (2) immersion, and (3) fluid-filled bag. Each technique can be performed using a stationary or a moving sound head.

Stationary Procedure

The stationary procedure involves directing the ultrasonic transducer so that the only area sonated is directly under the sound head. This technique is gen-

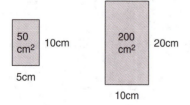

FIGURE 15–9 A comparison of ultrasound treatment areas. If the same amount of power and time are used for both areas, the larger area will receive only 25% of the energy per unit of tissue compared with the smaller area because the larger area is four times as big.

erally not recommended because of its potentially detrimental effects. Stewart et al[172] reported on the studies of Barth and Wachsman, which indicated that bone damage in dogs was produced by a stationary transducer at 0.5 W/sq cm to 1 W/sq cm compared with about 3 W/sq cm for a moving sound field. One might argue that treating with only low dosage (below 0.5 W/sq cm) should produce no detrimental effects. Unfortunately, the intensity of power indicated on many power meters is inaccurate.

Another disadvantage of the stationary technique is the development of "hot spots"—areas within the ultrasound field that are exposed to higher intensities than the surrounding tissue within the same sound field. (Refer to the preceding discussion of BNR.) Haar[173] emphasized the nonuniformity of the ultrasound field or beam. There are areas of peak intensity that are considerably higher than would be indicated by the spatial average intensity on the power meter. Haar recommended using a moving sound head technique so that no section of tissue is exposed to the peak intensity for a significant amount of time. Similarly, Allen and Barrye[174] as well as the U.S. Department of Health and Human Services[165] recommend using the moving sound head to compensate for the lack of uniformity of the ultrasound field.

Another reason to abandon the stationary technique is the possibility of impairing blood flow. Dyson and Pond[175] produced blood cell stasis in chick embryos exposed to therapeutic levels of ultrasound by the stationary sound head procedure. This outcome occurs only during the exposure period in vessels lying parallel to the direction of ultrasound propagation. This mechanism is believed to be associated with the production of standing waves that accompany the stationary technique. The stasis can be avoided by using a moving sound head.

We recommend avoiding the stationary technique for the preceding reasons. It should be noted, however, that others have used the technique at extremely low intensities. Griffin and Karselis[14] recommended this technique for treating small, localized areas of pain, spasm, or organized hematoma. They recommended intensities of 0.02 to 0.1 W/sq cm for 5 min or more. However, they cautioned that even at these extremely low intensities, overheating, particularly of the periosteum, can occur because one small area receives all the energy. Thus, a hot spot might develop within that area.

As clinicians replace old ultrasound units with new units that have lower BNR (2:1) and have higher output accuracy, stationary technique at low intensities may be safely used. This author suggests waiting until the clinical research has been done that establishes clear guidelines for this technique.

Moving Sound Head Procedure

Technique. When using the moving procedure, the sound head must be moved over the intervention area in a smooth, rhythmical pattern. It is important to keep the rhythm constant throughout the intervention and during each consecutive intervention. If the sound head is moved too slowly, the patient will be unable to tolerate as high an intensity. A consistent movement is required to ensure the even distribution of energy and to avoid hot spots. The choice of movement pattern is based on the contour of the area treated. The pattern can be either small overlapping circles or small overlapping strokes. The circular technique is desirable when treating an area with irregular contours; either technique can be used when treating a large flat area.

The circular method requires the therapist to make circles of small diameter, about the size of the sound head, that glide just far enough for the subsequent circle to overlap the preceding circle by half. The stroking method requires the therapist to glide the sound head slowly and longitudinally in one direction, then slide it laterally one-half the width of the sound head before returning longitudinally. The pattern chosen is repeated over the involved area for the desired intervention time. The pressure of the sound head against the body part is important for adequate coupling and efficient transmission. Gann et al[176] determined that when physical therapy students were trained to apply the optimal pressure of 600 grams, they retained this skill for a least 7 months as shown in their retesting. The untrained group used a mean pressure of only 321.92 g. Some authors have recommended that a large area should be treated in subdivisions so that the energy covers the area long enough to have an additive effect. For example, Lehmann[177] suggested exposing the area no more than 75 sq cm at a time to allow for effective heating. Oakley[178] recommended treating sections about 1.5 times the size of the transducer for 30-sec periods. This procedure is repeated over the entire intervention area until the total prescribed intervention time is reached.

Coupling Agents. A coupling agent must always be used between the sound head and the patient to enhance transmission. Most clinicians use a commer-cially prepared thixotropic gel for applications involving direct contact. Although thixotropic gel is the most expensive type of coupling agent, it is the most convenient to use. Warren et al[179] compared the degree of transmissiveness of four commercially available coupling agents—gels, mineral oil, glycerin, and degassed water—and found that, except for glycerin, which had the lowest transmissiveness (60%), the mean levels of transmissivity were within 10% of the reference: degassed water. Transmissiveness was measured through 1 mm films of the couplant, similar to the amount used in applications involving direct contact. Refer to the Phonophoresis section of this chapter for further discussion of transmissivity.

Tepid degassed water is the ideal medium for the immersion technique because it does not allow the formation of bubbles that can interfere with transmission. Tap water is used most commonly because of its ease of access and low cost. Investigations into the effective TTR obtained by underwater techniques compared with transmission through gel showed the immersion technique to be significantly less effective.[180,181] Klucinec et al[182] showed that only 31% of the acoustic energy was delivered during a tapwater bath. According to Griffin,[183] water transmits ultrasound more efficiently than does glycerin or mineral oil. If glycerin or mineral oil is used, it must be kept cooler than water. The coolness reduces the amount of surface heating that seems to impair deep heating by ultrasound when the immersion technique is used. Lehmann et al[184] suggested that water is an effective coupling medium at 75° F (24° C) but that mineral oil is not. Mineral oil may be no warmer than 64°F (18° C) to allow for heating at the level of a deep-set joint capsule.

Hydrogel sheets and semipermeable film membranes have become available for the application of ultrasound over open wounds. Klucinec et al[185] demonstrated that the effectiveness for ultrasonic transmission through these media varied significantly from product to product.

Direct-Contact Procedure

Technique. The most common, convenient, and efficient method of applying ultrasound is by direct contact: the sound head glides on the surface of the skin. Three basic requirements must be met to use this technique correctly. First, the contour of the part being treated must allow good contact of the sound head for the duration of the intervention. If total contact does not exist, the area of the transducer that is in contact with the air will be unable to dissipate its energy, and the transducer may overheat or the unit will shut off. Partial contact also will reduce the total amount of energy the patient receives.

Second, the skin or soft tissue must not be so sensitive to pressure that moving the sound head along the skin causes pain. This condition can be minimized by 5 to 7 min of ice massage immediately before the ultrasound. In our experience, the icing reduces the sensitivity of the skin without impairing the responsiveness of the deeper thermal receptors that are needed to prevent overexposure.

Third, the skin must be intact. If skin eruptions, blisters, or infection are present in the treated area, the movement of the sound head may irritate the area further or spread the infection. Therefore, ultrasound should not be applied over these areas.

Preparation for Intervention.   Before the intervention is initiated, the following procedures must be carried out:

1. Place the ultrasound unit, a coupling agent, and toweling in an area easily accessible to the therapist, but one that does not interfere with the patient.

2. Explain the procedure in a manner appropriate for each patient's intellect and interest. Inform patients that a mild sensation of warmth is acceptable but that they must tell the therapist if they feel even the slightest degree of heat, pain, or discomfort so that the intensity of the intervention can be reduced.

3. Position the patient so that the area to be treated is exposed, the patient is relaxed and comfortable, and stretching can be done if desired.

4. The sound head, which should not be turned on at this point, can be used to spread the coupling agent over the area to be treated. The couplant should cover the entire area with a thin film. (Note: If the patient reports a prickling, tingling, or superficial burning sensation during the intervention, the cause may be an inadequate amount of couplant. If this problem occurs, reduce the intensity to zero, and apply more couplant before continuing the intervention. If the patient continues to feel these sensations, check the machine.)

5. Switch the unit on with the power switch or by turning on the timer. Adjust the timer as required to bring the intensity to the desired level.

6. Check the meter to ensure that the intensity is at zero and that the desired mode (continuous or pulsed) is selected. If your machine allows, you may preset the intensity to the desired output level.

7. Place the sound head firmly on the patient. Move the sound head back and forth, maintaining total contact with the skin as the intensity gradually rises to the desired level. The sound head *must be moved continuously;* if not, the patient may report a sudden strong ache or a stabbing pain that resembles being struck by a needle as the intensity of the dose increases. These sensations are probably caused by periosteal overheating or a too-rapid rise in temperature locally in the soft tissue. This is obviously not the way to establish a good rapport and to gain your patient's confidence. At no time should the sound head be exposed to the air while the power is on.

8. At the end of the intervention, the timer should run out and stop the output of power. Turn the intensity control to zero before removing the sound head from the patient; many machines will now do this automatically. Wipe the couplant from the sound head, and place the head in its holder. Remove the couplant from the patient's skin with soft toweling. Most coupling gels are water soluble and do not stain clothing. If necessary, alcohol can be used to cleanse the skin and the sound head.

Immersion Procedure

Technique.   The next-most common method of applying ultrasound is to immerse the body part in a fluid medium. This technique is indicated when none of the three criteria for the direct-contact method are met. The immersion procedure is especially useful for treating small irregular surfaces such as joints of the hands and feet. It is also indicated for intervention of areas that are too sensitive to be touched or that have broken skin.

Preparation for Intervention.   The therapist must carry out the following preparatory procedures before initiating the intervention:

1. Prepare the immersion medium, and position the ultrasound unit in an easily accessible position.

2. Explain the procedure to the patient.

3. Position the patient so that the area to be treated is exposed and the patient is comfortable and relaxed.

4. Immerse the nonenergized sound head in the basin, and direct it toward the target about 0.5–1 inch from the skin.

5. Begin a slow, rhythmic pattern of movement similar to the one described for the direct-contact procedure, and slowly raise the intensity to the desired level. It is extremely important to direct the ultrasound waves perpendicular to the skin surface to reduce surface reflection. As the angle of incidence increases, less energy will be directed to the target structure and be available for penetration and absorption. Air bubbles on the skin or sound head also will increase reflection and reduce transmission. If air bubbles develop during the intervention, simply brush them away from the sound head or skin with a quick light stroke, using a piece of gauze attached to a tongue depressor.

6. When the intervention is finished, reduce the intensity to zero before removing the sound head from the medium, and then dry the head before replacing it in its holder.

Precautions. The ultrasound generator should be plugged into a receptacle that is protected by a *ground fault interrupter (GFI)*. This will protect both the patient and the therapist from a potential shock associated with leakage of low-level current that would not trip a standard circuit breaker. The GFI is recommended for use in areas where large amounts of moisture accumulate. The National Electrical Code requires a GFI for all newly built outdoor structures, bathrooms, and garages where electrical appliances are used.[186]

The therapist should avoid placing the hands in the path of the direct or reflected ultrasound waves. Poor technique will expose the therapist's hands to excessive amounts of ultrasound during repeated immersions.

Fluid-Filled Bag or Cushion Procedure

Technique. The fluid-filled bag, or fluid cushion, procedure, although not widely used, provides an alternative method of treating areas that have irregular contours or are overly sensitive. This procedure is more practical than immersion for treating a proximal body part such as a shoulder, scapula, or trochanter, which would require a large tank. The technique requires only a thin-membrane bag, such as a condom or a surgical glove, and a coupling medium such as degassed water, mineral oil, or glycerin. It is important

to use degassed water rather than tap water because clearing bubbles that form within the bag is difficult.

Preparation for Intervention. Before initiating the intervention, the therapist must carry out the following procedures:

1. Fill the condom or surgical glove with the fluid, and put the mouth of the bag around the sidewalls of the sound head. Squeeze the bag gently to force out the air until the sound head is in full contact with the fluid. Seal the bag with a rubber band or tape. Remember that air between the sound head and fluid will reduce transmission.

2. Apply the bag to the patient. Ideally, the medium used in the bag should be used on the skin and the outside of the bag to ensure good contact and to eliminate air bubbles from the skin surface.

3. With the bag in firm contact with the skin, begin moving the sound head within the bag rhythmically and gently as the intensity increases to the desired level. Keep the sound head at a 90° angle to the intervention surface, and avoid sliding the bag on the skin.

A variation of this procedure is the use of a fluid cushion, made by filling a bag with fluid and sealing it. The cushion is placed on the body part with a coupling medium between the bag and skin and between the bag and the sound head. While firmly holding the bag over the part, slowly stroke the top surface of the bag with the sound head. The major drawback of this technique is that it creates an extra interface between the sound head and the skin. Even the fluid-filled bag procedure creates one more interface than does the direct-contact method. The membrane of the bag and the couplant form an interface that attenuates sound waves.

INTERVENTION PROTOCOL

The intervention protocol for ultrasound is established by (1) the size of the area to be sonated, (2) the duration of the intervention, and (3) the intensity used. The frequency and total number of interventions must also be considered. **Box 15–3** summarizes the ultrasound intervention parameters and guidelines for choosing the most appropriate settings based on desired clinical effects.

Box 15–3 *Guidelines for Selecting Ultrasound Intervention Parameters*

Intensity	>1.0 wts/cm^2 for thermal effects (ie, for increasing soft tissue extensibility and decrease joint viscosity)	<1.0 wts/cm^2 for nonthermal effects (ie, during acute inflammation to promote tissue healing)
Frequency	1 MHz for targeting deep tissue (ie, to sonate the deep gluteal muscles such as the piriformis)	3 MHz for targeting superficial tissue (ie, to sonate the wrist extensor tendons distal to the lateral epicondyle of the elbow)
Duty Cycle	100% for thermal effects (ie, to significantly alter blood flow to the target tissue and elevate tissue temperature)	20% for nonthermal effects (ie, to prevent the buildup of heat in individuals with acute inflammation
Treatment Time	*Treatment Area* .4 × ERA Longer treatment time to get maximal heating, treating chronic conditions	*Treatment Area* >.67 × ERA Shorter treatment time for acute conditions

Size of Area and Duration of Intervention

The therapist determines the size of the area to be sonated. This determination is based on the area required to produce a healing effect or to relieve pain. The clinician must choose a small enough area to allow the therapeutic effect of the ultrasound. Ultrasonic energy is transmitted through the tissues of the body and absorbed along its path. The physiologic effects are initiated and prolonged during this application. When the energy source is removed, the body begins to restore its preultrasound state. If too large an area is sonated, the energy will be dispersed to such a degree that the threshold of tissue stimulation may never be reached. For a reaction to occur, energy must be applied at an adequate concentration for an adequate amount of time. Therefore, all considerations concerning time of application should be for areas two times the ERA, or approximately two times the size of the soundhead. This is adequate for the conditions treated by most physical therapists. An area too commonly treated that does not meet this size criterion is the paravertebral musculature, which the author feels should not be routinely ultrasounded. Paravertebral trigger points would be appropriate because of their small size.

In determining duration of intervention, the therapist should consider the following guidelines: (1) the first intervention may be shorter than subsequent interventions, (2) acute conditions may be treated for shorter periods than chronic conditions, and (3) smaller areas require less time than larger areas. To produce a maximally safe thermal response, the same intensity can be applied for a longer period to prolong the physiologic response.

These general principles have been stated because no definitive, objective standard exists for the duration of intervention. We suggest the following formulas for determining the duration of interventions. The formulas are general guidelines based on values recommended by others[13,19,20,21,22] and by clinical experience.

For subacute conditions:

$$\frac{\text{Area to be treated}}{0.67 \times \text{ERA}} = \text{Minutes of ultrasound}$$

where ERA is the effective radiating area.

For example, if you are treating an area of 50 sq cm with a transducer that has an ERA of 10 sq cm,

$$\frac{50}{0.67 \times 10} = \frac{50}{0.67 \times 10} = 7.5 \text{ minutes}$$

For chronic conditions:

$$\frac{\text{Area to be treated}}{0.5 \times \text{ERA}} = \text{Minutes of ultrasound}$$

For example, if you are treating an area of 50 sq cm with a transducer that has an ERA of 10 sq cm,

$$\frac{50}{0.5 \times 10} = \frac{50}{5} = 10 \text{ minutes of ultrasound}$$

For maximal thermal effect:

$$\frac{\text{Area to be treated}}{0.4 \times 10 \text{ ERA}} = \text{Minutes of ultrasound}$$

For example, if you are treating an area of 50 sq cm with a transducer that has an ERA of 10 sq cm,

$$\frac{50}{.4 \times 10} = \frac{50}{4} = 12.5 \text{ minutes of ultrasound}$$

Intensity of Intervention

When determining the intensity of intervention, the therapist should consider the following guidelines:

- A superficial lesion, including one near a bony prominence, should be treated with a higher frequency and lower intensity than a deep lesion.
- A subacute lesion, or any lesion where thermal effects are undesirable, should be treated with a lower intensity than is the case for a chronic lesion.
- A slightly lower-than-estimated "ideal" intensity should be used for the first intervention so that the patient's response can be assessed.
- The patient's feedback should be obtained both during and after the intervention to determine the appropriate intensity. (If the therapist decides to treat a patient with deficient sensory or thermal awareness, only a low intensity should be used.)

In the absence of any other deficits such as circulatory impairment, ultrasound can be applied to the part with the sensory deficit after establishing a safe dosage. This procedure can be done by determining the dosage that the patient can tolerate on the similar contralateral body part. Patients can tolerate (1) a higher intensity of pulsed ultrasound than continuous ultrasound and (2) a higher intensity during an immersion procedure than a direct-contact procedure. Forrest and Rosen[187] demonstrated that the temperature of pig extensor tendon did not rise to nearly the same degree when sonation was done under tap water compared with sonation by direct contact. Because of the reduced efficiency of energy transmission by the immersion technique, these authors suggested an increase in dosage. Hayes[188] recommended an increase

of 0.5 W/sq cm in the intensity for immersion versus direct contact. This is only a general guideline. The ultimate guide is the patient's response and clinical signs. Patients should not experience discomfort at any time. If they complain of an ache or a sudden stabbing pain, the intensity should be reduced, or the sound head should be moved more quickly.

It is difficult to prescribe precise values for different situations. Part of the problem relates to the individual differences in the output of the many ultrasound units in use. The power output of many units is extremely inefficient, and many demonstrate inaccurate metering. Thus, clinicians must be familiar with the characteristics of their particular ultrasound units.

Although estimates of intervention intensities are based on a scale of 0 to 2 W/sq cm, the key is to rely on the patient's response and clinical signs. If the patient experiences pain during the intervention, reduce the intensity immediately.

Patients may report several types of pain or discomfort. A sharp, stabbing pain is usually a sign of periosteal overheating caused by moving the sound head directly onto a bony prominence or by stroking it slowly over bone. This type of pain can be prevented by (1) reducing the intensity, (2) avoiding direct sonation over bony prominences, or (3) moving more quickly over bony prominences. A dull, aching pain is probably the result of an intensity that is too high, which causes a too-rapid TTR from prolonged application. In the latter case, intervention should be terminated.

A prickling, tingling, stinging, or vibrating sensation under the sound head may indicate an inadequate amount of couplant or inadequate contact with the skin. This problem can be corrected by (1) applying more couplant, (2) repositioning the part to allow adequate skin contact, or (3) changing to the immersion or fluid-filled-bag procedure.

The following suggestions for determining intensity are based on an ultrasound generator with a range of 0 to 2 W/sq cm on continuous mode using a moving sound head and the direct-contact procedure:

- For acute conditions, use 0.1–0.5 W/sq cm to reduce the production of thermal effects. The patient should feel no warmth. The therapist must be discreet and cautious when treating an acute condition.
- For subacute conditions, use 0.5–1.0 W/sq cm. If minimal thermal effects are desired, the patient

should feel no warmth or only minimal warmth on the skin.

- For chronic conditions, use 1.0–2.0 W/sq cm. If maximal safe thermal effects are desired, the patient should feel a strong sensation of warmth but no discomfort.

The preceding suggestions represent a common-sense perspective derived from a review of studies on the physiologic effects of ultrasound and from clinical experience. Refer to previous sections for more suggestions based on the parameters used in studies of the conditions in which you are interested.

Frequency and Number of Interventions

The documentation regarding optimal frequency and number of interventions is inadequate. However, the following suggestions have been fairly well accepted in clinical practice:

- Ultrasound is commonly applied once a day or every other day.
- The course of interventions depends on how quickly the desired effects are obtained.
- Intervention should be discontinued (1) when complete relief of symptoms and restoration of function is achieved, (2) if no positive results are achieved after three or four interventions, and (3) after a course of 12 to 15 interventions. (After 12 to 15 interventions, which in most cases produce the desired effects, the patient should be observed for 2 weeks without ultrasound. If the condition regresses during that period, another series of ultrasound interventions should be initiated. In special cases, eg, Dupuytren's contracture, interventions may continue for many months but with only one or two interventions per week.)
- The intervention should be modified immediately if the patient reports an exacerbation of symptoms. The symptoms must be evaluated

carefully to determine the cause of the exacerbation and to make the appropriate modifications in intervention.

Clinical experience indicates that a significant number of patients may report a mild increase in symptoms several hours after the first or second ultrasound intervention. This discomfort lasts for only a few hours, and the original symptoms improve by the following day. This pattern is not an indication that ultrasound should be discontinued. It appears to be a type of "soreness" that may be the result of increased activity in the tissue. The patient should be informed in advance that this soreness may occur and can be relieved by applying ice. This information should be presented to the patient in a manner that will not cause alarm. However, if the patient's symptoms increase immediately after the intervention and persist for 24 to 48 hours after the intervention, ultrasound should be discontinued. If ultrasound interventions are reinitiated later, they should be given at a lower intensity and only after the symptoms have subsided.

Discontinuation after 12 to 15 interventions is recommended to reduce the possible risk of excessive exposure to ultrasound. Only one case of clinical overexposure has been documented in the scientific literature. In this case, a woman who treated herself, unsupervised, over multiple body parts several times a day had many physical complaints that may or may not have been aggravated by the ultrasound.[189] Therefore, the recommendation to limit exposure to ultrasound is made from a perspective of caution. An ethical issue also may be involved. If a patient has not made significant progress after several interventions, another form of intervention should be considered. Another related issue is psychological addiction to ultrasound. Certain patients become dependent on ultrasound because of its immediate soothing effect. The therapist is responsible for discouraging or eliminating this dependency.

REVIEW QUESTIONS

1. What influences the depth of penetration of therapeutic ultrasound? How does the type of coupling agent influence the overall effectiveness?

2. What are attenuation, reflection, and refraction? What is the significance of these terms?

3. What are the four factors that contribute to the total tissue temperature rise (TTR)?

4. What is cavitation, and how can a therapist control for its occurrence?

5. List some therapeutic indications for US as an appropriate component of a PT intervention. Give a specific example.

6. List contraindications to continuous US. List contraindications to pulsed US.

7. What is the best application technique for phonophoresis?

8. How can a clinician perform a test of a US head to determine whether it is producing sound waves?

9. What is a ground fault interrupter? When must one be used?

10. In determining an intervention protocol, what variables must be known by the therapist? Give an example, and determine the appropriate time duration for the intervention.

11. During the application of an US intervention, what types of feedback from a patient would indicate the need to reassess the parameters being used?

KEY TERMS

ultrasound
piezoelectric effect
longitudinal (compression) wave
Fresnel zone
Fraunhofer zone
shear (transverse) wave
attenuation
scattering
micromassage

membrane permeability
cavitation
motor nerve conduction velocity (MNCV)
sensory nerve conduction velocity (SNCV)
phonophoresis
time average power
spatial average intensity

continuous-wave ultrasound
pulsed-wave ultrasound
duty cycle
temporal average intensity
spatial average intensity
beam nonuniformity ratio (BNR)
effective radiating area (ERA)

REFERENCES

1. Stewart HF, Absug JL, Harris GR: Considerations in ultrasound therapy and equipment performance. *Phys Ther* 1980; 60:425.

2. Robinson AJ, Snyder-Mackler L: Clinical application of electrotherapeutic modalities. *Phys Ther* 1988; 68:1235–1238.

3. Turner PA, Whitfield TW: A multidimensional scaling analysis of the techniques that physiotherapists use. *Physiother Res Int* 1997; 2(4):237–54.

4. Turner P: Multidimensional scaling analysis of techniques used by physiotherapists in Southeast Australia: A cross-national replication. *Aust J Physiother* 2002; 48(2):123–30.

5. Roebroeck M, Dekker J. Oostendorp R: The use of therapeutic ultrasound by physical therapists in dutch primary health care. *Phys Ther* 1998; 78:5.

6. Lindsay DM, Dearness J, McGinley CC: Electrotherapy usage trends in private physiotherapy practice in Alberta. *Physiother Can* 1995; 47(1):30–34.

7. Halliday D, Resnick R: *Physics*. New York: Wiley; 1990.

8. Ter Haar G: Therapeutic ultrasound. *Eur J Ultrasound* 1999; 9(1):3–9.

9. Schwan HP: *Therapeutic Heat and Cold*. Elizabeth Licht; 1965.

10. Williams AR: *Ultrasound: Biological Effects and Potential Hazards*. New York: Academic; 1983.

11. Carlin B: *Ultrasonics*, 2nd ed. New York: McGraw-Hill; 1960.

12. Lehmann J, Warren C, Guy A: *Ultrasound: Its Applications in Medicine and Biology*. New York: Elsevier; 1978.

13. Lehmann JF: *Therapeutic Heat and Cold*. Baltimore: Waverly; 1972.

14. Griffin J, Karselis T: *Physical Agents for Physical Therapists*. Springfield, IL: Charles C Thomas; 1982.

15. Allen KGR, Battye CK: Performance of ultrasonic therapy instruments. *Physiotherapy* 1978; 6:176.

16. Piersol GM, Schwan HP, Penwell RB, et al: Mechanism of absorption of ultrasonic energy in blood. *Arch Phys Med Rehabil* 1952; 33:327.

17. Wells PNT: Ultrasonics in medicine and biology. *Phys Med Biol* 1977; 22:629–69.

18. Frizzell LA, Dunn F: *Therapeutic Heat and Cold*. Baltimore: Williams & Wilkins; 1982.

19. Lehmann JF, Johnson EW: Some factors influencing the temperature distribution in thighs exposed to ultrasound. *Arch Phys Med Rehabil* 1958; 39:346.

20. Lehmann JF, DeLateur B, Stonebridge J, et al: Therapeutic temperature distribution produced by ultrasound as modified by dosage and volume of tissue exposed. *Arch Phys Med Rehabil* 1967; 664–66.

21. Draper D, Castel J, Castel D: Rate of Temperature Increase in Human Muscle During 1 MHz and 3 MHz Continuous Ultrasound. *JOSPT* 1995; 22:4.

22. Kimura I, Gulick D, Shelly J, Ziskin M: Effects of Two Ultrasound Devices and Angles of Application on the Temperature of Tissue Phantom. *JOSPT* 1998; 27:(1)27–31.

23. Licht S, Kamenetz H: *Therapeutic Heat and Cold.* 2nd ed. Baltimore: Waverly; 1972.

24. Lota M, Darling R: Changes in permeability of the red blood cell membrane in a homogeneous ultrasound field. *Arch Phys Med Rehabil* 1955; 36:282–87.

25. Dyson M, Pond JB, Joseph J, et al: The stimulation of tissue regeneration by means of ultrasound. *Clin Sci* 1968; 35:238.

26. Coble AJ, Dunn F: Ultrasonic production of reversible changes in the electrical parameters of isolated frog skin. *I Acoust Am* 1976; 60:225–29.

27. Mortimer AJ, Bresden B, Forester GV, et al: System for measurement of the effects of ultrasound on the membrane properties of the myocardium. *Med Biol Eng Comp* 1984; 22:22–27.

28. Mortimer AJ, Trollope BJ, Villeneuve EJ: Ultrasound enhanced diffusion of oxygen through isolated frog skin. *I Med Ultrasound* 1988; 6(suppl).

29. Mortimer AJ, Dyson M: The effect of therapeutic ultrasound on calcium uptake in fibroblasts. *Ultrasound Med Biol* 1988; 6:499–506.

30. Hogan RD, Franklin TD, Fry FJ: The effect of ultrasound on microvascular hemodynamics in skeletal muscle: Effect on arterioles. *Ultrasound Med Biol* 1982; 8(1):44–55.

31. Hogan RD, Burke KM, Franklin TD: The effect of ultrasound on microvascular hemodynamics in skeletal muscle: Effects during ischemia. *Microvas Res* 1982; 23:370–79.

32. Carlin B: *Ultrasonics.* 2nd ed. New York: McGraw-Hill; 1960.

33. Wells PNT: *Biomedical Ultrasonics.* London: Academic Press; 1977.

34. Baker KG, Robertson VJ, Duck FA: A review of therapeutic ultrasound: Biophysical effects. *Phys Ther* 2001; 81:1351–58.

35. Reid PC, Redford SB, King P: *Training: Scientific Basic and Application.* Springfield, IL: Charles C Thomas; 1972.

36. Wyke B: *The Lumbar Spine and Back Pain.* London: Sector; 1976:188.

37. Lehmann JF, Brunner GD, Stow RW: Pain threshold measurements after therapeutic application of ultrasound. *Arch Phys Med Rehabil* 1958; 39:560.

38. Szumski AJ: Mechanisms of pain relief as a result of therapeutic application of ultrasound. *Phys Ther Rev* 1960; 117.

39. Anderson TP, Wakim KG, Herrick JF: An experimental study of the effects of ultrasonic energy on the lower part of the spinal cord and peripheral nerves. *Arch Phys Med Rehabil* 1951; 32:71.

40. Zankel HT: Effect of physical agents on motor conduction velocity of the ulnar nerve. *Arch Phys Med Rehabil* 1966; 47:787–92.

41. Farmer W: Effect of intensity of ultrasound on conduction velocity of motor axons. *Phys Ther* 1968; 48:1233–37.

42. Paul WD, Imig CJ: Temperature and blood flow studies after ultrasonic irradiation. *AmPhys Med Rehabil* 1955; 34:370.

43. Abramson DI, Clier LSW, Tuck S: Effect of tissue temperature and blood flow on motor nerve conduction velocity. *JAMA* 1966; 198:10:156–62.

44. Currier DP, Greathouse D, Swift T: Sensory conduction: Effect of ultrasound. *Arch Phys Med Rehabil* 1978; 59:181–85.

45. Halle JS, Scoville CR, Greathouse D: Ultrasound's effect on the conduction latency of the superficial radial nerve in man. *Phys Ther* 1981; 61:345–50.

46. Consentino AB, Gross DL, Harrington RJ: Ultrasound effects on electroneuromyographic measures in sensory fibers of the median nerve. *Phys Ther* 1983; 62:1788–92.

47. Hong CZ: Reversible nerve conduction block in patients with polyneuropathy after ultrasound thermotherapy at therapeutic dosage. *Arch Phys Med Rehabil* 1991; 71:132–37.

48. Middlemast S, Chattergee DC: Comparison of ultrasound and thermotherapy for soft tissue injuries. *Physiotherapy* 1978; 64:331–32.

49. White L, Schweitzer M, Ryan S, Lombardi J, et al: Arthrographic effect induced by therapeutic ultrasound in magnetic resonance imaging of the wrist: A preliminary investigation. *Can Assoc Radiol J* 1997; 48(5–6):348–52.

50. Vanharanta H, Eronen I, Videman T: Effect of ultrasound on glycosaminoglycan metabolism in the rabbit knee. *Am J Phys Med Rehabil* 1982; 61:221–28.

51. Stratton SA, Heckmann R, Francis RS: Therapeutic ultrasound: Its effects on the integrity of a non-penetrating wound. *J Ortho Sports Phys Ther* 1984; 5:278–81.

52. Young SR, Dyson M: Macrophage responsiveness to therapeutic ultrasound. *Ultrasound Med Biol* 1990; 8:809–16.

53. Young SR, Dyson M: Effect of therapeutic ultrasound on the healing of full-thickness excised skin lesions. *Ultrasonics* 1990; 28:175–80.

54. Young S, Dyson M: The effect of therapeutic ultrasound on angiogenesis. *Ultrasound Med Biol* 1990; 16(3):261–69.

55. Byl N, McKenzie A, Wong T, et al: Incisional wound healing: A controlled study of low and high does ultrasound. *JOSPT* 1993; 18(5):619–28.

56. Byl N, McKenzie A, West J, et al: *Arch Phys Med Rehabil* 1992; 73(7):656–64.

57. Taskan I, Ozyazgan I, Tercan M, et al: A comparative study of the effect of ultrasound and electrostimulation on wound healing in rats. *Plast Reconstr Surg* 1997; 100(4):966–72.

58. Paul BJ, Lafratta CW, Dawson AR: Use of ultrasound in the treatment of pressure sores in patients with spinal cord injury. *Arch Phys Med Rehabil* 1960; 39:439–40.

59. Shamberger RC, Talbot T, Tipton H: The effect of ultrasonic and thermal treatment on wounds. *Plast Reconstr Surg* 1981; 68:860–70.

60. Dyson M, Suckling J: Stimulation of tissue repair by ultrasound: A survey of mechanisms involved. *Physiotherapy* 1978; 64(4):105–08.

61. Ferguson N: Ultrasound in the treatment of surgical wounds. *Physiotherapy* 1981; 67(2):43.

62. Peschen M, Weichenthal M, Schopf E, Vanscheidt W: Low-frequency ultrasound treatment of chronic venous leg ulcers in an outpatient therapy. *Acta Derm Venereol* 1997; 77(4):311–14.

63. Eriksson SV, Lundebert T, Malm M: A placebo controlled trial of ultrasound therapy in chronic leg ulceration. *Scand J Rehabil Med* 1991; 23:211–13.

64. Lundeberg T, Nordstom F, Brodda-Jansen G, et al: Pulsed ultrasound does not improve healing of venous ulcers. *Scand J Rehabil Med* 1990; 22(4):195–97.

65. Ter Riet G, Kessels A, Knipschild P: A randomized clinical trial of ultrasound in the treatment of pressure ulcers. *Phys Ther* 1996; 76(12):1301–11.

66. Cambier D, Vanderstraeten G: Failure of therapeutic ultrasound in healing burn injuries. *Burns* 1997; 23(3):248–49.

67. Enwemeka CS: The effects of therapeutic ultrasound on tendon healing. *Am J Phys Med Rehabil* 1989; 6:283–87.

68. Enwemeka CS, Rodriquez O, Mendosa S: The biomedical effects of low-intensity ultrasound on healing tendons. *Ultrasound Med Biol* 1990; 8:801–07.

69. Da Cunha A, Parizotto NA, Vidal BC: The effect of therapeutic ultrasound on repair of the achilles tendon (tendocalcaneus) of the rat. *Ultrasound Med Biol* 2001; 27(12):1691–96.

70. Jackson BA, Schwane JA, Starcher BC: Effect of ultrasound therapy on the repair of Achilles tendon injuries in rats. *Med Sci Sports Med* 1991; 2:171–76.

71. Gan BS, Huys S, Sherebrin MH, Scilley CG: The effects of ultrasound treatment on flexor tendon healing in the chicken limb. *J Hand Surg (Br)* 1995; 20(6):809–14.

72. Gum SL, Reddy GK, Stehno-Bittel L, Enwemeka CS: Combined ultrasound, electrical stimulation, and laser promote collagen synthesis with moderate changes in tendon biomechanics. *Am J Phys Med Rehabil* 1997; 76(4):288–96.

73. Karnes JL, Burton HW: Continuous therapeutic ultrasound accelerates repair of contraction-

induced skeletal muscle damage in rats. *Arch Phys Med Rehabil* 2002; 83(1):1–4.

74. Turner SM, Powell ES, Ng CS: The effect of ultrasound on the healing of repaired cockerel tendon: Is collagen cross linkage a factor? *J Hand Surg* 1989; 4:428–33.

75. Roberts M, Rutherford JH, Harris D: The effect of ultrasound on flexor tendon repairs in rabbits. *Hand* 1982; 14(1):17–20.

76. Bickford RH, Duff RS: Influence of ultrasonic irradiation on temperature and blood flow in human skeletal muscle. *Circ Res* 1953; 1:534–68.

77. Paul WD, Imig CJ: Temperature and blood flow studies after ultrasonic irradiation. *Am J Phys Med Rehabil* 1955; 34:370.

78. Buchan JB: The use of ultrasonics in physical medicine. *Practitioner* 1970; 305:319.

79. Imig CJ, Randal BF, Hines HM: Effect of ultrasonic energy on blood flow. *Am J Phys Med Rehabil* 1954; 3:100–02.

80. Abramson DI, Burnett C, Bell Y: Changes in blood flow, oxygen uptake, and tissue temperatures produced by the therapeutic physical agents, pt. 1. Effect of ultrasound. *Am J Phys Med Rehabil* 1960; 39:51.

81. Lota M: Electronic plethysmographic and tissue temperature studies of effect of ultrasound on blood flow. *Arch Phys Med Rehabil* 1965; 44:315–22.

82. Rubin MJ, Etchison MR, Condra KA, et al: Acute effects of ultrasound on skeletal muscle oxygen tension, blood flow and capillary density. *Ultraound Med Biol* 1990; 16(3):271–77.

83. Robinson SE, Buono MJ: Effect of continuous-wave ultrasound on blood flow in skeletal muscle. *Phys Ther* 1995; 75(2):145–49.

84. Fabrizio P, Schmidt J, Clemente F, et al: Acute effects of therapeutic ultrasound delivered at varying parameters on the blood flow velocity in a muscular distribution artery. *JOSPT* 1996; 25(5):294–302.

85. Lehmann JF, DeLateur BJ, Warren CG: Heating of joint structures by ultrasound. *Arch Phys Med Rehabil* 1968; 49:28–30.

86. Lehmann JF, Masock AJ, Warren CG: Effect of therapeutic temperature on tendon extensibility. *Arch Phys Med Rehabil* 1970; 51:481–87.

87. Knight CA, Rutledge CR, Cox ME, et al: Effect of superficial heat and active exercise warmup on the extensibility of the plantar flexors. *Phys Ther* 2001; 81:1206–14.

88. Ward R, Hayes-Lundy C, Reddy R, et al: Evaluation of topical therapeutic ultrasound to improve response to physical therapy and lessen scar contracture after burn injury. *Journal of Burn Care and Rehabilitation* 1994; 15(1):74–79.

89. Moll MJ: A new approach to pain: Lidocaine and decadron with ultrasound. *USAF Med Serv Digest*, May 8–11, 1977.

90. Kassan D, Lynch A, Stiller M: Phsycial enhancement of dermatologic drug delivery: Iontophoresis and phonophoresis. *Journal of the American Academy of Dermatology* 1996; April; 657–66.

91. Newman M, Kill M, Frompton G: The effects of ultrasound alone and combined with hydrocortisone injections by needle or hypospray. *Am J Phys Med Rehabil* 1958; 37:206–09.

92. Mune O: Ultrasonic treatment of subcutaneous infiltrations after injections. *Acta Orthop Scand* 1963; 33:346.

93. Novak FJ: Experimental transmission of lidocaine through intact skin by ultrasound. *Arch Phys Med Rehabil* 1964; 64:231–32.

94. Griffin JE, Touchstone JC: Ultrasonic movement of cortisol into pig tissues. *Am J Phys Med Rehabil* 1963; 43:77–85.

95. Griffin JE, Touchstone JC, Liu AC: The ultrasonic movement of cortisol into pig tissues, 11. Movement into paravertebral nerve. *Am J Phys Med Rehabil* 1965; 44:20–25.

96. Griffin JE, Echternach JL, Price RE, et al: Patients treated with ultrasonic-driven hydrocortisone and with ultrasound alone. *Phys Ther* 1967; 47:594–601.

97. Kleinkort JA, Wood F: Phonophoresis with 1 percent versus 10 percent hydrocortisone. *Phys Ther* 1975; 12:1320–24.

98. Ciccone C, Leggin B. Callamara J: Effects of ultrasound and trolamine salicylcate phonophoresis on delayed-onset muscle soreness. *Phys Ther* 1991; 71(9):666–78.

99. Griffin JE, Touchstone JC: Low-intensity phonophoresis of cortisol in swine. *Phys Ther* 1968; 12:1336–44.

100. Bare A, McAnaw M, Pritchard A, et al: Phonophoretic delivery of 10% hydrocortisone through the epidermis of humans as determined by serum cortisol concentrations. *Phys Ther* 1996; 76(7):738–49.

101. Benson HAE, McElnay JC, Harland R: Use of ultrasound to enhance percutaneous absorption of benzydamine. *Phys Ther* 1989; 69:113–18.

102. Cameron M, Monroe L: Relative transmission of ultrasound by media customarily used for phonophoresis. *Phys Ther* 1992; 72(2):142–48.

103. Cameron M, Monroe L: Reliable ultrasound transmission (response to letter to the editor). *Phys Ther* 1992; 72(8):611.

104. Johnson M, Mitragotri S, Patel A, et al: Synergistic effects of chemical enhancers and therapeutic ultrasound on transdermal drug delivery. *J Pharm Sci* 1996; 85(7):670–79.

105. Byl N: The use of ultrasound as an enhancer for transcutaneous drug delivery: Phonophoresis. *Phys Ther* 1995; 75(6):539–53.

106. Asano J, Suisha F, Takada M, et al: Effect of pulsed output ultrasound on transdermal absorption of indomethacin from an ointment in rats. *Biol Pharm Bull* 1997; 20(3):288–91.

107. McElnay J, Benson H, Harland R, Hadgraft J: Phonophoresis of methyl nicotinate: A preliminary study to elucidate the mechanism of action. *J Pharm Res* 1993; 10(12):1726–31.

108. Benson H, McElnay J, Harland R, Hadgraft J: Influence of ultrasound on the percutaneous absorption of nicotinate esters. *J Pharm Res* 1991; 8(2):204–09.

109. Franklin M, Smith S, Chenier T, Franklin R: Effect of phonophoresis with dexamethasone on adrenal function. *JOSPT* 1995; 22(3):103–07.

110. Mitragotri S, Blankschtein D, Langer R: Transdermal drug delivery using low-frequency sonophoresis. *J Pharm Res* 1996; 13:411–20.

111. Mitragotri S, Blankschtein D, Langer R: Ultrasound-mediated transdermal protein delivery. *Science* 1995; 269(5225):850–53.

112. Ueda H, Ogihara M, Sugibayashi K, Morimoto Y: Difference in the enhancing effects of ultrasound on the skin permeation of polar and nonpolar drugs (Abstract). *Chem Pharm Bull (Tokyo)* 1996; 44(10):1973–76.

113. Singer A, Homan C, Church A., McClain S: Low-frequency sonophoresis: Pathologic and thermal effects in dogs. *Acad Emerg Med* 1998; 5(1):35–40.

114. Falconer J, Hayes K, Chang R: Therapeutic ultrasound in the treatment of musculoskeletal conditions. *Arthritis Care and Research* 1990; 3(2):85–91.

115. Brosseau L, Casimiro L, Robinson V, et al: Therapeutic ultrasound for treating patellofemoral pain syndrome. *Cochrane Database Syst Rev* 2001; (4):CD003375.

116. Ogilvie-Harris DJ, Gilbert M: Treatment modalities for soft tissue injuries of the ankle: A critical review. *Clin J Sport Med* 1995; 5(3):175–86.

117. Van der Windt DA, van der Heijden GJ, van der Berg SG, et al: Ultrasound therapy for musculoskeletal disorders: A systematic review. *Pain* 1999; 81(3):257–71.

118. Gray RJ, Quayle AA, Hall CA, Schofield MA: Physiotherapy in the treatment of temporomandibular joint disorders: A comparative study of four treatment methods. *Br Dent J* 1994; 176(7):257–61.

119. Van der Windt DA, van der Heijden GJ, van der Berg SG, et al: Ultrasound therapy for acute ankle sprains. *Cochrane Database Syst Rev* 2002; (1):CD001250.

120. Van der Heijden GJ, van der Windt DA, de Winter AF: Physiotherapy for patients with soft tissue shoulder disorders: A systematic review of randomized clinical trials. *BMJ* 1997; 315(7099):25–30.

121. Welch V, Brosseau L, Peterson J, et al: Therapeutic ultrasound for osteoarthritis of the knee. *Cochrane Database Syst Rev* 2001; (3):CD003132

122. Robertson VJ, Baker KG: A review of therapeutic ultrasound: Effectiveness studies. *Phys Ther.* 2001; 81:1339–50.

123. Draper DO: Letter to editor. *Phys Ther* 2002; 82:190.

124. Lehmann JF, et al: Comparison of ultrasonic and microwave diathermy in the physical treatment of periarthritis of the shoulder. *Arch Phys Med Rehabil* 1954; 35:627.

125. Casimiro L, Brosseau L, Robinson V, et al: Therapeutic ultrasound for the treatment of rheumatoid arthritis. *Cochrane Database Syst Rev* 2002; (3):CD003787.

126. Bhatia R, Sobti VK, Roy KS: Gross and histopathological observations on the effects of therapeutic ultrasound in experimental acute chemical arthritis in calves (Abstract). *Zentralbl Veterinarmed [A]* 1992; 39(3):168–73.

127. Huang, MH, Tsau JC, Ding HJ, et al: The role of mucopolysaccharide induction in treatment of experimental osteoarthritis in rats by ultrasound (Abstract). *Kao Hsiung I Hsueh Ko Hsueh Tsa Chih* 1997; 13(11):661–70.

128. Ebenbichler GR, Resch KL, Nikolakis P, et al: Ultrasound treatment for treating the carpal tunnel syndrome: Randomized "sham" controlled trial. *Brit Med J* 1998; 316:731–35.

129. Markam DE, Wood MR: Ultrasound for Dupuytren's contracture. *Physiotherapy* 1980; 66:2:55–58.

130. Bierman W: Ultrasound in the treatment of scars. *Arch Phys Med Rehabil* 1954; 35:209.

131. Miller H, Ardrizzone J: Peyronie disease treated with ultrasound and hydrocortisone. *Urology* 1983; 21:584–85.

132. McBride A, Varghese G, Arthur D: Peyronie's disease: Treatment with long-term ultrasound (Abstract). *Arch Phys Med Rehabil* 1982; 63.

133. Culibrk MS, Culibrk B: Physical treatment of Peyronie disease. *Am J Phys Med Rehabil* 2001; 80(8):583–85.

134. Echternach JC: Ultrasound: An adjunct treatment for shoulder disability. *Phys Ther* 1965; 45:865.

135. Bearzy HJ: Clinical applications of ultrasonic energy in the treatment of acute and chronic subacromial bursitis. *Arch Phys Med Rehabil* 1953; 34:228.

136. Ebenbichler G, Resch K, Graninger W: Resolution of calcium deposits after therapeutic ultrasound of the shoulder. (letter to the editor). *Journal of Rheumatology* 1997; 24(1):235–36.

137. Fountain FP, et al: Decrease in muscle spasm produced by ultrasound, hot packs and infrared. *Arch Phys Med Rehabil* 1960; 41:294.

138. Portwood MH, Lieberman JS, Taylor RG: Causalgia of the foot: Successful management by simple conservative measures (Abstract). *Arch Phys Med Rehabil* 1981; 62:502.

139. Vaughn DT: Direct method versus underwater method in the treatment of plantar warts with ultrasound. *Phys Ther* 1973; 53:396–97.

140. Cherup N, Urben J, Bender LF: Treatment of plantar warts with ultrasound. *Arch Phys Med Rehabil* 1965; 44:602–04.

141. Rowe RJ, Gray JM: Ultrasound treatment of plantar warts. *Arch Phys Med Rehabil* 1965; 46:600.

142. Shin SM, Choi JK: Effect of indomethacin phonophoresis on the relief of temporomandibular joint pain. *The Journal of Craniomandibular Practice* 1997; 15(4):345–48.

143. Oakley EM: Dangers and contraindications of therapeutic ultrasound. *Physiotherapy* 1978; 64(6):173–74.

144. Sicard-Rosenbaum L, Lord D, Danoff J, et al: Effects of continuous therapeutic ultrasound on growth and metastasis of subcutaneous murine tumors. *Phys Ther* 1995; 75(1):3–12.

145. Sicard-Rosenbaum L, Danoff J, Guthrie J, Eckhaus M: Effects of energy-matched pulsed ultrasound on tumor growth in mice. *Phys Ther* 1998; 78(3):271–77.

146. Marmour JB, Pounds D, Hahn N, et al: Treating spontaneous tumors in dogs and cats by ultrasound-induced hyperthermia. *Int J Radiat Oncol Biol Phys* 1978; 4:967–73.

147. Chen L, ter Haar G, Hill CR: Influence of ablated tissue on the formation of high-intensity focused ultrasound lesions. *Ultrasound Med Biol* 1997; 23(6):921–31.

148. Worthington AE, Thompson J, Rauth AM, Hunt JW: Mechanism of ultrasound enhanced porphyrin cytotoxicity, part I: A search for free radical effects. *Ultrasound Med Biol* 1997; 23(7):1095–1105.

149. Botros YY, Volakis JL, VanBaren P, Ebbini ES: A hybrid computational model for ultrasound phased-array heating in presence of strongly scattering obstacles. *IEEE Trans Biomed Eng* 1997; 44(11):1039–50.

150. Hynynen K, Jolesz FA: Demonstration of potential noninvasive ultrasound brain therapy through an intact skull. *Ultrasound Med Biol* 1998; 24(2):275–83.

151. Orenberg, EK, Deneau DG, Farber EM: Response of chronic psoriatic plaques to localized

heating induced by ultrasound. *Arch Dermatol* 1980; 116:893–97.

152. DeForest RE: Effects of ultrasound on growing bone: Experimental study. *Arch Phys Med Rehabil* 1953; 34:21.

153. Wiltink A, Nijweide P, Oosterbaan W, et al: Effect of therapeutic ultrasound on endochondrial ossification. *Ultrasound Med Biol* 1995; 21(1):121–27.

154. Bradnock KB, Law HT, Roscor K: A quantitative comparative assessment of the immediate response to high-frequency ultrasound and low-frequency ultrasound (long wave therapy) in the treatment of acute ankle sprains. *Physiotherapy* 1996; 82:78–84.

155. Tsai C, Chang W, Liu T: Preliminary studies of duration of intensity of ultrasonic treatments on fracture repair. *Clin J Physiol* 1992; 35:21–26.

156. Reher P, Elbesher E, Harvey W, et al: The stimulation of bone formation in vitro by therapeutic ultrasound. *Ultrasound Med Biol* 1997; 23(8):1251–58.

157. Kristiansen TK, Ryaby JP, McCabe J, et al: Accelerated healing of distal radial fractures with the use of specific, low-intensity ultrasound. A multicenter, prospective, randomized, double-blind, placebo-controlled study. *J Bone Joint Surg Am* 1997; 79(7):961–73.

158. Dyson M, Brookes M: Stimulation of bone repair by ultrasound. *Ultrasound Med Biol* 1983; Suppl 2:61–66.

159. Heckman JD, Ryaby JP, McCabe J, et al: Acceleration of tibial fracture-healing by non-invasive, low intensity pulsed ultrasound. *J Bone Joint Surg* 1994; 76:26–34.

160. Pilla AA, Mont MA, Nasser PR, et al: Non-invasive low-intensity pulsed ultrasound accelerates bone healing in the rabbit. *J Ortho Trauma* 1990; 3:246–53.

161. Lehmann JF, Lane KE, Bell JW, et al: Influence of surgical metal implants on the distribution of the intensity in the ultrasound field. *Arch Phys Med Rehabil* 1958; 39:756–60.

162. Lehmann JR, Brunner GD, McMillan J: Influence of surgical metal implants on the temperature distribution in thigh specimens exposed to ultrasound. *Arch Phys Med Rehabil* 1958; 37:692–95.

163. Gersten JS: Effect of metallic objects on temperature rises produced in tissues by ultrasound. *Am J Phys Med Rehabil* 1958; 37:75–82.

164. Skoubo-Kristensen E, Sommer J: Ultrasound on internal fixation with a rigid plate in dogs. *Arch Phys Med Rehabil* 1982; 63:371–73.

165. Stewart HF, et al: Survey of use and performance of ultrasonic therapy equipment in Pinellas County, Florida. *Phys Ther* 1974; 54:707–14.

166. Fyfe MC, Parnell SM: The importance of measurement of effective transducer radiating area in the testing and calibration of "therapeutic" ultrasonic instruments. *Health Phys* 1982; 43:377–81.

167. Hekkenberg R, Oosterbaan W, van Beekum W: Evaluation of ultrasound therapy devices. *Physiotherapy* 1986; 72:390–94.

168. Lloyd J, Evans J: A calibration survey of physiotherapy ultrasound equipment in North Wales. *Physiotherapy* 1988; 74(2):56–61.

169. Artho PA, Thyne JG, Warring BP, et al: A calibration study of therapeutic ultrasound units. *Phys Ther* 2002; 82(3):257–63.

170. Pye SD, Milford C: The performance of ultrasound physiotherapy machines in Lothian Region, Scotland, 1992. *Ultrasound Med Biol* 1994; 20(4):347–59.

171. Ferguson B: A practitioner's guide to the ultrasonic therapy equipment standard. HHS Publication No. 85-8240; 1985.

172. Stewart HF, Abzug J, Harris G: Considerations in ultrasound therapy equipment and performance. *Phys Ther* 1980; 60:427.

173. Haar GT: Basic physics of therapeutic ultrasound. *Physiotherapy* 1978; 64(4):102.

174. Allen KGR, Barry CK: Performance of ultrasonic therapy instruments. *Physiotherapy* 1978; 64(6):179.

175. Dyson M, Pond JB: The effects of ultrasound on circulation. *Physiotherapy* 1973; 59:284–87.

176. Gann N, Rogers C, Dudley A: A comparison of physical therapy students with and without instructions in ultrasound pressure application. *J Allied Health* 2002; 31(2):103–05.

177. Lehmann JF, McMillan JA, Brunner SD, et al: Comparative study of the efficiency of short-wave, microwave and ultrasonic diathermy in heating the hip joint. *Arch Phys Med Rehabil* 1959; 40:510.

178. Oakley EM: Application of continuous beam ultrasound at therapeutic levels. *Physiotherapy* 1978; 64(6):170.

179. Warren GC, Koblanski JN, Sifelmann R: Ultrasound coupling media: Their relative transmissivity. *Arch Phys Med Rehabil* 1976; 57:218–22.

180. Forrest G, Rosen K: Ultrasound: Effectiveness of treatments given under water. *Arch Phys Med Rehabil* 1989; 70:28–29.

181. Forrest G, Rosen K: Ultrasound treatments given in degassed water. *J Sports Rehabil* 1992; 1:284–89.

182. Klucinec B, Scheidler M, Denegar C, et al: Transmissivity of coupling agents used to deliver ultrasound through indirect methods. *J Orthop Sports Phys Ther* 2000; 30:263–69.

183. Griffin J: Transmissiveness of ultrasound through tap water, glycerin, and mineral oil. *Phys Ther* 1980; 60:1010–16.

184. Lehmann J, DeLateur BJ, Silverman DR: Selective heating effects of ultrasound in human beings. *Arch Phys Med Rehabil* 1966; 47:331–39.

185. Klucinec B, Scheidler M, Denegar C, et al: Effectiveness of wound care products in the transmission of acoustic energy. *Phys Ther* 2000; 80:469–76.

186. Frankel W: *Basic Wiring*. Chicago: Time-Life Books; 1980.

187. Forrest G, Rosen K: Ultrasound: Effectiveness of treatments given under water. *Arch Phys Med Rehabil* 1989; 70:28–29.

188. Hayes KW: *Manual for Physical Agents*. 2nd ed. Evanston, IL: Northwestern University Medical School, 1979.

189. Levenson JL, Weissberg MP: Ultrasound abuse: Case report. *Arch Phys Med Rehabil* 1983; 64:90–91.

16

Diathermy

MARY JOAN DAY, PT, MS

JOANNE S. KATZ, PHD, PT

Chapter Outline

Diathermy is a physical agent used to increase temperature in deep tissues in order to (1) increase delivery of nutrients to the area by increasing blood flow; (2) promote resolution of inflammatory infiltrates, edema, and exudates; (3) diminish pain; (4) relieve muscle spasms; (5) decrease joint stiffness; or (6) increase the extensibility of tissues in musculoskeletal disorders.[1] Diathermy utilizes nonionizing electromagnetic energy from the radio-frequency portion of the electromagnetic spectrum.[2] To determine whether its application in patient management is theoretically and therapeutically sound, it is important to understand both the scientific basis and the effects of diathermy.

Two major types of diathermy, shortwave and microwave, have been used by physical therapies to increase the temperature in tissues below the surface of the skin. The frequency ranges allocated by the Federal Communications Commission (FCC) for microwave diathermy (MWD) include 2,456 MHz and 915 MHz.[1] Equipment operating at 2,456 MHz is more commonly used; however, research has shown that 915 MHz is more effective.[1,3] With MWD, tissues with high-water content absorb greater amounts of energy. Direct-contact applicators that air-cool the superficial tissue layers are used to obtain better coupling and less stray radiation.[1] These microwave applicators cover a smaller area, but they heat muscle more selectively and to a greater depth than does shortwave diathermy.[3] **Shortwave diathermy (SWD)** is currently the only type that is in common use in the United States today and is therefore the type discussed in this chapter.

Like MWD units, the frequency ranges at which SWD devices may operate are rigorously controlled by the FCC. The frequencies that are approved for SWD by the FCC include 13.56 MHz, 27.12 MHz, and 40.68 MHz.[2] Most of the commercially available equipment for SWD operate at a frequency of 27.12 MHz.[1]

The electromagnetic energy generated by devices available to physical therapists is assumed to travel at a constant velocity, the velocity of light (about 300×10^6 m/s). Thus, the wavelength of electromagnetic energy (ie, the distance between the apex of two successive waves) is inversely related to the frequency of its output and may be calculated according to the formula $\lambda = c/F$, where λ represents the wavelength, $c =$ the velocity of light, and $F =$ the frequency of oscillation.[1] The frequency of oscillation is the number of wavecycles produced per unit of time and is expressed as cycles per second, which is sec^{-1}, or Hz^4 (see **Fig. 7–3**). According to the formula $\lambda = c/F$, the wavelength of a SWD unit that has a frequency of 27.12 MHz will be calculated as follows:

$$\lambda = \frac{c}{F}$$

$$\lambda = \frac{3 \times 10 \text{ m (sec}^{-1})}{27.12 \times 10 \text{ sec}^{-1}}$$

$$\lambda = 11.06 \text{ m}$$

Thus, a SWD unit that operates at a frequency of 27.12 MHz will have a corresponding wavelength of approximately 11 m. Since SWD has a longer wavelength and lower frequency than infrared, it will penetrate body tissues more deeply than infrared.[5] Because SWD is characterized by a long wavelength (11 m), theoretically its most potent thermal effect is not on skin and subcutaneous tissues but on the underlying musculature and associated connective tissues.

BIOPHYSICS AND PHYSIOLOGIC EFFECTS

The shortwave diathermy unit can be viewed as having a *primary* and a *secondary* circuit. The primary circuit is connected to the power supply and is also called a **power** or **machine circuit.** The secondary circuit, a parallel resonant circuit with variable tuning,[6] is also called the **patient circuit,** because the patient is positioned to be part of that circuit. The machine circuit converts 110 V–60 Hz house current into high-voltage, high-frequency (27.12 MHz), low-amp current to be used in the patient circuit (**Fig. 16–1**). This machine circuit is then coupled to the patient circuit. This high-frequency energy is conveyed from the primary oscillating circuit of the machine circuitry into a secondary oscillating circuit in the patient circuitry, which then transfers energy into the patient's tissues.

The tissue type, the position of the body part, and the position of the SWD electrodes influence the oscillation frequency in the patient circuit. The electrodes used in SWD are metallic drums through which current and voltage are conveyed to induce heating in the patient.[2] For maximum efficiency, the oscillating

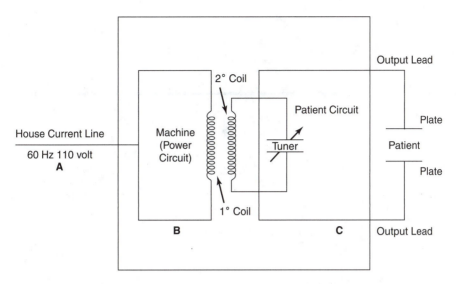

FIGURE 16–1   A simplified diagram of a shortwave diathermy unit with a patient positioned between condenser plates. (**A**) A representation of AC house current for the machine circuit. (**B**) The machine circuit which includes the transformers, rectifier, power amplifiers and primary (1°) radio-frequency oscillator of the machine circuit. (**C**) The patient circuit, which includes the secondary (2°) transformer coil, the tuner, high-frequency output leads, and condenser plates.

frequency of the patient circuit must be in resonance with that of the machine circuit; this is achieved by matching the frequency of the patient circuit with that of the machine circuit. The outcome is similar to what occurs when a radio is *tuned* to receive a clear signal from a specific station—meaning that the bandwidth or frequency of the radio is adjusted to match with that of the primary output from the radio station.

Most current-day SWD units are designed so that tuning is adjusted automatically. After appropriately positioning the patient within the eletromagnetic field of the primary or patient circuit, the adjustment required on the unit is that of the *output* indicator and timer control, with the rate indicator as an additional adjustment in the pulsed models (Fig. 16–2). The rate indicator shows the on/off bursts provided by the pulsed diathermy machine. The timer control indicates the exposure time of the patient.[6] The output indicator gauges the *average current*, or power output (in watts), passing through the patient circuit. However, the output indicator does not accurately indicate the amount of energy actually passing through the treated body parts. Following manufacturer's guidelines, the therapist must then rely on patient report of heat sensation to determine the level at which to set

the output indicator. Lehmann and Delateur[1] recommend the following guidelines for SWD dosage (dosimetry):

1. For mild intervention, the shortwave diathermy application is used to produce a feeling of warmth in the patient.
2. For vigorous intervention, a feeling of warmth may be accompanied by reaching the pain threshold. At the moment pain is experienced, the therapist reduces the output of the equipment, adjusting it to maintain a level just below the maximally tolerated output.[1]

When the oscillating frequency of the patient circuit is tuned and is in resonance with that of the machine circuit, the resultant output is high-frequency (>10 MHz), low-amp electromagnetic energy. As a consequence of this extremely high frequency, nerve depolarization does not occur because the rapid rate of change in current direction does not allow time for ions to flow across the nerve membrane. Rather, elevation of tissue temperature occurs with SWD, which must be in the therapeutic range of 40–45°C for intervention to be effective.[7]

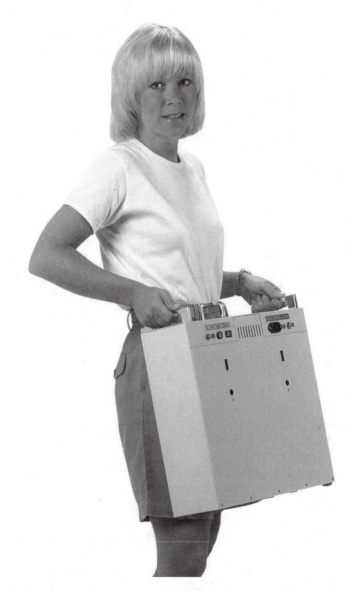

FIGURE 16–2   A portable pulsed SWD unit. (*Courtesy of International Medical Electronics, LTD., Kansas City, MD.*)

Shortwave diathermy is subdivided into condenser (capacitor) field diathermy and induction field diathermy. Guy et al[6] have shown that condenser field diathermy produces greater power absorption in subcutaneous fat than in deeper muscle tissues. Inductive field diathermy has been shown to produce higher power absorption in the deeper, high-water-content tissues such as muscle, than in subcutaneous fat.[1] Most manufacturers of SWD in the United States today produce induction field diathermy; however, there are still condenser field diathermy units that may be found in clinics.

Condenser (Capacitor) Field Diathermy

In condenser field diathermy, a high-frequency alternating-current (AC) generator emits electromagnetic energy from a pair of oppositely charged electrodes called **condensers** or **capacitor plates,** which are part of the secondary oscillating circuit. The charge on each electrode alternates in accordance with the frequency of the alternating current. As a result, a strong electrical field is generated between the plates.[2] **Figure 16–3** is an illustration of this strong electrical field. Note that the strength of the field is not homogeneous; it is strongest near the plates but spreads or diverges farther from the plates and according to the type of tissue in the electromagnetic field. Because the strength of the field is greatest near the plates, it might overheat skin and subcutaneous fat if placed too close; thus, the condensers are positioned a slight distance from the skin (about 2–3 cm) to allow some divergence before contact with the skin. When a body part is positioned properly between the oppositely charged condensers (ie, within the **electric field** of the plates), the electrical energy will cause ions and dipole molecules (molecules that behave as if they had oppositely charged ends) within the tissues to change direction every time the charge on the plates and the direction of the electric field change. The faster the current changes direction (ie,

the higher its frequency), the smaller the actual movement of the particles from their original position. The frequency of the back-and-forth oscillation of the ions matches the output frequency of the generator.

Ordinarily, dipole molecules tend to be randomly situated within tissue; however, when subjected to the energy emitted from the diathermy unit, they rotate in the direction dictated by their polar charge **(Fig. 16–4).** The rate of rotation is tightly coupled with the frequency of the energy emitted from the diathermy unit.[8] Thus, the high-frequency oscillatory movement of ions and dipoles results in increases in molecular kinetic energy, which leads to increased tissue temperature. However, dipole rotation is not a significant source of heating with condenser field SWD.

The tissue response to the high-frequency oscillatory field is somewhat analogous to the response of any conductor when electrical current passes through it. According to Joule's law, the amount of energy converted to heat (H) is proportional to the square of the current intensity (I^2), the impedance of the conductor (R), and the duration of current flow (t). This law is often expressed as

$$H = I^2Rt$$

By applying this law and assuming that the strength of the current is equal throughout the tissues within the electric field, it is theoretically possible to predict the location of the tissues having the greatest temperature increases. If the condenser field plates and the tissues are arranged in series with one another **(Fig. 16–5),** with one plate on the dorsal surface and one on the ventral surface of a body part, the heat produced will be proportional to the impedance of the tissue. (See **Chapter 18** for a more detailed discussion of series circuits.) Because the current intensity is the same in all parts of a series circuit, the temperature of the tissue having the greatest impedance to the molecular activity is elevated to the greatest degree. For example, fat has a significantly higher impedance than does muscle or bone; therefore, more heating occurs in fatty tissues than occurs in more conductive tissues such as muscle.[9]

The relative heating pattern is similar to that depicted in **Fig. 16–6.**[10,11] This heating pattern of the tissues can be changed so that the temperature of muscle is elevated but the entire cross section of the part is *not*, as it is when plates and tissue are in series with each other (see **Chapter 18**). This is

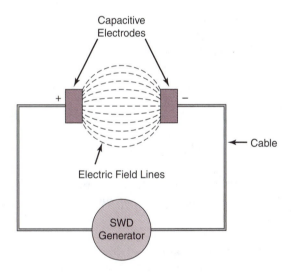

FIGURE 16–3 With condenser field diathermy, an electric field occurs between two oppositely charged electrodes (dashed lines). The distance between lines indicates the relative strength of the field. Note that the field is stronger near each electrode. (*Modified from HHS Publication FDA 85–8237. Kloth L, Morrison MA, Ferguson BH: Therapeutic Microwave and Shortwave Diathermy: A Review of Thermal Effectiveness, Safe Use, and State of the Art: 1984, Food and Drug Administration,* U.S. Department of Health and Human Services.)

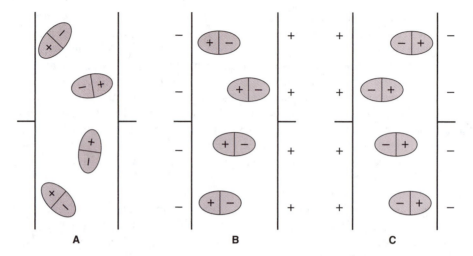

FIGURE 16–4 Dipole molecules. **(A)** Random arrangement when condenser plates are not charged, **(B, C)** Direction toward which dipoles rotate according to the change in polarity of the plates. The positive end of the dipole is always toward the negatively charged plate. (*Modified from* Clayton's Electrotherapy Theory and Practice, *Forster A, Palastanga N. 9th ed. 1985, Bailliere Tindall.*)

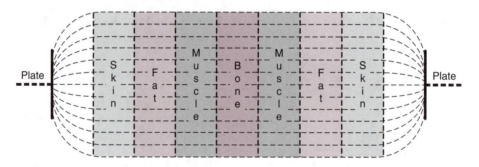

FIGURE 16–5 Theoretical example of an high-frequency oscillatory field, assuming that the strength of the electric current is uniform through the tissues within the electric field. The condenser plates are in series with the cross section of a body part. Note the field spread in the space between the plates and the skin, indicating that the field density is less at the skin than it would be if the plates were on the skin.

accomplished by positioning the plates so that deeper tissues are in parallel with more superficial tissues. This configuration is easily achieved by placing the part to be treated under, rather than between, the two condenser plates **(Fig. 16–7)**. In this configuration, the heat produced is more dependent on the intensity of current because the density of the current varies throughout a parallel circuit. In a parallel circuit, the current could follow a number of paths, but it will always follow the path of least resistance. To the extent that this parallel position of plates produces a parallel circuit, more current

will flow through tissues of low impedance, and more heat will be generated in those tissues.

Muscle tissue has low impedance properties and thus will be heated selectively when the two plates are placed in parallel on the body part to be treated. This application may be useful when treating areas such as the mid- and low back **(Fig 16–8)**. This more selective heating of muscle is clearly advantageous when treating problems of muscular origin.

In clinical practice, both arrangements of condenser plates are used. **Contraplanar positioning** (also called *transverse positioning*) of plates uses the

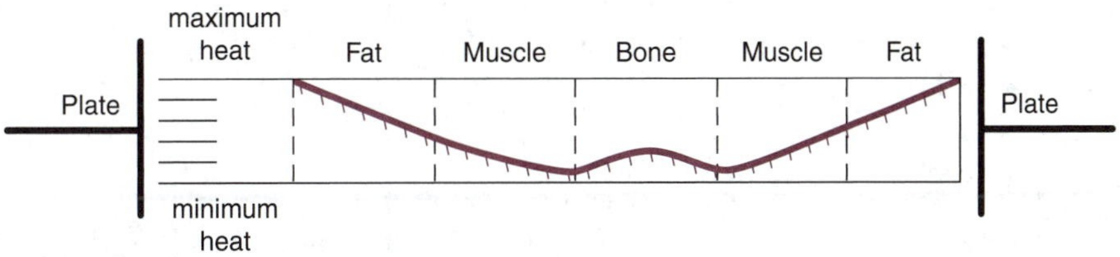

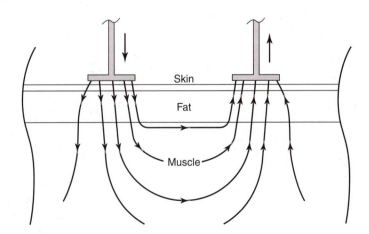

FIGURE 16–6   In this schematic rendition of inner tissues of a body part, with the tissues in series with the condenser plates, note that although the temperature of the entire cross section has increased, the temperature of the fatty-tissue is higher than that in muscle tissue when the condenser plates are in series. (*Adapted with permission from* Introduction to Shortwave and Microwave Therapy. *H Thom 1966, Charles C Thomas.*)

"series" arrangement, whereas **coplanar positioning** of plates uses the "parallel" arrangement. Although the analogy of series versus parallel electrical circuits is useful to explain the heating patterns of SWD, clinically the situation is more complex.

Essential differences exist between electrical line circuits and body tissues in series. Within the body, the strength of the electric field, and therefore the amount of current flow, is not uniform throughout. The lines of force of the electric field diverge with increasing distance from the plates and according to the electrical properties of the various tissues. For example, there is less divergence in fat than in tissues with a higher fluid content (eg, muscle). In narrow body parts such as an ankle or a wrist, the lines of force converge, and the field is much stronger **(Fig. 16–9).**

In addition, unlike "phantom model" tissue layers, tissues in the body are seldom found in precisely layered arrangements.

Although coplanar positioning is comparable to parallel electrical circuits, this electrode positioning in fact produces within the body a combination of series and parallel circuits. All current must first pass through the skin and fat layers in series before selecting the course of least resistance through deeper tissues (see **Fig. 16–9**). A parallel arrangement of electrodes will allow more selective heating of deep muscle tissue than a series arrangement; however, all current must first pass through skin and fat layers, even with parallel placement of electrodes. This process implies that with either form of condenser field diathermy, heating of subcutaneous fat will occur.

FIGURE 16–7   Schematic drawing of condenser plates in parallel with a longitudinal section of a body part. (*Modified with permission from* Therapeutic Heat and Cold *Lehmann J, ed. 3rd ed. 1982, Williams & Wilkins Co.*)

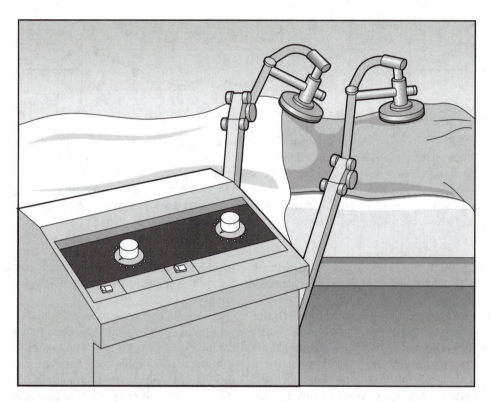

FIGURE 16–8 Condenser plates positioned in the parallel position to treat muscle in the mid- and lower back. Although not shown, one thin layer of toweling over the skin is recommended to absorb moisture.

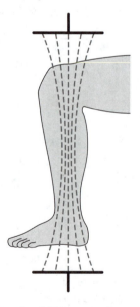

FIGURE 16–9 The field must converge when in a narrow part of the body such as the lower leg.

With either series or parallel positioning, any metal on or within the body, or metal anywhere within the electric field, will alter the heating pattern. The field can concentrate in metal and may overheat adjacent tissues.[1]

Induction (Coil) Field Diathermy

The second type of SWD is referred to as induction (coil) field diathermy. The principal difference between condenser field and induction field diathermy is that, with induction field diathermy, as current flows through the coil inside the drum, a strong **magnetic field** is produced about the coil in the patient circuit, which then induces an electrical current within the body part. In condenser field diathermy, the body part is positioned in an electrical field generated between two condenser plates. In induction field diathermy, a single induction field electrode is used that is made of coil-shaped metal **(Fig. 16–10)** and has properties of high conductivity. **Figure 16–11**

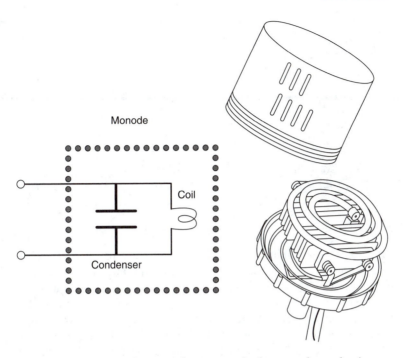

FIGURE 16–10   Inductive shortwave diathermy electrode (monode): arrangement of preshaped coils used for induction shortwave diathermy. (*Reproduced with permission from* Therapeutic Heat and Cold. *Lehmann J, ed. 3rd ed. 1982, Williams & Wilkins Co.*)

shows the typical arrangement of coils: the *monode*, with the coil arranged in one plane, and the hinged *diplode*, which permits the electrode to be positioned on 1 to 3 sides of a body part. Then high-frequency electrical energy is applied to the coil, which generates a fluctuating magnetic field around the coil. As with any current-conducting wire, a coil shape increases the strength of the magnetic field along the concave side. The direction of the magnetic field changes with each change in the direction of current passing through the coil.

When a low-impedance conductor such as a body part is placed *within the magnetic field*, electric currents are induced within that conductor. Within the body part, these are small *eddies* (circular-shaped currents) that alternate in direction in concert with the changes in the direction of the magnetic field.

Although the strength of the magnetic field fluctuates in phase with the high-frequency current that produced it, it is uniform throughout the various tissues at any given distance from the inductor. However, the amount of current density that is induced by the magnetic field in tissues is not uniform throughout various tissues because the current density varies

according to each tissue's impedance. In accordance with Joule's law, the greatest heat generated is within low-impedance tissues. The higher the electrolyte content of the tissue, the lower the impedance. Blood has the highest electrolyte content of all tissues (0.9%); therefore, muscle, which is rich in blood, can be heated more easily than fat, bone, or collagen tissues.[2,8,10,11] This pattern of heat distribution is shown in **Figure 16–12**. Note that the magnetic field is strongest near the coil; thus, skin and subcutaneous tissues are also affected, but not as much as in muscle. In general, the heating that occurs depends on the type of tissue and its depth.

Metal on, or implanted in, tissues must be considered. Because metal is a better electrical conductor than body tissues, the magnetic flux will induce more eddy currents in the metal. Thus, in accordance with Joule's law, the metal will heat—and may overheat—adjacent tissues.

Although coplanar parallel positioning of plates in condenser field SWD produces more effective heating of muscle than contraplanar series positioning, condenser field SWD still does not increase muscle tissue temperature as effectively—and possibly

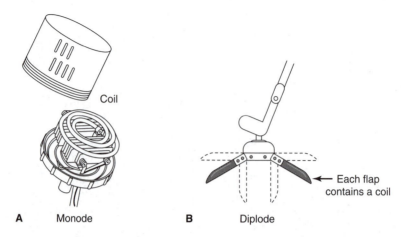

A   Monode   **B**   Diplode

FIGURE 16–11   Inductive shortwave diathermy (drum) electrodes. Two arrangements of preshaped coils used for induction shortwave diathermy. (**A**) The monode sends energy to tissues in the same plane as the surface of the drum. (**B**) The diplode has coils in each flap. The three-section hinged arrangement permits heating at various angles around three sides of the body part or in one plane. (*Modified with permission from* HHS Publication FDA 85–8237. *Kloth L, Morrison MA, Ferguson BH:* Therapeutic Microwave and Shortwave Diathermy: A Review of Thermal Effectiveness, Safe Use, and State of the Art: *1984. December 1984 Food and Drug Administration, U.S. Department of Health and Human Services.*)

as safely—as induction field SWD (**Fig. 16–13**). This is the case because condenser field SWD electrodes create an electric field that is predominantly absorbed in the skin and subcutaneous fat (because of divergence of the electric field), thus decreasing the amount that goes to the muscle.[2] This in turn may lead to an increased danger of superficial burns.[12] Induction field diathermy will be absorbed more readily in the muscle tissue without risk of overheating the subcutaneous fat because inductive SWD causes a greater increase in temperature in tissues with high conductivity, such as muscle, than it does in tissues with low conductivity, such as fat.[13]

Pulsed Shortwave Diathermy

On the basis of the belief that nonthermal benefits can be derived from high-frequency electromagnetic energy, some advocate the use of **pulsed shortwave diathermy.** Units such as Magnatherm® and Diapulse® are available that permit on-off cycles so that the energy is absorbed in the tissues but the blood

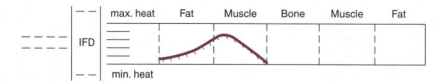

FIGURE 16–12   Pattern of depth of heat distribution in induction field shortwave diathermy (IFD). The temperature in muscle is elevated to a greater degree than the temperature in fatty tissue, but no temperature change occurs in bone. (*Adapted with permission from* Introduction to Shortwave and Microwave Therapy. *H Thom 1966 Charles C Thomas.*)

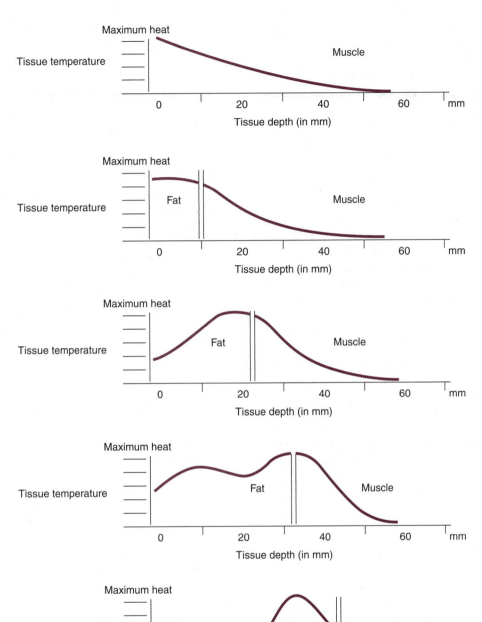

FIGURE 16–13   Influence of the thickness of the fat layer on heat distribution in muscle and fat during microwave diathermy. As the thickness of the fatty layer increases, its absorption of the heat increases and the absorption of heat by muscle decreases. (*Adapted with permission from* Introduction to Shortwave and Microwave Therapy. *H Thom 1966, Charles C Thomas.*)

flow during the off cycle prevents tissue temperature rise (TTR). The therapeutic effect of pulsed SWD is thought to be due to electromagnetic changes. These changes may restore cell membrane potentials, leading to physiochemical changes of osmosis secondary to the passage of ions.[14] Pulsed SWD, also known as **pulsed electromagnetic fields (PEMF),** was developed in the early 1960s and has a pulse duration of 20–400 msec, with an intensity of up to 1,000 watts per pulse.[15] The literature is equivocal regarding the therapeutic efficacy of pulsed SWD with patients who have various diagnoses. Pulsed SWD, or **pulsed electromagnetic energy,** has been shown to relieve pain at trigger points more effectively than moist heat,[16] significantly reduce the number of medications and length of stay for foot surgery patients,[17] improve the rate of healing following trauma[18,19] and surgery,[20] decrease pain and swelling in acutely sprained grade I and II ankle injuries,[21] and promote healing of Stage II and III ulcers.[22] Pulsed SWD was not found to be effective in treating perineal edema following childbirth,[23] nor to enhance healing of minimally displaced humeral neck fractures.[14] The ability of pulsed SWD to promote healing of skeletal muscle injury in rabbits was inconclusive.[24] In this study, Brown and Baker[24] found no significant difference in healing rate between treated and controlled animals after 8 days. It may be possible that the intervention dosages were too low.[24] Brown and Bakers's study[24] may be contrasted with the work by Schurman et al,[19] which demonstrated that maximum heat application with pulsed SWD promoted fibular fracture healing in rabbits. The varying results in these studies may have been due to differing pulse durations, intensities, intervention times, as well as differently pulsed SWD models. Further controlled trials are needed on patients with various diagnoses to determine the effects of pulsed SWD and optimal dosages with various diathermy units.

INTERVENTIONS

Preparation

Before initiating the intervention, the therapist should carry out the following steps:

1. Remove all clothing, jewelry, coins, and electronic devices from the area. Magnetic fluctuation may demagnetize watches or other electronic devices such as hearing aids.

2. Inspect the area to be treated, checking carefully for any metal on or around the patient, and ask the patient whether any metals (eg, prosthetic implants, sutures, pacemaker, intrauterine devices) are within the body. Note that **pacemakers constitute an absolute contraindication** because the electromagnetic field of the SWD may cause interference with the pacemaker frequency.

3. Cleanse the area to remove all dirt and oils.

4. Place the patient in a seated, prone, supine, or side-lying position, depending on the particular condition or body part to be treated. The patient should be relaxed and comfortable. Use pillows as needed to promote comfortable positioning. Be sure no zippers are present in the pillows.

5. Elevate an extremity to be treated to encourage fluid drainage.

6. Position the patient so that the musculature in the area to be treated is at the physiologic resting length or slackened, whenever possible, unless the goal is to increase the extensibility of tissues during heating. In such cases, position to encourage elongation of involved tissues.

7. Place the electrodes over the body part to be treated, according to the manufacturer's directions. When using the condenser field diathermy method, nonconductive tissues such as fat are treated more effectively with contraplanar positioning of plates. Conductive tissues such as muscle are treated with coplanar positioning. The electrodes must be placed 1–3 inches from the patient and must be placed parallel to the skin to prevent excessive heating of tissues.[25] If the electrodes are not housed in a prespaced drum, dry toweling of 1–3 inch thickness must be placed between the electrodes and the patient's skin to provide appropriate spacing. Today, with induction field diathermy, a drum in which the coil of wire is prespaced within a plastic encasing is most often used. The drum is placed directly over the body part, with one layer of toweling for hygienic purposes and to absorb and prevent pooling of perspiration.

8. Instruct the patient about the expected heat sensation and to notify you in case of any discomfort or if "it gets too hot."

9. Instruct the patient not to move after the unit is positioned for intervention because any changes in the arranged position may increase or decrease the amount of heat received. Movement can

change the tuning, either improving or reducing the frequency resonance between primary and secondary circuits.

The patient must **not** be positioned on a metal bed or plinth, on a mattress with metal springs, or in a metal chair such as a wheelchair when receiving diathermy intervention. In addition, the presence of any indwelling metal devices in the effective field represent contraindications. **In short, any metal in the effective area of the diathermy unit must be removed, or diathermy is contraindicated** because the heat generated can burn tissues or objects.

When positioning the patient, dry toweling is applied to body surfaces for sanitary purposes and to absorb perspiration. If perspiration is allowed to accumulate, it may cause a strong concentration of energy leading to excessive heating of the skin and possible burns. Absorbent material must be inserted whenever two skin surfaces such as the axilla are likely to make contact.

With diathermy, as with other electrical devices, the patient is positioned so that he or she cannot touch anything connected to the ground (eg, a radiator, a water pipe, an electrical outlet). Although the energy in the patient circuit was induced from the primary circuit and thus is "ground free," dangerously excessive current may flow through the body should the patient become grounded.

Dosage

Because the actual amount of energy that the patient received during the intervention cannot be monitored directly, the patient's own subjective sensation of heat is the most important indicator. A dose that produces a mild but pleasant sensation of heat is believed to be beneficial for subacute inflammatory processes, whereas chronic conditions respond to a more vigorous dose that leads to a sensation of heat that is just below the patient's maximum tolerance.[1,26] It is recommended that pulsed SWD may be used at very low settings to promote wound healing and to reduce pain and edema in acute soft tissue injuries, whereas moderate to vigorous heating may be used for a variety of subacute and chronic musculoskeletal conditions.[27] Clinicians generally assume that the sensation of heat on the skin is correlated with the degree of heating in deeper-lying tissues; however, the existence of a correlation between heat sensation on the skin and the degree of heating of deeper tissues has not been determined experimentally. Obviously, **the patient**

must be alert and able reliably to report sensations of heat. If the integrity of the peripheral nervous system is suspect, the therapist must test the patient's sense of temperature before initiating intervention.

In addition, it is prudent in a first intervention to take the extra precaution of using slightly lower intensities. A more subtle point is the need to monitor the patient's report of heat sensation at the initial phase of intervention and again during the intervention. When the output of the diathermy unit is adjusted, a "lag" of several seconds occurs between the time the output is changed and the time that the patient will be aware of a change in the sensation of heat. Therefore, the patient must be given sufficient time to perceive this change before further adjustments are made.

The duration and frequency of intervention and the use of pulsed versus continuous mode depend on the intervention goals (decreased pain or increased tissue extensibility) and the status of the condition treated (acute, subacute, or chronic). Lehmann[1] has shown that 20 to 30 min interventions are usually long enough to be therapeutically beneficial. It may take 3 to 8 min for the tissue temperature to rise to desired levels. After the temperature reaches the plateau caused by the diathermy application, an additional 10 to 20 min should be sufficient to achieve therapeutic gains. The TTR is an important consideration when the goal is to elongate tissues at high temperatures. For example, if the intent is to heat and stretch for 20 min and the TTR requires 8 min, the intervention should continue for about 30 min.[1] The specific absorption rate (SAR) and guidelines for dosages based on the SAR are given in **Chapter 8 and Table 8–2.**

Techniques

The therapist should be familiar with and follow the manufacturers' recommendations for the proper application of specific diathermy units. This section presents general recommendations for condenser and induction field SWD.

Condenser Field Diathermy. Placing the condenser plates parallel to the body part to be treated is recommended to heat superficial muscle. If this is not possible or if it is desirable to treat two sides of a body part such as a shoulder, knee, or ankle, the plates should be placed in a contraplanar position with the body part to be treated. The plates themselves, usually located within plate guards, can be moved a predetermined distance to vary the spacing between plate and skin. The guard can contact the skin or overlying towel, but the metal plate itself must not contact the towel or skin. Power output is dictated by the patient's subjective sensation of heat. At any given energy output, the closer the plates are to the skin, the greater the sensation of heat. As the distance between the plate and the skin increases, the sensation of heat decreases; thus, the power output can be increased and more energy can be provided to promote greater heating of deep-lying tissues.[5] A plate-skin distance of 1 inch is suggested to provide maximum heating at maximum depths with minimum risk to the patient (see **Figs. 16–9** and **16–14**).[28]

Induction Field Diathermy. Depending on the manufacturer, this current conductor may be pre-shaped into a coil (sometimes referred to as a drum) designed as a diplode or monode (see **Fig. 16–11**). The induction field SWD units most frequently used today have a monode (**Fig. 16–15**). The space between the coiled conductor and the surface of the drum is fixed, so a single layer of toweling laid on the body part provides adequate spacing **(Fig. 16–16)**.

Shortwave diathermy had decreased in clinical popularity for many years because it was complicated to set up, because its safety was questioned, and because other electroanalgesia such as TENS, electroacupuncture, and lasers were discovered.[29] Today there are induction field diathermy units that are easy to set up, have automatic tuning and easily movable drums, emit predominantly magnetic field output without the electric field, and are relatively safe for the patient and clinician.

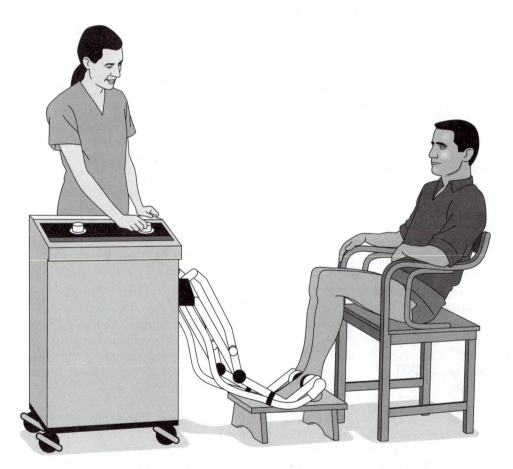

FIGURE 16–14   Contraplanar (transverse) position of condenser plates. The plates are in series with body tissues.

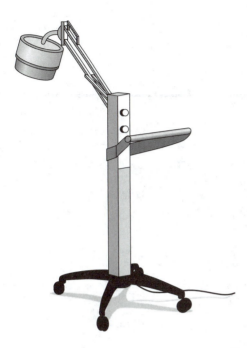

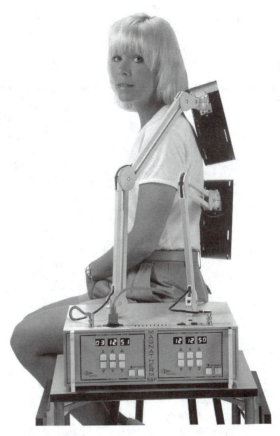

FIGURE 16–15   This is a single-drum unit with automatic turning, as shown on p. 13 of J. Kahn's book. Autotherm is the brand name.

FIGURE 16–16   Inductive shortwave diathermy with dual monode drum coil electrodes. (*Courtesy of International Medical Electronics, LTD., Kansas City, MD.*)

Reflex Heating.   As described in **Chapter 9 reflex heating** is a technique of applying heat to one area of the body that results in an increase in cutaneous circulation in a remote area of the body. Because the effect occurs almost immediately, before systemic changes have had the opportunity to occur, it is referred to as reflex heating. Shortwave diathermy has been used to invoke reflex heating by heating the axilla to promote distal heating of the upper extremity, or heating the anterior thigh or lumbosacral plexus to produce distal heating of the lower extremity. However, the literature is controversial concerning the potential for SWD to produce reflex heating. Hoeberlein et al[30] did not find evidence of increased cutaneous blood flow peripherally, as measured with a laser Doppler monitor, during 20-min SWD interventions to the lumbosacral plexus or anterior thigh of normal, healthy young individuals. Santoro et al[31] administered SWD for 20 min at a high setting and 10 min at a low setting to the anterior thigh of 10 volunteers with a diagnosis of arterial peripheral vascular disease. They measured transcutaneous partial pressure of oxygen ($tcpO_2$) on the dorsum of the feet and found a significant increase in $tcpO_2$ in the untreated lower extremity. They attributed this finding to reflex vasodilation.[31] The discrepancies between the results of these two studies may have been due to the use of different diathermy equipment and different power settings, as well as the application of different outcome measuring tools.

Box 16–1 contains the common clinical uses for shortwave diathermy. More detailed information related to indications and contraindications follow within the text of this chapter.

Indications and Contraindications (see Boxes 16–2 and 16–3)

Indications.   Box 16-1 lists the common indications for shortwave diathermy. It has been well documented that the application of shortwave diathermy can lead to therapeutically useful elevations of deep-tissue

Box 16–1   *Clinical Uses of Continuous and Pulsed Shortwave Diathermy*

Reflexive vasodilatation for individuals with peripheral arterial occlusive disease	Concentration of heat proximally on an extremity or the trunk to cause vasodilatation into a distal area with diminished blood flow.
Subacute and chronic inflammation (ie, bursitis, tendonitis)	Increased blood flow and cellular activity to assist in the inflammatory and healing process following injury or overuse.
Musculoskeletal pain and associated muscle spasm	Increased thermal sensory input. Increased blood flow to wash out inflammatory chemicals associated with pain and muscle spasm.
Tightness in soft tissue (ie, joint restrictions, adaptive muscle shortening, scar tissue)	Elevate tissue temperature to increase soft tissue extensibility during stretching.
Wound healing	To increase activity in those cells involved in the inflammatory and proliferative phases of healing.

temperature.[1,5,6,32] Diathermy is especially effective when treating tissues and joints that lie up to 2.0 cm below the skin surface.[1,33,34] Diathermy has been used to help clear inflammatory exudates in subacute conditions; however, it is most frequently used in the intervention of musculoskeletal disorders. The use of SWD to decrease pain due to musculoskeletal trauma has been shown to be effective as a short-term method of analgesia, but it may not be as effective for long-term pain control.[35] Further research is required to determine what methods of SWD administration may be beneficial for long-term analgesia.

Diathermy is used by therapists to promote wound healing; however, open wounds and wounds with

Box 16–2 *Indications for Diathermy*

Treatment of musculoskeletal disorders, including the following specific applications:

Short-term analgesia for musculoskeletal disorders[35]

Wound healing[36,37]

Muscle spasm or pain due to osteoarthritis, sprains, and strains[28]

Stretching of collagenous tissue[34,39,40]

Adjunct to treatment of neck and low-back pain[41,42]

Adjunct to treatment of osteoarthritic knees[44]

Temporomandibular joint pain dysfunction syndrome[49]

Other indications for diathermy:

Pelvic inflammatory disease[29]

Primary dysmennorrhea[51]

Herpes zoster[54]

Sinusitis[55]

Pneumonia[53]

Box 16–3 *Contraindications for Continuous Diathermy*

Over an area of acute inflammation

Over an area of hemorrhage or active bleeding

Over an area with poor circulation

Inability to perceive or report heat sensation accurately

Fever

Over an area of metal or an implant

Cardiac pacemakers or any pacing devices[5,25,57]

Menstruation (precaution)[51]

Pregnancy[1,59,60]

Testes

Eyes

Epiphyses[2]

Malignancies[10]

occlusive dressing are contraindicated for diathermy. It has been demonstrated that heat increases blood perfusion and oxygenation of local cells in subcutaneous wounds.[36] This increased perfusion and oxygen tension in turn facilitates healing through increased collagen deposition and tensile strength in wounds.[37] Although the physiologic process by which heat promotes healing in wounds is known, reports by therapists of wound healing through the use of diathermy are mainly anecdotal. It is imperative that controlled clinical trials be implemented to determine the efficacy of diathermy in wound healing.

Diathermy is desirable with skin conditions that may be aggravated by moisture and is also indicated with patients who are sensitive to the weight of a hot pack.[38] It is especially effective when treating secondary muscle spasms or pain associated with pathologies such as degenerative joint disease, sprains, and strains.[28] Furthermore, the extensibility of collagenous tissue is increased when the tissue temperature is elevated.[28] Therefore, when stretching is the goal of the physical therapy program, positioning that elongates the tissues to be stretched while diathermy is applied, and stretching or exercising the part while the temperature is still elevated, will enhance the results of the stretching techniques.[34,39,40]

When treating these disorders, selection of a heating modality depends on the depth of the penetration of each modality, the depth of the tissue to be treated,

the size of the area to be treated, and the amount of heating required. The depth of penetration of SWD is greater than the infrared modalities and less than ultrasound. The size of the body part that can be heated may be a small circumscribed area or a relatively large area, depending on the type of diathermy and electrodes used. When diathermy is applied to deep-seated joints covered by a thick layer of tissue (eg, the hip joint), the temperature of that joint does not increase appreciably. The highest temperatures occur in the superficial to deep musculature.[2]

When treating patients with nonspecific back and neck complaints, Koes et al[41] found that manipulative therapy and physical therapy (which included SWD) were significantly more effective than general practitioner (analgesic) intervention and placebo intervention in decreasing pain and improving function. Manipulative therapy also yielded slightly better results than physical therapy that did not include manipulation.[41] Davies et al[42] investigated the effect of SWD in the intervention of patients with low back pain and found that SWD combined with exercise was more effective than SWD alone in relieving pain; however, the difference between the two intervention groups was not significant. A larger sample size might have yielded a significant difference.[42] These studies demonstrate that SWD alone may not be effective in relieving pain and improving function in patients with back pain. Using SWD to improve extensibility of shortened joint tissues and relieve pain followed by manipulative therapy and therapeutic exercise may be an effective means of improving function.

When instructing patients in a therapeutic exercise program after an SWD intervention, it is important to be cognizant of the time frame. Many clinicians will instruct patients in exercise within a short period following therapeutic heat application in order to take advantage of the analgesic and soft-tissue lengthening effects of heat. Chastain[43] has found, however, that immediately following an SWD intervention, mean isometric strength in the quadriceps muscle decreased in normal, healthy young adults. Thirty minutes after the cessation of the SWD intervention, mean strength would then increase to levels above preintervention readings. This increase in strength then persisted for 90 min. Chastain recommends, therefore, that there be a 30-min rest period between heat interventions and strengthening exercise.[43] More research is required to determine the effect of deep heat on exercise performance with different age groups and patients with different diagnoses.

When treating joints with minimal soft-tissue coverage, such as the knee or ankle, diathermy can significantly elevate the temperature in the joint and surrounding musculature. The therapist should therefore consider the desirability of heating within a joint in light of a patient's specific condition. Jan and Lai[44] demonstrated a significant improvement in functional capacity and peak torque in knee musculature following a course of ultrasound and SWD in patients with osteoarthritic knees. They found no significant difference between ultrasound and SWD, and combining an exercise program with the physical agents was found to be more effective than using the physical agents alone.[44] Oosterveld et al[45] found an increase in knee-joint cavity temperature from 32.5°C to 36.0°C following SWD intervention in healthy subjects. Because destructive enzyme activity occurs during active synovitis when joint temperature is found to be 35° to 36°C,[46,47] Oosterveld et al.[45] suggest that interventions that raise intraarticular temperature should be used with caution in patients with arthritis. On the basis of these studies, it seems that deep-heating agents may work well as adjuncts to a comprehensive intervention program with patients with osteoarthritis, but should be used judiciously because of the possibility of activating destructive enzymes in the synovium. More information is needed to determine the short- and long-range effects of vigorously heating joint synovium.

SWD has been found to be significantly better than placebo intervention in the relief of pain due to temporomandibular joint pain dysfunction syndrome (TMJPDS).[48] Although SWD was found to be effective, its success rate was not significantly different from other modalities examined, including megapulse, ultrasound, and soft laser.[48] When pulsed SWD was compared with ultrasound and galvanic currents for pain relief, however, there was no significant difference demonstrated between the methods.[49] Since a number of modalities may be effective in treating musculoskeletal conditions such as TMJPDS and osteoarthritis, the clinician may want to consider other factors (eg, cost effectiveness and long-term pain relief) when choosing a modality for treating musculoskeletal conditions.

Diathermy has been shown to be helpful in pelvic inflammatory disease (PID)[29] and primary dysmenorrhea.[50] Balogun and Okonofua[29] administered SWD to a woman with an 8-year history of PID to address her chronic abdominal and back pain. After 9 interventions, and for a least 67 months following discharge from the therapy, the woman remained pain free. SWD is capable of causing a slight rise in intrauterine temperature;[51] however, the mechanism by which SWD relieves pain due to PID is unknown. Vance et al[50] administered MWD to a woman with primary dysmenorrhea who had experienced severe monthly pain for 18 years. Intervention involved the use of MWD as needed for pelvic pain that began at the onset of menses each month. They found that diathermy effected an almost-immediate and long-lasting relief of symptoms. After the 7-month course of diathermy, the patient was able to manage any pain with ibuprofen and no longer lost workdays because of primary dysmenorrhea.[50] These case studies are promising and point out the need for further research to determine the efficacy of diathermy in gynecological conditions.

Physical therapists should be aware of their indications for SWD for which supporting literature exists. Shortwave diathermy has been used to (a) resolve small pneumothoraces in significantly shorter time than in controls,[52,53] (b) relieve pain associated with herpes zoster through daily intervention to the spinal cord at the level of the involved dermatome,[54] (c) increase circulation to mucous membranes to resolve chronic sinusitis,[55] and (d) be related to a reduction in mortality in patients with pneumonia when compared with controls.[56] The study on SWD with pneumonia was conducted long before the introduction of antibiotics. With the advent of these drugs, interventions such as SWD fell into disuse for diagnoses such as pneumonia. However, with the new drug-resistant strains of bacteria that now exist, SWD may be found to be effective in treating resistant infections. More controlled research is needed to demonstrate the efficacy of SWD in the intervention of pneumonia, as well as other diseases such as herpes zoster and sinusitis.

Contraindications.   Box 16–3 lists the commonly recognized contrainoication for shortwave diatherm. The general contraindications associated with any modality that elevates tissue temperature must be observed. The application of diathermy is always avoided if inflammation is acute, hemorrhage is likely, the vascular system is compromised, the patient cannot perceive or report heat sensation accurately, or the patient has a fever.

The contraindications associated specifically with diathermy are numerous. As was mentioned earlier, any metal in the field is clearly a contraindication. Furthermore, cardiac pacemakers or other pacing devices are of special concern because their presence is a contraindication in itself.[56] In addition, the **energy emanating from the diathermy unit may disrupt the operation of a pacemaker in any person in proximity to the diathermy unit.**[5,25] Although metal in the field is a contraindication, there is evidence to show that the presence of a copper-bearing intrauterine device (IUD) seems to be safe during an SWD intervention.[57] There is only a slight increase in intrauterine temperature of approximately 0.5°C, which falls within normal diurnal variation[58] and therefore will not affect the IUD nor the surrounding tissue.[51,57]

Because the application of diathermy to the low back has been reported to increase menstrual flow, menses may represent a contraindication in some cases. However, Vance et al[50] were able to successfully decrease a female patient's pain due to dysmenorrhea through administration of MWD at the onset of menses. Diathermy use during menstrual flow may therefore be a precaution and not an absolute contraindication.

The evidence that high-frequency current has a negative effect on the pregnant uterus when the low back or abdomen are treated is equivocal; therefore, pregnancy remains a contraindication to diathermy. Furthermore, Lehmann and DeLateur[1] recommend that pregnant therapists avoid operating the unit. Imrie[58] reported that of three women who received SWD inadvertently during the early weeks of pregnancy, one woman experienced a spontaneous abortion. This outcome was attributed to the timing of the SWD intervention, which took place close to the day of expected ovulation, which is near the time of fertilization.[58] A more recent epidemiological study by Ouellet-Hellstrom and Stewart[59] concluded that the operation of MWD equipment by pregnant physical therapists was associated with an increased risk of miscarriage. However, they found that use of SWD equipment did not pose such a risk.[59]

It is always wise to avoid direct diathermy heating of the testes, the area near the eyes, and the epiphyses in growing children. Although bone is not effectively heated when covered by an adequate layer of soft tissue, the size of the SWD drum in relationship to the size of a growing child may prevent the unit from being applied in such a way as to avoid superficial epiphyses.[2] Direct heating of malignancies is contraindicated because the increased vascularity may increase blood flow to the extent that metastases may occur.[10] Although hyperthermia is a form of cancer therapy, the diathermy equipment and the techniques used for cancer therapy are not the same as the equipment and techniques commonly used in physical therapy clinics.[60]

The evidence that stray radiation from diathermy units constitutes an occupational hazard is equivocal. Silverman[61] and Michaelson[62] reviewed studies on the possible deleterious effects of microwaves and concluded that the results of the studies were not compelling.[61,62] Two separate groups of investigators studied the effects of exposure to shortwave and MWD respectively.[63,64] Both groups concluded that ordinary prudent practice (remaining within 1 m of an operating unit for only short periods) makes it unlikely that therapists would be exposed to harmful levels of radiation. A more recent report by Martin et al[65] also recommended that therapists remain at least 1 m from continuous-wave SWD units, and 0.5 m from microwave units and pulsed SWD machines. Tzima and Martin[66] found that the highest electric and magnetic field strengths with continuous SWD extended for 1 m from the electrodes and cables. They recommended that operators remain at least 1 m from continuous SWD units, 0.5–0.8 m from pulsed condenser field

SWD, and 0.2 m from pulsed inductive field SWD.[66] A study by Brown-Woodman et al[67] illustrates the importance of avoiding close proximity to the SWD unit by the operator. They exposed female rats to radio-frequency radiation by placing them 0.5 m from the center of the electromagnetic field during intervention. This experiment led to a reduction in the number of rats that mated and became pregnant as compared with controls.[67] Other researchers are investigating the possible development of brain cancer due to radio-frequency exposure that occurs with portable cellular telephones,[68] but no definite relationship has been proven.

Hamburger[69] reported an association between heart disease in male physical therapists and the use of SWD. However, of the 3,004 male therapists who responded to the survey, only 73 reported heart disease, and most of them were in the age group frequently associated with heart disease. In addition, information about smoking habits, alcohol consumption, and the like was not gathered. Thus, more rigorously designed studies are needed.

SUMMARY

At the frequency commonly found in clinics, SWD and pulsed SWD, if properly applied, increase the temperature of skeletal muscle to varying degrees. The greatest elevations in temperature will occur in skeletal muscle that is close to the surface, while virtually no changes in temperature occur in muscles surrounding a deep-seated joint such as the hip joint. Like other modalities, diathermy will result in some transference of heat to other tissues by conduction and by local circulation of warmed blood, but its greatest effect is mild-to-moderate heating of superficial musculature. The distribution pattern of temperature resulting from a diathermy intervention is influenced by the type of diathermy and the method of its application. If properly executed, intervention with induction field and condenser field diathermy can increase temperatures in skeletal muscle. The actual amount of energy absorbed by specific tissues and the dosage required to elicit maximum therapeutic benefits have not been elucidated. More investigations similar to those undertaken by Lehmann et al[70] are needed. With further research, physical therapists can make more precise decisions about the efficacy of this modality and other modalities in the management of musculoskeletal disorders. As with any modality, the decision to use diathermy for a particular intervention situation depends on a number of variables: the type of diathermy unit employed; the depth of penetration of the modality; the depth of tissue to be treated; the size of the area to be treated; whether vigorous, moderate, or mild heating is desired,[1] and whether the primary intervention goals include tissue nutrition, extensibility, and/or pain relief. Another important consideration includes intervention cost to the therapist and the patient. Shortwave diathermy may be a cost-effective modality for the physical therapist because the therapist is free to perform other duties during the SWD intervention. Shortwave diathermy may also be cost effective for patients and their employers if it promotes healing that results in an earlier return to work following injury. There is anecdotal evidence to support this possibility; however, research needs to be done to ascertain the cost effectiveness of SWD.

REVIEW QUESTIONS

1. What is the relationship between diathermy frequency and depth of heating?
2. Describe the lines of force as they refer to the strength of magnetic or electric fields.
3. Describe the role of a tuner in SWD.
4. What is the difference between a condenser field and an induction field in a diathermy application?
5. Can induction field diathermy increase the temperature of superficial or deep muscles? Explain your answer.
6. List three indications for which deep heat might be more helpful than superficial heat.
7. What are the contraindications for use of diathermy?

KEY TERMS

diathermy
shortwave diathermy (SWD)
machine (power) circuit
patient circuit
condenser (capacitor) field
  diathermy

condensers
capacitor plates
electric field
contraplanar positioning
coplanar positioning
induction (coil) field diathermy

magnetic field
pulsed shortwave diathermy
pulsed electromagnetic fields
  (PEMF)
pulsed electromagnetic energy
reflex heating

REFERENCES

1. Lehmann JF, Delateur BJ: Therapeutic Heat. In: Lehmann JF (ed). *Therapeutic Heat and Cold.* 4th ed. Chapter 9. Baltimore: Williams & Wilkins, 1990; 417–581.

2. Kloth L, Morrison MA, Ferguson BH: *Therapeutic Microwave and Shortwave Diathermy: A Review of Thermal Effectiveness, Safe Use, and State of the Art: 1984.* Food and Drug Administration, U.S. Department of Health and Human Services; December 1984. HHS Publication FDA 85-8237.

3. Jackins S, Jamieson A: Use of Heat and Cold in Physical Therapy. In: Lehmann JF (ed). *Therapeutic Heat and Cold.* 4th ed. Chapter 9. Baltimore: Williams & Wilkins, 1990; 645–73.

4. Diamond SR: *Fundamental Concepts of Modern Physics.* New York: Amsco School Publications, Inc, 1970; 224.

5. Griffin JE, Karselis TC: *Physical Agents for Physical Therapists.* Springfield, IL: Charles C Thomas; 1982.

6. Guy AW, Lehmann JF, Stonebridge JB: Therapeutic applications of electromagnetic power. *Proc IEEE* 1974; 62:55–75.

7. Lehmann JF. Diathermy. In: Krusen FH, Kottke FJ, Ellwood PM Jr (eds). *Handbook of Physical Medicine and Rehabilitation.* 2nd ed. Chapter 11. Philadelphia: Saunders, 1971; 273–45.

8. Thom H: *Introduction to Shortwave and Microwave Therapy.* Springfield, IL: Charles C Thomas; 1966.

9. Lehmann JF, Guy AW, Stonebridge JB, et al: *Review of Evidence for Indications, Techniques of Application, Contraindications, Hazards, and Clinical Effectiveness of Shortwave Diathermy.* Food and Drug Administration, U.S. Department of Health and Human Services; 1974. Report No. FDA/HFK-71-1.

10. Paetzold J: Physical laws regarding distribution of energy for various high frequency methods applied in heat therapy. *Ultrasonics Biol Medi* 1964; 9(3):58–67.

11. Kebbel W, Krause W, Paetzold J: Composition of energy distribution in fat muscle layers of long-decimeter waves and high-frequency waves. *Elektromedizin Band* 1964; 9:171–79.

12. Brown G: Diathermy: A renewed interest in a proven therapy. *Phys Ther Today* Spring 1993; 78–80.

13. Kloth LC, Ziskin MC: Diathermy and Pulsed Electromagnetic Fields. In: Michlovitz SL (ed). *Thermal Agents in Rehabilitation.* 2nd ed. Chapter 8. Philadelphia: Davis, 1990; 170–99.

14. Livesley PJ, Mugglestone A, Whitton J: Electrotherapy and the management of minimally displaced fracture of the neck of the humorus. *Injury* 1992; 23:323–27.

15. Lipsky J. Diathermy: What the heck is it anyway? *Rehab Ther Products Rev* July/August 1992; 20–21.

16. McCray RE, Patton NJ: Pain relief at trigger points: A comparison of moist heat and shortwave diathermy. *J Orthop Sports Phys Ther* 1984; 5:175–78.

17. Santiesteban AJ, Grant C: Post-surgical effect of pulsed shortwave therapy. *J Am Podiatr Med Assoc* 1985; 75:306–09.

18. Bassett CA, Mitchell SN, Gaston SR: Treatment of united tibial diaphyseal fractures with pulsing electromagnetic fields. *J Bone Joint Surg* 1981; 63A:511.

19. Schurman DJ, Piziali R, Swenson L, et al: Shortwave diathermy and fracture healing in rabbit fibula model: preliminary report. Transactions of the 26the Annual Meeting, Orthopaedic Research Society. 1980; 5:160.

20. Arghiropol M, Jieanu V, Paslaru L, et al: The stimulation of fibronectin synthesis by high peak power electromagnetic energy (Diapulse). *Rev Roumaine Physiol* 1992; 29:77–81.

21. Pennington GM, Danley DL, Sumko MH: Pulsed, non-thermal, high-frequency electromagnetic energy (DLAPULSE) in the treatment of grade I and grade II ankle sprains, *Military Med* 1993; 158:101–04.

22. Itoh M, Montenmayor JS Jr, Matsumoto E, et al: Accelerated wound healing of pressure ulcers by pulsed high peak power electromagnetic energy (Diapulse). *Decubitus* 1991; 4:24–25.

23. Grant A, Sleep J, McIntosh J, Ashurst H: Ultrasound and pulsed electromagnetic energy treatment for perineal trauma. A randomized placebo-controlled trial. *Br J Obstet Gynaecol* 1989; 96:434–39.

24. Brown M, Baker RD: Effect of pulsed shortwave diathermy on skeletal muscle injury in rabbits. *Phys Ther* 1987; 67:208–13.

25. Hayes K: *Manual for Physical Agents*. Norwalk, CT: Appleton & Lange; 1993.

26. Avery WR: Cell membranes: The electromagnetic environment and cancer promotion. Neurochem Res 1988; 68:710–12.

27. Goats GC: Continuous shortwave (radio-frequency) diathermy. (Review). *Br J Sport Med* 1989; 23:123–27.

28. Shore RE: Electromagnetic radiations and cancer. *Cancer* 1988; 62(suppl):1747–54.

29. Balogun JA, Okonofua FE: Management of chronic pelvic inflammatory disease with short-wave diathermy: A case report. *Phys Ther* 1988; 68:1541–45.

30. Hodberlein TS, Katz JS, Balogun JA: Does indirect heating using shortwave diathermy over the abdomen and sacrum affect peripheral blood flow in the lower extremities? (Abstract). *Phys Ther* 1996; 76:S67.

31. Santoro D, Ostrander L, Lee BY, et al: *Inductive 27.12 MHz: Diathermy in arterial peripheral vascular disease*. 16th International IEEE/EMBS Conference. IEEE Press, 1994.

32. Guy AW: Biophysics of high frequency currents and electromagnetic radiation. In: Lehmann JF (ed). *Therapeutic Heat and Cold*. Baltimore: Williams & Wilkins; 1990.

33. Cassvan A: Rehabilitative measures in arthritis and related conditions. *Osteopath Ann* February 1977; 78–87.

34. Lehmann JF, Warren CG, Scham SM: Therapeutic heat and cold. *Clin Orthop Rel Res* 1974; 99:207–45.

35. Comorosan S, Vasilco R, Arghiropol M, et al: The effect of diapulse therapy on the healing of decubitus ulcer. *Rom J Physiol* 1993; 30:41–45.

36. Seaborne D, Quirion-DeGirardi C, Rousseau M, et al: The treatment of pressure sores using pulsed electromagnetic energy (PEME). *Physiother Can* 1996; 48:131–37.

37. Stiller MJ, Pak GH, Shupack JL, et al: A portable pulsed electromagnetic field (PEMF) device to enhance healing of a recalcitrant venous ulcers: A double-blind, placebo-controlled clinical trial. *Br J Dermatol* 1992; 127:147–54.

38. Tood DJ, Heylings DJ, Allen GE, McMillin WP: Treatment of chronic varicose ulcers with pulsed electromagnetic fields: A controlled pilot study. *Ir Med J* 1991; 84:54–55.

39. Mayrovitz HN, Larsen PB: A preliminary study to evaluate the effect of pulsed radio frequency field treatment of lower extremity peri-ulcer microcirculation of diabetic patients. *Wounds* 1995; 7:90–93.

40. Warren CG, Lehmann JF, Koblanski JN: Elongation of rat tail tendon: Effect of load and temperature. *Arch Phys Med* 1971; 54:465–74.

41. Koes BW, Bouter LM, van Mameren H, et al: Randomised clinical trial of manipulative therapy and physiotherapy for persistent back and neck complaints: results of one-year followup. *Brit Med J* 1992; 304(6827):601–05.

42. Davies JE, Gibson T, Tester L: The value of exercises in the treatment of low back pain. *Rheumatol Rehabil* 1979; 18:243–47.

43. Chastain PB: The effect of deep heat on isometric strength. *Phys Ther* 1978; 58:543–46.

44. Jan MH, Lai JS: The effects of physiotherapy on osteoarthritic knees of females. *Formosan Med Assoc* 1991; 90:1008–13.

45. Oosterveld FGI, Rasker JJ, Jacobs JWG, Overmars HJA: The effect of local heat and cold therapy on the intraarticular and skin surface temperature of the knee. *Arthritis Rheum* 1992; 35:146–51.

46. Harris ED, McCroskery PA: The influence of temperature and fibril stability on degradation of cartilage collagen by rheumatoid synovial collagenase. *N Engl J Med* 1974; 290:1–6.

47. Wolley DE, Evanson JM: Colagenase and its natural inhibitors in relation to the rheumatoid joint. *Connect Tissue Res* 1977; 5:31–35.

48. Gray RJ, Quayle AA, Hall CA, et al: Physiotherapy in the treatment of temporomandibular joint disorders: A comparative study of four treatment methods. *Brit Dent J* 1994; 176:257–61.

49. Svaroova J, Trnavsky K, Zvarova J: The influence of ultrasound, galvanic currents and shortwave diathermy on pain intensity in patients with osteoarthritis. *Scand J Rheumatol* 1988; Suppl 67:83–85.

50. Vance AR, Hayes SH, Spielholz JI: Microwave diathermy treatment for primary dysmenorrhea. *Phys Ther* 1996; 76:1003–08.

51. Heick A, Espersen T, Pedersen HL, Raahauge J: Is diathermy safe in women with copper-bearing IUDs? *Acta Obstet Gynecol Scand* 1991; 70:153–55.

52. Ma W, Li J, Liu Y: Shortwave diathermy for small spontaneous pneumothorax. *Thorax* 1997; 52:561–62.

53. Allberry J, Manning FRC, Smith EE: Shortwave diathermy for herpes zoster. *Physiother* 1974; 60:386.

54. Cash JE: *Physiotherapy in Some Surgical Conditions.* London: Faber & Faber, 1977.

55. Stewart HE: *Diathermy and Its Application to Pneumonia.* New York: Paul B. Hoeber, Inc., 1923.

56. Jones SL: Electromagnetic field interference and cardiac pacemakers. *Phys Ther* 1976; 56:1013–18.

57. Neilsen NC, Hansen R, Larsen T: Heat induction in copper-bearing IUDs during shortwave diathemy. *Acta Obstet Gynecol Scand* 1979; 58:495.

58. Imrie AH: Pelvic shortwave diathermy given inadvertently in early pregnancy. *J Obstet Gynaecol Br Commonwealth* 1971; 78:91–92.

59. Oueller-Hellstrom R, Stewart WF: Miscarriages among female physical therapists who report using radio- and microwave-frequency electromagnetic radiation. *AM J Epidemiol* 1995; 41:273–74.

60. Shimm DJ, Gerner E: Hyperthermia in Treatment of Malignancies. In: Lehmann JF, ed. *Therapeutic Heat and Cold.* Baltimore: Williams & Wilkins; 1990.

61. Silverman C: Epidemiologic studies of microwave effects. *Proc IEEE* 1980; 68:78–84.

62. Michaelson SM: Bioeffects of High-Frequency Currents and Electromagnet Radiation. In: Lehmann JF, ed. *Therapeutic Heat and Cold.* Baltimore: Williams & Wilkins; 1990.

63. Stuchly MA, Repacholi MH, LeCuyer DW, et al: Exposure to the operator and patient during shortwave diathermy treatments. *Health Physics* 1982; 42:341–66.

64. Moseley H, Davison M: Exposure of physiotherapists to microwave radiation during microwave diathermy treatment. *Clin Phys Physiol Meas* 1981; 2:217–21.

65. Martin CJ, McCallum HM, Heaton B: An evaluation of radiofrequency exposure from therapeutic diathermy equipment in the light of current recommendations. *Clin Phys Physiol Meas* 1990; 11:53–63.

66. Tzima E, Martin CJ: An evaluation of safe practices to restrict exposure to electric and magnetic fields from therapeutic and surgical diathermy equipment. *Physiol Meas* 1994; 15:201–16.

67. Brown-Woodman PDC, Hadley JA, Richardson L, Bright D, Porter D: Evaluation of reproductive function of female rats exposed to radiofrequency fields (27.12 MHz) near a shortwave diathermy device. *Health Physics* 1989; 56:521–25.

68. Rothman KJ, Oho CK, Morgan R, et al: Assessment of cellular telephone and other radiofrequency exposure for epidemiologic research. *Epidemiology* 1996; 7:291–98.

69. Hamburger S, Logue JN, Silverman PM: Occupational exposure to non-ionizing radiation and as association with heart disease: An exploratory study. *J Chron Dis* 1983; 36:791–802.

70. Lehmann JF, McDougall JA, Guy AW, et al: Heating patterns produced by shortwave diathermy applicators in tissue substitute models. *Arch Phys Med Rehabil* 1983; 64:575–77.

17

Safety Considerations
for Thermal Modalities

BERNADETTE HECOX, PT, MA

JOHN P. SANKO, PT, EdD.

Chapter Outline

- MONITORING SIGNS AND SYMPTOMS
- EFFECTS OF AMBIENT CONDITIONS
- CONSIDERATIONS FOR THERAPISTS
- REACTIONS CAUSED BY EXCESSIVE EXPOSURE TO HEAT
  OR COLD
  Cardiovascular Reactions
  Sudomotor Reactions
  Metabolic Reactions

- PROBLEMS CAUSED BY OVEREXPOSURE TO HEAT
  Prickly Heat
  Dehydration
  Heat Cramps
  Heat Exhaustion
  Heat Stroke
- REVIEW QUESTIONS
- KEY TERMS

Earlier chapters in Part 2 have shown that the application of thermal modalities can produce systemic as well as local responses. Both ambient conditions and the patient's activity level can augment or diminish these systemic responses. For example, an extremely warm day or swimming rather than just soaking in a heated pool can place greater demands on body systems that are affected by temperature changes. Although healthy adults can usually tolerate these demands, they may be excessive for many of the patients seen in physical therapy (ie, young children, older adults, or individuals who are debilitated). Therefore, the physical therapist must constantly be alert to the reactions that may occur in these patients.

This chapter briefly discusses the monitoring of signs and symptoms that may indicate overstressed systems. It then reviews ambient conditions that may place extra stress on patients but are unlikely to affect a healthy, working therapist. Finally, the chapter turns to heat-related problems, their causes, related signs and symptoms, and appropriate interventions.

MONITORING SIGNS AND SYMPTOMS

Observing the condition of the patient's skin, as well as being aware of the status of all vital signs, is essential when applying thermal modalities. In simple cases, when the patient has no systemic involvement, visual observation is sufficient.

The skin reveals changes in blood flow, body temperature, the patient's general health, and the autonomic nervous system's reactions to pain or to emotions such as fear. The general condition and color of the skin must always be observed, and any abnormalities noted in the patient's chart.

Depending on the dosage (intensity, duration, and area of the body to which the modality is applied), changes in vital signs may occur. Therapists should know what changes in vital signs to expect and recognize those that are within the normal range for the amount of stress produced by the specific intervention. For example, with a 20-min, very warm Hubbard tank treatment, a rise in core temperature of 2°F is expected, as are temporary fluctuations in blood pressure and pulse rate (see **Chapter 11**).

Therapists may be treating people who already have elevated body temperature (hyperpyrexia), rapid or slow heart rate (tachycardia or bradycardia), high or low blood pressure (hypertension or hypotension),

or a combination of symptoms. In many physical therapy departments (eg, acute-care hospitals, nursing homes), a high percentage of patients may have some form of heart disease. When intervening for patients with these problems, the therapist should do the following:

- Consult with a physician if cardiac or other problems are such that they might be exacerbated by a thermal treatment.
- Proceed cautiously with or discontinue the treatment if the patient complains or shows signs of general discomfort, displays a notable increase in respiration, or has a marked increase or decrease in pulse rate.
- Always take the pulse rate before a vigorous or prolonged heat treatment, and do so often during the treatment.

Because debilitated patients can experience cardiac stress from thermal treatments, safety guidelines adapted from those prescribed for exercise and for cardiac rehabilitation are presented here.[1-5]

During any normal 20 to 30 min heat treatment, the therapist should discontinue the treatment and make a note in the patient's chart if any of the following signs are observed:

- If the pulse rate of a young adult approaches double the resting rate. For deconditioned people, use the age-rate formula: ie, subtract the patient's age from 220; the pulse rate should not exceed 50% of that number.

$$\text{Pulse rate limit} = (220 - \text{age}) \times 0.5$$

- If the strength of the patient's pulse diminishes.
- If the patient's blood pressure changes from pretreatment resting levels, according to the following guidelines:
  1. if a nonwell adult's systolic pressure declines more than 15–20 mm Hg or increases more than 30 mm Hg; the decrease in systolic pressure is a major sign of danger;
  2. if the diastolic pressure increases more than 20 mm Hg or goes above 110 mm Hg or if it decreases more than 20 mm Hg;[6]
  3. if extreme increases in systolic and diastolic pressures are accompanied by headache or blurred vision; or

4. if the systolic pressure and the pulse rate decrease progressively, **stop treatment immediately and summon a physician.**

Vigorous generalized heat treatments should not be given if the patient's systolic pressure is less than 90 mm Hg. Cardiologists commonly advise patients with ischemic heart disease to avoid extremes in ambient temperature, either hot or cold.

Effects of Ambient Conditions

When considering the physiologic changes that occur with application of heat or cold, the therapist should pay attention to the ambient conditions in which the thermal treatments are given. Although wind velocity and atmospheric pressure are important ambient factors, this chapter's discussion is limited to ambient temperature and humidity.

In general, healthy people who are accustomed to living in any given climate function well and maintain a constant internal temperature despite day-to-day changes in the weather. Whenever such changes cause the body temperature to deviate even slightly, most people maintain thermal homeostasis by adjusting their behavior—by changing their activity level and the amount of clothing worn and by appropriate alterations in physiologic effector responses such as shivering or sweating.[7] However, if a person is suddenly exposed to different climatic conditions, although the usual effector responses may operate, they may be inadequate for safe and comfortable thermoregulation.

We have all experienced or observed the behavioral and physiological reactions occurring after a flight to a climate that differs from the climate to which we are accustomed. For example, if a New Yorker flies to Florida on a February day that is 25°F in New York and 88°F and humid in Florida, he feels hot and sweaty even though he puts on summer clothes and moves slowly when outdoors. Meanwhile, Floridians are comfortably engaging in their normal activities.

A few days later, a Texan leaves home where the temperature is 88°F and arrives in New York City, where the temperature is 50°F, an unusually mild February day. Despite putting on two pairs of warm-up pants and a sweater under her coat, she is extremely uncomfortable, shivering, complaining about the cold, and preferring to stay indoors. Meanwhile, New Yorkers are strolling with open coats and enjoying the unseasonably warm day.

In both cases, the travelers' behavioral responses are appropriate. Because their physiologic systems are not "set" to maintain homeostasis in the new environment, the adaptations in their clothing, shelter requirements, and activities protect them from excessive shivering or sweating until their systems are "reset." Each day they become more comfortable as physiologic changes occur during the process of acclimatization.

Acclimatization can be defined as the means by which humans, when placed in a different climatic environment, gradually make physiologic adjustments that enable them to function comfortably and maintain homeostasis.[8] The terms *artificial acclimatization* and *acclimation* are often used to describe adjustments that occur under laboratory conditions where an artificial change in climate has been created.[9,10] However, all three terms are used interchangeably.

During the process of acclimatization, the activities of the thermoregulatory systems of the body adjust to cope with the new environment. These adjustments occur only if exposure to the changed climatic conditions is sufficient to place a stress on these systems. Such stress is referred to as *heat stress* or **cold stress.**[8]

Unfortunately, heat and cold stress can overload the thermoregulatory systems of many patients seen in physical therapy unless the patients are carefully monitored. Patients who are susceptible to systemic breakdowns include those who have recently arrived from other climates, those who are debilitated and attempt therapeutic exercise at the onset of unexpected seasonal changes such as a sudden heat wave, and those who receive prolonged or intense heat treatments to large areas of the body. It has been reported that people with borderline heart conditions may experience severe heart failure in hot weather because the increase in blood flow to the skin necessary for cooling puts an extra load on the heart. When the weather cools again, the cardiac condition reverts to its borderline status.[11] Children also are at high risk for heat-related illnesses. Physiologically, their thermoregulatory systems are less well controlled than adult systems, and their capacity to sweat and convect heat from core to body surface is not as great. Morphologically, the ratio of their surface area per volume is greater than that of adults; thus, heat is transferred more easily from the environment to their bodies.[12]

In many treatment situations, especially home care, minimally equipped nursing homes, and heated pool areas, therapists are concerned about reactions caused by an increase rather than a decrease in ambient temperature. Therefore, this discussion of heat acclimatization is limited to the major points that may help clinicians gauge the intensity of interventions given when patients are suddenly exposed to hot ambient conditions.

In the past, tolerance for certain climates was attributed to physiologic and anatomic factors inherent to the peoples who had survived in those climates and was thought to be related to skin pigmentation and thus to race. Although racial factors have not been ruled out, the results of several studies indicate that peoples other than natives can achieve much the same tolerance because humans have the ability to make appropriate adjustments when placed in a different climate.[13–15]

Studies in which young healthy men, who were adjusted to working in temperate climates, were required to do moderate exercise under hot climatic conditions illustrate the acclimatization process.[16,17] On Day 1, their heart rates increased markedly while stroke volume decreased; thus, their cardiac output remained about the same as it was in temperate conditions. Although the men sweated profusely, their rectal temperatures rose, on the average, 2°F higher than when they performed the same work in temperate conditions. Over a period of days, adjustments occurred. The men's sweat volume increased, whereas the concentration of sodium in the sweat decreased. Their heat rate and rectal temperatures declined to levels similar to those under temperate conditions.

In general, studies have shown that adequate adjustment occurs in 4–7 days and that acclimatization is nearly complete in 12–14 days.[18,19] These physiologic adaptations can occur with as little as 1 hour per day of heat stress, but a greater adaptation occurs if an individual is stressed for approximately 2 hours. A single 100-min period of work in heat is shown to be more effective than two 50-min periods.[16] For children, the rate of acclimatization is slower than that for adults.[12]

Although passive acclimatization has some benefits,[13] investigators generally agree that a person who is sedentary during the acclimatization period is adjusted only to sedentary conditions in the hot climate.[20] In the hot climate, the individual must do sufficient work to cause heat-work stress during the acclimatization period. Thus, if a soccer team from Chicago plans to play safely and efficiently in tropical West Africa, the players should not only live in that West African climate for at least 5 days but also prac-

tice to the point of stress each day. Adjustments to heat are relative to the amount of stress experienced. Because each person will display individual reactions throughout the adjustment period, heart rate, temperature, and sweat volume must be carefully monitored.[21]

How long acclimatization will be maintained once a person is removed from the heat stress situation has not been determined. Some investigators believe that the physiologic adjustments will be maintained for 2 weeks or more,[22] whereas others believe that some decline occurs even over a weekend without heat-work stress.[23]

When an individual experiences a sudden increase in ambient temperature, the behavioral adjustments, apparently made to alleviate discomfort, are in fact extremely important for maintaining homeostasis. Because the cardiovascular and sudomotor systems are not yet "set," the individual may sweat a great deal, but the sudomotor system is not prepared to provide enough sweat to maintain thermal homeostasis for the hotter conditions. If this loss of fluid continues with the usual salt concentration, dehydration and a severe electrolyte imbalance could result. Much of the fluid required for sweat is furnished by blood plasma. Thus, when the cardiovascular system acts to cool (by dilation of peripheral vessels and increased heart rate, which send more blood to the periphery), it not only brings internal heat to the surface for radiation but also provides fluid for sweat. If cardiac output remains constant but the peripheral blood flow increases, blood must be shunted from visceral systems such as the renal system. If this situation continues, vital organs will be deprived of their blood supply. The increased heart rate that occurs can fatigue heart muscles that have not been trained for such activity.

Fortunately, within a few days, the following adjustment mechanisms occur:

- Total plasma volume increases.
- There is an increase in blood flow to the skin, which allows more heat dissipation, and to muscles, which increases their ability to do work.
- The adrenal system adjusts to allow more sweating, which enables more cooling by evaporation.
- With these increases in cooling mechanisms, vital signs stabilize.
- The salt concentration in sweat decreases; thus, the electrolyte balance is maintained.

CONSIDERATIONS FOR THERAPISTS

The information in this section of the chapter has direct application to clinical situations.

1. Patients who are suddenly exposed to a hotter or more humid environment should do some exercise daily, with careful monitoring of vital signs and other symptoms of distress. The patient cannot be expected to rest for 5 days and then be adjusted for normal activities.

2. The therapist must consider the status of each patient because of individual differences in physiologic responses.

3. The therapist should consider a modality other than heat rather than superimpose hot weather, a heat modality, and therapeutic exercise on a patient.

4. The therapist must be aware that patients with cardiac problems are unable to tolerate new cardiovascular demands and that patients with Addison's disease or other adrenal problems are unable to tolerate excessive sweating.

5. The therapist must be aware that children, debilitated people, and older adults, if unable to tolerate the overload of heat, may have a breakdown in one or more of the many systems involved in thermoregulation and can experience a "heat accident," as described later in this chapter.

REACTIONS CAUSED BY EXCESSIVE EXPOSURE TO HEAT OR COLD

Excessive ambient heat does not "burn up" a body. Rather it causes system burnout as a result of overload—in other words, the heat loss mechanisms cannot work hard enough to balance the heat gain. With excessive cold, the body's attempt to increase heat production through shivering and exercise may lead to exhaustion.

Cardiovascular Reactions

If the heart rate, stroke volume, or both are unable to increase sufficiently to maintain cardiac output, the blood pressure will drop, which in turn may increase the amount of blood pooling in the veins. People who stand in one position in hot weather frequently become faint because blood has pooled in their legs,

thus depriving the brain of its supply.[5,20] Increased venous pooling also decreases cardiac filling. When less blood reaches the heart, the ultimate result is less blood for cardiac emptying, which causes a further drop in blood pressure.[24] The heart responds by increasing the pulse rate, which results in a greater decrease in stroke volume. In turn, the heart rate increases even more in a an attempt to rectify the decrease in blood pressure. This vicious cycle continues until the attempts of the heart are beyond its capability. If the heart rate increases beyond 140–200 beats per min, depending on the individual, the time for cardiac filling is insufficient even in healthy individuals.[25] The result may be cardiac arrest.

Sudomotor Reactions

Because evaporation of sweat is the primary means by which the body loses heat in hot weather, the importance of an intact sudomotor system in maintaining thermal homeostasis cannot be overemphasized. If people are acclimatized to the heat conditions to which they are exposed, the adrenal and endocrine systems can usually regulate the fluid-electrolyte balance provided that the body maintains ample fluids and electrolytes to meet the demand. The output of sweat must be balanced by the intake of fluid and food. However, when a nonacclimatized person is exposed to high temperatures for prolonged periods, the demands on the systems that regulate fluids and pH balance may be too great. Excessive sweating without changes in the concentrations of salt and other electrolytes can lead to serious heat-related problems ranging from heat cramps to heat stroke. These problems are discussed later in this chapter.

Metabolic Reactions

Because the metabolic rate is temperature related, excessive heating may increase the rate to the point that the other systems cannot clear metabolic wastes adequately. Consequently, the normal pH balance is disturbed. If an excessive amount of acid escapes with sweat and the blood alkaline level increases, the systems usually react by periodical reversing of the pH in the sweat and blood fluids. However, with extreme demands, the systems may become deregulated.

The metabolic response to a decrease in the temperature of local tissues differs from the response to general body cooling. When the temperature of local tissues drops, the metabolic rate of those tissues decreases. However, if the central thermoregulating areas receive information that the internal temperature of the body is decreasing, the metabolic rate will increase. Although this increased rate is in part chemically induced, it is primarily the result of shivering and other movements made to keep warm. But both the movements and the shivering, if prolonged, may lead to physical exhaustion. **Figure 17–1** illustrates which thermoregulatory system is primarily responsible for maintaining thermal homeostasis when a person is exposed to different ambient temperatures. Physical therapists can use this information to make decisions about treating people with borderline systemic problems. The temperatures given are approximate, and the reactions are relative to the severity and duration of the exposure.

An ambient temperature ranging from approximately 71.6°F to 86°F (22° to 30°C) is considered to be the **zone of thermal neutrality.** This is the range in which vasomotor regulation provides sufficient heat loss to balance the metabolic heat gain. The range for a nude resting man is 82.4° to 86°F (28° to 30°C); if the man is wearing light clothes, doing mild exercise, or both, the range may be lowered to between 71.6°F and 75.2°F (22° and 24°C).[10] When the temperature exceeds this range, the vasomotor activity will increase, but the system will be incapable of maintaining a constant core temperature because the effectiveness of radiation diminishes as the temperature gradient between the environment and skin decreases. Thus, the sudomotor system must act to maintain homeostasis. Even when resting, a man's sensible sweating begins when the ambient temperature rises to about 85°F (29°C), and a woman's sensible sweating begins when the temperature reaches approximately 89.6°F (32°C). Sweating increases as the temperature increases. When the ambient temperature equals or is higher than the body surface temperature (approximately 96°F) (35.5°C), radiation ceases or reverses direction. The temperature range above approximately 86°F (30°C) is considered to be the **zone of sudomotor regulation.** Because the vaporization process is what cools the body, the environment must allow this sweat to evaporate. If the temperature-humidity index is high, evaporation cannot occur, and the core temperature and metabolic rate will increase. Thus, the **apparent temperature,** which is based on the relationship between temperature and humidity rather than temperature alone, provides a better description of ambient conditions. **Table 17–1** illustrates the differences. If the ambient temperature is 90°F and the humidity is only 20%, the apparent temperature is 87°F. If the humidity is 60%, however, the apparent temperature is 100°F. If the temperature is 85°F but the humidity is 90%, the apparent temperature is 102°F; but if the humidity is 40%, the apparent temperature is 86°F.

In general, disabled people can exercise safely when the ambient temperature is 80°F if the humidity is 40% (apparent temperature 79°F). However, exercise is unsafe if the humidity is 70% (apparent temperature 85°F).[26] Because of the humidity, apparent

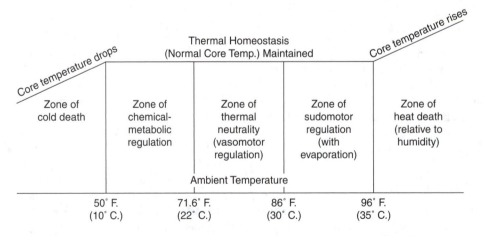

FIGURE 17–1 Systems maintaining thermal homeostasis in various ambient temperatures denoted by zones. Relative to the duration of exposure, humans cannot maintain a normal internal (core) temperature if the ambient temperature is lower than 50°F or higher than 96°F relative to the humidity.

TABLE 17–1   *Examples of Apparent Temperatures*

Ambient Temperature	Relative Humidity	Apparent Temperature
90°F	60%	100°F
90°F	20%	87°F
85°F	90%	102°F
85°F	40%	86°F
80°F	70%	85°F
80°F	40%	79°F

Adapted from a table compiled by the National Weather Service. *Utica Observer Dispatch*, August 4, 1988.

temperatures are commonly within the range where caution should be used in hydrotherapy.

With continued increase in ambient temperature, the danger of system breakdowns increases. Neither the vasomotor nor sudomotor system is capable of functioning adequately to maintain thermal equilibrium. Excessive increases in body temperature and metabolic rate can cause serious problems, or death. If the body temperature is higher than about 106°F (41.1°C) for long enough, brain damage occurs. If the body temperature is higher than about 110°F for even brief periods, the result may be death. If the increase in metabolic rate is excessive, severe disturbances in pH balance can lead to tetany or death.[9,10]

The range of ambient temperature from approximately 71.6° to 50°F (22° to 10°C) is considered to be the **zone of chemical-metabolic regulation.** The first systemic reactions that occur to preserve the constant internal temperature are cutaneous vasoconstriction and pilo erections. Although some production of chemical-metabolic heat may begin at ambient temperatures 86° to 77°F (30° to 25°C), it increases markedly at temperatures below 68°F (20°C). These chemical-metabolic reactions are the shivering and nonshivering thermogenesis mentioned in **Chapter 11.**[27]

PROBLEMS CAUSED BY OVEREXPOSURE TO HEAT

The following section outlines the adverse reactions that the clinician needs to be aware of not only when using thermal modalities but also when treating patients who are engaging in therapeutic exercise or functional activities and in those individuals with compromised thermoregulation. Exposure to exces-

sive heat can cause a variety of problems. Dermatologic problems such as prickly heat (miliaria) or temporary dehydration are minor problems, but they can lead to more serious disorders, or heat accidents: heat cramps, heat exhaustion, and heat stroke. Many patients seen in physical therapy are susceptible to these problems and require the precautionary measures discussed next. (Numerous studies are available.[28–33])

Prickly Heat

Prickly heat is a minor skin infection caused by obstructions in the ducts of the active sweat glands. It is seen in areas of the body that remain moist because of sweating and a lack of exposure to air (eg, areas constantly covered by hot compresses, clothes, or diapers. This infection is characterized by pinpoint-sized lesions and prickly itching sensations.[34] To prevent prickly heat from developing, the therapist should always allow the patient's skin to dry completely after removing a modality that produces sweating. Knochel[32] reported that any form of sweat gland malfunction or entrapment, including prickly heat, renders people with diseases such as scleroderma or cystic fibrosis more susceptible to heat stroke.

Dehydration

Dehydration is a net decrease in body fluids and electrolytes resulting in hyponatremia, which occurs when fluid intake is insufficient to compensate for fluids lost normally through sweat, respiration, urine, and feces. In general, the fluid lost per day can be replaced by consuming about 2 quarts of fluids in drink and food each day.[35] The amount of fluid intake required increases with increases in heating and the activity level. During the Gulf War of 1991, active American military personnel were instructed to drink 6 or more gallons of water per day.[36] Vomiting, diarrhea, or intestinal drainage—conditions often experienced by patients seen in physical therapy—result in loss of both fluid and electrolytes.[37] Such patients can be encouraged to sip fluids during or soon after exercise periods. If a therapist suspects that a patient's electrolyte balance is in jeopardy, however, the therapist should consult the patient's physician. Although temporary dehydration is not a serious problem, it may precipitate a more serious heat-related disorder. Ranging from least to most severe, these heat accidents include heat cramps, heat exhaustion, and heat stroke.

Although the heat accidents are discussed separately, more than one component of the thermoregulatory system often breaks down, and early symptoms of heat distress may include characteristics of each component. Thus, the symptoms of these conditions are not as clear-cut as may appear from the discussions.

Heat Cramps

Heat cramps are believed to result from either an imbalance of electrolytes (primarily reduced salt in muscles) or water depletion.[30,34] The precise cause is not completely understood. This imbalance of electrolytes can occur in hot weather and is the result of either insufficient salt intake or excessive salt output. Insufficient salt intake can occur if a person drinks an excessive amount of nonsalty fluids such as plain water, thus disturbing the fluid or salt balance, or if the person's diet provides an insufficient amount of salt. Excessive salt output can occur when a normal output of sweat contains a high salt concentration or when the salt concentration is normal but sweating is excessive.

Laborers and athletes who sweat profusely and replace the water but not the salt often experience heat cramps. The primary symptoms are severe cramps in the extremities, the abdomen, or both areas. Vital signs are usually unchanged with heat cramps. However, death can result from hyponatremia.

Treatment includes rest and immediate but gradual replacement of fluid balance by drinking fluids, which perhaps contain a small amount of salt, and by increasing the amount of salt in the diet. The type of fluid that should be ingested, especially its salt and sugar content, is subject to much debate. Some researchers have shown that increasing the amount of salt in the diet is sufficient to balance the amount lost in fluids.[38] Other studies have shown that hypertonic drinks may be more effective in maintaining normal plasma volume and electrolyte balance.[18,39] Since plasma supplies fluid for sweat, a decreased volume of plasma will reduce the rate of sweating. In general, the subjects in these studies were healthy young adults or animals, not debilitated individuals or older adults; thus, extrapolating the results to patients may be questionable. Salt tablets are not recommended, since their hypertonicity may cause fluid shift into the gastrointestinal (GI) tract.[29] According to the current definition of heat cramps, findings or symptoms other than muscular cramps automatically categorize the problem as some form of heat exhaustion.[32]

Heat Exhaustion

Heat exhaustion occurs when a person is exposed to more heat than the thermoregulatory mechanisms are capable of controlling. Although heat exhaustion rarely occurs in pure form, in order to differentiate the causes, it can be categorized as exercise-induced heat exhaustion (heat syncopy), water-depletion heat exhaustion, or salt-depletion heat exhaustion.[8]

A form of heat exhaustion called **heat syncopy** is characterized by fainting or collapse when standing or exercising in extreme heat. The peripheral dilation and tachycardia resulting from the heat, the exercise, or both can cause an increase in venous pooling, which in turn results in hypotension, a loss of blood flow to the brain, and fainting.

Water-depletion heat exhaustion may occur in people who do hard work in a temperate climate or moderate work in a hot climate, in children, and in feeble adults who are unable to ask for or obtain water—for example, in residents of marginally staffed nursing homes. Early symptoms include intense thirst, fatigue, weakness, discomfort, anxiety, or impaired judgment. The body temperature is elevated slightly.[29] If the condition is not treated, more serious symptoms or heat stroke can develop.

Salt-depletion heat exhaustion usually afflicts nonacclimatized people who have a high concentration of salt in sweat or who sweat excessively. The symptoms may differ from those resulting from water depletion. The victims do not complain of thirst; they are likely to complain of headaches or nausea and may experience giddiness, vomiting, or diarrhea. The skin will be pale and clammy. The body temperature may be normal or subnormal. The major symptoms are hypotension and tachycardia.[29]

Although heat exhaustion caused by water and that caused by salt depletion have been differentiated, the causes and symptoms frequently overlap. The symptoms of heat exhaustion may actually indicate the early stage of heat stroke.[33]

Treatment includes cooling the patient gradually, positioning the patient's head level with or lower than the trunk to encourage blood flow to the brain, and elevating the patient's legs to encourage venous return from the lower extremities. Massaging the lower extremities also reduces venous pooling. The lost fluid or salt should be replaced **gradually.**

Heat Stroke

Heat stroke, the most dangerous of all heat accidents, may result in coma or death if not treated immediately. Heat strokes occur most commonly during hot, humid weather, when sweat does not evaporate, and during exposure to excessive, uninterrupted heat (eg, during a heat wave without cooling periods at night). The body temperature increases, and the cardiovascular system responds excessively in an attempt to bring more blood to the periphery.[32]

Three factors that predispose a person to heat stroke are dehydration, lack of acclimatization to a hot, humid environment, and poor physical fitness. Healthy adults who work hard for prolonged periods in heat (eg, road workers laying tar in extremely hot, humid weather), older adults, and the debilitated are susceptible to heat stroke. In addition, people who suffer from malnutrition, diabetes mellitus, or cardiac problems are vulnerable.[31] Finally, drugs such as benztropine mesylate, atropine, and other anticholinergics; phenothiazine; and antihistamines may increase vulnerability.[32]

Heat waves in the United States, even in recent years, have caused many heat stroke–related deaths among older adults who did not have air conditioners or adequate cooling devices. Because some physical therapy departments and home care settings are not air-conditioned, therapists must be aware of their susceptible patients, those who are elderly or have cardiac problems, especially if they are doing exercise.

Although a variety of factors are involved in the etiology of heat stroke, the three prevalent ones are elevated body temperature, metabolic acidosis, and hypoxia. Victims of heat stroke usually have body temperatures higher than 107°F (41.6°C), but if temperatures as low as 104 < °F (40°C) are maintained long enough, heat stroke can result.[2,40] Heat strokes can occur even in young adults who are experiencing intense heat and in people who are experiencing great heat stress without physical exertion, for example, while in a sauna or a Turkish bath.[33]

Time is of the essence when treating heat strokes. Unless the body temperature is lowered quickly, metabolic acidosis and tissue hypoxia develop.[31] Early symptoms may be similar to those related to heat exhaustion and may or may not include headache, light-headedness, vertigo, and abdominal distress. However, the major sign is a rapid increase in body temperature, which may lead to delirium, coma, brain damage, or death. The pulse will be fast—130 to 160 beats per minute—and breathing will be rapid. The skin will be hot but not necessarily dry. The common belief that the major symptom of heat stroke is cessation of sweating is misleading because many victims maintain the sweating function.

Treatment begins by using any possible, even drastic, means of cooling the body in an attempt to lower the body temperature rapidly. Move the person out of the sun, expose the person's entire body to a cool breeze, and elevate the person's head to avoid increased blood flow to the brain. Use whatever means of cooling are available (eg, immerse the body in cool water or wrap it in cold wet towels). Some authors recommend that the rectal temperature should be reduced 0.54°F (0.3°C) every 5 min for the first 30 min.[31] Cooling the body at a rate faster or slower than this reduces the chance of survival. Cooling should continue until the person's temperature has been reduced to 102°F (38.9°C).

Table 17–2 includes the major causes, symptoms, and immediate treatments for the three major types of heat accidents. Any person who treats or cares for elderly or disabled people or treats patients with heat or exercise, especially in a hot environment, should be familiar with the information in the table.

REVIEW QUESTIONS

1. What precautionary steps should a physical therapist take when treating a patient who has a cardiac problem?

2. How does the therapist determine the pulse-rate limit of a deconditioned 35-year-old man during a 30-min heat treatment? What should the therapist do if his pulse rate exceeds that limit?

3. What changes in blood pressure should cause a physical therapist to discontinue a heat treatment?

TABLE 17–2 *Factors Associated with Heat Accidents*

Factor	Heat Cramps	Heat Exhaustion			Heat Stroke
		Exercise Induced Exhaustion Syncopy	Water Depletion Exhaustion	Salt Depletion	
Etiology	Electrolyte imbalance Negative salt balance in muscles. Caused by drinking excessive amounts of nonsalt fluids or food, excessive sweating with normal salt content, or normal sweating with high salt content.	Peripheral vascular dilatation, tachycardia, or both causing venous pooling.	Insufficient water intake for amount of exercise per temperature-humidity performed.	Insufficient salt intake to replenish (1) excessive salt in normal amount of sweat or (2) excessive sweat.	Exposure to excessive heat/humidity, usually for prolonged periods or for short periods of strenuous exercise.
Those susceptible in excessive heat	The very active and the ill or debilitated.	People doing excessive exercise or prolonged standing.	Healthy adults doing prolonged or strenuous exercise in heat without replenishing water; children; nonexercising feeble adults unable to obtain water.	Nonacclimatized people.	People in poor physical condition; those suffering from conditions such as cardiac problems, diabetes mellitus, malnutrition, and healthy people doing strenuous exercise.
Symptoms	If active, severe cramps in extremities or abdomen. If ill, minor discomfort and muscle weakness. No change in vital signs.	Fainting or collapse.	Thirst, fatigue, weakness, discomfort, anxiety, impaired judgment. Temperature may be slightly elevated.	Headache, giddiness, nausea, vomiting, pale and clammy skin. Temperature may be normal or subnormal. Hypotension, tachycardia.	In early stages, may be similar to heat exhaustion. EXTREMELY HIGH TEMPERATURE: 102–107°F or more. Rapid pulse and respiration; skin hot; cessation of sweating (usually but not always).
Treatment	Rest; immediate but gradual replacement of salt intake in fluids and in diet.	Rest. Cooling the patient. Place head level with or lower than trunk. Elevate and massage legs. Begin gradual replacement of fluids or salt in drinks and food. The heat exhaustion problems may overlap.			Keep head elevated. Begin cooling immediately by using cool towel wraps, immersing in cool water, ice massage, or whatever means available. Reduce rectal temperature approximately 0.54°F (0.3°C) every 5 min until 102°F.

What changes in blood pressure are extremely dangerous?

4. What temperature range defines the zone of thermal neutrality?

5. If a physical therapist is treating a disabled 55-year-old woman with heat modalities and the ambient temperature is 80°F (26°C) and the humidity is 40%, is it safe to proceed? Why?

6. While visiting Miami, where the temperature is 88°F, a healthy woman from Montana sprains her ankle and needs physical therapy. Is it safe to use heat modalities? Why?

7. Three months after a back injury, a football player returns to football practice on a hot and humid August day. How long should he practice on Day 1?

8. After 2 hours of practice on Day 2, the football player complains of nausea, his pulse rate is fast, and his blood pressure has dropped. How should the physical therapist begin treatment?

9. Describe the differences between water-depletion and salt-depletion heat exhaustion. Include major symptoms for each.

10. What should be the immediate treatment intervention for an individual experiencing heat stroke?

KEY TERMS

acclimatization
cold stress
zone of thermal neutrality
zone of sudomotor regulation
apparent temperature

zone of chemical-metabolic
  regulation
prickly heat
dehydration
heat cramps

heat exhaustion
heat syncopy
water-depletion heat exhaustion
salt-depletion heat exhaustion
heat stroke

REFERENCES

1. Amundsen L, ed: *Cardiac Rehabilitation.* New York: Churchill Livingstone: 1981.

2. Blair S, Gibbons L, Painter P, et al: *Guidelines for Exercise Testing and Prescription.* 3rd ed. *Amer Col of Sports Med* Philadelphia: Lea & Febiger; 1986; 8–21.

3. Ellestad M: *Stress Testing,* 3rd ed. Philadelphia: Davis; 1986; 31:116–18.

4. Irwin S: *Cardiopulmonary Physical Therapy.* St. Louis: Mosby; 1985; 51.

5. Pollock M, Wilmore J, Fox S: *Exercise in Health and Disease.* Philadelphia: Saunders; 1984; 315.

6. McArdle WD, Katch FI, Katch VL: *Exercise Physiology,* 4th ed. Baltimore: Williams & Wilkins; 1996; 276–79.

7. Hensel H: *Thermoreception and Temperature Regulation.* New York: Academic; 1981; 199.

8. Leithead C, Lind A: *Heat Stress and Heat Disorders.* Philadelphia: Davis; 1964; 16:20–21.

9. Clark R, Edholm O: *Man and His Thermal Environment.* London: Edward Arnold; 1985; 136, 155.

10. Houdas Y, Ring E: *Human Body Temperature: Its Measurement and Regulation.* New York: Plenum; 1982; 59, 97, 108–09, 112, 118, 179–81.

11. Guyton A: *Textbook of Medical Physiology.* 6th ed. Philadelphia: Saunders; 1981; 353, 623, 894.

12. American Academy of Pediatrics: Climatic heat stress and the exercising child. *Physician and Sports Med* 1983; 11(8):155–59.

13. Fox R, Budd G, Woodward P, et al: A study of temperature regulation in New Guinea people. *Phil Trans Roy Soc London* 1974; 268:375–91.

14. Hammel H: Effect of race on response to cold. *Fed Proc* 1963; 22:795–800.

15. Strydom N, Wyndham C: Natural state of heat acclimatization of different ethnic groups. *Fed Proc* 1963; 22:801–09.

16. Lind A, Bass D: Optimal exposure time for development of acclimatization to heat. *Fed Proc* 1963; 22:704.

17. Senay L, Mitchell D, Wyndham C: Acclimatization in a hot, humid environment: Body fluid adjustment. *J Appl Physiol* 1976; 40:786–96.

18. Greenleaf J, Brock P: Na⁺ and Ca⁺⁺ ingestion: Plasma volume-electrolyte distribution at rest and exercise. *J Appl Physiol* 1980; 48:838–47.

19. Pichan G, Sridharan K, Swamy Y, et al: Physiological acclimatization to heat after a cold conditioning in tropical subjects. *Aviat Space Environ Med* 1985; 56:436–40.

20. Rowell L: Human cardiovascular adjustments to exercise and thermal stress. *Physiol Rev* 1974; 54(1):75–159.

21. McArdle W, Katch F, Katch V: Exercise Physiology, 2nd ed. Philadelphia: Lea & Febiger; 1986; 448–49.

22. Nadel E, Pandolf K, Roberts M, et al: Mechanisms of thermal acclimation to exercise and heat. *J Appl Physiol* 1974; 37:515–20.

23. Wyndam C, Jacobs G: Loss of acclimatization after six days of work in cool conditions on the surface of a mine. *J Appl Physiol* 1957; 11:197–98.

24. Nielson B, Rowell L, Bonde-Petersen F: Heat stress during exercise in water and in air. In: Hales J, ed. *Thermal Physiology*. New York: Raven Press; 1984; 395–98.

25. Caldroney R: Heat induced illness. *J Kentucky Med Assoc* 1982; 80:671–74.

26. National Weather Service table. *Utica Observer Dispatch*, August 4, 1988.

27. Stanier M, Mount L, Bligh, J.: *Energy Balance and Temperature Regulation*. Cambridge, UK: Cambridge University Press; 1984.

28. Borrell R, Parker R, Henley E, et al: Comparison of in vivo temperatures produced by hydrotherapy, paraffin wax treatment, and fluidotherapy. *Phys Ther* 1980; 60(10):1273–76.

29. Gollehon D, Drez D: Heat syndromes: A review. *J Louisiana State Med Soc* 1982; 134(6):9–11.

30. Johnson L: Preventing heat stroke. *Am Fam Physician* 1982; 26(7):137–40.

31. Khogali M, Mustafa M: Physiology of heat stroke: A review. In: Hales J, ed. *Thermal Physiology*. New York: Raven Press; 1984; 503–10.

32. Knochel J. Environmental heat illness. *Arch Intern Med* 1974; 133:841–64.

33. Shibolet S, Lancaster M, Danon Y: Heat stroke: A review. *Aviat Space Environ Med* 1976; 47:280–301.

34. Wyngaarden J, Smith L Jr, eds: *Cecil's Textbook of Medicine*, 17th ed. Philadelphia: Saunders; 1985; 358, 2229, 2304–06.

35. Guyton A: *Human Physiology and Mechanisms of Disease*, 4th ed. Philadelphia: Saunders; 1987; 130, 190.

36. Environment adds to challenge facing Desert Shield physicians. Medical News and Perspectives. *JAMA* 1991; 265:435, 439–40.

37. Anthony C, Thibodeau G: *Textbook of Anatomy and Physiology*, 11th ed. St. Louis: Mosby; 1983; 567.

38. Costill D, Cote R, Miller E, et al: Water and electrolyte replacement during repeated days of work in heat. *Aviat Space Environ Med* 1975; 46:795–800.

39. Fox R, Woodward P, Exton-Smith A, et al: Body temperatures in the elderly: A national study of physiological, social, and environmental conditions. *Br Med J* 1973; 1:200–06.

40. Assia E, Yoram E, Shapiro Y: Fatal heat stroke after short march at night: A case report. *Aviat Space Environ Med* 1985; 56: 441–42.

PART III

Electrotherapy

The use of electrotherapy can be traced back to ancient times. Its application has passed through periods of popularity and controversy. The following highlight a few of the important historical milestones. A detailed account of this interesting history can be found in *Therapeutic Electricity and Ultraviolet Radiation* (GK Stillwell, ed. Baltimore: Williams & Wilkins; 1983).

In 48 A.D. Scribonius Largus, a Roman physician, used shock from torpedo fish to treat chronic headache and gout. In 1791 Luigi Galvani stimulated frog nerves and muscles with electrical charges from lightning and reported that the animals spontaneously developed electricity. In 1796 Alessandro Volta proved that the electrical charges in Galvani's experiment were the result of current between two dissimilar metals in contact with each other and were not spontaneously produced by the animals.

Throughout the 19th century, a variety of medical conditions were routinely treated with electrical stimulation: for example, hemiplegia, epilepsy, kidney stones, sciatica, gout, rheumatism, and angina pectoris. In 1849 Guillaume B. Duchenne used "induced current" to treat atrophy and paralysis. He reported that he could apply this current to a patient in a less painful manner by using moistened surface electrodes and concluded that induced current was better than galvanic current. In 1870 L. Erb recommended the use of both induced and galvanic currents to stimulate nerve and muscles in the belief that these currents stimulated nutrition to atrophied muscles. During the polio epidemic of 1920, electrical stimulation was routinely used to treat paralysis. Some of the basic techniques used today were developed during that time. In subsequent years, electrotherapy went through periods of rising and declining interest.

At present, there is a renewed interest in the use of therapeutic electricity to stimulate nerve and muscle tissues. In addition, its application has been extended to interventions for pain, the healing of wounds and fractured bones, and the introduction of ions to tissue. Electrical stimulation is also used as an evaluative tool.

Numerous electrotherapeutic devices are available today that offer a wide range of choice with respect to current type, frequency, mode, and ease of application. The selection of an electrotherapeutic device with the appropriate type of current, voltage, frequency, and intensity for effective use is a difficult task. To simplify the task and to use this physical agent appropriately, physical therapists must have a good understanding of basic electricity and its effect on the body and be thoroughly familiar with the devices. Furthermore, therapists should remember that the intervention goal is the most important guide to the choice electrical device and its appropriate setup.

The electrotherapy and electrophysiologic testing section of this text consist of six chapters. **Chapter 18** covers basic electricity and some of the background information necessary to understand the topic. **Chapters 19 and 20** discuss the effects of electrical stimulation on the body and the clinical application of this physical agent. **Chapter 21** presents the use of transcutaneous electrical nerve stimulation (TENS) and point locator-stimulation for pain modulation. **Chapter 22** describes the use of iontophoresis for therapeutic interventions and **Chapter 23** addresses the topics of electrophysiologic tests, nerve conduction velocity, and electromyography.

18

Therapeutic Electricity

TSEGA ANDEMICAEL MEHRETEAB, PT, MS
THOMAS HOLLAND, PT, PhD

Chapter Outline

Electrical stimulation is used to assess and treat nerve and muscle tissues and to manage various neuromuscular conditions. For example, it is used to evaluate the integrity of neuromuscular tissues with tests such as nerve conduction velocity, electromyography, and the strength-duration test. Electrical stimulation is commonly used in physical therapy to treat neuromuscular conditions, enhance local circulation and tissue healing, decrease pain, and increase range of motion (ROM). This chapter looks at the basic physical concepts of electric current, voltage, resistance, and waveforms. It applies these concepts to the various types of electrical stimulators and presents the body's response to electrical stimulation. Later chapters detail the uses of electrical stimulation in normal and pathologic conditions.

ATOMIC STRUCTURE

The atom is primarily composed of electrons, protons, and neutrons. The **electron** has a negative charge (−), the **proton** has a positive charge (+), and the **neutron** has no charge. The amount of positive charge carried by the proton is equal to the amount of negative charge carried by the electron. A neutral atom has an equal number of electrons and protons. If an atom gains or loses an electron, it is no longer neutral and is referred to as an **ion.** When an atom gains an electron, the number of its electrons becomes greater than the number of its protons, and the atom becomes a negatively charged ion. Conversely, if an atom loses an electron, the number of its electrons will be less than the number of its protons, and it becomes a positively charged ion. Superscripts (−) and (+) are used to designate the charge of the ion. When more than one electron is transferred to or from an atom, a number next to the + or − signs is used to indicate the number of electrons transferred. For example, Cu^{2+} indicates the loss of two electrons from copper. SO_4^{-2} indicates the gain of two electrons by sulfate. The amount of charge carried by any substance is proportional to the number of charged individual atoms or molecules. For example, Cu^{+2} or SO_4^{-2} has twice as much charge as Cu^+ or NO_3^-, respectively. Similarly, a substance containing eight ions of Cu^+ has twice the amount of charge as the same amount of substance containing only four ions of Cu^+. The unit used for charge is the coulomb. The **coulomb (C)** is equivalent to the combined charge of 6.29×10^{18} electrons.

ELECTRICITY

The movement or flow of charged particles such as electrons or ions from one place to another constitutes an **electrical current.** In metals, electricity is conducted by the flow of electrons; in solutions, electricity is conducted by the flow of ions. The amount of electrical current depends on the number of electrons or ions passing a given point per unit of time. The unit of current is an **ampere** (A). One ampere represents particles with a total charge of 1 C flowing every second through a given point. Thus, 1 A = 1 C per second (C/sec). Smaller units are the milliampere (mA) = 10^{-3} A and the microampere (A) = 10^{-6} A.[1] The following discussion of the electrolytic cell demonstrates the role of ions and electrons in the generation of electricity.

Electrolytic Cells

Figure 18–1 represents an example of an electrolytic cell, a simple circuit containing a solution of copper chloride ($CuCl_2$) and water (H_2O), two metallic rods known as **electrodes,** and a battery. Each electrode is

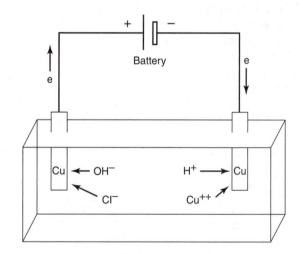

FIGURE 18–1   An electrolytic cell containing a solution of copper chloride ($CuCl_2$) in water (H_2O), two electrodes, and a battery. The two copper electrodes are connected to the battery with wire. As the battery is turned on, the negatively charged ions, OH^- and Cl^-, are attracted toward the anode (+ charged electrode) and the positively charged ions (anions), H^+ and Cu^{2+}, are attracted toward the cathode (− charged electrode). The electrolytes in this solution are $OH-$, $Cl-$, H^+, and Cu^{2+}. The battery is represented by ⊣⊢.

connected with a wire to the battery on one end and is immersed in the electrolytic solution on the other end. The positively and negatively charged ions in solution that conduct current are called **electrolytes.** In this circuit, the electrolytes are copper (Cu^{2+}), chloride ($Cl-$), hydronium (H^+), and hydroxide ($OH-$) ions.

The electrode attached to the positive side of the cell is called the **anode,** and the electrode attached to the negative side of the cell is called the **cathode.** Thus, the cathode ($-$) is electron rich, and the anode ($+$) is electron deficient. The positive ($+$) and the negative ($-$) signs are used to designate the anode and the cathode, respectively. In this circuit, the ions (Cu^+, H^+, $Cl-$, and $OH-$) are responsible for carrying the electrical charges through the solution. However, the electrical current flowing through the electrodes and through any wires in the circuit is the result of the flow of electrons.

At the metal-solution interface (see **Fig. 18–1**), electrons are exchanged between the electrodes and the ions in the solution. The negatively charged ions are attracted and flow toward the anode. These ions are called **anions.** At the anode, the anions give up their excess electrons to the electron-deficient electrode. At the same time, electrons are leaving the negative side of the battery and flowing toward the cathode. In solution, the positively charged ions, called **cations,** are attracted to and flow toward the cathode, where they pick up excess electrons.

Electricity passes through the solution circuit as long as the excess of electrons in the cathode and deficiency of electrons in the anode are maintained. That is, a **difference in potential** exists between the two ends of the circuit. In an electrolytic solution, the ions migrate in opposite directions: cations ($+$) toward the cathode, and anions ($-$) toward the anode. A two-way migration of ions in solution is known as **convection current.**[2] Because body fluids contain electrolytes, the electrical current through tissue fluids involves convection.

Figure 18–2 represents a typical electrical circuit; it is a diagrammatic representation of the basic components for electrical current. The circuit must be completed, that is, a continuous loop is required for charges to flow. In such a circuit, the electrical current continues until the battery is no longer charged or the electrolytes in the solution are depleted. In other words, all the cations are reduced or pick up electrons ($Cu^{++} + 2e \rightarrow Cu$), or all the anions are oxidized or lose their excess electrons ($2Cl \rightarrow Cl_2 + 2e$). Note that

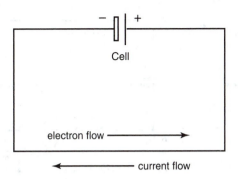

FIGURE 18–2 **(A)** A schematic representation of a complete electrical circuit. The arrows depict the direction of electron and current flow. Electrons flow from the cathode ($-$) toward the anode ($+$), but, by arbitrary convention, the direction of current is designated to be from the positive electrode (anode) toward the negative electrode (cathode). Current continues to flow until the battery is turned off or the electrolytes are depleted. The battery is represented by ⊣⊢.

electrons flow from the negative electrode (cathode) to the positive electrode (anode). However, historically, the direction of current has been designated as from the positive to the negative electrode.

Body fluids such as blood, sweat, interstitial fluid, and urine all contain electrolytes including potassium (K^+), sodium (Na^+), calcium (Ca^{2+}), chloride (Cl^-), and sulfate (SO_4^{-2}). As electrical current passes through such electrolytic solutions, a number of chemical reactions occur. The magnitude of these electrochemical reactions depends on how long the current is applied and on what the current density is. **Current density** is the amount of current per unit of electrode area and is proportional to the **current amplitude** (intensity). Current amplitude, electrode size, and current duration are important factors in the safe application of electrical stimulation.

Therapeutic Current Classification

Therapeutic electrical currents can be classified into one of three categories: direct current (DC), alternating current (AC), and pulsatile current (PC). Direct current flows continuously in one direction (**Fig. 18–3**) and has a pulse duration that is > 1 second. Alternating current flows continuously in two directions (**Fig. 18–4**) and has a pulse duration measured in milliseconds. Pulsatile currents can flow in one (monophasic) or two (biphasic) directions, but they do not flow continuously because they have regular

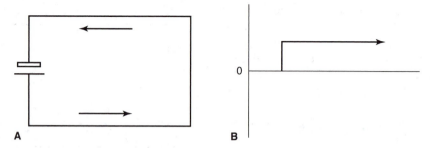

FIGURE 18–3 (A) schematic representation of a direct current circuit, where the current flows in only one direction and the two ends of the circuit maintain their positive or negative charges. (B) The line with an arrow represents a continuous flow of direct current beginning at the isoelectric line. Current flows continuously until the circuit is disconnected or the battery is turned off. The battery is represented by ⊣⊢ .

intervals of no electrical activity between individual pulses. The pulse duration for PC is measured in microseconds, and the space between pulses is termed an interpulse interval. Most therapeutic stimulators employ PC because it produces improved neuroexcitation with less discomfort for patients. The extremely narrow pulse duration of PC allows better discrimination among the sensory, motor, and pain fibers.

In DC circuits, the electrodes maintain their positive or negative polarity; therefore, when these electrodes are used to stimulate tissues, positive and negative fields will be established and maintained under the electrodes. Unlike AC, where the electrode polarity changes, DC will always maintain one electrode as positive (anode) and the other electrode as negative (cathode). Direct current has the greatest potential to cause tissue damage if used incorrectly because of its electrochemical reactions (**Table 18–1**). Direct current's long pulse duration and strong polarity can cause skin irritation and possible burns. The maintained polarity attracts the body's ions to the electrodes. The anode will attract negative ions (anions) such as chloride. Chloride ions will in turn bind to hydrogen ions from water, resulting in the accumulation of hydrochloric acid (HCl) under the anode. Hydrochloric acid accumulation creates an acidic chemical reaction on the skin under the anode. The cathode will attract positive ions (cations) such as

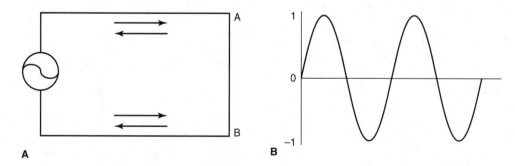

FIGURE 18–4 (A) A schematic representation of an alternating current circuit, where the current changes direction. This occurs as the polarity (field charge) of the two ends of the circuit, A and B, changes from positive to negative. (B) Each cycle of the current is graphically represented by a sine waveform. One complete cycle contains both positive and negative phases. The source of the alternating current is represented by ⊘ .

TABLE 18–1   *Polar Reactions under Each Electrode*

Anode (+)	Cathode (−)
Attraction of anion (−ions)	Attraction of cations (+ions)
Acidic reactions	Alkaline reactions
Example: formation of HCl	Example: formation of NaOH
Solidification of protein	Liquification of protein
Hardening of tissue	Softening of tissue
Hyperpolarization	Hypopolarization
Increased nerve excitability	Increased nerve excitability

(Davis, RB (ed). *Pediatric Neurology for the Clinician.* Norwalk, Conn.: Appleton & Lange; 1992, with permission.)

sodium. Sodium ions will bind to hydroxyl ions from water, resulting in the accumulation of sodium hydroxide (NaOH) under the cathode. An alkaline reaction occurs under the cathode because of the accumulation of NaOH. The clinician will usually notice redness under the electrodes after using DC. This redness can be attributed to the chemical reactions that arise from the maintained electrode polarities. Monophasic pulsed current (PC) creates weak chemical reactions because they flow in one direction as does DC. The PC chemical reactions are much weaker than those of DC because of their short pulse durations (microseconds) and interpulse intervals. In stimulation protocols that require strong polarity, such as iontophoresis, a continuous unidirectional current (DC) is required (see **Chapter 22**).

Alternating currents (AC) are made up of cycles commonly represented by sine waves that move continuously in one direction and then change to the opposite direction in a time period that is less than 1 second. These currents do not create the same strong chemical effects on the skin as DC creates because the flow of charged particles constantly changes. Modulated AC is used in medium-frequency currents (interferential and Russian) for such clinical applications as pain modulation and muscle strengthening.

Pulsatile currents that flow in two directions can be classified as either biphasic symmetrical or biphasic asymmetrical. The positive polarity phase is equal to the negative polarity phase in biphasic symmetrical, whereas they are unequal in biphasic asymmetrical. In a way similar to monophasic pulsatiles, some weak chemical reactions occur with asymmetrical biphasic because of the ion attraction under the electrodes.

CHARACTERISTICS OF AN ELECTRICAL CIRCUIT

An electrical circuit is a pathway through which electrons or other charged particles move. **Figure 18–1** represents a circuit made up of electrodes, electrolytic solution, and battery. For a current to exist, all components of the circuit (eg, battery, electrodes, switches) must be in physical contact so that electrons or other charged particles can move from one area to another. The flow of electrons or charged ions is called **current.**

Electromotive Force

To have a continuous flow of charges, or current, in a circuit, a driving force is required. This driving force arises from a difference in potential between two ends or points of the circuit and is often called an **electromotive force (EMF).** However, this term is misleading because EMF is a measure of the maximum work per unit charge rather than a measure of force. A difference in potential is established when the amount of charges at one end of the circuit is greater than that at the other end or between any two points of the circuit. This difference in potential can be established by a motor or a battery. For example, the cathode end of a battery supplies excess electrons, whereas the anode end is deficient of electrons; therefore, if the two ends of the battery are connected, electrons will flow from the cathode to the anode, and an electrical current will be established in the circuit. The electrons or other charged particles will continue to flow as long as the difference in potential is maintained and the circuit is completed. The difference in potential is expressed in **volts (V);** smaller units are expressed in millivolts (mV, 10^{-3} V) and microvolts (V, 10^{-6} V).

Resistance

When electrons or ions flow through the circuit, they encounter **resistance (R)** by the medium through which they are made to flow. The unit used for resistance is the **ohm (Ω);** larger units are the kilo-ohm ($10^3\Omega$) and mega ohm ($10^6\Omega$). Materials that offer less resistance and readily allow electric current to pass through them are called **conductors.** For example, copper, silver, and tap water are good conductors. Materials that offer high resistance and impede the passage of current are called **insulators.** For example, glass, rubber, paraffin, and distilled water are good insulators. Materials that are neither good conductors nor insulators are called **semiconductors.** For example, silicon and germanium, which are used in solid-state circuits, are good semiconductors.

The resistance encountered in a circuit depends on the type, size, shape, and composition of the conductor material. In addition, other factors such as temperature may influence the resistance of a circuit. For example, increasing the temperature of a metal may decrease its conductivity, whereas increasing the temperature of a tissue may improve its electrical conduction because of an increase in body fluids (eg, blood or sweat) in the area. A moist piece of gauze or paper is used as a conductive medium between the skin and the electrode in transcutaneous electrical stimulation (TENS).

The type of conductor material determines the level of resistance to the current. For example, metals have less resistance than do nonmetals. Silver and copper have the least resistance among the metals; thus, they are good conductors. Copper wires are commonly used for house current. Nonmetals such as rubber, formica, and various other plastics have high resistance and are used to insulate electrical circuits. Even among good conductors and good insulators, differences in the degree of resistance are encountered. In liquids, the degree of resistance in the system is determined by the composition of the solution, ie, the materials that make up the medium through which current is passing. Solutions such as salt water, which has many electrolytes, offer less resistance than solutions such as tap water, which has few or no electrolytes. Body fluids such as blood, sweat, and interstitial fluid contain many electrolytes and therefore are good conductors.

The length (L), the cross-sectional area (A), and the **resistivity** (ρ) of the conductor also determine the resistance (R) of a circuit. These can be expressed by the following equation:

$$R = \frac{\rho \times L}{A}$$

For example, a thin copper wire offers higher resistance than a thick copper wire, and a long copper wire offers greater resistance than a short copper wire. As electrical current encounters resistance, heat is generated. According to Joules' law, the heat produced is proportional to the resistance, the intensity, and the duration of the current. The electrical-to-thermal energy conversion can be expressed by the following equation:

$$H = 0.24 \times I^2 \times R \times t$$

where 0.24 is a constant, H is heat in joules (gram-calories), I is current intensity in amperes, R is resistance in ohms, and t is time in seconds. To avoid hazardous consequences, the appropriate type and size of wiring should be used in electrical devices. Otherwise, heat buildup may lead to breakage of machinery and even electrical fire.

Electrical circuits are represented in **Figure 18–5.** These resistors are physical elements that are placed in the circuit or may represent hindrance offered by various components of the circuit. The two resistors are represented by R_1 and R_2, and the driving force, or

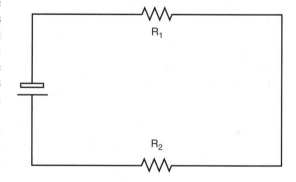

FIGURE 18–5   Electrical circuit with resistance. This schematic diagram illustrates an electrical circuit with two resistors, R_1 and R_2. The ⌁ represents the resistors and ⊣⊢ represents the battery, the electromotive force, or the voltage.

voltage, is represented by the symbol for battery. The amount of electrical current or intensity I through the circuit depends on the voltage or potential difference, usually symbolized by E or V and the resistance R. The greater the voltage (difference in potential), the higher the intensity. On the other hand, for a given voltage, the greater the resistance, the lower the rate of electrical flow. This relationship is shown by the following equation called **Ohm's law:**

$$I = E/R \text{ or } E = IR$$

where I is the current intensity in amperes, E is the potential difference in volts, and R is the resistance in ohms.[3]

If any two of the preceding electrical quantities are known, the third can be calculated. For example, in a circuit with a 10 Ω resistor and a 45 V potential difference, what is the amount of electric current flowing through the circuit? The answer is

$$I = E/R, I = 45/10 = 4.5 \, A$$

Arrangement

The components of an electrical circuit can be arranged in series or parallel to each other. Most electrical circuits consist of a combination of series and parallel components.

Series Circuits.   When several resistors, such as R_1, R_2, and R_3 in **Figure 18–6** are arranged so that the same current flows through each of them, they are said to be in series with each other. When electrical stimulation is administered *transcutaneously* (through the skin), the skin and fat layers can be considered to be in series. The total resistance (R_T) is the arithmetic sum of the resistors in series: that is,

$$R_T = (R_1 + R_2 + R_3 \ldots \ldots R_n.)$$

The same amount of current (I_T) flows through each resistor; thus,

$$I_T = I_1 = I_2 = I_3$$

From Ohm's law,

$$I_T = E/R_T$$

Note that voltage E must be sufficient to overcome the total resistance R for current I to exist. For example, in the preceding series circuit, if $R_1 = 100$ Ω, $R_2 = 200$ Ω, and $R_3 = 300$ Ω, and the voltage = 60, what is the intensity through this circuit?

$$R_T = 100 \, Ω + 200 \, Ω + 300 \, Ω = 600 \, Ω$$

$$I_T = E/R_T = 60V \, / \, 600 \, Ω = 0.1 \, A$$

Parallel Circuits.   In **Figure 18–7**, resistors R_4, R_5, and R_6 are arranged so that the current has multiple alternative pathways. This circuit is said to be arranged in parallel. In a parallel circuit, the reciprocal of the total resistance R_T is equal to the sum of the reciprocals of each resistor in parallel $1/R_T$: that is,

$$1/R_T = (1/R_4 + 1/R_5 + 1/R_6 + \ldots \ldots 1/R_n)$$

For example, in the preceding parallel circuit, if $R_4 = 100$ Ω, $R_5 = 200$ Ω, and $R_6 = 200$, then the total resistance (R_T) can be calculated as follows:

$$1/R_T = 1/R_4 + 1/R_5 + 1/R_6 = 1/100 \, Ω + 1/200 \, Ω + 1/200 = 1/50 \, Ω$$

$$R_T = 50 \, Ω$$

With a voltage of 250 V across the resistors, the total current I_T across all the resistors can be calculated as follows:

$$I_T = E/R_T = 250V \, / \, 50 \, Ω = 5 \, A$$

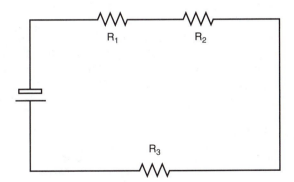

FIGURE 18–6   Resistors in series. This schematic diagram illustrates a circuit with three resistors, R_1, R_2, and R_3, in series. The –∿∿– represents a resistor, and –⊣⊢ represents the battery, the electromotive force, or the voltage.

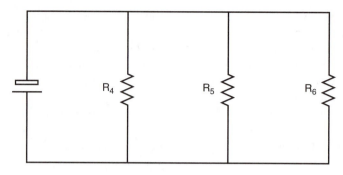

FIGURE 18–7   Resistors in parallel. This schematic diagram illustrates a circuit with three resistors, R_4, R_5, and R_6, in parallel. The ⌇W⌇ represents the resistors, and ⊣⊢ represents the battery, the electromotive force, or the voltage.

In a parallel circuit, the voltage across each resistor is the same. Because current takes the path of least resistance, the current I through each resistor in parallel is inversely proportional to their resistance. The current across the individual resistors is calculated as follows:

$$I_1 = 250/100 = 2.50 \, A$$

$$I_2 = 250/200 = 1.25 \, A$$

$$I_3 = 250/200 = 1.25 \, A$$

Therefore

$$I_T = I_1 + I_2 + I_3 = 2.5 \, A + 1.25 \, A + 1.25 \, A = 5 \, A$$

the same answer as that obtained by first calculating the total resistance (R_T) in the earlier example.

Note that for a parallel circuit, the resistance is effectively reduced. In fact, the total resistance ($R_T = 50 \, \Omega$) of the circuit is less than the resistor, which offers the least resistance ($R_4 = 100 \, \Omega$). The circuit also can be arranged with a mixture of series and parallel components. In such an arrangement, the components must first be resolved segment by segment before the values of the total circuit can be calculated.[1] In the body, the resistive components are arranged in series *and* in parallel. As shown in **Figure 18–8**, skin and fat are arranged in series. In the deeper tissues, the electrical current takes the path of least resistance; thus, muscle, blood, tendon, and bone can be considered to be resistors in a parallel circuit.

In addition to the circuit arrangement just discussed, other physical characteristics of a circuit influence the pattern and magnitude of current flow. Three such characteristics are capacitance, inductance, and impedance.

Capacitance

The characteristic that enables a device or circuit to store electrical charges in an electrostatic field is called **capacitance,** which is based on the voltage of the circuit. Capacitance is measured in units of **farads (F).** One farad is the amount of capacitance of 1 C of charges stored in a circuit with difference in potential of 1 V (F = C/V). Because a farad is an enormously large unit, capacitance is measured in microfarads (10^{-6} F) and picofarads (10^{-12} F). An electronic device called a **capacitor** is used to store electrical charges and to release them at a later time. It is made up of two conductors with a dielectric (insulating) material in between. A capacitor does not allow direct current to pass through it, whereas it does allow alternating current to pass.

Inductance

The characteristic that enables a circuit or device to store electrical energy in an electromagnetic field is called **inductance,** which is a function of current intensity. Inductance is measured in **henries (H).** Smaller units are the millihenry (mH, 10^{-3}H) and microhenry (μH, 10^{-6}H). The symbol for inductance is L. An inductor is a device that stores electrical energy

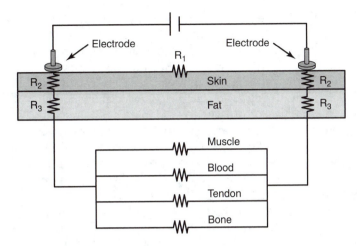

FIGURE 18–8 Resistive components of tissue. This schematic diagram represents the flow of current through a biologic tissue. The resistive components representing the skin and fat are arranged in series, and muscle, blood, tendon, and bone are arranged in parallel. Muscle tissue and blood offer less resistance to current than do skin and fat. R_1 = resistance along skin. R_2 = resistance through skin. R_3 = resistance through fat.

in an electromagnetic field. Both capacitors and inductors impede or limit alternating current flow in a circuit. These hindrances are called capacitive reactance (X_C) and inductive reactance (X_L), respectively.

Impedance

Similar to the resistance in a direct current circuit, the hindrance to current flow encountered in an alternating current circuit is call **impedance (Z),** which is measured in units of ohms. Biological tissues, because of their complex composition, present various factors and interactions that limit current flow. Body tissue such as muscle, nerve, fat, and skin offer various degrees of impedance to electrical current passed through them. Impedance is composed of resistance (R), capacitive reactance (X_C) and inductive reactance (X_L), and is expressed by the following equation:

$$Z = \{sqrt\}\ \{R^2 + (X_L - X_C)^2\}$$

where R^2, X_L and X_C are static resistance, inductive reactance, and capacitive reactance, respectively.

As shown in the following equation, capacitive reactance (X_C) is inversely proportional to the frequency of the alternating current. In general, the higher the frequency of the stimulating current, the lower the impedance of the tissue:

$$X_C = \frac{1}{2\pi fC}$$

where $\pi = 3.14$, f is the frequency of applied voltage in hertz (cycles per second), and C is capacitance in farads. For a more detailed review of these concepts, the reader should consult a general physics text.[4] Skin contains keratin and offers the highest impedance to electrical current. If the skin is slightly abraded, the impedance can decrease by 50% to 100%. Although necessary for accurate electrical testing, abrading the skin is not usually necessary for routine electrical stimulation. Removing dirt, oil, and dead skin with alcohol or soap and water is usually sufficient for this procedure. In addition, the clinician should note that the tissue impedance may decrease as stimulation time progresses. Therefore, clinically, the body part should be stimulated a few times before setting up the final amplitude. Furthermore, the amplitude should be checked frequently during the first few minutes of stimulation.

Other factors that influence the effectiveness of electrical stimulation are current density and the composition and volume of the tissue stimulated. Current density (current/unit area) depends on the intensity, the size of the electrodes, and the site of the tissue stimulated. For example, the subcutaneous fat in obese people presents high resistance. Therefore, effective stimulation of the nerve or muscle requires an extremely high intensity, which the person may not tolerate. In addition, the body acts as a volume conductor, that is, the current spreads in all directions in the immediate vicinity of the electrode. This result may reduce the effective density of the stimulating current. In general, the more fluid and the greater the electrolyte content, the greater the conductivity of the tissue. The percentage of water in the various body tissues can be used as a guide for their relative conductivity. For example, muscle contains 72–75% water, whereas fat contains 14–15% water.[5]

CLASSIFICATION OF ELECTRICAL STIMULATORS

General Characteristics of the Stimulus Output

Numerous electrical devices can be used to achieve physical therapy intervention goals. The different designs of available electrical devices make it challenging to select the appropriate device for a desired objective. To simplify this task, the most common electrical stimulators can be classified according to the general characteristics of their stimulus output: namely, the waveform, duration, and frequency of the output. In addition, electrical stimulators have been classified according to their frequency and voltage. For example, low- versus medium-frequency and low- versus high-voltage are terms sometimes used to refer to a particular type of electrical device.

Waveforms.   **Waveform** is the geometric representation of an electrical wave or stimulus. The shape of the wave depicts the amplitude and pulse duration of each stimulus. Electrical stimulators may offer a choice of waveforms or may operate on only one preset waveform. The main variables of a waveform are the amplitude, duration, and rise and decay times.

Some typical waveforms available in electrotherapeutic devices are shown in **Figure 18–9**. Note that the monophasic waveforms do not transverse the **isoelectric line,** the line that crosses the zero point on the representative graph of the waveform. The waveforms above or below the isoelectric line are in the positive or negative phase, respectively. The **phase** is the flow of charges in one direction for a finite period of time. Waveforms representing direct current can be in either the positive or the negative phase and are called **monophasic.**

Waveforms representing alternating current cross the isoelectric line, contain a negative and a positive phase, and are called **biphasic.** Biphasic waveforms are symmetrical if the shape and area under the positive and negative phases are equal. Some biphasic waveforms are asymmetrical: that is, the shape and area under the positive and negative phases are not equal. The area under a phase represents a phase charge. In an asymmetrical biphasic waveform, the phase charge can be balanced or unbalanced. In a balanced asymmetrical biphasic waveform, the net positive and negative phase charges are equal, and the output is electrically neutral. On the other hand, in an unbalanced asymmetrical biphasic waveform, the net positive and negative phase charges are unequal, and the output is not electrically neutral. Typical names used to refer to waveforms are *faradic, sine, rectangular biphasic*, and *asymmetrical biphasic*. A single waveform representing a stimulus output is called a pulse. The **pulse duration** represents the time elapsed from the beginning to the end of the waveform and is given in units ranging from microseconds to seconds. The **interpulse interval** represents the time between two successive pulses. The rate at which these pulses occur in a second is the pulse frequency or frequency and is given in pulses per second (pps).

The amount of current used can be expressed as peak current amplitude, average current, or current density. **Peak current amplitude** is the maximum amplitude of the waveform. For some waveforms, such as the twin peak waveform of the high-voltage pulsed current stimulator, the peak current amplitude can be reached only for a brief period. **Average current** (the total current per unit of time), on the other hand, is the current amplitude averaged over the total duration of the waveform. This is determined by dividing the area under the waveform by the duration of the waveform. Another way of expressing current amplitude is the mathematically derived root mean

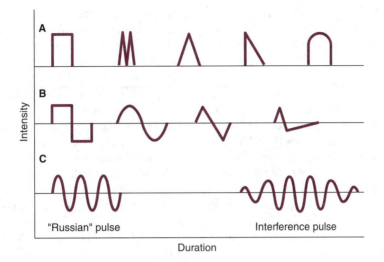

FIGURE 18–9   Basic waveforms. (**A**) monophasic, (**B**) biphasic, and (**C**) polyphasic. (*Adapted from* Clinical Electrotherapy, 3rd ed. *RM Nelson, K Hayes, DP Currier. 1999, Prentice Hall.*)

square (RMS). The current amplitude depends on the shape of the waveform (**Fig. 18–10**). For example, the RMS of a sinusoidal waveform is 0.70 of the peak amplitude, whereas the average current is 0.64 of the peak amplitude.[6] For electrical stimulators, the stimulus intensity or amplitude is usually given in units of milliamperes or microamperes.

Other characteristics of a waveform are its rise and decay times. The **rise time** (speed of rise) represents the time required to reach peak amplitude. Some waveforms, such as the square waveform, almost immediately rise to peak amplitude, whereas others, such as the triangular or saw tooth waveforms, have a slower rise time. The rise time may affect the response of tissues to the stimuli. For example, nerve tissue fails to respond to a slowly rising pulse, whereas denervated muscle tissue does not; the reason is that nerve tissue accommodates to the stimuli and muscle tissue does not. **Decay time** represents the amount of time the pulse takes to go from peak to zero amplitude.

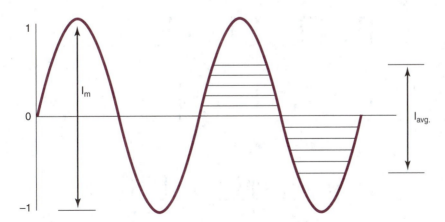

FIGURE 18–10   Peak and average current amplitude of a sinusoidal waveform. I_m is the peak current amplitude measured from the isoelectric point to the peak of the current waveform. I_{avg} is the amplitude of current averaged over the duration (t) of the waveform. $I_{avg} = 0.64 \times I_m$.

This also may affect the response of tissue to the stimuli. The frequency and duration of the waveform or pulse also can be modified to produce a variety of stimulus outputs.

Waveform Modulations.   The stimulus output, the waveform, can be modified to alter the quality of the response to the stimulation. This modification is called output modulation, which can be achieved in many ways. The most common modulations are phase duration modulation, phase amplitude modulation, and pulse frequency modulation. The duration, amplitude, or frequency of the waveform is modified to increase and decrease gradually. The quality of the response changes as the basic characteristics of the stimulus output change (**Fig. 18–11**).

Surged modulation is produced when the individual pulses within a series or train of pulses are programmed so that the peak amplitude of each sequential pulse is either gradually or abruptly increased to peak amplitude and is gradually or abruptly decreased to zero amplitude. The time required to reach a maximum amplitude of the surged mode is called **ramp time.** A train of pulses can be ramped up or down. The pulse duration can also be modulated by increasing or decreasing the duration of successive pulses. Because of the gradual recruitment of motor units, surged modulations elicit a muscle contraction that builds up gradually. The increasing intensity, or duration, recruits motor units with increasing stimulus thresholds. The surged mode rate is expressed in surges per minute. The gradual increase and fall in stimulus intensity may be better tolerated. Note that some authors use rise time and ramp time interchangeably. For the sake of clarity, the term *ramp time* is used for surged pulses, and the term *rise time* is used for a single waveform or pulse.

In addition to the amplitude, duration, and frequency modulation, the stimulus output can be delivered continuously or interrupted periodically. A continuous mode or pattern is an ongoing, nonmodified series or train of pulses. When the series of pulses commence and cease at regular intervals, an interrupted or **burst mode** is produced. The rate of bursts or interruptions per second determines the quality of muscle contraction. For example, an interruption rate of 10 pulses per second produces a twitch contraction, whereas an interruption of 50 pulses per second produces tetanic contractions. For example, the so-called Russian electrical stimulator delivers polyphasic waveforms at 2500 Hz. These pulses are patterned to deliver bursts of pulses 50 times per second, with each burst or envelope of pulses lasting 10 milliseconds (**Fig. 18–12**).

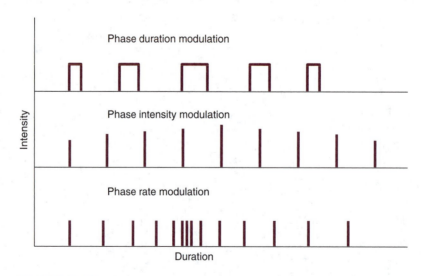

FIGURE 18–11   Dynamic modulations of pulse characteristics. Modulation of phase duration, intensity, pulse rate and duration, and combined amplitude. (*Adapted from* Clinical Electrotherapy, 3rd ed. *RM Nelson, K Hayes, DP Currier. 1999, Prentice Hall.*)

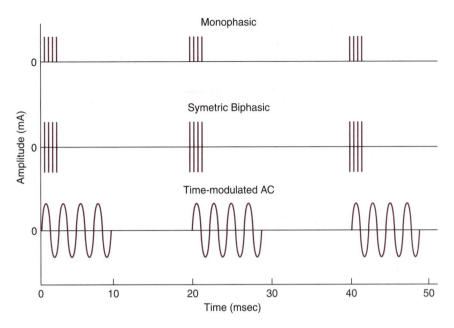

FIGURE 18–12   Burst modulation of various pulses. The stimulus output is modulated so that the pulses last for only a brief period. Monophasic pulsed bursts usually last only 1 millisecond, whereas biphasic bursts last 10 milliseconds. (*Adapted from* Clinical Electrotherapy, 3rd ed. *RM Nelson, K Hayes, DP Currier. 1999, Prentice Hall.*)

Duty Cycle.   In addition to the surged modulation, the pulse output can be modified by selecting patterns with different total on-versus-off periods of the output. This is referred to as the **duty cycle.** The duty cycle is the ratio of the on-time of the trains of pulses to the total period. It relates the net on-time of the stimuli to the total time period (on + off) of the stimuli. The duty cycle is usually expressed as the percentage of on-time to the total period (on + off). For example, when a train of stimuli is on for 10 seconds and off for 30 seconds, the duty cycle is 25% (10 ms/40 ms × 100%), or a ratio of 1:4. For a given duty cycle, the longer the on-time, the greater the possibility that the stimulated muscles will become fatigued.

Frequency.   The classification of therapeutic electrical devices can be based on the frequency of the stimuli output or the carrier frequency used. This classification includes devices that deliver low-frequency output (1–1,000 Hz), medium-frequency output (1,000–10,000 Hz), and high-frequency output (10,000 Hz or more). Devices with low-voltage direct and alternating current and those with high-voltage pulsed current are examples of low-frequency units.

The interferential current stimulators use two medium-frequency circuits in the range of 4000–5000 Hz. One circuit delivers a preset frequency of 4000 Hz; the second circuit delivers a variable frequency of 4,001–4,150 Hz (**Fig. 18–13**). The tissue is apparently stimulated by a net frequency of 1–150 Hz.[7]

The designation *high frequency* is reserved for electrical devices that use extremely high-frequency currents. Such high frequencies do not stimulate muscle or nerve tissues and are used for therapeutic heating of tissue. Examples of this category of intervention are the shortwave and microwave diathermies. Note that frequency as a basis for classification of electrical stimulators tends to be confusing because the terms *low frequency* and *medium frequency* are relative.

In addition to waveform and frequency, the type of current and the voltage are sometimes used to classify electrical stimulators. Type of current refers to direct current or alternating current (biphasic waveform), and voltage refers to the low-voltage versus so-called high-voltage designations of electrical stimulators.

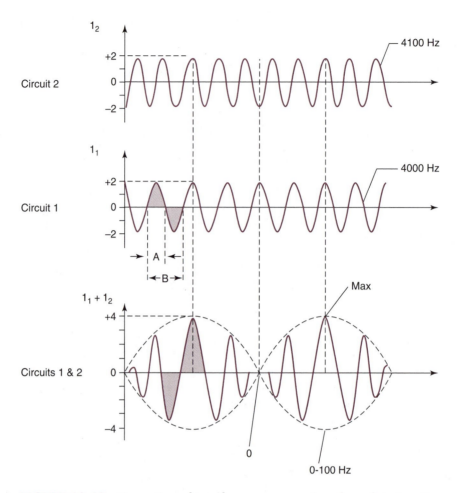

FIGURE 18–13   Generation of interference current. A = phase duration, B = pulse duration. Note that when the two circuits are in phase, the amplitude of the envelope is twice as high, thus providing an intensity that is adequate for excitation. (*Adapted from* Clinical Electrotherapy, 3rd ed. *RM Nelson, K Hayes, DP Currier. 1999, Prentice Hall.*)

The low-voltage stimulating devices use approximately 0–150 volts, and their stimulus amplitude or intensity is measured in terms of milliamperes. The stimulus output is displayed in current intensity rather than the actual voltage used to deliver such current. The so-called high-voltage pulsed current stimulator, on the other hand, displays voltages as high as 500 to deliver limited average current of 1.0–1.5 milliamps. The stimulus amplitude in such devices is given in terms of volts, as displayed on the voltmeter. The terms *low voltage* and *high voltage* are relative and should be used only to distinguish be-tween these two types of clinical devices. The term *high voltage*, when used in a nontherapeutic sense, represents devices carrying at least 2500 V. Relative to such devices, the clinical high-voltage pulsed-current units can be considered in the low-volt range.

Constant Current and Constant Voltage Stimulators

The stimulus output used to stimulate tissues en-counters an ever-changing environment because of changes in the impedance of electrodes, skin, and other tissue. To deliver a constant stimulus output, electrical devices are designed either as constant voltage or constant current units. This adjustment occurs in the output amplifier section of an electrical device and is a response to changing load (ie, the total impedance encountered by the stimulus output). Constant voltage generators are designed to adjust current so that the voltage of the stimulus output is maintained within a set amount. Constant current generators are designed to adjust the voltage so that the current amplitude is maintained within the preset amount. In addition, such devices limit the voltage changes within predetermined ranges to prevent skin burns when the load suddenly increases, as in the case of a dry electrode. (A more detailed discussion of this concept can be found elsewhere.[8])

PLACEMENT OF ELECTRODES

In general, for a given current amplitude, the smaller the electrode, the higher the current density and the stronger the stimulus. Current density, the amount of current concentrated under an electrode, is expressed in milliamperes per unit of area (mA/cm^2). For example, for a 2 cm^2 electrode that is delivering 10 mA, the current density directly under the electrode is 10 mA/2 sq cm^2 or 5 mA/cm^2. Current density is considered when choosing the appropriately sized electrode for stimulation or for current dispersion. In therapeutic electrical stimulation, the smaller electrode delivering higher current density is referred to as the active or stimulating electrode, and the larger electrode, which is mainly used to complete the circuit, is referred to as the dispersive electrode.

For any electrical stimulation to be effective, the circuit must be completed; that is, the two leads with at least two electrodes must be secured to the body part to be stimulated. Because the body is a good conductor, placing these electrodes on any part of the body would complete the circuit. For effective stimulation of the target tissue, however, the electrodes should be placed selectively. For the purposes of electrophysiologic testing and therapeutic application, electrodes of the same circuit are placed on the target area either in a monopolar or a bipolar arrangement. The designation *monopolar* or *bipolar* is based on the relative size and location of the electrodes used for stimulation.

Monopolar Placement

In a **monopolar placement,** a single small electrode (the active or stimulating electrode) is placed on the target area to be stimulated, the area where the greatest effect is desired (eg, the motor point). The second, larger electrode (the dispersive or reference electrode) is placed on the same side of the body and away from the target area. In this arrangement, the current density under the smaller electrode is higher than it is under the larger dispersive electrode (**Fig. 18–14**). Many wound-healing protocols use unipolar techniques in which a small electrode concentrates polarity in the wound bed and a large dispersive pad is placed more proximally.

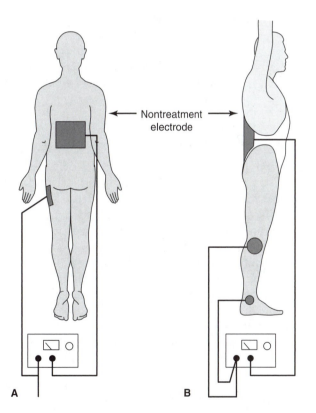

FIGURE 18–14 Monopolar technique of placing electrodes. (**A**) The simple method. (**B**) The method with a bifurcated lead so that both knee and ankle can be treated simultaneously. (*Adapted from* Clinical Electrotherapy, 3rd ed. *RM Nelson, K Hayes, DP Currier. 1999, Prentice Hall.*)

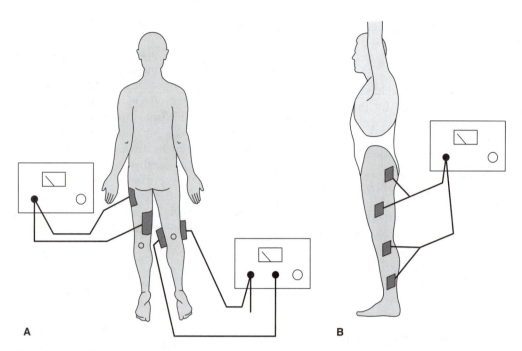

FIGURE 18–15   Bipolar technique of placing electrodes. (**A**) The simple method over a joint or muscle. (**B**) The bifurcated method along the dermatomal distribution. (*Adapted from* Clinical Electrotherapy, 3rd ed. RM Nelson, K Hayes, DP Currier. 1999, Prentice Hall.)

Bipolar Placement

In a **bipolar placement,** two electrodes of the same size are placed on the target area in such a way that the electrical current of the circuit efficiently stimulates the target tissues. In this arrangement, the electrical current is concentrated in the target area (**Fig. 18–15**). Note that more than two electrodes in a circuit (channel) can be used by bifurcating the leads of the circuit. The total electrode area is determined by adding the areas of all electrodes used in each lead of the circuit. More than one channel can be used to stimulate a large area of the body. Different areas of the body also can be stimulated at the same time using different channels. For example, two channels with four equal sized electrodes can be used to stimulate a large area such as the back. The electrode of each channel can be oriented parallel to (adjacent) or in a crossed pattern to each other. The interferential current stimulator uses a crossed pattern of electrode placement (**Fig. 18–16**).

Most stimulator electrodes are thin metals covered with a wet sponge or are carbon-rubber electrodes that are coupled to the skin with conductive gel or a wet sponge. For convenience, many clinics use pregelled electrodes that provide good conductivity and adherence to the skin. These electrodes have a conductive gum material that can be used with the same patient for multiple stimulation sessions.

CLINICAL INTEGRATION OF CURRENTS AND STIMULATION PARAMETERS

When working with a therapeutic stimulator, the clinician needs to understand the various types of currents and the stimulation parameters used to shape the current waveforms; intervention goals influence the choice of current type and stimulation parameters. **Table 18–2** summarizes the clinical applications for different current types, and **Table 18–3** describes the various stimulation parameters and their clinical significance. When working with a therapeutic stimulator, for example, in **neuromuscular electrical stimulation (NMES),** the clinician needs to be familiar with the stimulation parameter controls and be able to set them on the basis of intervention goals.

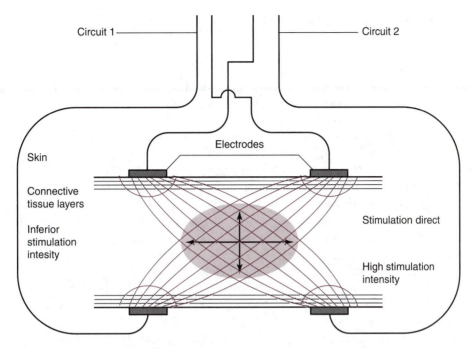

FIGURE 18–16   Interferential stimulation technique of placing electrodes. Electrodes of Circuit 1 are placed in a crossed pattern with the electrodes of Circuit 2. The maximum interference of current of the two circuits occurs where they cross. In this area, the modulated amplitude of the stimulus output is higher than it is under either electrode.(*Adapted with permission from* Traditional and Modern Aspects of Electrotherapy. *A Hansjorgens, HU May, 1982.*)

TABLE 18–2   *Commonly Used Therapeutic Currents and Recommended Clinical Use*

Current Type	Suggested Clinical Use
Direct current	Stimulation of denervated muscle
	Iontophoresis
	Wound healing (with very low intensity)
High-voltage current	Wound healing
	Pain modulation
	Acute edema (electro-osmosis)
Interferential current	Pain modulation
	Chronic edema (muscle pump)
Russian current	Muscle strengthening
	NMES for individuals with CNS lesions
Monophasic pulsatile	Wound healing
	Acute edema (electro-osmosis)
Biphasic pulsatile	Muscle strengthening
	NMES for individuals with CNS lesions
	Pain modulation

TABLE 18–3   *Commonly Used Stimulation Parameters and Clinical Relevance*

Stimulation Parameter	Clinical relevance
Pulse amplitude	Neural responses ranging from subsensory to painful stimulation are controlled by pulse amplitude. Muscle strengthening protocols will require strong motor intensity (higher amplitude), whereas conventional pain protocols will use comfortable sensory intensity (lower amplitude). Current amplitude can be described on the basis of neuroexcitation level (ie, subsensory, sensory, motor, and pain).
Pulse frequency	Less than 10 pps creates twitching contractions during NMES. Increasing the frequency causes increased twitching contraction rates. At frequencies greater than 35–50 pps, a rapid depolarization rate keeps the muscle in a sustained tetanic contraction. Tetanizing frequencies are used for muscle strengthening and neuromuscular facilitation protocols.
Pulse duration	An inverse relationship exists between pulse amplitude and pulse duration. Less pulse amplitude is required for peripheral nerve excitation at wide (high) pulse durations. As pulse intensity sets neuroexcitation level (ie, sensory, motor, pain), pulse duration further contributes to the particular level of neuroexcitation. A pulse duration increase during NMES results in stronger muscle contraction when compared with narrow pulse duration stimulation at the same pulse amplitude.
Pulse modulation	The way that current is delivered to the patient, either in an interrupted or in a continuous mode, is controlled by modulation. Interrupted stimulation requires on and off controls to be set on the basis of muscle endurance during muscle strengthening protocols. Ramping is also controlled by pulse modulation and provides a gradual current introduction (ramp-up) and withdrawal (ramp-down) during stimulation periods. Stimulation protocols that require high intensity are made more comfortable by ramping pulse intensity. Some stimulators ramp or modulate pulse frequency and width to make their current more "dynamic" and efficient during sensory and motor stimulation protocols.

REVIEW QUESTIONS

1. Explain why direct current used incorrectly has the most potential to harm the skin.

2. Explain the relationship between current intensity and (a) electrical voltage and (b) electrical resistance.

3. Draw a pictorial representation for the following currents: (a) direct current, (b) alternating current, (c) monophasic pulsatile current, and (d) biphasic pulsatile current.

4. What factors influence electrical conductivity in the tissues of the body?

5. Define capacitance and inductance. What is the significance of each in an electrical stimulator?

6. What are the differences between a monopolar and a bipolar electrode arrangement?

7. What is the relationship between electrode size and current density, and how does this relationship impact neuroexcitation?

8. What are the frequency ranges for the following types of stimulation: (a) low frequency, (b) medium frequency, and (c) high frequency?

9. Describe the difference between constant current and constant voltage stimulators.

10. Provide an outline of the significance of each of the following stimulation parameters: (a) pulse amplitude, (b) pulse frequency, (c) pulse duration, and (d) pulse modulation.

KEY TERMS

electron
proton
neutron
ion
coulomb (C)
electrical current
ampere (A)
electrodes
electrolytes
anode
cathode
anions
cations
difference in potential
convection current
current density
current amplitude
current

electromotive force (EMF)
volts (V)
resistance (R)
ohm (Ω)
conductors
insulators
semiconductors
resistivity (ρ)
Ohm's law
capacitance
farads (F)
capacitor
inductance
henries (H)
inductor
impedance (Z)
waveform
isoelectric line

phase
monophasic
biphasic
pulse duration
interpulse interval
peak current amplitude
average current
rise time
decay time
surged modulation
ramp time
burst mode
duty cycle
monopolar placement
bipolar placement
neuromuscular electrical
   stimulation (NMES)

REFERENCES

1. Tammes AR: *Electronics for Medical and Biology Laboratory Personnel.* Baltimore: Williams & Wilkins; 1971:8.

2. Scott PM: *Clayton's Electrotherapy and Actinotherapy.* Baltimore: Williams & Wilkins; 1975:42.

3. Karselis T: *Descriptive Medical Electronics and Instrumentation.* Thorofare, NJ: Charles B. Black; 1973:12.

4. Halliday D, Resnick R, Walker J: *Fundamentals of Physics.* 4th ed. New York: Wiley; 1993.

5. Shriber WA: *Manual of Electrotherapy*, 4th ed. Philadelphia: Lea & Febiger; 1975; 120.

6. Newton R: *Electrotherapeutic Treatment: Selecting Appropriate Waveform Characteristics.* A Preston; 1984; 5–6.

7. Savage B. *Interferential Therapy.* Boston: Faber & Faber; 1984; 19.

8. Stillwell K: *Therapeutic Electricity and Ultraviolet Radiation.* 3rd ed. Rehabilitation Medicine Library. Baltimore: Williams & Wilkins; 1983; 91.

19

Electrophysiology

TSEGA ANDEMICAEL MEHRETEAB, PT, MS

THOMAS HOLLAND, PT, PhD

Chapter Outline

Both nerve and muscle cells are excitable. For example, electrical stimulation of a normal peripheral motor nerve elicits a muscle contraction. This chapter reviews the normal physiologic responses of nerve and muscle tissue to electrical stimulation and discusses the use of electrophysiologic tests to determine the integrity of nerve and muscle tissue.

PHYSIOLOGIC RESPONSES

Action Potential

Electrical stimulation of a normal peripheral motor nerve elicits a muscle contraction. This response involves the excitation and conduction of a nerve impulse. **Excitation** refers to the events leading to the generation of an action potential, and **conduction** refers to the transmission or propagation of the action potential away from the site of stimulation.[1] Both nerve and muscle cells respond to different kinds of stimuli (eg, electrical, thermal, mechanical, and chemical). This excitability of nerve and muscle cells is caused by a change in their transmembrane potential, which is established by the unequal distribution of charged ions between the inside and the outside of the semipermeable membrane. The resting potential or the voltage difference between the inside and the outside of nerve or skeletal muscle fibers (cells) at rest is between 60 mV and 90 mV, the inside being more negative. Adequate stimulation of a nerve axon or a muscle cell causes an abrupt change of the resting membrane potential, leading to the development of an **action potential** (excitation of the cell).[2]

The action potential depicted in **Figure 19–1** is made up of sequential events. A stimulus initiates a **depolarization phase,** or a reduction of its negative charges, which also represents a reduction of the membrane potential of the cell. When the depolarization or excitation of the membrane reaches its peak, it is followed by a **repolarization phase** that reestablishes the resting potential. The nerve axon requires sufficient time to recover after one stimulus and before another stimulus can be effective. The repolarization phase includes a **refractory period,** during which the nerve axon either fails to respond to a subsequent stimulus (absolute refractory period) or requires more intensity (relative refractory period) to respond to a subsequent stimulus. This rest period may range from 0.5 to 1 millisecond.[1] When a nerve-muscle complex is electrically stimulated, the rest period should be at least equal to the refractory period of the nerve so that a subsequent stimulus can be just as effective.

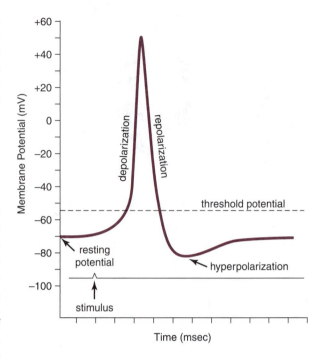

FIGURE 19–1 Changes in membrane potential during an action potential. A stimulus causes a cell membrane to undergo an action potential. The transmembrane potential is rapidly depolarized. When it reaches its maximum intensity, it dips below the resting potential and becomes even more negative, or hyperpolarized, then returns to its resting potential.

Impulse Propagation

The action potential, or impulse, self-propagates from the site of stimulation in all directions. For example, electrical stimulation of a peripheral motor axon causes the conduction of a nerve impulse from the point of stimulation toward the neuromuscular junction. There, the impulse causes the release of neurochemical transmitters that generate a muscle action potential and elicit muscle contraction. *Orthodromic conduction* and *antidromic conduction* are terms used to describe the direction of impulse conduction. When an impulse travels along its normal or physiologic direction, the conduction is referred to as **orthodromic conduction:** for example, a motor axon conducting an impulse from a proximal site of stimulation toward its neuromuscular junction. **Antidromic conduction** occurs when the impulse is conducted in the opposite direction of its normal or physiologic direction: for example, a motor axon conducting an impulse from a distal (peripheral) site of stimulation toward the cell body (proximally).

Effectiveness of Electrical Stimuli

The effectiveness of an electrical stimulus depends on its intensity (amplitude), duration, and rise time (speed of rise).

Intensity.   The intensity of a stimulus that is just sufficient to depolarize the cell membrane and cause an action potential is called a **threshold stimulus.** An intensity lower than threshold is called a subliminal or **subthreshold stimulus.** The subthreshold stimulus may cause some changes in the immediate environment of the tissue stimulated, but it does not depolarize the membrane sufficiently to trigger an action potential. Conversely, increasing the amplitude, duration, or both higher than threshold does not increase the magnitude of the action potential; thus, generation of an action potential follows the all-or-none principle of excitation. Because nerves usually contain many axons with different excitation thresholds, thus increasing the stimulus amplitude, they excite the axons with high stimulus thresholds in addition to those with low thresholds, resulting in a stronger response. Such a response is caused by the recruitment of more axons rather than by an increase in the magnitude of any individual action potentials.

Duration.   In addition to the stimulus amplitude, the duration of the stimulus must be long enough to excite the tissue. The minimum stimulus duration required by a tissue depends on the characteristics of the tissue. For example, nerve tissue is more excitable than muscle tissue and thus requires a shorter duration stimulus than does muscle tissue. Other factors such as the temperature and general condition of the tissue may influence the minimum duration required to excite the tissue. For example, increasing the temperature and local circulation of the tissue may decrease its resistance and thus require a shorter stimulus duration and less intensity.

Figure 19–2 presents the inverse relationship between stimulus intensity (strength) and duration for the different levels of neuroexcitation. Less stimulus intensity is required for peripheral nerve excitation at wide (high) pulse widths. If pulse duration is decreased during neuromuscular electrical stimulation (NMES), there is a need to increase the stimulus intensity to maintain the same contraction strength. The order of neural responses remains consistent at the different stimulus durations (1st sensory, 2nd motor, 3rd pain, 4th maximal tolerable pain) and will be more spread out at short pulse durations (see **Fig. 19–2**). The increased discrimination between the different neural responses at

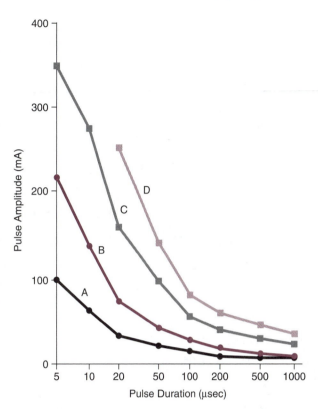

FIGURE 19–2   Strength-duration curves of the four major excitatory responses. (**A**) Sensory threshold. (**B**) Motor threshold. (**C**) Pain threshold. (**D**) Maximal tolerable painful stimulation. (*Austra J Physiother 29: 195–201, 1983*)

short durations has led to the use of more short duration currents (PC) to get sensory and motor excitation without creating a noxious response by avoiding the recruitment of nerve fibers that convey painful stimuli.

The quality of neuromuscular response to electrical stimulation also depends on the rate, or frequency, of the stimuli. For example, a low frequency of 1 or 2 stimuli per second will produce a single response referred to as a **twitch contraction.** This is followed by complete relaxation of the contractile elements of the muscle. At higher frequencies (eg, 15 pulses per second) there is not enough time for relaxation, and the action potentials begin to summate, giving rise to a partial or an incomplete contraction called an *unfused tetanus.* A **tetanus** is a sustained muscle contraction caused by a rapid succession of stimuli. As shown in **Figure 19–3**, at progressively higher frequencies—greater than 30 stimuli per second, for example—summation of the action potentials is more nearly complete and produces a fused tetanus. It should be

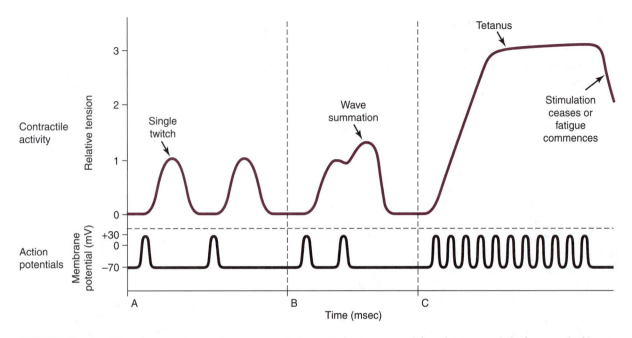

FIGURE 19–3   Wave summation and tetanus: twitch, partial tetanus, and fused tetanus. (**A**) If a muscle fiber is restimulated after it has relaxed completely, the second twitch is the same magnitude as the first twitch. (**B**) If a muscle fiber is restimulated before it has relaxed completely, the second twitch is added on to the first twitch, resulting in a wave summation and a partly fused muscle contraction or an incomplete tetanus. (**C**) If a muscle fiber is stimulated so rapidly that it has no opportunity to relax between stimuli, a maximal sustained contraction called *tetanus* occurs. (*Reproduced with permission from* Human Physiology: From Cells to Systems. *Sherwood L. 1989. St. Paul: West Publishing.*)

noted that higher stimulus frequencies, which produce tetanic muscle contraction and duty cycles with short rest periods, promote muscle fatigue. Therefore, to avoid fatigue, it is necessary to provide sufficient rest between stimuli.[3]

Rise Time.   The third criterion that a stimulus must meet to be effective is a sufficient rise time. *Rise time* is the time required for the stimulus to reach its maximum intensity or peak amplitude. This characteristic is dependent on the waveform of the stimulus. The rise time of a square waveform is virtually immediate compared with that of an exponential waveform. If the stimulus reaches peak amplitude slowly, nerve tissue accommodates to the passage of such current and fails to respond to it. *Accommodation* is the rise in the excitation threshold of nerve tissue resulting from a gradually increasing stimulus intensity. Clinically, the phenomenon of accommodation occurs only in nerve tissue, not in muscle tissues.

The three parameters—stimulus amplitude (intensity), duration, and rise time—can be used to measure the response of the tissue to a given stimulus and are

useful measurements in electrophysiologic tests. Comparision of the results of these tests with the results from the normal contralateral side may indicate whether the nerve axon is intact or whether the muscle is partially innervated or completely denervated.

ELECTROPHYSIOLOGIC TESTS

Nerve tissue is more excitable than muscle tissue. Thus, normal nerve tissue has a lower threshold than muscle tissue and is expected to respond to stimuli with a lower intensity and shorter duration than is required by muscle tissue. A number of classical and contemporary electrophysiologic tests based on this inherent difference in excitability help determine the excitability of nerve and muscle tissues. The classical electrodiagnostic tests include: (1) strength-duration (SD), (2) chronaxie, and (3) reaction of degeneration (RD). The more contemporary tests include (1) nerve . . . and (2) electro nerve conduction velocity (NCV), and (5) electromyography (EMG). The nerve conduction velocity and electromyography tests are described in **Chapter 23.**

Strength-Duration Test

The intensity and duration of a stimulus are inversely related. In general, the shorter the duration, the higher the intensity required for excitation. The relationship of intensity and duration is a quantitative measure of the excitability of muscle and nerve tissues. This relationship is demonstrated by the intensity-duration curve, commonly referred to as the **strength-duration (SD) curve** (**Fig. 19–4**). This curve is obtained by plotting on a graph the stimulus amplitude required to produce a minimally visible contraction of a muscle as the stimulus duration is varied. Note that there is a minimum stimulus duration below which the tissue ceases to respond regardless of the intensity available; similarly, there is a minimum intensity below which the tissue ceases to respond regardless of the duration available.

In addition to the relative position of the curve, two points on the SD curve, rheobase and chronaxie, should be noted. **Rheobase** is the minimum intensity required to elicit a minimally visible contraction when the duration is infinite. Clinically, duration of 100–300 milliseconds is used. **Chronaxie** is the duration required for a stimulus with twice the rheobase intensity to elicit a minimally visible contraction.

The SD test is a quantitative test because the intensity required to produce minimally visible contractions in response to a stimulus of a given duration is measured and is compared with the intensity, on the normal contralateral side. The intensity values obtained for different durations are then plotted on a graph with duration and intensity coordinates (see **Fig. 19–4**). For example, nerve tissue has a considerably lower chronaxie (approximately 0.03 millisecond) than a denervated muscle tissue (approximately 10 milliseconds). A chronaxie greater than 1 millisecond is considered to be abnormal for a nerve and may indicate muscle denervation. The excitatory response of nerve fibers depends on the inherent impedance of the tissue. The large-diameter nerve fibers such as the A-fibers are excited sooner than smaller-diameter fibers that transmit noxious stimuli.[4]

Procedure.   To conduct the SD test, a direct-current generator with a square waveform and a variable duration (300–0.01 millisecond) is used. An ampmeter is used to measure the required intensity. For the test results to be accurate, test conditions must remain as constant as possible. The body part must be positioned appropriately, and there must be proper lighting so that any changes in response can be observed easily and accurately. The position of the electrode on a given motor point is not changed as the test proceeds. Ideally, an assistant is present to record the results. Note that the test has some inconsistencies regarding contractions and possibly some experimental inconsistencies. Such limitations can be minimized by having the same person conduct the tests on the same patient.

The steps listed next should be followed when conducting the SD test:

1. Explain the test and what to expect to the patient. Position the patient comfortably, and prepare an SD or a chronaximeter for testing.

2. The body part to be tested is supported in a semistretched position. The area is well lit so that any response can be seen easily.

3. Set the instrument on automatic interruption mode so that stimulation occurs every 0.5–2 seconds.

4. Set the duration on 100–300 milliseconds. The 100 msec setting may be more comfortable for some patients.

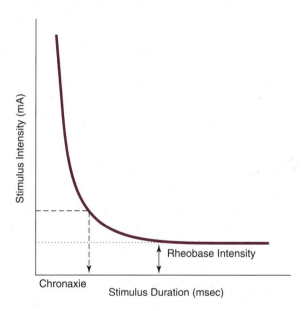

FIGURE 19–4 Strength/duration (SD) curve. This curve shows the stimulus amplitude (intensity) required to produce a minimally visible contraction (response) of a muscle as the duration of the stimulus is varied. There is a minimum duration below which the tissue does not respond regardless of the intensity of the stimulus. The rheobase is the minimal intensity of infinite duration that is required to elicit a response. The chronaxie is the duration of a stimulus that is twice the intensity of the rheobase and is required to elicit a response.

5. For the active, stimulating electrode, use a hand-held stimulator with an extremely small electrode tip. Place a dispersive pad on an appropriate area proximal to the area to be stimulated.

6. Locate a motor point of a muscle innervated by the peripheral nerve to be tested. At least one proximal and one distal muscle innervated by that nerve should be tested and compared with the contralateral side (if it has normal innervation), established normal values, or both.

7. To ensure consistent results after locating the motor point, decrease the intensity until observable contractions disappear, and then increase the intensity gradually until a minimally visible contraction is noted. Record the intensity used.

8. Sequentially decrease the duration from 100 to 0.01 millisecond. For example, set the duration at 100, 50, 30, 20, 10, 5, 3, 2, 1, 0.5, 0.2, 0.1, 0.05, and 0.01 milliseconds. For each duration, record the intensity used to produce the minimally visible contraction.

9. On a special SD log paper, plot the intensity versus the duration used. Connect the points on the graph to form a curve.

10. Compare the results of proximal versus distal muscles innervated by the peripheral nerve. Also compare the results with those of the normal side.

11. On the SD curve, identify the rheobase: the minimum stimulus amplitude required to elicit a minimally visible contraction when the stimulus duration is infinite (100–300 milliseconds).

12. On the SD curve, identify the chronaxie: the stimulus duration required to produce the minimally visible contraction when the stimulus intensity is twice that of the rheobase.

Interpretation. As shown in **Figure 19–5**, the SD curve of a denervated muscle requires a higher intensity for a given duration than does an innervated muscle. Therefore, the SD curve of a denervated muscle is shifted up and to the right on the SD coordinate. The relative position of the SD curve of the tested nerve and the progress or lack of progress in subsequent tests are useful to document the status of the nerve-muscle complex and to arrive at a prognosis for a given condition. In addition, the shape of the SD curve may indicate partial denervation or partial innervation in subsequent tests. For example, such curves may be discontinuous or may have a bend or kink on them.

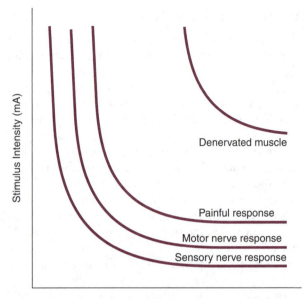

FIGURE 19–5 Strength/duration (SD) curves comparing the intensity and duration of stimuli necessary to elicit a response from various tissues. The relative position of the curves indicates that a normal sensory nerve responds more quickly than a motor nerve and requires a lower stimulus amplitude and duration. Sensory nerve fibers that transmit pain or noxious stimuli require a higher amplitude and a longer duration. Denervated muscle, although an excitable tissue, requires a stimulus of higher amplitude and longer duration than a normally innervated muscle.

Chronaxie Test

The chronaxie test is a quick means of obtaining a chronaxie value without having to test for every duration and plot a complete graph. Note that the procedures for setting up the test are the same as those for the SD test:

1. Explain the test and what to expect to the patient. Position the patient comfortably. Prepare an SD or a chronaximeter for testing.

2. The body part to be tested is supported in a semi-stretched position. The area is well lit so that any response can be seen easily.

3. Set the instrument on automatic interruption mode so that stimulation occurs every 0.5–2 seconds.

4. Set the duration on 100–300 milliseconds; 100 milliseconds may be more comfortable for some patients.

5. For the active, stimulating electrode, use a hand-held stimulator with an extremely small electrode tip. Place a dispersive pad on an appropriate area proximal to the area to be stimulated.

6. Locate a motor point of a muscle innervated by the peripheral nerve to be tested. At least one proximal and one distal muscle innervated by that nerve should be tested and compared with the normal contralateral side, established normal values, or both.

7. To ensure consistent results after locating the motor point, decrease the intensity until observable contractions disappear, and then increase the intensity gradually until a minimally visible contraction is noted. Record the intensity used.

8. Record the rheobase, and turn the duration to zero.

9. Set the instrument at double (2x) the rheobase intensity.

10. Gradually increase the duration until the minimally visible contraction is reproduced. This duration at double the rheobase intensity is the chronaxie value.

11. Compare the obtained value with normal established chronaxie values or with the chronaxie of the normal contralateral side.

Reaction of Degeneration Test

The **reaction of degeneration (RD) test,** or **faradic/galvanic test,** is a qualitative test based on a characteristic difference between the response of nerve and muscle tissues to a long- or short-duration electrical stimulus. To conduct the test, an electric generator is used that can produce both monophasic long-duration and biphasic short-duration pulses. To minimize the spread of current through volume conduction, a handheld electrode with a small area of stimulation is used. For long-duration stimuli, the test uses interrupted monophasic pulses with pulse durations of 100 milliseconds that are repeated approximately once a second. For short-duration stimuli, the test uses biphasic pulses with a duration of less than 1 millisecond that are applied at a frequency higher than 120 Hz. Such stimuli will elicit a tetanic contraction of a normally innervated muscle. The quality of muscle contraction in response to the short-duration versus long-duration stimuli is used to characterize the response as twitch versus tetanic, brisk versus sluggish, or diminished contractions. The presence or absence of a response also is indicative of the condition of the tissue. **Table 19–1** depicts the possible responses to short- versus long-duration stimuli. The possible results of an RD test are normal reaction, partial reaction of degeneration, full reaction of degeneration, or absolute reaction of degeneration.

Procedure.   Locate a motor point of a muscle innervated by the peripheral nerve to be tested. At least one proximal and one distal muscle innervated by that nerve should be tested and compared with the normal contralateral side. Begin the test on the normal side to establish a baseline.

Test for response to pulses of short duration. Follow these steps when conducting this test:

1. Explain the test and what to expect to the patient. Position the patient comfortably.

2. The body part to be tested is supported in a semi-stretched position. The area is well lit so that any response can be seen easily.

3. Select an electric generator that can produce both monophasic long-duration and biphasic short-duration pulses.

4. Test with the short-duration stimuli first. Set the generator on tetanizing frequency (> 35 Hz) and a stimulus duration less than 1 millisecond.

5. Place a dispersive electrode over an appropriate area proximal to the area to be stimulated. A large, smooth area such as the upper back or shoulder for the upper extremity tests and the lower back or buttocks area for the lower extremity test is recommended. Place the electrodes on the same side of the body to avoid stimulation across the heart.

6. For the active, stimulating electrode, use a hand-held electrode with an extremely small tip and a "make-or-break" switch for manual interruption of the stimulus output.

7. Locate and stimulate the motor point of the muscle to be tested. If the muscle responds, increase the intensity to obtain a strong contraction.

8. Note and record the quality of the muscle contraction in response to the short-duration tetanizing current. Short-duration, tetanizing stimuli elicit a tetanic contraction of a normally innervated muscle. Decrease the intensity back to zero.

9. Do not remove the stimulating electrode from the motor point. For consistent results, the same motor point should be used for the next segment of the test.

TABLE 19–1   *Reaction of Degeneration Test*

Reaction	Stimuli of Short Duration	Stimuli of Long Duration
Normal		
Nerve	Tetanic contraction	Brisk twitch contraction
Muscle	Tetanic contraction	Brisk twitch contraction
Partial		
Nerve	Diminished or partial	Diminished or partial individual contraction
Muscle	tetanic contraction	Sluggish contraction
Full		
Nerve	No contraction	No contraction
Muscle	No contraction	Sluggish contraction
Absolute		
Nerve	No contraction	No contraction
Muscle	No contraction	No contraction

Test for response to pulses of long duration. Follow these steps when conducting this test:

1. Maintain the same position of the stimulating electrode over the motor point tested.
2. Change to the long-duration stimulus current of the generator. Set the duration on 500 milliseconds. Set the instrument on the automatic interruption mode so that the stimulus output occurs once each second. If an automatic setting is not available, interrupt the current manually every 500 milliseconds with the "make-or-break" switch on the stimulating electrode.
3. Select the cathode for the stimulating (active) electrode and the anode for the dispersive electrode.

TABLE 19–2   *Classical Electrodiagnostic Tests Interpretation*

E/D Test	Normal	Abnormal
Chronaxie value	<1 millisec	> 1 millisec (wider pulse duration required to stimulate denervated muscle).
S/D curve	Slight slope until the duration approaches the chronaxie value.	Curve is shifted up and to the right (higher intensities required at each long pulse duration and a complete inability to respond to short pulse duration).
R/D test	Strong muscle contraction during short pulse duration (PC or AC) stimulation.	Partial R/D, diminished response with short pulse duration (PC or AC) stimulation.
		Full R/D, no response with short pulse duration (PC or AC) stimulation, a response observed with long pulse duration (DC) stimulation.
		Absolute R/D, no response to long pulse duration (DC) stimulation.

4. Stimulate the motor point of the muscle to be tested, and if the muscle responds, increase the intensity to get a strong, brisk twitch contraction.

5. Note and record the quality of the muscle contraction in response to the long-duration stimulus. If the muscle is normally innervated, a brisk

twitch contraction is elicited. Any variation of the observed response should be noted and compared with those in **Table 19–2**.

6. Decrease the stimulus output to zero intensity.

7. Repeat these procedures on the involved side.

REVIEW QUESTIONS

1. What are the different phases of an action potential? Describe the changes in ionic concentrations inside the nerve membrane throughout the action potential.

2. In order to create an action potential in a peripheral nerve, what must the stimulus have in terms of intensity and duration?

3. Define orthodromic and antidromic nerve conduction. Give examples of each as related to (a) sensory nerve and (b) motor nerve.

4. Describe the relationship between stimulus intensity and duration.

5. What is the normal order of neuroexcitatory responses when using therapeutic electrical stimulation?

6. What is the main purpose of stimulus frequency when performing neuromuscular electrical stimulation?

7. What is nerve accommodation? What stimulation parameters may influence nerve accommodation?

8. Define rheobase and chronaxie, and describe their position on the strength-duration curve.

9. What happens to the strength-duration curve and chronaxie value with denervation?

10. How can the reaction of the degeneration test be used to help differentiate between a central and a peripheral nervous system lesion?

KEY TERMS

excitation	orthodromic conduction	strength/duration (SD) curve
conduction	antidromic conduction	rheobase
action potential	threshold stimulus	chronaxie
depolarization phase	subthreshold stimulus	reaction of degeneration (RD) test
repolarization phase	twitch contraction	faradic/galvanic test
refractory period	tetanus	

REFERENCES

1. Sherwood LL: *Human Physiology from Cells to Systems.* St. Paul: West; 1989.

2. Nelson RM, Currier DP: *Clinical Electrotherapy.* Norwalk, CT: Appleton & Lange; 1991.

3. Benton LA, Baker LL, Bocoman BR, et al: *Functional Electrical Stimulation: A Practical Guide.* Downey, CA: Rancho Los Amigos Rehab

Engineering Center, Rancho Los Amigos Hospital; 1981.

4. Li CL, Bak A: Excitability characteristics of the A- and C-fibers in peripheral nerve. *Exp Neural* 1976; 50:67.

20

Clinical Applications of Electrical Stimulation

TSEGA ANDEMICAEL MEHRETEAB, PT, MS

THOMAS HOLLAND, PT, PhD

Chapter Outline

- MUSCLE STRENGTHENING AND PREVENTION OF ATROPHY
- MUSCLE SPASM
- CENTRAL NERVOUS SYSTEM LESIONS
- PERIPHERAL NERVOUS SYSTEM LESIONS
- EDEMA AND PERIPHERAL VASCULAR DYSFUNCTION
- WOUND HEALING
- INCONTINENCE
- REVIEW QUESTIONS
- KEY TERMS

Electrical stimulation has been used as an adjunct in the intervention of various clinical problems such as pain, muscle weakness, poor motor control due to central nervous system (CNS) lesions, edema, nonhealing wounds, and poor peripheral circulation. Electrical stimulation produces neuroexcitatory and physiologic effects on non-neural tissue that permit its use for therapeutic applications. Electrotherapy is most successful when used in conjunction with a comprehensive rehabilitation program. For example, pain modulation is best achieved when electrical stimulation is used while addressing the underlying causes of pain (eg, muscle imbalance, poor posture, repetitive stress). When treating wounds, pressure relief and an optimal wound environment with the most appropriate dressing are required to promote tissue healing with electrotherapy. Clinicians are encouraged to use electrotherapy as an adjunct that facilitates and augments the complete rehabilitation program. **The clinical uses and respective rationale for interventions with therapeutic electrical stimulation are outlined in Box 20–1.**

Before using electrotherapy, the clinician needs to be aware of the general contraindications and precautions for electrical stimulation **(Box 20–2)**. Knowledge of contraindications/precautions and good clinical judgment are necessary to ensure an effective intervention while maintaining patient safety.

Muscle Strengthening and Prevention of Atrophy

Muscle weakness and atrophy occur from immobilization or disuse in cases of prolonged casting, chronic pain, or postsurgical immobilization. Stressing disused muscles with exercise and functional activities are ways to increase strength following immobilization. Active assistive, active, and resistive exercise programs are chosen on the basis of present muscle strength. In some cases of weakness and atrophy, electrical stimulation will improve muscle fiber recruitment beyond what can be achieved with active recruitment.[1,2] In addition, **neuromuscular electrical stimulation (NMES)** creates muscle contractions by depolarization of motor nerves that serve both fast- and slow-twitch muscle fibers. Large-nerve axons that innervate fast-twitch muscle fibers are more sensitive to NMES and will become depolarized with low levels of NMES.[3] Active

Box 20–1 *Clinical Uses of Electrical Stimulation*

Clinical Use	Rationale
Pain modulation (Chapter 21)	Introduce more non-noxious sensory input. Promote release of endogenous opiates.
Muscle weakness and disuse atrophy	Enhance muscle fiber recruitment during active contractions. Increase recruitment of fast twitch muscle fibers.
Paralysis due to CNS lesion	Enhance cortical output to paretic muscles. Minimize disuse atrophy and maintain ROM. Temporarily reduce spasticity. Integrate into functional activities and exercise regimes (FES).
Edema	Mobilize edema with mechanical forces from electrically induced muscle contractions.
Wounds	Add electrical potential into a poorly healing wound. Attract cells involved in the inflammatory and proliferative phases of wound healing.
Enhance transdermal delivery of ions (Chapter 22)	Repulsion of topical ions through the skin with the polarity of direct current (iontophoresis).
Increase peripheral circulation	Increase venous return with an electrically induced muscle pump. Increase release of vasoactive byproducts of muscle metabolism.

Box 20–2 *Contraindications and Precautions for the Use of Electrical Stimulation*

Contraindications/Precautions	Rationale
In the area of a demand-type pacemaker	May interfere with the conduction pacing from the pacemaker.
Directly over a pregnant uterus during the first trimester	Effect on embryo is unknown.
In the area of the head in individuals with epilepsy	Has potential to induce a seizure
Over the carotid sinus	Has potential to induce a hypotensive response.
Across the chest of patients with cardiac disease	May interfere with normal cardiac conduction.
Over thrombotic or embolic blood vessels	Motor levels of stimulation may dislodge a blood clot.
Over tissues or blood vessels that are vulnerable to hemorrhage	Motor levels of stimulation may cause active bleeding.
Over the eyes	Effects on the eye are unknown.
On mucosal surfaces	Increases current concentration and sensitivity.
Over wounds or skin breaks	Increases sensitivity to current.
	Motor levels of stimulation may traumatize a healing wound.
In individuals with significant impaired mentation	May create possible decreased tolerance and feedback during stimulation interventions.
Over areas of impaired and absent sensation	Decreased feedback and increased chance of unreported skin irritation.
Over areas where active movement must be avoided	Motor levels of stimulation may disrupt healing bone and soft tissue.
Over areas with active cancer	Stimulation may increase tissue metabolism.

contractions will not recruit fast-twitch fibers as easily as NMES, especially in individuals with weakness and atrophy. Therefore, NMES can augment therapeutic exercise by enhancing the recruitment of muscle fibers and by increasing fast-twitch fiber recruitment.

Well-documented clinical studies demonstrate that electrical stimulation is effective in retarding disuse atrophy as measured by limb girth measurements and the maximum voluntary isometric torque. Electrical stimulation promotes early active range of motion (ROM) in postsurgical and cast-immobilized limbs.[4–6] For example, Morrissey et al.[7] compared the use of electrical stimulation of the quadriceps of immobilized patients following anterior cruciate ligament reconstruction with unexercised patients. They used 350-microsecond, monophasic pulsed current at 50 pulses per second (pps) to stimulate the quadriceps. Their results showed a less pronounced decrease in thigh circumference and maximum voluntary isometric torque in the immobilized group as compared with the unexercised group. In another study, an alternating current of 2500 Hz, delivering 50 bursts per second, was used to stimulate the quadriceps and hamstrings of patients following anterior cruciate ligament reconstruction. The results indicated increase in the maximum voluntary isometric torque of knee extension and flexion.[1]

To create strong muscle contractions, a high *motor* intensity should be used during NMES. Tetanic muscle contractions are achieved by raising the pulse rate to create a rapid succession of motor nerve depolarizations that hold innervated muscle fibers in a sustained contraction. Most NMES strengthening protocols use 50 pps or slightly less. An excessively high pulse rate may contribute to rapid fatigue, whereas low pulse rates create twitching contractions and are not recommended during muscle-strengthening protocols. The pulse duration should be relatively *wide* (≥ 300 microseconds) to enhance motor nerve recruitment within a tolerable level. Small muscles (eg, wrist, hand or ankle, foot) require lower durations when compared with large muscles (eg, upper arm, shoulder girdle, upper leg, pelvis and trunk).

An interrupted modulation is required when using NMES for muscle strengthening. A sufficient rest period between NMES-induced contractions is necessary because of the selective fast-twitch fast-fatigue fiber recruitment. Fatigue is avoided by using high stimulation on:off ratios (on:off ≥ 1:3). A low on:off ratio may be used as muscle endurance improves (ie, 1:1). A ramped intensity is another consideration for pulse modulation. Ramping will gradually introduce peak intensity to create smoother and more comfortable contractions (**Fig. 20–1**).

Electrodes are commonly placed on the stimulated muscles' motor points. These points represent areas of increased motor innervation and usually correspond to the muscle belly. Clinicians can easily find motor points by using electrodes that can be moved along the targeted muscle during motor stimulation. The areas that produce the strongest muscle contraction at a low motor intensity should be used for electrode placement during NMES muscle strengthening. If a muscle group innervated by the same nerve is targeted for stimulation, then an electrode can be placed on the peripheral nerve. For example, ankle dorsiflexion and eversion can be achieved if at least one electrode is placed on the common peroneal nerve by the fibula head. One electrode can stimulate both muscle groups because the nerve is excited before it divides into its various motor points. Strong contractions can thus be achieved with reduced need for multiple electrode placements.

Neuromuscular electrical stimulation effects are enhanced when individuals are asked to contract with the stimulation. Research literature supports the notion that strength gains are greater when an individual works with NMES-induced contractions rather than being a passive recipient.[8,9] Clinically, the authors have found that active muscle contraction of stimulated muscles also improves NMES tolerance and comfort for strong motor stimulation.

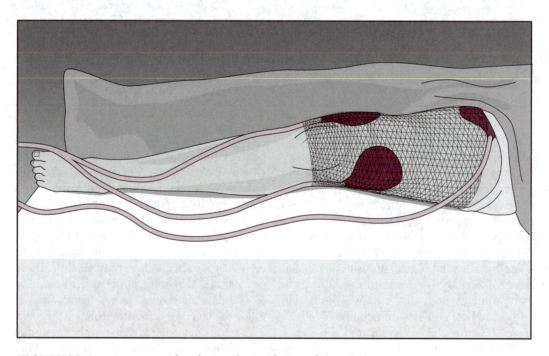

FIGURE 20–1   Neuromuscular electrical stimulation of the quadriceps.

Muscle Spasm

Trauma, pain, and muscle weakness may lead to irritation and pain; this condition is commonly referred to as **muscle spasm** or **muscle-holding state** (see **Chapter 6**). The cause and mechanism of this condition are not clearly understood. The possible causes include microtrauma, accumulation of metabolic irritants, and pain. Anxiety and tension seem to increase the occurrence or severity of this condition. Regardless of the original cause, pain and discomfort result in more pain and protective muscle holding; thus, a vicious cycle of "pain-spasm-pain" is established. Electrical stimulation, by increasing the circulation in large vessels[10,11] and enhancing nutrition, may be an effective means of disrupting this cycle and thus facilitating normal function. The goals of intervention are to relieve pain, promote relaxation of the involved muscles, and restore normal motion to the area of pain.

There are two methods for treating muscle spasm with electrical stimulation: (1) intermittent electrical stimulation and (2) high-frequency stimulation to elicit a sustained and continuous contraction of the muscles in spasm.

Intermittent electrical stimulation causes alternating muscle contraction and relaxation. Such rhythmic activation of the muscles causes an increase in the local circulation, helps remove metabolic irritants from the area, and provides a mechanical stimulation to muscle fibers.

High-frequency stimulation is used to elicit sustained and continuous muscle contractions of the muscles in spasm. The goal is to induce fatigue in the muscle. The patient's tolerance and the predisposition of the muscle to local ischemia should be carefully assessed before this approach is used. Because sustained muscle contractions may impede normal blood flow to the area, low stimulating frequencies are used.

Central Nervous System Lesions

Provided that the peripheral nervous system is intact, NMES can induce muscle contractions when there is a loss of volitional control due to a central nervous system (CNS) lesion (**Fig. 20–2**). Neuromuscular electrical stimulation can be used in conjunction with therapeutic exercise and functional retraining to enhance motor control following cerebral vascular accident (CVA) or traumatic brain injury (TBI).[12,13] As individuals with hemiparesis work with NMES-induced contractions, the goal is to facilitate reconnection from the lesioned and surrounding areas of the brain to the affected muscles. In addition, the NMES may increase sensory input and in some cases provide a temporary reduction in spasticity.[14]

Varying rationales have been posed to explain the mechanism responsible for reducing spasticity by electrical stimulation. Walker et al,[15] demonstrated that a 20-pps spike waveform stimulation of the radial, median, and saphenous nerves, applied for 1 hour twice a day for 1 week, suppressed clonus via spinal reflexes. The effect was reported to have lasted approximately 3 hours. Stimulation of the spastic muscles resulted in a generalized decrease of abnormal tone and the flexion-reflex response. One possible mechanism involved in reducing spasticity is sensory habituation of cutaneous reflexes. High-frequency stimulation of spastic muscles to produce tetanic muscle contraction and an amplitude adjusted to produce the maximum tolerable contraction has also been shown to reduce spasticity in patients with spinal cord injuries.[16–18] The reduction in tone lasted approximately 30 min after stimulation. A possible rationale for the decrease in tone may be the antidromic activation of the axon of an alpha motor neuron. The antidromic stimulation of the alpha motor neuron activates the motor unit and, through recurrent collaterals, excites a pool of Renshaw cells. In turn, the Renshaw cells inhibit the alpha motor neurons of the activated pool and the motor neurons of synergistic muscles. A thorough discussion of motor neurons and the role of Renshaw cells can be found elsewhere.[19]

Electrical stimulation of the antagonist muscle has been associated with concomitant inhibition of the spastic agonist muscle. Baker et al[14] reported a reduction of flexor spasticity in hemiplegic patients following bipolar stimulation of wrist and finger extensors. They used a monophasic stimulus of 200 microseconds duration at a rate of 33 pps, with a 7 seconds on, 10 seconds off, duty cycle and an amplitude high enough to produce a sustained isotonic muscle contraction through the full range of motion. Alfieri[20] demonstrated a reduction in spasticity lasting from 10 to 15 minutes to 2 hours in 96 hemiplegic patients when muscles antagonistic to those with spasticity were stimulated.

Electrical stimulation of spastic muscles and their antagonists with a rhythmical reciprocal pattern of stimulation, activating agonist and antagonists alternately, has effectively reduced spasticity. Vodovnic et al[21] reported a reduction in the hypertonicity of knee flexors and extensors of patients with spinal cord

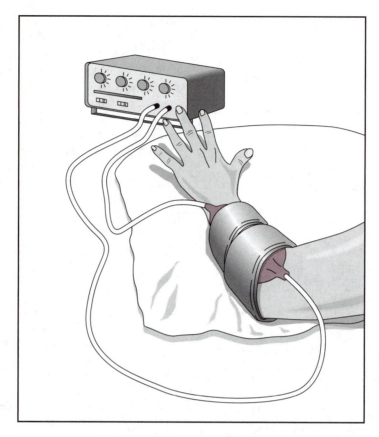

FIGURE 20–2   Neuromuscular electrical stimulation to activate paretic wrist extensors.

injuries following a reciprocal pattern of bipolar stimulation of quadriceps and hamstrings. The stimulus used was asymmetrical biphasic pulses of 300 microseconds duration at a rate of 30 pps and 100 mA current amplitude. Stimulation lasted for 30 min.

In summary, three methods of electrical stimulation are used to decrease spasticity: (1) direct stimulation of the spastic muscles, (2) stimulation of muscles antagonistic to the spastic muscles, and (3) reciprocal stimulation of spastic muscles and their antagonists.

Individuals with CNS lesions are prone to joint and soft-tissue restrictions arising from paralysis and spasticity. Muscle and joint tightness can be prevented when NMES is used in conjunction with passive ROM and soft-tissue stretching.[22] Electrically evoked muscle contractions help move associated joints through their available ROM when active motion is not possible because of paralysis and spasticity. This type of application works best on smaller joints such as the wrist or ankle. In addition to working on ROM,

repetitive NMES activation helps prevent disuse atrophy by creating contractions in the paretic muscle.

Neuromuscular electrical stimulation is also used to provide functional joint movements and stabilization when there are motor control deficits. This type of application is termed **functional electrical stimulation (FES)** and is used during activities such as standing, walking (**Fig. 20–3**), and reaching. Muscle activation required for the stance and swing phase of gait can be programmed in the NMES unit. Pressure sensors can be placed in the shoe to trigger NMES-induced contraction in antigravity muscles during stance (eg, quadriceps) and dorsiflexor muscles during swing (eg, anterior tibialis). The FES on and off times are dictated by the functional activity.

Hemiplegic shoulder subluxation and overstretching of shoulder muscles have been treated with NMES.[23,24] Deltoid and supraspinatus stimulation during standing and upright activities help support the shoulder without the use of a constricting arm sling. Daily stimulation

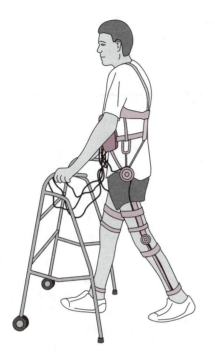

FIGURE 20–3 Multichannel functional electrical stimulation for ambulation in an individual with quadriparesis.

with a motor intensity and frequency lasting up to *6 hours* a day has been shown to reduce the abnormally large suprahumeral space and improve volitional muscle activation following cerebrovascular accident (CVA).[24]

Individuals with spinal cord injury (SCI) use NMES to prevent disuse atrophy and strengthen muscles with full peripheral nervous system (PNS) and partial CNS innervation.[25] Patients are able to increase muscle-fiber recruitment as they work along with the NMES. In addition, repetitive lower extremity NMES has been used for general conditioning, with the paretic muscle stimulated to allow cycling on a modified stationary bicycle. A significant increase in peripheral circulation, cardiovascular work performance, and maximal oxygen consumption in individuals with SCI is reported when utilizing electrically induced cycling programs.[26,27]

Neuromuscular electrical stimulation used with assistive devices, such as rolling walkers and lower leg bracing, increases standing and walking independence for individuals with SCI.[28,29] Stimulation is programmed to excite required muscles throughout the normal gait cycle. Although movements tend to be robotic and fatiguing, the option for standing and walking and its associated health benefits are made available for the individual with SCI.

PERIPHERAL NERVOUS SYSTEM LESIONS

In cases of peripheral nerve denervation, muscle must be directly stimulated because there is no motor nerve present to depolarize for muscle contraction. Muscle is not as excitable as nerve to electrical stimulation, as evidenced by an inability to respond to short-duration currents (pulsatile or alternating current). Most NMES units use short-duration currents and cannot be used for denervated muscle stimulation. Direct muscle stimulation requires long-duration direct current (DC) to produce a muscle contraction. Interrupted DC stimulation may be beneficial by producing muscle contraction and increasing circulation and nutrition in the denervated muscle. These effects may help slow down the changes resulting from the lack of physical activity of the denervated muscles. Animal model studies have indicated that electrical stimulation of denervated muscles retards atrophy.[30–32] However, other studies have shown that electrical stimulation of denervated muscles may actually interfere with peripheral nerve regeneration.[33–35]

The controversy over the benefits and disadvantages of this approach is supported by numerous conflicting studies. (A thorough review of this topic appears elsewhere.[36]) In light of the controversial results and the possible disadvantage of electrical stimulation in denervated muscles, the physical therapist's primary goal of maintaining joint mobility and function in patients with peripheral nerve injury resulting in denervation can be better accomplished by other therapeutic approaches such as soft-tissue mobilization, therapeutic exercise, bracing, and positioning.

PERIPHERAL VASCULAR DYSFUNCTION

Trauma may cause an excessive amount of body fluids to accumulate in the interstitial spaces. Congestion of body fluids also may occur because of compromised peripheral vascular function such as venous insufficiency and reduced lymphatic reabsorption. Muscle contractions during routine daily activities such as walking provide pumping action, which aids venous and lymphatic return. Individuals are encouraged to perform exercises such as ankle pumps, quadriceps isometrics, and gluteus maximus isometrics to maintain good venous return and to help mobilize postoperative edema. Individuals with postmasectomy edema can elevate their involved upper extremity and create a muscle pump by repetitively opening and closing the hand. Interference with the pumping action of muscles can occur as a result of trauma; decreased activity, as in prolonged bed rest; or weakness, pain, or other neuromuscular problems. Electrical stimulation of these muscles may improve the pumping action and thus improve circulation by increasing venous return and mobilizing edema.[37]

Muscle contractions must be closely monitored for individuals with severe peripheral arterial occlusive disease (PAOD) because of increased risk for muscle ischemia and claudication. As with active contractions, the individual with PAOD may not be able to transport the required oxygen and nutrients to the contracting muscle. Increased rest periods between electrically induced contractions and decreased pulse amplitude and frequency are effective ways to minimize ischemic pain. Electrodes can be placed at the motor points in the major muscle groups of the lower extremity in order to create a muscle pump. Electrically induced contractions, much like pneumatic external compression, are also beneficial to prevent stagnation of venous blood flow and associated risks for thrombus formation.

WOUND HEALING

Electrotherapy can be integrated in the intervention of poorly healing wounds. Normally, wounds will heal as they pass through the different phases of inflammation, proliferation, and maturation.[38] There are barriers that impede normal healing—arterial insufficiency, venous insufficiency, prolonged pressure in and around the wound, and peripheral neuropathy—with associated abnormal sensory, motor, and autonomic changes in the foot and lower leg. Protective footwear, pressure relief, edema reduction, and promotion of an optimal wound environment with proper dressings are essential in the prevention and intervention of wounds.

Wounds demonstrate a subtle difference in electrical potential when compared with surrounding intact tissue.[39] A positive potential has been identified in the wound, and it is considered necessary to initiate the healing process. As the wound progresses through proliferation, the potential will become less positive and will eventually match the negative charge seen in the intact epidermis after maturation. Electrical stimulation delivered through a conductive dressing has been hypothesized to add the electrical potential required for healing.

The healing process of wounds also begins with the formation and migration of epithelial cells, the activation of phagocytes, an increase in the number of polymorphonuclear leukocytes and lymphocytes, and an increase in the synthesis of fibroblast and collagen. Electrical stimulation, especially at the positive electrode, has been shown to increase the number of polymorphonuclear leukoctyes, increase collagen synthesis, and accelerate wound epithelialization.[40] Clinicians generally agree that the positive electrical field is more effective for tissue healing.

Chemical changes (eg, altering wound pH) are believed to create an environment that kills certain types of bacteria. In vitro and in vivo studies have supported the bactericidal effects of electrical stimulation. In vitro electrical stimulation of *Staphylococcus aureus*[41] and *Escherichia coli*[42] with continuous low-intensity DC have been shown to have bactericidal effect either by retarding or inhibiting bacterial growth. Furthermore, Rowley et al[43] stimulated ischemic skin ulcers of humans with low-intensity direct current (200–1000 uA) using the negative electrode, and found that the stimulation retarded the growth of *Pseudomonas aeruginosa*. The bacterial count in their study either decreased or remained stable, whereas the count for the control group increased. Kincaid and Lavoie[44] reported that the growth of three species of bacteria was inhibited by stimulation with high-voltage monophasic pulses.

The precise mechanism for the bactericidal effect is not clearly understood. One plausible rationale is the depletion of substrates as a result of continued cell membrane excitability as the microorganism attempts to maintain homeostasis. Another plausible rationale is that the electrical fields alter the internal processes of the microorganism and thus cause its death.[45] These mechanisms may work together or separately. For the bactericidal effect, a negative electrical field, with high voltage pulsed current (HVPC) and low-amplitude direct current are used. The negative electrode is recommended to create the bactericidal effects during wound stimulation. Negative polarity with low intensity direct current (LIDC) has also been reported to increase the strength and density of surgical scars during maturation.[46] Nalty et al[47] provide a review of intervention time, waveform/polarity choice, and stimulation parameters in the various studies using electrical stimulation for wound healing.

Polarity is the essential element when using electrical stimulation for direct wound healing. The current should flow in one direction so that the electrical field can be maintained under the electrodes. The waveforms most commonly used are monophasic pulsatile (high-voltage galvanic stimulation) and low-intensity direct current (LIDC). Sterile technique and universal precautions to protect the patient and health care provider need to be followed as a conductive dressing such as a hydrogel or saline-soaked gauze is loosely packed into the wound (**Fig. 20–4**). A unipolar technique is indicated, in which a small disposable electrode is placed over the wound dressing, and a large dispersive electrode is placed at a remote proximal site. The positive electrode is used for tissue healing. If a bacterial infection is evident, the negative electrode is used first until the infection clears up, then followed by positive electrode stimulation for tissue

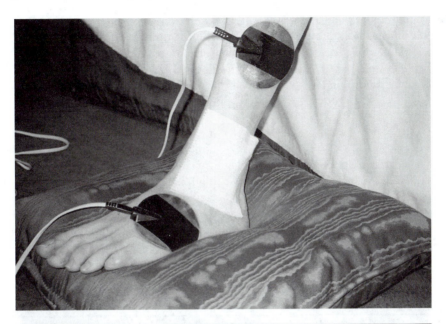

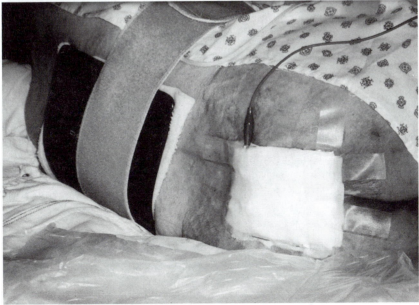

FIGURE 20–4 Electrode setups for wound healing interventions. (*Reproduced with permission from Nelson RM, Clinical Electrotherapy, 3rd ed., Prentice Hall, Upper Saddle River, NJ.*)

healing. Wound size and depth measures and photographs should be taken before and periodically after the intervention to document progress. Polarity may be switched if it appears that there has been a plateau in the healing process.

To further facilitate healing, pressure at the wound site must be avoided and excessive necrotic tissue removed. Direct stimulation to the wound should never be so high as to create a motor response that may disrupt or traumatize the fragile granulation tissue. Patient positioning is based on the type of wound receiving electrical stimulation. A venous wound is treated with the leg elevated and an arterial wound with the leg in a dependent position.

INCONTINENCE

Skeletal and smooth-muscle contraction of the pelvic floor can be achieved with NMES. **Pelvic floor electrical stimulation (PFES)** is used to treat stress and urge incontinence as surface electrodes and indwelling probes are placed in and around the anal/vaginal areas to depolarize the pudendal nerve.[48,49] Pelvic floor muscles and the anal and external urethral sphincter will contract as sufficient current intensity depolarizes the pudendal nerve.

Stress incontinence, seen in many postmenopausal women, is marked by bladder leakage due to sphincter and pelvic floor muscle weakness. When treating stress incontinence, integrating high-frequency electrical stimulation (20–50 pps) with active exercise (eg, Kegel exercises) and biofeedback helps increase pelvic floor awareness and an individual's ability to volitionally recruit pelvic floor musculature.[49] An increase in pelvic floor fast-twitch muscle fibers and slow-twitch fiber strength needed for resting urethral closure is reported following training regimes with high frequency PFES.[50]

Pelvic floor electrical stimulation is also indicated for detrusor (bladder smooth muscle) inhibition.[51] Inhibitory neurons that promote bladder relaxation are activated with low-frequency PFES (5–20 pps). Inhibitory low-frequency PFES is indicated for urge incontinence, in which the bladder is hyperactive and the individual has difficulty reaching the bathroom because of poor general mobility. For more on pelvic floor rehabilitation, see **Chapter 30.**

REVIEW QUESTIONS

1. Identify the precautions and contraindications for using electrical stimulation.

2. Provide the rationale and stimulation parameters for using electrical stimulation for muscle strengthening.

3. Provide the rationale and stimulation parameters for using electrical stimulation for the temporary reduction of spasticity.

4. Provide the rationale and stimulation parameters for using electrical stimulation for increasing venous return and edema mobilization.

5. What types of electrical current are recommended for wound healing protocols?

6. What types of electrical current are recommended for stimulation of peripherally denervated muscle?

7. Provide some examples of how neuromuscular electrical stimulation can be used during functional activities.

8. How can fatigue with neuromuscular electrical stimulation be minimized?

9. Describe the electrode management when using electrical stimulation for wound healing.

10. What are the recommended stimulation parameters for pelvic floor electrical stimulation?

KEY WORDS

neuromuscular electrical stimulation (NMES)
muscle spasm

muscle-holding state
functional electrical stimulation (FES)

pelvic floor electrical stimulation (PFES)

REFERENCES

1. Delito A, Rose SJ, et al: Electrical versus voluntary exercise in strengthening the thigh musculature in patients after anterior cruciate ligament surgery. *Phys Ther* 1988; 68:660–63.

2. Eriksson E, Haggmark T: Comparison of isometric muscle training in the recovery after major knee ligament surgery. *Am J Sports Med* 1979; 7:169–71.

3. Delitto A, Snyder-Mackler L: Two theories of muscle strength augmentation using percutaneous electrical stimulation. *Physical Therapy* 1990; 70:158–64.

4. Knight KL: Electrical muscle stimulation during immobilization. *Phys Sport Ed* 1980; 8:147.

5. Godfrey CM, Jayawardena H, et al: Comparison of electrostimulation and isometric exercise in strengthening the quadriceps muscle. *Physiother Cana* 1979; 31:265–67.

6. Gould N, Donnermeyer D, et al: Transcutaneous muscle stimulation to retard disuse atrophy after open meniscectomy. *Clin Orthop Rel Res* 1983; 178:190–97.

7. Morrissey MC, Brewster CE, et al: The effect of electrical stimulation on the quadriceps during postoperative knee immobilization. *Am J Sports Med.* 1985; 13:40–45.

8. Alon G, McCombe SA, Koutsantonis S, et al: Comparison of the effects of electrical stimulation and exercise on abdominal musculature. *J Orthop Sports Phys Ther* 1987; 8:567–73.

9. Grove-Lainey C, Walmsley RP, Andrew GM: Effectiveness of exercise alone versus exercise plus electrical stimulation in strengthening the quadriceps muscle. *Physiother Can* 1983; 35:5–11.

10. Randall BF, Imig CJ, Hines HM: Effect of electrical stimulation upon blood flow and temperature of skeletal muscle. *Am J Phys Med* 1953; 32:22.

11. Currier D, Petrilli C, Threlkeld J: Effect of medium frequency electrical stimulation on local blood circulation to healthy muscles. *Phys Ther* 1986; 66:937.

12. Bogataj U, Gros N, Malezic M, et al: Restoration of gait during two to three weeks of therapy with multichannel electrical stimulation. *Physical Ther* 1989; 69:319–27.

13. Baker LL, Parker K, Sanderson, D: Neuromuscular electrical stimulation for the head injured patient. *Physical Ther* 1983; 63:1967–74.

14. Baker LL, Yeh C, et al: Electrical stimulation of wrist and fingers for hemiplegic patients. *Phys Ther* 1979; 59:1495–99.

15. Walker JB: Modulation of spasticity: A prolonged suppression of spinal reflex by electrical stimulation. *Science* 1982; 216:203–04.

16. Lee WJ, McGovern JP, Duval EN: Continuous tetanizing currents for relief of spasm. *Arch Phys Med* 1950; 31:766–71.

17. Bowman B, Bajd T: Influence of electrical stimulation on skeletal muscle spasticity. In: *Proceedings of the International Symposium on External Control of Human Extremities.* Belgrade, Yugoslavia: Committee for Electronics and Automation; 1981; 561–76.

18. Vodovnik L, Bowman BR, Hufford P: Effects of electrical stimulation on spinal spasticity. *Scand J Rehabil Med* 1984; 16:29.

19. Somjen G: *Neurophysiology: The Essentials.* Baltimore: Williams & Wilkins, 1983.

20. Alfieri V: Electrical treatment of spasticity. *Scand J Rehabil Med* 1982; 14:177–82.

21. Vodovnic L, Stanic U, et al: Functional electrical stimulation for control of locomotor systems. *Crit Rev Bioeng* 1981; 6:63–131.

22. DeVahl J: Neuromuscular electrical stimulation in rehabilitation. In: Gersch MR, ed. *Electrotherapy in Rehabilitation.* Philadelphia: Davis; 1992; 237–39.

23. Baker LL: Neuromuscular electrical stimulation of the muscles surrounding the shoulder. *Phys Ther* 1986; 66:1930–34.

24. Faghri PD, Rodgers MM, Glaser RM: The effects of functional electrical stimulation on shoulder subluxation, arm function recovery, and shoulder pain in hemiplegic stroke patients. *Arch Phys Med Rehabil* 1994; 75:73–79.

25. Nalty T, Sabbahi MA: Electrical stimulation of the spinal cord injured person. In Nalty T, Sabbahi MA, eds. *Electrotherapy: Clinical Procedures Manual.* New York: McGraw-Hill; 2001:229–51.

26. Mohr T, Andersen J, Biering-Sorensen F, et al: Long-term adaptation to electrically induced cycle training in severe spinal cord injured individuals. *Spinal Cord* 1997; 35:1–6.

27. Nash MS, Montalvo BM, Applegate, B: Lower extremity blood flow and responses to occlusion

ischemia differ in exercise-trained and sedentary tetraplegic persons. *Arch Phys Med Rehabil* 1996; 77:1260–65.

28. Gallien P, Brissot R, Eyssette M, et al: Restoration of gait by functional electrical stimulation for spinal cord injured patients. *Paraplegia* 1995; 33:660–64.

29. Stein RB, Gordon T, Jefferson J, et al. Optimal stimulation of paralyzed muscle after human spinal cord injury. *J. Appl. Physiol* 1992, 72:1393–1400.

30. Davis H: Is electrostimulation beneficial to denervated muscles? A review of results from basic research. *Physiother Can* 1983; 35:306–10.

31. Harada Y, Nakano K, Fujiwara M: Effects of electrical stimulation on the denervated rat muscle. *Acta Med Hypogoensia* 1979; 4:129.

32. Pachter BR, Eberstein A, Goodgold J: Electrical stimulation effect on denervated skeletal myofibers in rats: A light and electron microscopic study. *Arch Phys Med Rehabil* 1982; 63:427.

33. Girlanda R, Dattola R, Vita G, et al: Effect of electrotherapy on denervated muscles in rabbits: An electrophysiological and morphological study. *Exp Neurol* 1982; 77:483.

34. Brown MC, Holland RL, Ironton R: Nodal and terminal sprouting from motor nerves in fast and slow muscles of the mouse. *J Physiol* 1980; 306:493.

35. Ironton R, Brown MC, Holland RL: Stimuli to intramuscular nerve growth. *Brain Res* 1978; 156:351.

36. Spielholz N: Electrical stimulation of denervated muscle. In: Nelson R, Currier D, eds. *Clinical Electrotherapy*, 3rd ed. Norwalk, CT: Appleton & Lange; 1999:411–46.

37. Alon G, DeDomenico G: *High Voltage Stimulation: An Integrated Approach to Clinical Electrotherapy*. Chattanooga, TN: Chatanooga Corporation; 1987.

38. Kloth L, McCulloch J, Feedar: *Wound Healing: Alternatives in Management*. Philadelphia: Davis; 1990.

39. Becker RO, Murray DG: Method for producing cellular differentiation by means of very small electrical currents. *Trans NY Acad Sci* 1967; 29:606.

40. Carley P, Wainapel S: Electrotherapy for acceleration of wound healing: Low intensity direct current. *Arch Phys Med Rehabil* 1985; 66:443–46.

41. Barranco S, Berger T: In vitro effect of weak direct current on *Staphylococcus Aureus*. *Clin Orthop* 1974; 100:250–55.

42. Rowley B: Electrical current effects on *E. coli* growth rates. *Proc Soc Exp Biol Med* 1972; 139: 929–34.

43. Rowley B, et al: The influence of electrical current on an infecting microorganism in wounds. *Ann NY Acad Sci* 1974; 238:543–51.

44. Kincaid C, Lavoie K: Inhibition of bacterial growth in vitro following stimulation with high voltage, monophasic pulse current. *Phys Ther* 1989; 69:651–55.

45. Wolcott L, et al: An accelerated healing of skin ulcer by electrotherapy: Preliminary clinical results. *South Med J* 1969; 62:795–801.

46. Dunn MG, Doillon CJ, Berg RA, et al: Wound healing using a collagen matrix: Effect of DC electrical stimulation. *J Biomed Mater Res* 1988; 22:191–206.

47. Nalty T, Sabbahi MA: Electrical stimulation to promote wound healing. In Nalty T, Sabbahi MA, eds. *Electrotherapy: Clinical Procedures Manual.* New York: McGraw-Hill; 2001:105–29.

48. Fall M: Advantages and pitfalls of functional electrical stimulation. *Acta Obstet Gynecol Scand* 1998; 168:16–21.

49. Bo, K: Effect of electrical stimulation on stress and urge urinary incontinence: Clinical outcome and practical recommendations based on randomized controlled trials. *Acta Obstet Gynecol Scand* 1998; 168:3–11.

50. Fall M, Lindstrom S: Electrical stimulation: A physiological approach to the treatment of urinary incontinence. *Urol Clin North Am* 1991; 18:393–407.

51. Yaminishi T, Yasuda K, Sakakibara, R., et al: Randomized, double-blind study of electrical stimulation for urinary incontinence due to detrusor overactivity. *Urology* 2000; 55:353–57.

21

Transcutaneous Electrical Nerve Stimulation (TENS)

JOSEPH WEISBERG, PT, PhD
ROBERT TROIANO, MS, DPT, CHT

Chapter Outline

Transcutaneous electrical nerve stimulation (TENS) is the procedure of applying controlled, low-voltage electrical impulses to the nervous system by passing electricity through the skin via surface electrodes.[1] Its primary purpose is to control or alleviate pain. Treating both acute and chronic pain by use of TENS has been widely used in both the medical and rehabilitative communities over the past three decades.[2–23] Transcutaneous electrical nerve stimulation was originally developed as a byproduct of the Dorsal Column Electrical Stimulator, a device formerly used to control pain by directly stimulating the nerves in the dorsal column of the spinal cord. The Dorsal Column Electrical Stimulator needed to be surgically implanted to provide pain relief. Transcutaneous electrical nerve stimulation was used to screen patients and to test the effects of such stimulation before the implantation procedure. Investigators soon realized that TENS alone was producing the desired analgesic effects. Intervention with this surface device was sufficient to reduce the patient's pain and avoid surgical implantation. Increasing clinical use of TENS was seen during the 1970s. The 1980s and 1990s brought more convenient machines and a wealth of documented cases of pain relief using this modality.

The user-friendly application of TENS has made it a popular choice for treating many postsurgical and painful conditions.[2–23] Transcutaneous electrical nerve stimulation appears to be surviving the onset of managed care because of its efficacy, simplicity, and its availability to patients in their homes. Similarly, TENS has survived the scrutiny of the Food and Drug Administration (FDA) because it is a safe and an effective method of treating pain. Transcutaneous electrical nerve stimulation has few contraindications and minimal side effects. According to the FDA's medical device regulations, TENS is considered to be a Class II device whose distribution and application to patients must be prescribed by a licensed physician.

PAIN SUPPRESSION THEORIES

Several theories have been postulated to explain why TENS changes the perception of pain. The first theory, and the one responsible for the development of TENS, is the gate theory. This theory states that stimulation of non-nociceptors or their axons can interfere with the relay of sensation from the nociceptors to higher centers in the brain where pain is perceived.[24] According to the theory, TENS stimulates large sensory a-beta fibers with high-frequency stimulation. The impulses of this stimulation flood the pathway to the brain and close the "gate" to transmission of pain. This type of stimulation seems to manage the pain threshold.[25] The gate theory, proposed by Melzack and Wall, has recently undergone refinement to include the influence of descending pain control mechanisms on the "gating" effect.[26]

The second theory is based on the existence of natural opiates, (pain suppressors), in the body. These opiates are produced by the pituitary gland (beta endorphins) and in the spinal cord (enkephalins). Stimulation of sensory nerves with low-frequency TENS stimulates the release of these opiates, thus affecting the perception of pain.[27] Other investigators have proposed that the release of these natural opiates are the result of sympathetic nervous system and brainstem nuclei stimulation.[28]

A third theory relates to the findings of several investigators that TENS stimulation induces local vasodilation in patients with myofascial symptoms or other painful conditions,[29–31] targeting pain that is caused by trigger points. These trigger points may be the result of tissue ischemia. Fassbender[31] demonstrated that the trigger points are in fact related to ischemic areas in the connective tissue and/or muscle. The vasodilatation produced by the TENS intervention possibly alters the ischemic area, thus decreasing the pain.

Another means of affecting vasodilatation is through sympathetic nervous system stimulation. TENS may activate the sympathetic nervous system, causing vasomotor responses, with the resultant increase in blood flow dissipating pain-producing substances.[28]

A fourth theory relates to acupuncture, the practice of which is based on energy lines (meridians) and entry points (acupuncture points). The theory is that TENS can be used to stimulate acupuncture points that affect the flow of energy (chi) through the meridians, thus altering the condition that caused the pain. Several studies indicate that stimulating acupuncture points as an intervention for pain may be as effective, or even more effective, than using TENS on other somatic points.[32,33]

In looking at all possible mechanisms in which TENS may affect pain perception, it is important to consider its role at other sites in the nervous system in addition to the dorsal horn. Transcutaneous electrical nerve stimulation may mediate pain responses at several levels of the CNS or PNS. Antidromic stimulation of the afferent neurons may be a possible mechanism of TENS action that is proposed to block the transmission of impulses from the nociceptors to the spinal cord.[28] By creating antidromic stimulation, substance P is thought to be released from sensory neurons, leading to vasodilation. It was demonstrated by Levin et al[34] that both acupuncturelike and conventional TENS stimulate similar afferent fibers.

It is important to briefly mention here the role of the **placebo effect** on pain suppression. Lewis et al[35] demonstrated that active TENS resulted in no clear benefit compared with placebo TENS in a 9-week crossover study on 36 patients. Other investigators have demonstrated similar results.[36,37]

Treating pain with TENS is never a simple matter because patients and their conditions present the clinician with many variables. Furthermore, clinical use of TENS is itself varied, and each practitioner claims success with particular protocols. The therapist must realize that the key to clinical effectiveness lies in understanding the uses of TENS and its limitations—not in any specific formula that seemed to work for someone else. Transcutaneous electrical stimulation, like many other intervention techniques, must be patient-specific.

INDICATIONS AND CONTRAINDICATIONS

Indications

Indications for TENS intervention include, but are not limited to, the various pain syndromes:

- acute pain
- chronic pain
- phantom limb pain
- postoperative pain
- obstetric pain
- menstrual pain
- cardiopulmonary pain
- arthritic pain
- peripherally based neurologic pain (eg, shingles)
- preceding potentially painful interventions (eg, stretching a contracture, wound debridement) to elevate the patient's pain threshold[38]

Contraindications

The contraindications for TENS are listed at the beginning of Chapter 20. In general, TENS is a safe modality. Very few negative effects have been reported in the literature. One adverse reaction reported has been skin irritation. The source of this irritation may be an allergic reaction to the gel or adhesive, poor application technique (eg, lack of gel, inadequate cleansing of the skin, or uneven electrode contact), excessive intervention time, or rough removal of electrodes. Electrically induced thermal burns are possible, but rare. A burn would be the result of elevated current density either beneath or between electrodes. The therapist must also consider that if the current is unevenly distributed in areas under the electrodes, micropunctate electrothermal burns can occur.[28] Uneven current distribution may be the result of poor skin-electrode contact.

INSTRUMENTS

Figure 21–1 displays a typical transcutaneous electrical nerve stimulator being used for pain modulation. Although many different TENS units are available, most have the following features:

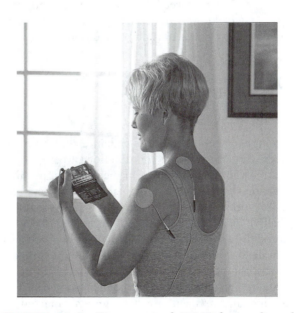

FIGURE 21–1 Home use of TENS for neck and shoulder pain. (*Courtesy of Empi, Inc., St. Paul, MN.*)

- solid-state generators, for durability;
- rechargeable battery, for convenience and economy;
- single, dual, or multiple channels, for multiple electrode placement;
- intensity control; large myelinated fibers require less current than small unmyelinated fibers;
- pulse frequency control; large myelinated fibers respond to a high rate (more than 100 pps), whereas small unmyelinated fibers respond more effectively to a low rate (less than 100 pps);
- pulse duration control; large myelinated fibers respond to impulses with shorter duration (50 ms), whereas small unmyelinated fibers respond to impulses of longer duration (200 ms);
- a variety of waveforms; the waveform generated is usually of constant current, asymmetric, and biphasic;
- modulation control, which allows the therapist to vary the current characteristics by at least 10%; varying the parameters (usually frequency or pulse duration) will delay accommodation of the nervous system to the TENS;
- electrodes; the most commonly used types are discussed later;
- weight of unit; portable, with an average weight of about 8 oz.; and
- size of unit; approximately 3 × 5 inches.

According to the weight and size of these units, patients are able to wear the device and move about during sessions, which is an added convenience.

Procedure

Initial Assessment

A complete assessment of the patient includes a medical history, the etiology and duration of pain, previous interventions, current pain medications, pending litigation that is related to the pain, employment status, as specific a description of the pain as possible (quality, location, frequency, duration, etc.), and a thorough physical examination. It may be beneficial in evaluating the interventions' ultimate effectiveness to have the patient fill out a standardized pain questionnaire, including a visual analogue pain scale.[39,40] A baseline measurement of vital signs is obtained to evaluate any effects that the TENS intervention may have on these values.

Approach to the Patient

After deciding that TENS is the appropriate intervention, the therapist explains the procedure to the patient to allay any anxiety about electrical modalities, describing the type of sensation usually associated with TENS. The therapist explains that the patient controls the intensity and can terminate the procedure at any time. Furthermore, **the therapist needs to emphasize the fact that TENS will not cure the underlying problem.** TENS treats the symptom of pain much as pain medication does. When TENS is planned for postsurgical pain relief, the therapist must explain the procedure to the patient *before* surgery. After the surgery, the therapist ascertains that the patient fully comprehends the instructions and is applying the device appropriately. Continual monitoring of patient's use of the device and reaction to the intervention is vital. Adjustment in the mode of application may be necessary to optimize results. Once it is clear that the patient fully understands the use of the TENS device, the unit may be taken home.

As stated earlier in this chapter, pain can be of various origins and can be managed in several ways. It is important that patients understand that pain—especially constant pain of long duration—may be a sign of more serious pathology. It is important to address the use or abuse of TENS to mask the pain of more serious illnesses and to educate patients to pursue the proper medical intervention for more serious conditions.

Modes of Application

There are several commonly used modes of application. Four will be discussed here: (1) high-rate conventional, (2) low-rate acupuncturelike, (3) bursts of pulse trains, and (4) brief and intense.

High-rate conventional TENS is the most commonly used mode. It affects primarily the large afferent a-beta fibers, which are the pathway of segmental inhibition in the gate theory. Utilizing this mode of application, the clinician would use a high pulse frequency of 75–100 pps and a pulse duration of less than 200 sec. Pulse amplitude or intensity is set to a level at which the patient will experience a comfortable paresthesia with no muscle contraction. Intervention time is usually 30 to 60 min in the home setting and can be repeated several times a day on the basis of patient response. The authors do not recommend using this modality for extended periods of time (hours). Pain suppression effects may be of shorter duration than other modes.

Low-rate acupuncturelike TENS is directed toward the small-diameter (C) fibers. This type of stimulation affects both sensory and motor nerves in the area of pain or their corresponding segmental myotomes. Suprasegmental pain suppression via endorphin release has been suggested as the means of action of low-rate TENS. The stimulation characteristics are low-frequency (1–4 pps) and long-pulse duration (200–300 ms). The pulse amplitude is set at a level to produce visible muscle twitches. The intensity should be strong but within the patient's comfort level. Intervention time is usually 45 min, and the pain-relieving effects are usually of longer duration, lasting several hours and, at times, days.

Burst of pulse trains is a mode of TENS application wherein each burst contains a higher-frequency wave ranging from 5 to 100 Hz. These bursts are delivered at a low rate of 1–4 per second. Because of the low-burst delivery rate and the potential high frequency of pulses within the burst, this type of TENS can offer the benefits of both high-rate conventional TENS and low-rate acupuncturelike TENS (pain relief via the gating mechanism and the endorphin-mediated response).[28] The clinician can expect to see a visible muscle contraction with use of the mode.

Brief and intense TENS is a technique for inducing pain suppression in preparation for and during potentially painful medical procedures including wound debridement, friction massage, joint mobilization, passive stretching, and more. The parameters for this technique are a high rate (above 100 pps) and a long pulse duration (above 200 ms) current. The pulse amplitude should be at a level to achieve strong intermittent muscle fasciculation. This type of TENS stimulation results in surface analgesia lasting for 5 to 10 min.

Research has been conducted regarding the relevance of TENS to pain suppression, but investigators have produced varying results.[34,41,42] Clinically, patients also have varying degrees of success with the various modes of TENS. Therapists need to be flexible, exploring which mode of TENS is suitable for a particular patient. One approach is to begin with high-rate conventional TENS because it is the mode that the patient usually tolerates the best. If the patient's initial response is poor, the therapist first tries varying the placement of the electrodes, and then manipulating the parameters. Other modes may be used with this same patient only if these two strategies have failed. Finally, the patient should be told in advance that it may be necessary to change the parameters to achieve optimal results.

Selection of the TENS Unit

Many TENS devices are available on the market, and most permit the manipulation of three variables: (1) the amplitude (intensity) of the stimulus, (2) the pulse frequency, and (3) the pulse duration. Most TENS units employ a symmetric biphasic waveform. Several of the TENS units offer a modulation feature that will automatically alter the parameters during a given intervention session to avoid or delay accommodation by the patient.

Once the patient understands and can follow intervention protocols, the therapist selects the appropriate unit for that patient. The following questions should be answered before deciding which device the patient should rent or buy:

- Did the patient respond well to intervention with a particular unit?
- Do the characteristics of the unit encompass all that is required for effective intervention?
- Is the unit easy to operate, specifically by the patient with poor vision or dexterity?
- Is the unit durable and serviceable? (These units are expensive and therefore should serve the therapist or patient for many years.)
- Are rental units available for patients who need the unit for a relatively brief period?
- Is the size and weight of the unit appropriate for a particular patient?
- How will the cost of the unit be covered? Will you need a less sophisticated unit to keep costs down?

Selection of the Electrodes

Many different types of electrodes are available to meet patients' needs. The advantages of some electrodes are their disposability and ease of application; the advantages of others are that they are reusable, more economical, and more durable.

One type of electrode used is the fabric-covered orthopedic felt electrode that is soaked in water. This type of electrode causes the least amount of skin irritation; however, it must be rewet every 2 to 3 hours. Patients who are wearing their electrodes for longer periods of time may find this type very inconvenient.

Another type of electrode is the carbon-impregnated rubber electrode, or carbon-silicone electrode. This type requires the application of a gel for good conductivity. It has the advantage of allowing more continuous wear time by the patient (24 hours or more). The carbon-rubber electrode is a very popular electrode because it is reusable and therefore less expensive in the long run. One negative aspect of this electrode is that it must be held in place by adhesive tape or patch, and it requires conducting gel. Self-adhesive electrodes are convenient and popular for both clinic and home use. They are made of karaya gum or synthetic polymers.[28] These type of electrodes do not require conductive gel to be effective, but they are less durable and more expensive.

When selecting electrodes, the therapist should consider the relative size of the electrodes and its relationship to current density (amp/area)—the larger the electrodes, the less the current density. In most situations, the size of the two electrodes should be equal to permit equal current density under both. Finally, the therapist must consider the patient's mental ability, dexterity, financial situation, and the location of the sites to be stimulated

Placement of the Electrodes

To date, the literature has shown no optimal electrode placement that applies to all patients. The clinician bases electrode placement on several commonly used techniques, including the following:

- skin overlying the painful region
- superficial point of the peripheral nerve
- dermatomal distribution of the nerve involved
- trigger points
- acupuncture points
- segmentally related myotomes
- motor points (points on the skin where the least current activates the muscle)
- course of a peripheral nerve[28,43]

Selecting the site for stimulation depends on the etiology, location, and character of the pain. In addition, the clinician must consider the patient's initial response to the selected site. If desired results are not achieved by the initial placement, another site should be tried. Patients who are using the TENS unit at home may be instructed to change electrode placement to achieve the desired effect. Patients given the

clearance to change electrode placement must clearly understand all the contraindications and precautions that apply to the TENS device.

When electrode placement is changed, the intensity of the current that the patient can tolerate also may change, especially if the distance between the electrodes is changed. This is the case because skin resistance to the flow of current varies with the distance between the electrodes; the closer the electrodes, the more superficial and concentrated the stimulus. When electrodes are moved further apart, the converse is true. Accordingly, electrodes should be placed 1 cm or more from each other to avoid blistering or burning.

Electrodes can be placed unilaterally or bilaterally and can be bracketed or crossed. The electrodes can be placed along a peripheral nerve or along a dermatome. They can also be placed transcranially unless that method is contraindicated. The stimulation sites for acupuncturelike TENS are most commonly (1) acupuncture points, (2) superficial aspects of peripheral nerves, and (3) segmentally related myotomes.

Application of the Electrodes

After the appropriate sites have been selected, the conducting gel is applied uniformly on the electrodes. Each electrode should be secured to the skin to ensure total contact. If the clinician is using self-adherent electrodes, no gel or securing tape is required. Remember that poor skin contact may cause burning, rather than the desired paresthesia, in the area surrounding the electrode.

Stimulation Parameters

Adjustment of the stimulating parameters depends on the patient's condition, the mode being used, and the patient's tolerance. The primary purposes for adjusting stimulation parameters are (1) to avoid accommodation to the stimulus and (2) to substitute for the first set of parameters if they proved to be ineffective.

Optimal stimulation parameters for differing clinical conditions have not been clearly defined. However, Walsh et al[42] conducted a study in which their results demonstrated the importance of coupling certain pulse frequencies with certain pulse durations. They showed that a pulse frequency of 110 pps coupled with a pulse duration of 200 μsec was the most effective of the four combinations they tested.

Intervention time can range from minutes to hours. Usually, the intervention is given daily for about a week before the results are evaluated. If the results are positive, as determined by the patient's subjective response, the patient is asked to rent the device on a 30-day trial basis to evaluate its long-term effectiveness. As stated earlier, it may be beneficial to have the patient fill out a pain questionnaire or survey both before beginning the trial and at the end of the 30 days.

Postintervention Evaluation

It is critical that the patient fully demonstrate an understanding of the TENS device and application procedure before its effectiveness can be evaluated. Close monitoring during the 30-day period of TENS usage will ensure that the patient is adhering to the planned procedure.

The postintervention evaluation is necessarily imprecise because of the subjective nature of pain. Nonetheless, a clinician can assess the effectiveness of the intervention by the following:

- objective measures of improved function (eg, functional outcome measures, functional surveys, increased ROM, increased tolerance to an activity, increased strength).
- a descriptive pain scale (ranging from no pain through mild, moderate, severe, and very severe pain)
- a pain rating index from 1–10 (where 1 equals no pain and 10 equals excruciating pain)
- the patient's verbal description of the pain experience
- a visual analog scale by which the patient records pain intensity
- a combination of any of the preceding

POINT LOCATOR AND STIMULATOR

A **point locator/stimulator** is a device that identifies trigger or acupuncture points and is then used in interventions to stimulate the points. Trigger points and acupuncture points are often associated with myofascial and visceral pain and dysfunction. Many clinical approaches have been developed to treat pain and dysfunction, including the stimulating of these points

either electrically or with a cold laser beam. The effectiveness of trigger or acupuncture point therapy has recently been the subject of some research;[44–47] however, the effectiveness of electrical stimulation or cold laser stimulation is not well established.[5] The question of intertester reliability when identifying trigger points by manual means has also had recent study.[48,49,50]

Travell and Simons[51] have defined **trigger points** by four major criteria:

1. Palpable firm area of muscle, referred to as the taut band;
2. Within the taut band, a localized spot of exquisite tenderness to manual pressure, the TrP;
3. A characteristic pattern of pain, tingling, or numbness in response to sustained pressure on the TrP within the taut band; and
4. A local twitch of the taut band when the TrP is distorted transversely.

The impedance of the skin over a trigger point is also lower than that of most of the surrounding skin.[52] Stimulating the trigger point reduces its sensitivity and reduces the referred pain.

An **acupuncture point** is a point located on a meridian (a line of energy described in Chinese medicine). Acupuncture points are considered the entry points into the body's energy system. They are usually tender to palpation in the presence of pathology or dysfunction ("disharmony"). Stimulating these points helps to "rebalance" the disharmony in the body's energy system, thus reducing the "pathology of the dysfunction." The skin impedance of the acupuncture points is lower than the impedance of the surrounding skin.[53,54] Stimulating either a trigger point or an acupuncture point causes the impedance of these points to increase temporarily to the level of the surrounding tissue.[55]

STIMULATION OF POINTS

Skin impedance varies significantly among individuals. Moreover, skin impedance in one person varies from area to area. For example, the impedance of the skin in the palm of the hand is much less than it is in the dorsal aspect of the hand.[56] In addition, the impedance of the skin at any site may change over time as conditions affecting the physiology of the skin change. For example, pathology—especially hypothyroidism or hyperthyroidism,[56] sympathetic hyperactivity or hypoactivity,[57,58] and mental state—can cause physiologic changes in the skin that affect its impedance.

As was mentioned earlier, acupuncture and trigger points have lower impedance values relative to their surrounding tissue, and the lower impedance value at these points is constant.[52,59,60] However, once these points are stimulated (eg, with a cold laser beam), the skin impedance may increase to the level of the surrounding tissue. This change in impedance may be associated with improvement in a patient's symptoms.[48]

The point locator portion of a point locator/stimulator produces extremely low-voltage current, which is enough to flow only through points of low impedance. This current activates visual signals, auditory signals, or both in the unit, thereby indicating the sites of the points. Some units use a low-voltage current only to locate the site and then use the cold laser beam to stimulate the trigger or acupuncture points. One cold laser has now been approved for carpal tunnel syndrome. Most of the other types of units are currently accepted as therapeutic modalities, and their mode of stimulation is electrical current. Clinicians who use these devices claim clinical success. However, 5% of patients report an increased sensitivity to pain after the initial stimulation; this sensitivity then subsides after the second or third treatment.[61]

Technique

Figure 21–2 displays point stimulation to a trigger point. When treating patients, the therapist carries out the following steps:

- Cleanse the skin in the suspected area, preferably with 70% isopropyl alcohol to reduce the impedance of the skin.
- Place a handheld electrode in the patient's hand to complete the electrical circuit.
- Palpate for the pain-sensitive area, and identify the general location of the trigger or acupuncture point.
- Turn on the point locator of the unit, and adjust the sensitivity knob.
- Move the probe tip over the area to pinpoint the spot, and apply just enough pressure to ensure good contact. When the probe tip is immediately over the point, the therapist will hear a signal or see a display of lights or a moving needle, depend-

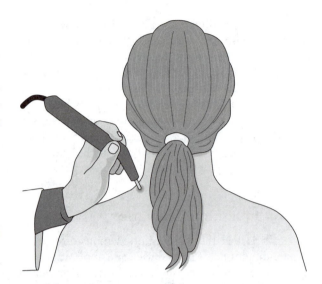

FIGURE 21–2   Point stimulation to a trigger point in the upper trapezius muscle.

ing on the type of unit. This device indicates that the impedance of the spot that the probe is touching is lower than that of the surrounding tissue.

- Stimulate the spot with electrical stimulation. The probe should remain in contact with the skin over the spot while the therapist switches the control from the point locator to the point stimulator and increases the current to the highest level that the patient can tolerate. If a cold laser beam is used, it is best to pull the probe away from the skin about 1 mm and to focus the beam at the site of low impedance.[62] For both electrical and laser stimulation, the duration of stimulation is 15–60 seconds per site.

For indications and contraindications to these modalities, see the indications and contraindications for TENS and laser treatments in **Chapters 19 and 28**. Finally, consult the manufacturer of the unit for more specific information.

Need for Further Research

Although more studies have been conducted regarding clinical effectiveness of TENS, many of them have produced conflicting results. Double-blind experiments have shown TENS to be effective; however, other studies show strong placebo effects. The bottom line is that, as with all therapeutic interventions, TENS usage needs to be challenged and investigated further. New studies should be undertaken to look at type of stimulator used, condition treated, mode of stimulation, specific parameters used (pulse duration, pulse frequency), placement of electrodes, type of electrodes, duration of intervention, and frequency of intervention.

As clinicians we strive to provide effective and efficient health care to our patients. We are continually faced with the changes in the current health care environment. TENS may be a more attractive option for both patients and third-party payers when compared with other costly medical procedures. We look forward to further investigation of this mode of intervention.

REVIEW QUESTIONS

1. Describe the gate theory of pain and the way that TENS can be used to modulate pain in line with the theory.

2. Describe the endogenous opiate theory of pain modulation and the way that TENS can be used to modulate pain in line with this theory.

3. Identify the possible electrode placements when using TENS for pain modulation.

4. Provide a list of general indications for the use of TENS for pain modulation.

5. When using TENS with motor intensity stimulation, why is it important to use a low-pulse frequency?

6. Identify the common features found in most small portable TENS units.

7. What are the criteria commonly used to determine a trigger point?

8. What is skin impedance, and how does it differ at trigger and acupuncture points?

9. Why is a monopolar technique used during point stimulation?

10. What are the usual treatment times for TENS and point stimulation when attempting to modulate pain?

KEY TERMS

transcutaneous electrical nerve
   stimulation (TENS)
placebo effect
high-rate conventional TENS

low-rate accupuncturelike TENS
burst of pulse trains
brief and intense TENS

point locator/stimulator
trigger points
acupuncture point

REFERENCES

1. Manheimer JS, Lampe GN: *Clinical Transcutaneous Electric Stimulation.* Philadelphia: Davis; 1984

2. Klin B, Uretzky G, Magora F: Tanscutaneous electrical nerve stimulations (TENS) after open heart surgery. *J Cardiovasc Surg* 1984; 25:445–48.

3. Lagas H, Zuurmond W, Rietschoten W, et al: Transcutaneous nerve stimulation for the treatment of postoperative pain. *Acta Anesthsiol Belg* 1984; 35:253–57.

4. Navarathnam R, Wang Y, Thomas D, et al: Evaluation of the transcutaneous electrical nerve stimulator for postoperative analgesia following cardiac surgery. *Anaesth Intensive Care* 1984; 12:345–50.

5. Ticho U, Olshwang D, Magora F: Relief of pain by subcutaneous electrical stimulation after ocular surgery. *Am J Ophthalmic* 1983; 89:803–08.

6. Arvidsson I, Eriksson E. Postoperative TENS pain relief after knee surgery. Objective evaluation. *Orthopedics* 1986; 9:1346–51.

7. Jensen JE, Conn RR, Hazelrigg G, et al: The use of transcutaneous neural stimulation and isokinetics testing in arthroscopic knee surgery. *Am J Sports Med* 1985; 13:27–33.

8. Smith MJ, Hutchins RC, Hehenberger D: Transcutaneous neural stimulation used in postoperative knee rehabilitation. *Am J Sports Med* 1983; 11:75–82.

9. Evron S, Schenker J, Olshwang D, et al: Postoperative analgesia by percutaneous electrical stimulation in gynecology and obstetrics. *Eur J Obstet Gynecol* 1981; 12:305–13.

10. Hollinger J: Transcutaneous electrical nerve stimulation after cesarean birth. *Phys Ther* 1986; 66:36–38.

11. Aubin M, Marks R: The efficacy of short-term treatment with electrical stimulation for osteoarthritic knee pain. *Physiotherapy* 1995; 81(11):669–75.

12. Fedorczyk J: The role of physical agents in modulating pain. *Journal of Hand Therapy* 1997: 110–21.

13. Nitz J, Cheras F: Transcutaneous electrical nerve stimulation and chronic intractable angina pectoris. *Australian Physiotherapy* 1993; 39(2):109–113.

14. Minor M, Sanford M: Physical instructions in the management of pain in arthritis. December 1993; 6 (4):197–206.

15. Nicholas J: Physical modalities in rheumatological rehabilitation archives of physical medicine and rehabilitation. September 1994; 75:1994–2001.

16. Bauer W: Electrical treatment of severe head and neck cancer pain. *Arch Otolaryngol* 1983; 109:382–83.

17. Magora F, Aladjemoff L, Tannenbaum J, et al. Treatment of pain by transcutaneous electrical stimulation. *Acta Anaesth Scand* 1978; 22:2–8.

18. Olahgang, D, Aladjemoff L, Magora A: Five years' experience with transcutaneous electrical stimulation (TENS) in a pain clinic. Jerusalem, Israel, Department of Anesthesiology. *Hadassah University Hospital* 1978; 227–31.

19. Peled I, Wexler M, Rousso M, et al: Electrical stimulation in the treatment of the painful hand. *Ann Plast Surg* 1982; 8:434–37.

20. Schuster G, Marsden B: Treatment of pain by transcutaneous electric nerve stimulation in general practice. *Med J Aus* 1980; 1:137–41.

21. Thurin E, Meehan P, Gilbert B: Treatment of pain by transcutaneous electric nerve stimulation in general practice. *Med J Aus* 1980; 1:70–71.

22. Bending J: TENS in a pain clinic. *Physiotherapy* 1989; 75:292–94.

23. Longobardi AG, Clelland JA, Knowles CJ, et al: Effects of auricular transcutaneous electric nerve stimulation: A pilot study. *Phys Ther* 1989; 69:10–17.

24. Melzack, R. Wall PD: Pain mechanisms: A new theory. *Science* 1965; 150:971–77.

25. Singer K, D'Ambrosia R, Graf B, et al: Electrical Modalities. In: Drez P Jr, ed. *Therapeutic Modalities for Sports Injuries.* Chicago: Yearbook; 1989.

26. Jessel TM, Kelly DD: Pain and Analgesia. In: Kandel ER, Schwatz JH, Jessel TM, eds. *Principles of Neural Science*, 3rd ed. New York: Elsevier; 1991; 385–89.

27. Salar G, Job I, Mingrino S, et al: Effect of transcutaneous electrotherapy on CSF beta-endorphin content in patients without pain problems. *Pain* 1984; 10:169–72.

28. Gersh, MR: *Electrotherapy in Rehabilitation.* Philadelphia: Davis; 1992.

29. Leandri M, Brunetti O, Parodi CI: Telethmographic findings after transcutaneous electrical nerve stimulation. *Phys Ther* 1986; 66:210–13.

30. Milsom I, et al: A comparative study of the effect of high intensity transcutaneous nerve stimulation and oral naproxen on intrauterine pressure and menstrual pain in patients with primary dysmenorrhea. *AM Journal Ostet. Gynecol* Vol. 170; Part 1:123–29.

31. Fassbender HG: Nonarticular Rheumatism. In: Fassbender HE, ed. *Pathology of Rheumatic Diseases.* New York: Springer-Verlag; 1975; 313–14.

32. Lein DH Jr, Clelland JA, Knowles CJ, et al: Comparison of effects of transcutaneous electric nerve stimulation of auricular, somatic, and the combination of auricular somatic acupuncture points on experimental pain threshold. *Phys Ther* 1989; 69:671–78.

33. Noling LB, Clelland JA, Jackson Jr, et al: Effect of transcutaneous electrical nerve stimulation at

auricular points on experimental cutaneous pain threshold. *Phys Ther* 1988; 68:328–32.

34. Levin MF, et al: Conventional and acupuncture-like trancutaneous electrical nerve stimulation excite similar afferent fibers. *Arch. Phys Med Rehabil* 1993; 74:54–60.

35. Lewis B, et al: The comparative analgesic efficacy of transcutaeous electrical nerve stimulation and nonsteroidal anti-inflammatory drug for painful osteoarthritis. *Brit J Rheumatol* 1994; 33:455–60.

36. Deyo R, et al: A controlled trial of TENS and exercise for chronic low back pain. NEJM 1990; 322:1627–34.

37. Craig JA, et al: Lack of effect of transcutaneous electrical nerve stimulation upon experimentally induced delayed-onset muscle soreness in humans. *Pain* 1996; 67:285–89.

38. Wang B, Tang J, White PF, et al: Effect of the intensity of transcutaneous acupoint electrical stimulation on the postoperative analgesic requirement. *Anesth Analg* 1997; 85(2):406–13.

39. Melzack R: The McGill Pain Questionnaire: Major properties and scoring methods. *Pain* 1975; 1:277–89.

40. Huskisson EC: Pain: Mechanism and measurement. In: Hart FD, ed. *The Treatment of Chronic Pain*. Philadelphia: Davis; 1974; 24–53.

41. Wang SF, et al: The effect of electrical stimulation on nocieptive responses in the rat. *Phys Ther* 1997; 77(8):839–47.

42. Walsh DM, et al: Transcutaneous electrical nerve stimulation, relevance of stimulation parameters to neurophysiological and hypoanalgesic effects. *Am J Phys Med Rehabil* 1995; 74(3):199–206.

43. Kahn J: *Principles and Practices of Electrotherapy*, 3rd ed. New York: Churchill Livingstone; 1994; 107–25.

44. Kovacs FM, Abraira V, Pozo F, et al: Local and remote sustained trigger point therapy for exacerbations of chronic low back pain. A randomized, double-blind, controlled, multi-center trial. *Spine* 1997; 22:786–97.

45. Bendtsen I, Jensen R, Jensen NK, et al: Muscle palpation with controlled finger pressure: New equipment for the study of tender myofascial tissues. *Pain* 1994; 59:235–39.

46. Wolfe F, Simons DG, Fricton J, et al: The fibromyalgia and myofascial pain syndromes: A preliminary study of tender points and trigger points in persons with fibromyalgia, myofascial pain syndrome and no disease. *J Rheumatol* 1992; 19:944–51.

47. Jensen K: Quantification of tenderness by palpation and use of pressure algometers. In: Fricton JR and Awad EA, eds. *Myofascial Pain and Fibromyalgia: Advances in Pain Research and Therapy*. Vol. 17. New York: Raven Press; 1990; 165–81.

48. Paris DL, Baynes F, Gucker B: Effects of neuroprobe in the treatment of second-degree ankle inversion sprain. *Phys Ther* 1983; 63:35–40.

49. Gerwin RD, Shannon S, Chang-Zern H, et al: Interrater reliability in myofascial trigger point examination. *Spine* 1997; 69:65–73.

50. Nice DA, Riddle DL, Lamb RL, et al: Intertester reliability of judgments of the presence of trigger points in patients with low back pain. *Arch Phys Med Rehabil* 1992; 73:893–98.

51. Travell JG, Simons DG: *Myofascial Pain and Dysfunction: The Trigger Point Manual*. Vol. 1. Baltimore: Williams & Wilkins; 1983.

52. Snyder-Mackler L, Bork C, Bourbon B, et al: Effect of helium-neon laser on musculoskeletal trigger points. *Phys Ther* 1986; 66:1087–90.

53. Hyrarinen J, Karisson M: Low-resistance skin points that may coincide with acupuncture loci. *Med Biol* 1977; 55:88–94.

54. Reichrnanis M, Marino AA, Becker RO: Electrical correlates of acupuncture points. *IEEE Trans Biomed Eng* 1975; 22:533–35.

55. Brown ML, Ulett GA, Stern JA: Acupuncture loci: Techniques for location. *Am J Clin Med* 1974; 2:67–74.

56. Richter CP: Physiological factors involved in the electrical resistance of the skin. *Am J Physiol* 1929; 88:596–615.

57. Van Metre TE Jr: Low electrical skin resistance in the region of pain in painful acute sinusitis. *Bull Johns Hopkins Hosp* 1949; 85:409–415.

58. Riley LH, Richter CP: Uses of electrical skin resistance method in the study of patients with neck and upper extremity pain. *Johns Hopkins Med* 1975; 137:69.

59. Hyrarinen J, Karisson M: Low-resistance skin points that may coincide with acupuncture loci. *Med Biol* 1977; 55:88–94.

60. Reichmanis M, Marino AA, Becker RO: Electrical correlates of acupuncture points. *IEEE Trans Biomed Eng* 1975; 22:533–35.

61. Roy S. R, Richard I:*Sports Medicine: Prevention, Evaluation and Rehabilitation.* Englewood Cliffs, NJ: Prentice-Hall; 1983:103.

62. Kahn J: *Low Volt Technique (Clinical Electrotherapy),* 4th ed. Syosset, NY: Joseph Kahn; 1985:2.

22

Iontophoresis

TSEGA ANDEMICAEL MEHRETEAB, PT, MS

THOMAS HOLLAND, PT, PhD

Chapter Outline

- DOSAGE AND DENSITY
- CONTRAINDICATIONS
- PROCEDURE
- CLINICAL APPLICATIONS
- REVIEW QUESTIONS
- KEY TERMS

Iontophoresis is the treatment technique in which an electric current is used to drive ions of various substances through the skin and into underlying tissues. Continuous direct current (DC) is used to transfer the charged ions into the tissues. The substances must dissociate into their charged ionic form and be readily available for transfer into the skin under the electrode. Although some studies are available on the use and effects of some therapeutic ions, there is a dearth of material on standard clinical procedures and of published studies supporting the efficacy of iontophoresis. This chapter presents general guidelines and procedures for application as well as a chart listing sample ions with their sources, therapeutic effects, recommended dosages, and references that will provide additional information.

Continuously flowing DC from an electric generator that provides constant current is used to drive ions into the skin and other tissues. The ions are delivered to the tissue as they are repelled by an electrode with the same polarity; therefore, the polarity of the ion must be known before the appropriate polarity of the active electrode can be determined. For example, a positively charged ion such as zinc (Zn^{2+}) is applied under the positive electrode (the anode), and chloride ion (Cl^-) is applied under the negative electrode. In other words, matching the ion and the appropriate electrode is an extremely important step in the procedure. To determine the polarity of the ion, consult a pharmacist, refer to established literature, or use the periodic table of elements found in most chemistry books. In cases of ionic compounds composed of two elements, the first element is positively charged, and the second is negatively charged. For example, in sodium chloride (NaCl), sodium is positive and chloride is negative.

DOSAGE AND DENSITY

The ion to be applied must be available in its charged form and should be soluble in either water or lipid medium. For example, the ion can be prepared in water or be suspended in an inert base (eg, as ointment). Because the concentration of the ions as well as the physical size of each ion may vary, the dosage must be carefully determined before the ion is applied. Dosage for the selected ionic concentration is expressed as a product of the intensity in milliamperes and the duration of the treatment in minutes. For example, a dosage of 20 mA-min may

represent a current with an intensity of 4 mA applied for 5 min or an intensity of 2 mA applied for 10 min.

For safety, the density of the current should be considered. *Current density* is determined by dividing the current amplitude by the total area of the electrode. The range of density used for iontophoresis is between 0.1 and 0.5 mA per cm^2. The maximum safe current density is approximately 1 mA per square inch. The therapist must exercise caution to avoid an allergic reaction to the direct current, commonly referred to as a **galvanic rash.** This reaction is usually the result of hypersensitivity to a direct current. A galvanic rash may develop within 5 min of electrical stimulation. In addition, possible allergies or sensitivities to the substances used for iontophoresis should be carefully and thoroughly investigated before they are applied.

A commercially prepared electrode with a DC generator is also available for iontophoresis. This type of unit contains an electrode unit with a cavity for the ionic solution, a portal for filling the cavity with the solution, a semipermeable membrane that is placed directly over the skin, and a lead that connects the electrode unit to the current generator. A second lead and a dispersive electrode complete the circuit.

The net amount of ions deposited in the tissue is affected by a variety of factors. For example, the local circulation may move ions away from the local area of application, or other ions in the area with a similar charge may compete with the ions to be applied. In addition, the higher the concentration of ions, the lower the uptake by the tissue. This phenomenon has been shown by measuring the uptake of different concentrations of radioactive phosphorus through iontophoresis.[1]

CONTRAINDICATIONS

The therapist thoroughly investigates for possible allergies or sensitivities to the substances and direct current to be applied. The skin offers a significant impedance to current flow. An area devoid of its skin covering lacks this natural protection. In addition, current tends to concentrate in areas of least resistance; therefore, avoid current application over areas with broken skin, cuts, or bruises. Iontophoresis is contraindicated when there is acute injury and bleeding in the area to be treated. Box 20–2 provides the contraindications and precaution for using electrical stimulation.

PROCEDURE

Figure 22–1 displays an example of an iontophoresis application. The following are the basic procedures for setting up an iontophoresis intervention.

1. Clean the skin, and inspect it for cuts or bruises; check for sensation.

2. Explain to the patient both the procedure and what to expect from the treatment.

3. Position the patient and the area to be treated appropriately.

4. Use a DC generator with constant-current output and well-calibrated controls (the ammeter should indicate the exact intensity delivered in milliamperes).

5. Follow the manufacturer's suggested procedures if using a commercially prepared electrode (**Fig. 22–2**) and a DC generator. The electrode comes with a cavity and portal system; the premeasured medication is directly injected into this cavity.

6. Use two electrodes (if the electrodes are self-prepared), an active electrode with the same polarity as the ion to be applied, and a larger dispersive electrode. The dispersive electrode should be at least 4 times the size of the active electrode and should be placed on a distant area. Electrodes should be made of a flexible metal such as tin, copper, aluminum, or aluminum foil that is cut to the appropriate size. Contemporary iontophoresis units use flexible electrodes that conform easily to the body's contours and provide better contact.

7. If the traditional iontophoresis intervention is used secure several layers of gauze or sponge saturated with the solution containing the ion over the area to be treated. Place the flexible metal electrode over the gauze. If the ion is in a topical form, spread a thin layer of the ointment over the area to be treated, and apply several layers of gauze moistened with distilled water over the ointment. To keep the metal from contacting the skin, the size of the electrode should be slightly smaller than the gauze preparation, and the other side of the electrode should be covered with insulating material. Contemporary iontophoresis units minimize the electrode preparation time and chance of skin irritation.

8. Connect the electrodes to the current generator. Apply the electrode evenly, and avoid air bubbles.

9. Use nonmetallic straps or weights to ensure firm and even contact of the electrode with the body part.

10. Determine the dosage by taking the area of the electrodes into consideration; the maximum safety limit is 1 mA per square inch. The dosage should be increased gradually over time and must be consistent with the results sought. When the current is turned on or off, the intensity should be gradually increased or decreased to avoid a twitch response.

11. Pay special attention when the cathode ($-$) is used as the treatment electrode. The chemical or polar effects of the cathode include alkaline reactions that may cause a burn, commonly referred to as a **negative electrode burn.**

12. Gradually turn the current intensity up or down to avoid an abrupt interruption of the direct current.

13. Observe the skin every 3 to 5 min during treatment for any adverse reactions such as a galvanic rash or negative electrode burn. Also observe the skin after treatment, and instruct the patient to observe and report any adverse reactions.

14. Ensure that the antidote ion or substance is readily available.

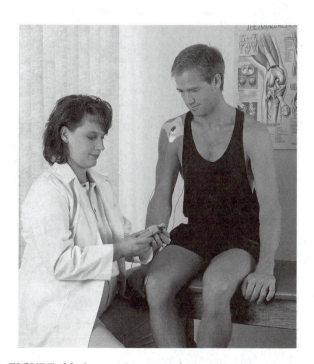

FIGURE 22–1   Application of iontophoresis to the shoulder. (*Courtesy of Empi, Inc., St. Paul, MN.*)

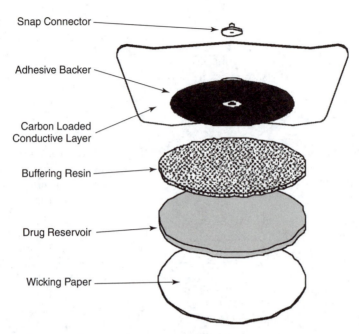

FIGURE 22–2 A buffered electrode for iontophoresis. (*Courtesy of Empi, Inc., St. Paul, MN.*)

The ions available for clinical use may vary in concentration and in the type of carrier used (ie, an aqueous solution or an ointment base). To avoid undesirable ions of the same charge from being delivered, the aqueous solution or the ointment carrier should not contain competing ions. The carrier substance should be chemically stable. There are recommended concentrations for various ions; however, a standard guide for concentration and dosage is lacking. See **Table 22–1** for recommended dosages for some ions that are used in physical therapy.

CLINICAL APPLICATIONS

Table 22–1 lists the applications of sample ions and their clinical use. The names and charges of the ions are listed in Column 1; the main sources of the ions and the concentration of the desired substances are listed in Column 2; and the therapeutic uses and effects, the recommended dosages, and references are listed in Columns 3, 4, and 5, respectively. (The table references provide additional information on these ions.)

REVIEW QUESTIONS

1. What type of current is required for iontophoresis?
2. What are the recommended safe ranges for current density when performing iontophoresis?
3. Identify the contraindications for use of iontophoresis.
4. Identify the commonly used topical agents and their respective ionic charges.
5. Identify the commonly used topical agents and their therapeutic use.
6. What factors will influence transport and absorption of topical medicines during an iontophoresis treatment?
7. To maintain a dosage of 40 milliamp-min, how long should the treatment session be if the stimulation intensity is (a) 1 mA, (b) 2 mA, (c) 3mA, and (d) 4 mA?
8. Why should the negative electrode (cathode) be larger than the positive electrode (anode) during an iontophoresis treatment?
9. Identify the ways in which skin irritation can be minimized during an iontophoresis treatment.
10. Describe the different electrode systems used during iontophoresis.

TABLE 22–1   *Sample Ions and Their Clinical Uses*

Ion/Charge/Electrode	Main Source	Therapeutic Use	Recommended Dosage	References
Acetate/(−) cathode	Acetic acid, 2% solution	Calcified tendonitis; decreases calcium deposits	3–4 mA for 10–20 min.	2, 3
Copper/(+) anode	Copper sulfate 1% solution	Fungicidal; athlete's foot	10 mA for 15 min for 2 weeks. Bath method.	4
Dexamethasone/(−) cathode	Dex NA_2PO_3	Anti-inflammatory; arthritis, bursitis, tendonitis	1–4 mA for 15–20 min.	5–7
Hyoluronidase/(+) anode	150 USP units in 250 cc of 0.1 M acetate buffer solution at 5.4 pH wydase	Reduce edema	1–2 mA per 2.5 sq cm electrode for 20–40 min.	8, 9
Lidocaine/(+) anode	Lidocaine hydrochloride	Analgesia; bursitis, neuritis	2 mA for 1 min. and 4 mA for 5 min. Current density < 0.65 mA/sq cm.	10
Salicylate/(−) cathode	1% sodium salicylate 2% sodium salicylate	Analgesia; myalgia Plantar warts	4 mA for 45 min 10 mA for min. 1/wk.	11, 12
Tap water/(+) or (−) anode or cathode	Tap water	Hyperhidrosis of palms or feet	15–29 mA for 10–15 min, 2–3 wk.	13, 14
Zinc/(+) anode	01. M zinc oxide ointment	Bactericidal; ischemic ulcer	4 mA for 15 min, 2x/day.	15

KEY TERMS

iontophoresis   galvanic rash   negative electrode burn

REFERENCES

1. O'Malley EP, Oester YT: Influence of some physical chemical factors on iontophoresis using radioisotopes. *Arch Phys Med Rehabil* 1955; 36:310–16.

2. Psaki C, et al: Acetic acid ionization: A study to determine the absorptive effects upon calcified tendonitis of the shoulder. *Phys Ther Rev* 1955; 35:84.

3. Khan J: Acetic acid iontophoresis for calcium deposits. *Phys Ther* 1977; 57(6):658–59.

4. Haggard H, et al: Fungous infections of hand and feet treated by copper iontophoresis. *JAMA* 1939; 112:1229.

5. Glass J, et al: The quantity and distribution of radio-labeled depamethasone delivered to tissues by iontophoresis. *Int J Dermatol* 1980; 19:519.

6. Harris PR: Iontophoresis: Clinical research in musculoskeletal inflammatory conditions. *J Orthop Sports Phys Ther* 1982; 4:109.

7. Bertolucci L: Introduction of anti-inflammatory drugs by iontophoresis: Double blind study. *J Orthop Sports Phys Ther* 1982; 4:103.

8. Shwarth M: Hyaluronidase by iontophoresis in the treatment of lymphodema. *Arch Intern Med* 1955; 95:662.

9. Russo J, et al: Lidocaine anesthesia: comparison of iontophoresis, injection, and swabbing. *Am J Hosp Pharm* 1980; 37:843–47.

10. Magistro C: Hyaluronidase by iontophoresis. *Phys Ther* 1964; 44:169.

11. Garzione J: Salicylate iontophoresis as an alternative treatment for persistent thigh pain following hip surgery. *Phys Ther* 1978; 58:570.

12. Gordon A, Weinstein M: Sodium salicylate iontophoresis in the treatment of plantar warts. *Phys Ther* 1969; 49:869–70.

13. Levit F: Simple device for treatment of hyperhidrosis by iontophoresis. *Arch Dermatol* 1968; 98:505.

14. Shrivastava S, Sing G: Tap water iontophoresis in palm and plantar hyperhidrosis. *Br J Dermatol* 1977; 96:189.

15. Cornwall M: Zinc iontophoresis to treat ischemic ulcers. *Phys Ther* 1981; 61:359.

16. Banta C: A prospective nonrandomized study of iotophoresis, wrist splinting, and anti-inflammatory medication in the treatment of carpal tunnel syndrome. *J Occup Med* 1994; 36:166.

17. Gudeman S, et al: Treatment of plantar fasciitis by iontophoresis with 0.4 % dexamethasone: A randomized, double-blind, placebo-controlled study. *Am J Sports Med* 1997; 25:312.

23

Clinical Electroneuromyography

ARTHUR W. NELSON, JR., PT, PhD, FAPTA

Chapter Outline

The comprehensive evaluation of a patient referred for physical therapy includes clinical **electroneuromyography (ENMG)** when a patient presents with flaccid paralysis, atrophy of muscles, and sensory loss or pain radiating to limbs. Any pattern of progressive weakness may call for an ENMG examination. The ENMG exam is used to differentiate between disorders of the central nervous system (CNS) and peripheral nervous system. It is also regularly used in the comprehensive evaluation of individuals with cervical and lumbar pain syndromes to search for evidence of nerve root compromise. Serial studies may be used to identify progression or regression of a neuropathy, myopathy, or a neuromuscular junction. Finally, the ENMG may be used to predict the time of recovery of function in selected patients.

The ENMG examination typically consists of two components: (1) nerve conduction studies, or evoked response component, and (2) electromyographic examination of the muscles, or the electromyography (EMG) component. A **nerve conduction** study entails electrical stimulation of a peripheral nerve at a number of sites along its course. This involves the selective stimulation of motor or sensory components of the peripheral nerve. **Electromyography** involves the insertion of needle electrodes into a muscle to identify the nature of the electrical discharges when the electrode is inserted, when the muscle is at rest, and when the muscle contracts with various intensities.

This chapter is divided into three sections. The first section provides information about the ENMG examination that is required before embarking on discussions about nerve conduction studies and the EMG examination. Before conducting the actual ENMG examination, the examiner must review the patient's medical history, carry out a clarifying neurologic assessment, and inspect the patient's skin, nails, and hair distribution. The patient's medical history includes pertinent medical information, medications taken over the past several months, laboratory data, radiologic and other reports, and a detailed description of the onset of symptoms, their duration and constancy, their intensity, and the factors that alter those symptoms. A summary of this history is typically contained in the ENMG report.

On the basis of the findings of the medical history and the patient's complaints, further clarification is obtained by assessing the sensory system, manual muscle testing, reflex responsiveness at selected areas, and other procedures appropriate to the patient's history and complaints. It is useful for the examiner to have disposable pins, cotton wads, and a tendon hammer for this clarifying assessment.

The purpose of evaluating the sensory system is to uncover a pattern of loss or distortion that conforms to some recognizable distribution that would be ultimately compared with the findings of the ENMG examination. It might be surprising to uncover sensory loss in the area where a person is experiencing pain. Patients often cannot discern sensory loss until the examiner pinches them. Many times patients will say a limb is "numb" when in actuality they are describing a sensory **dysesthesia** of "pins and needles," not **hypoesthesia** or loss of sensation. The distribution of sensory change may help distinguish between a nerve root, a peripheral nerve, or another pattern. This information will be used later to correlate with the ENMG findings.

The manual muscle test differs from the conventional one in that it is frequently performed bilaterally to assess differences from side to side. In some instances, the clinician must perform a definitive muscle test on individual muscles, but generally this assessment is to obtain an overview of groups of muscles. During this testing, the examiner observes for atrophy, wasting, or trophic changes in the skin. These are noted in the report along with muscle test findings.

Deep-tendon jerk responses are elicited at the major sites associated with the suspected problem of the patient. These would be recorded as absent, brisk, or exaggerated, using a numerical scale on the report form. Any other responses such as the plantar (Babinski) reflex should be reported as well. Some examiners use tuning forks to assess response to vibratory stimuli. The special tests for vision, hearing, taste, smell, and equilibrium (caloric test) may not be conducted unless they are pertinent to or are absent from the patient's records.

The purpose of the clarifying examination is to provide the examiner with a clearly focused direction for the testing. Rather than following a set procedure, it may be advantageous first to examine the body part that exhibits the clinical findings. This will help to ensure that relevant information is obtained should the patient abort the test before reaching the most essential area.

ELECTRONEUROMYOGRAPHIC EXAMINATION

Purpose

The ENMG examination can be viewed as an extension of the manual muscle test that permits a more detailed look at the internal electrical state of the muscle during varying states of activity as well as the responsiveness of nerves to stimuli at various sites along the nerve path. When an individual has a peculiar feeling of heaviness but does not exhibit gross loss of strength, it may be possible to uncover changes within the muscle that are not visible without the EMG. Similarly, total paralysis from a nerve injury may reveal early, subtle changes that signal the return of innervation.

The ENMG examination is helpful in distinguishing between CNS disorders and peripheral disorders. For instance, a patient suffering from sensory disturbances in one leg and one arm can be evaluated to determine whether this indicates a problem in the cerebral hemisphere or a cervical or lumbar nerve root disorder.

Identifying the severity of a lesion is an important goal of this test, and serial studies can be used to form a prognosis for recovery. The monitoring of progressive disorders such as muscular dystrophy may help primary caregivers determine the rate of progression and its distribution. This information contributes to program planning, the appropriateness of surgical intervention, or the use of orthoses, and to other critical decision making.

It is also necessary to determine whether a more acute disturbance has been superimposed on a chronic one—for example, if someone with a chronic cervical radiculopathy has had another injury to the neck and is now complaining of additional symptoms. How much acute change beyond the chronic findings has occurred? The answer can have important legal and liability implications.

The ENMG findings may provide information regarding the optimal time to begin intervention. A study by Brown and Ironton[1] suggests that if initiated too early after denervation, electrical stimulation may retard reinnervation; therefore, it is probably wise to wait until a significant reduction has occurred in fibrillation within the muscle. Similarly, the effectiveness of intervention can be monitored with ENMG to determine whether there is objective evidence of improvement.

The ultimate purpose of the ENMG examination is to identify what the problem actually is, what structures are involved, and to what extent. Some typical problems confronting the physical therapist include weakness, numbness and tingling, pain, dizziness or light-headedness, loss of equilibrium, fatigue, inability to perform tasks previously accomplished, and loss of skill. These complaints are reviewed in the context of the patient's history, laboratory findings, the clarifying neurological assessment, and other information pertinent to forming a statement of the problem. Patients often tell the examiner what the problem is, but the examiner has already reached a conclusion and does not listen with an open mind.

Suppose the patient complains of dizziness. Where does the therapist begin?

The history is reviewed to determine when the dizziness occurs:

- Does the dizziness occur upon first arising in the morning or after straining to have a bowel movement?
- Has the patient had a significant cardiac or respiratory problem?
- Has there been a history of middle ear infections?
- Do other family members have similar problems?
- What does the person do to alleviate the symptoms?
- Does activity improve or worsen the problem?
- What happens to the person's blood pressure when he or she rises from a sitting position?

If the therapist finds that none of the previous questions provides any clues, then perform a sensory examination. If there is a stockinglike loss of sensation from midcalf to the toes to stimulation with a wisp of cotton, this finding indicates the direction that the ENMG examination should take: looking for changes compatible with peripheral neuropathy, caudae equinae lesions, or compromise of the lumbosacral nerve roots.

A peripheral neuropathic disorder results in changes that are generally correlated anatomically with it. Determine the following:

- Does the person have peculiar, unexplained sensations in the feet and lower legs?
- Does the person experience more dizziness when in a dark room?

- Have the toenails changed?
- Do the feet "go to sleep" easily?
- Do the legs tire more easily than they used to?
- Is there significant back pain?
- Does the patient have radiation of pain to the legs?
- Does the patient have "pins and needles" in the lower legs and feet?

Lumbosacral nerve root compression can produce numbness of legs and weakness of selected lower extremity muscles.

The examiner then conducts a neuromuscular evaluation to delineate which nerves and muscles will be examined, and in what order. If the neuromuscular examination reveals sluggish jerk responses in the Achilles tendon and a loss of response to light touch with a wisp of cotton in a stockinglike distribution of both legs, the impression of peripheral neuropathy is supported. However, these findings may be caused by lumbosacral nerve root or plexus compression, or a caudae equinae lesion. With these alternative conditions in mind, the examiner conducts the ENMC to delineate and thereby rule out two of the four possibilities.

Therefore, the structure of the ENMG examination will include study of the peripheral nerves of the lower legs and feet. The study of a peripheral nerve involves stimulating the nerve at two sites and measuring the velocity with which it conducts the stimuli. A distal muscle is used to determine the response of the nerve to stimuli. The magnitude of its response, known as the **amplitude,** is also an important bit of information. The distal portion of the conduction also is helpful. This examination process continues to the other major nerve in each leg to provide a basis of comparison both with the nerve in question and with normal values. Special studies of the proximal segment of the nerve are conducted to determine its status and thereby assess the lumbosacral plexus and the nerve roots. Electromyography follows a similar line of reasoning: evaluating the distal musculature of a given peripheral nerve, looking at a proximal muscle of that nerve, and then examining muscles that are innervated by nerve roots or components of the lumbosacral plexus. For instance, the paralumbar muscles can be examined to reveal a more proximal problem such as a lumbar or sacral nerve root compression.

Principles

The principles involved in conducting a proper ENMG examination include the following:

1. Examine both a distal and a proximal muscle in a given peripheral nerve. A distal and a proximal muscle innervated by a particular nerve root also should be examined to delineate the lesion. This principle is known as the **proximal and distal rule.**
2. Examine muscles that are innervated by the same nerve roots but different peripheral nerves to localize the changes to one or the other.
3. Keep examining muscles until normal values are uncovered because it is impossible to delineate the level of involvement until the findings are within normal limits.

In summary, the first principle is proximal versus distal, the second is nerve root versus peripheral nerve, and the third is to keep going until normal values are found.

To understand the findings obtained in an ENMG examination, it is imperative to explore some anatomic and physiologic correlates such as the motor unit, the fascicular organization of nerve and muscle, the resting membrane potential, the junctional potentials, the action potential, neuromuscular transmission, and electromechanical coupling. For a more complete treatment of these subjects, consult a neurophysiology text.

Anatomic Correlates

The motor unit is the most fundamental element of neuromuscular control. A **motor unit** consists of the motor neuron and its axon, which extends from the anterior horn region of the spinal cord to the muscle fibers innervated by that axon. The ratio of muscle fibers innervated by a single axon has been identified by Weddell et al[2] as ranging from as few as 7 to 9 muscle fibers per axon in extraocular muscles to as many as 1400 muscle fibers per axon in the medial gastrocnemius muscle. Obviously, the lower the ratio, the greater the control of that muscle. The muscle fibers innervated by an axon are distributed throughout a fascicle in a checkerboardlike configuration. This arrangement ensures that the tension of the motor unit will be evenly distributed throughout the muscle-tendon unit. Buchthal[3] estimated that the motor unit detected by an electrode will occupy between 5 and 15 sq mm of a muscle and will be mixed with 3 to 6 other motor units. If the tip of the exploring electrode can effectively determine 2–3 sq mm, it is clear that this electrode must be shifted to a number of sites within the muscle to survey adequately the motor units within the muscle in question.

The axons are collected into bundles, and those bundles are collected into larger bundles that finally accumulate in the nerve trunk. Each collection of bundles has a sheath of connective tissue with the nerve trunk having a covering of perineural connective tissue that encloses the entire structure. Note also that these fascicles are not found in a parallel arrangement but in a loose "braid" within the nerve trunk. For this reason, stimulation applied to the nerve trunk must be of sufficient intensity to ensure that 100% of the axons are stimulated; a lesser stimulus may not stimulate the same fibers at another level of the nerve. This intense stimulus is known as a **supramaximal stimulus.**

Physiologic Correlates

The cell membrane of nerve as well as muscle possesses an electrical charge known as the **resting membrane potential.** If a micropipette electrode is inserted into this membrane and connected to a voltmeter, it will register a negative charge of 70–90 mV. The membrane in a resting state acts as a type of storehouse of electrical charge, much like a battery. This resting charge requires an ionic imbalance of excess sodium on the outside of the membrane and excess potassium on the inside of the membrane. In addition, a metabolic pump must maintain this imbalance using an adenosine triphosphate (ATP) energy source. The membrane is thereby relatively impermeable to sodium and less so to potassium. The resting membrane potential is close to the equilibrium potential of potassium.

When an electrical stimulus is delivered to a nerve membrane, it apparently discharges the capacitance of that portion of the membrane, resulting in a dramatic change in the permeability of the membrane to sodium. This process leads to a dramatic reversal of the membrane potential so that the inside of the membrane becomes positive. This reversal of the potential is called a **depolarization.** Because this depolarization occurs three-dimensionally in a progression from the point of stimulation, it is called the wave of depolarization. Once this depolarization reaches its peak, the sodium egress is maximal, while potassium has been

exiting the membrane at a slower rate. A repolarization then takes place with the membrane potential returning to a negative value. The actual value reached is more negative than the resting potential. This overshoot is called **hyperpolarization.** This hyperpolarization makes the membrane refractory to stimuli at this instant; it ensures a set frequency of discharge of nerve and muscle membrane so that the motor neurons designed for high-frequency firing will have short after-hyperpolarization periods, and low-frequency-firing motor neurons will have longer ones.

If an electric current is applied with an extremely slow increase of intensity, there may be no change in the resting membrane potential, which is termed **accommodation.** However, if the slow increase in current has resulted in no response, the sudden cessation of the current will result in a change in the resting membrane potential. Therefore a response may be elicited by turning the current off.

It is clear that proper electrolyte balance will be necessary for the optimal function of these reversal depolarization and repolarization potentials. Moderate increases in extracellular potassium reduces the concentration gradient and lowers the resting potential of the nerve and muscle membranes. Small increases in extracellular potassium produce partial depolarization, and the cell will fire easily and sometimes spontaneously. This outcome is recognized as an abnormality on the ENMG examination of a muscle. Large increases in potassium concentration can produce a depolarization block, resulting in profound paralysis and the danger of cardiac failure. These electrolyte imbalances may be encountered in kidney disease and in hyperkalemic periodic paralysis. Anoxia and hypoxia resulting in a decreased oxygen concentration produce an accumulation of potassium extracellularly, which results in transient signs and symptoms. These symptoms may be reflected in the sensory system as tingling, loss of vision, or "seeing stars." In the motor system, it may be manifested as loss of strength, twitching of muscles, or lack of endurance.

If sodium conductance is interfered with (eg, in tetrodotoxin poisoning), the wave of depolarization, the **action potential,** will be blocked. Structural changes in the nerve membrane brought on by disease, injury, or ischemia may lead to a leakage of sodium, which could increase excitability or, if extreme, a complete block in conduction. An increase in extracellular sodium will increase the amplitude, and the rise time of the action potential will be faster.

Conversely, a decrease in sodium outside the membrane results in a reduced action potential amplitude and a slower rise time of the action potential. If the decrease of sodium is severe, it may block the action potential formation entirely.

Calcium ions act as a membrane stabilizer, and if they are absent, the result is a decreased concentration gradient of sodium and potassium. For example, hypocalcemia will reduce the resting membrane potential, resulting in increased excitability, which is seen on the EMG as spontaneous firing of motor units called **fasciculations.** The most common symptoms of hypocalcemia will be twitching, tingling, or both. It also is likely that synaptic transmission will be interfered with, which would result in weakness. Excess calcium tends to reduce the action potential and enhance synaptic transmission but is difficult to determine clinically.

Drugs (eg, cocaine) that interfere with sodium conductance in the axon membrane will block the action potential, starting with the thinnest fibers first—hence their value for blocking pain conduction. Vincristine affects the neurotubule system and therefore results in deterioration of the delivery of substances such as transmitters to the terminal axon. This outcome may result in a deterioration of the distal axon known as a *dying-back neuropathy.*

When nerves have been injured and the axons have degenerated, a supersensitivity of the postsynaptic terminus of those axons will develop. In the case of muscle fibers innervated by a degenerated axon, the muscle fibers will become supersensitive to acetylcholine, and if any of this transmitter is near those fibers, they will spontaneously fire. The muscle fibers will be irritated by mechanical stimulation such as the insertion of the needle electrode during the ENMG examination. The irritability can then be represented as increased insertional activity, fibrillation potentials at rest, or positive sharp waves while the muscle is at rest.

Variables Influencing Conduction Velocity of Nerve.

The velocity of nerve conduction is proportional to the diameter of the axons within the nerve trunk and the degree of myelinization around each axon. The amount of myelin is significant because it enhances the conduction seven times more than would occur without myelin sheathing. Therefore, if demyelination occurs, it will severely reduce conduction velocity. The thickest axons and the most richly myelinated ones are the primary afferents derived from the muscle spindles that are responsible for the tendon jerk response. Because thick axons are more vulnerable to compressive lesions, the tendon jerk will be among the first deficits observed.

Conduction of Evoked Stimuli in the Nerve Trunk.

When short-duration pulses of current (0.1–0.2 milliseconds) are delivered to a nerve trunk, more and more axons are added to those thickest fibers that respond earliest. Electrical stimulation elicits responses in the thickest axons first; and then, as the intensity increases, smaller and smaller diameter fibers are brought in. Because all the pulses of current are arriving simultaneously in all the axons, the result is a compilation of all the individual motor units firing in a confined period of time. The result is a single response known as a **motor action potential (MAP).** To be certain that all the axons are responding and none are left out, the response is observed on the oscilloscope screen while the intensity of the pulses of stimuli is slowly increased until there is no further increase in the amplitude of the MAP. This is then a supramaximal stimulus because no further increase in amplitude has taken place despite the 10% increase in the intensity of the stimuli (**Fig. 23–1**).

Voluntary Recruitment of Motor Units.

The final determiner of whether muscular action will occur is the excitation of the anterior horn cell, also known as the alpha motor neuron. Once the anterior horn cell is activated at the axon hillock, the action potential is conducted at either maximum amplitude or not at all throughout its course. This property is known as the **all-or-none law,** which ensures that whatever firing frequency is established in the anterior horn cell will be the frequency that is applied to the neuromuscular junction and subsequently to the muscle membrane, assuming no disorder of the neuromuscular junction or muscle membrane—this means all muscle fibers supplied by each axon, which can be as many as 1400 muscle fibers in the medial head of the gastrocnemius or as few as 5 or 6 in the extraocular muscles. Because these individual muscle fibers are spread through the fascicle, the needle electrode of the EMG will act as a type of averager, and there will be an amalgamation of the individual action potentials from the many muscle fibers into a **compound motor unit potential (cMUP) (Fig. 23–2).**

Duration of the Motor Unit Potential.

The duration of the compound motor unit potential (cMUP) is determined by the spread of the endplate zone in

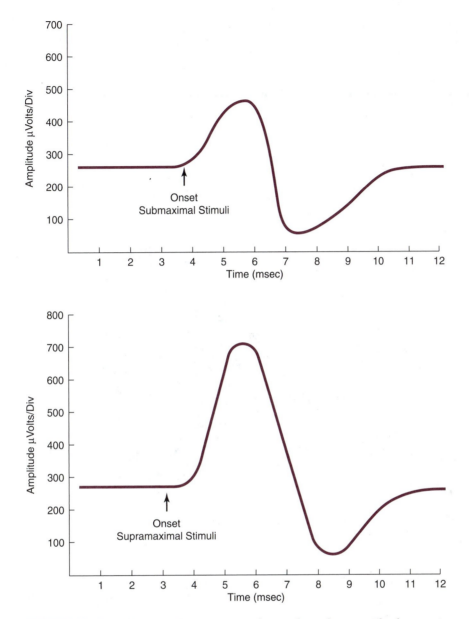

FIGURE 23–1   Influence of supramaximal stimuli on latency. The latency is 2.7 milliseconds with supramaximal stimuli and 3.4 milliseconds with submaximal stimuli.

relation to the total length of the muscle fibers. For example, the abductor pollicus brevis muscle has an endplate zone that is 50% of the total length of the fibers of the muscle. Conversely, the biceps brachii has an endplate zone that is only 10% of the total length of the muscle fibers. This arrangement results in a longer duration of the cMUP of the abductor pollicis brevis muscle than the biceps brachii muscle.

Amplitude of the Motor Unit Potential.   The size or amplitude of the cMUP is determined by the circumference of the muscle fibers with respect to the total cross section of the muscle. Therefore, larger diameter fibers in a relatively small muscle will result in a higher-amplitude cMUP in that muscle when sampled with EMG. For example, the abductor pollicis brevis will have a higher amplitude MUP than

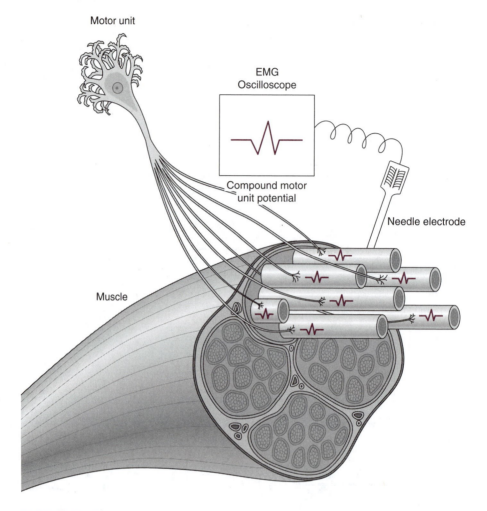

FIGURE 23–2   Formulation of a compound motor unit potential. The action potentials from each muscle fiber are amalgamated into an averaged potential.

does the biceps brachii. As noted earlier, the extracellular sodium can influence the amplitude of the cMUP as well.

Recruitment of Motor Units. The final common pathway is the anterior horn cell and its axon and all the muscle fibers attendant to it. The all-or-none law assures that once the anterior horn cell is activated by threshold stimuli, the axon also will be fired with the same all-or-none response, and, presuming that there is no neuromuscular junction deficit, the action potential will be transmitted to the muscle membrane, resulting in the activation, or **recruitment,** of all (8–1400) muscle fibers of that particular motor unit. The spread of the endplate zones on the skeletal muscles will be varied and, in some muscles, will represent

a wide distribution when comparing the end-plate zone with the total length of the muscle fibers. When an EMG electrode is inserted within a muscle and it detects action potential sweeping along the course of the muscle membranes, it actually blends the individual action potentials together and forms a type of average called the **motor unit potential (MUP).** The duration of the MUP is determined by the spread of the endplate zone in relation to the total length of the muscle fiber. For example, the abductor pollicis brevis muscle has an endplate zone that is 50% of the total length of the fibers of that muscle. Conversely, the biceps brachii has an endplate zone that is only 10% of the total length of the muscle fibers, which results in a shorter duration of the MUP than in the abductor pollicis brevis muscle (**Fig. 23–3**).

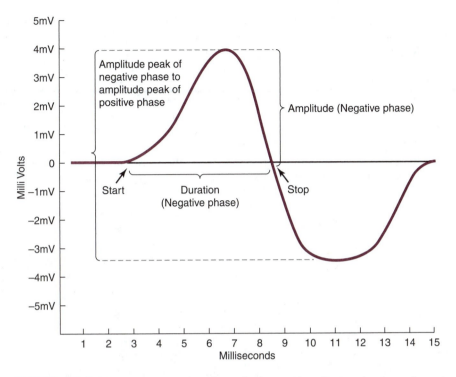

FIGURE 23–3   Motor unit potential; evoked response. Determination of amplitude and duration as seen on the oscilloscope.

The amplitude or size of the MUP is determined by the circumference of the muscle fibers with respect to the cross section of the total muscle. Therefore, larger diameter fibers in a small muscle will result in a higher amplitude MAP in that muscle when sampled electromyographically.

During voluntary contraction of a muscle, the small motor units within the muscle are activated first and will increase their frequency of firing from approximately 5 per second to 10–15 per second. As the smaller unit increases its rate of firing and more force is being called for, larger and larger motor units are added, and they in turn increase their rate of firing. This process is referred to as the **size principle of motor unit recruitment,** as identified by Hennemann et al.[4] Observing the increased rate of firing, the therapist can estimate the degree of effort. If a person has only a few motor units available to fire actively and if they are "asked" to contract the muscle with greater and greater force, the frequency of firing will increase in those available motor units. But if a person is feigning weakness, the rate of firing remains stable. Confusing the person with reciprocating motions usually reveals increased rates of firing in

the muscle in question. De Luca et al[5] believed that the highest rate of firing of motor unit potentials would range from 35 to 45 per second during maximal effort.

Neuromuscular Transmission.   The axon does not conduct the action potential directly to the muscle fibers but must release chemical transmitters at the neuromuscular junction. The wave of depolarization releases calcium from the neuroplastic reticulum. In the presence of calmodulin, the calcium ruptures the vesicles containing acetylcholine, which spills out into the synaptic cleft between the nerve and the muscle membrane. The acetylcholine molecules bind to the receptor sites on the muscle membrane, thus changing the permeability of the membrane to sodium and potassium. The change in permeability leads to an increase in the positive charge on the inside of the membrane that is proportional to the number of activated gates. The new potential is referred to as a **graded junctional potential** or an **endplate potential** because it is proportional to the amount of acetylcholine binding to the membrane. Once that graded potential reaches threshold, an action potential is formed on the muscle membrane that is subsequently conducted along the surface of the muscle membrane at a rate of 3–5 meters per second.

Electromechanical Coupling. Once the muscle action potential reaches the openings of the transverse tubule system, it enters the depths of the muscle fiber. There, the action potential activates calcium in the sarcoplasmic reticulum in the presence of calmodulin. The released calcium bonds to troponin, which is wrapped around the actin molecules and bound to tropomyosin, which is released by the calcium binding to troponin. When this process occurs, an electrostatic inhibition between actin and myosin is released, permitting actin and myosin to bind. The hinge of the myosin molecule bends, thereby exerting tension when this actin-myosin binding takes place. This tension is exerted by a new molecule called myosin-actin-ATPase. The energy is provided by the breakdown of adenosine triphosphate for the formulation of the bond. To release the bond, energy is required through the breaking down of ATP in the presence of magnesium. This process is accompanied by an active pumping of calcium back into the sarcoplasmic reticulum. If calcium remains in the region of the actin and troponin, the bond will not release, and a rigor will remain within the sarcomere that does not require an action potential. Thus it is possible, under this special circumstance, to have contraction of a muscle without EMG potentials being in evidence.

Instrumentation

All electroneuromyographs used in clinical investigations have two basic components: the nerve conduction mode and the electromyography mode. The two components are contained within a single device called an **electromyograph (EMG).** The essential elements of the EMG consist of the oscilloscope, the stimulate mode, the EMG mode, the manual modes and gain-and-sweep speed controls, and a printer mode with buffer. Attendant to this EMG are a preamplifier with a long cable and a stimulator with another cable attached to the body of the stimulate mode. An essential element within the EMG is the **differential amplifier,** which is essential to distinguish extremely small voltages from larger ones that surround us in every environment. The electrodes are attached to the preamplifier to complete the circuit (**Fig. 23–4**).

The examiner's choice of the proper electrodes to bring the small signals from the patient's body to the EMG is crucial. The current recommendation is to use disposable needle electrodes for EMG, metal-disk electrodes for motor nerve conduction studies, and ring or clip electrodes for sensory nerve conduction studies. The electrodes are the most critical link in the entire system and are subject to many sources of error. The electrodes are used to transfer the essential physiologic information from the subject to the EMG preamplifier and the differential amplifier, which expands the information and displays it on an oscilloscope, as well as converting it to sound that can be heard on speakers. The interaction of metal needles with the biologic tissue is a complex one and varies in many circumstances, producing distortions of the tiny electrical signals.

Considering the tiny contact of a needle electrode within a muscle, which moves and twists the electrode during contraction, it is possible to sense the larger problem of obtaining reliable information from the electrode. The purpose of the electrode within the muscle is to pick up the microvolt level potentials while there are much larger electrical influences in the adjacent area such as electric power wiring, appliances, and lighting. The trick is to distinguish between the tiny biologic signals within the body and the rather large electrical signals surrounding the body. Most electrical interference is handled by applying an appropriate ground that effectively nullifies the larger currents or isolates the biologic signals from the larger ones. It is helpful to disconnect all equipment that may be plugged into the wall socket in the vicinity of the EMG. The design of the amplifier is an important factor in providing a dependable signal-to-noise (information-versus-error) ratio.

The electrodes and the ground plate are connected to the preamplifier, a boxlike structure with pin receptacles labeled for the input of cathode, anode, and ground. The purpose of the preamplifier is to increase the magnitude of the signals taken from the electrodes without requiring long leads (wires) from them. In place of long unshielded wires or leads, the preamplifier has a shielded cable of sufficient length to reach the subject being tested and not incur the distortions of long leads and the influences of surrounding currents that would distort the signals. A good preamplifier must have low electronic noise levels and should have high input impedance and differential amplification with high common mode rejection. The latter will be discussed later.

Electronic noise (unwanted electrical messages) is always a part of any instrument, and it does not con-

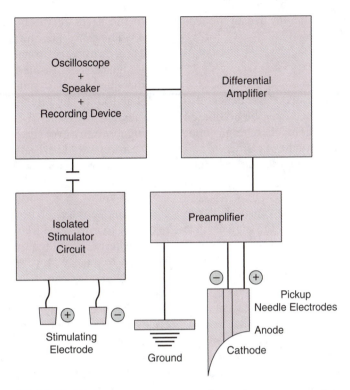

FIGURE 23–4 Block diagram of an electromyographic circuit.

tribute to the identification of useful biologic data. Electronic noise may develop from within the instrument, and the better the design of the amplifier, the less noise there will be. External sources of noise are called interference or artifacts. These may arise from fluorescent lighting, wall power outlets, dimmer switches, poor grounding within the electrical circuits in the building, and broadcast radio signals within range of the patient. When internal noise is smaller than the biologic signal, the distortion may not prevent accurate recognition of the biologic EMG signal. This becomes critical when the signal is extremely small (such as, a sensory evoked response, which will be less than 10 µV. The internal electronic noise may be 20 µV, thereby overshadowing the sensory response and making it invisible. A technique known as averaging is used to record only the signal that is always taking place at the same time and rejecting the signals that are occurring randomly. Once the small signals leave the electrodes and are conducted to the amplifier, their power and size is such that the smaller internal noise is no longer a major source of distortion. Thus, the electrodes used and the quality of the pre-

amplifier are the most important factors for minimizing the distortion of the biologic signal.

Another important property of the preamplifier is the proper match between the impedance of the electrode system and the impedance of the preamplifier. **Impedance** is defined as the combined effect of resistance capacitance and inductance of any circuit. It is desirable for the electrodes to have low impedance at the site of the signal pickup; however, at the terminals of the preamplifier, it is essential to have an extremely high impedance. In simpler words, the signal should be conducted, unhampered, from the source to the amplifier, where it should not be conducted but stopped from conducting. It also is important for the impedance of the two terminals to be well matched. If there is a mismatch, the current will move into the terminal of lower impedance and thereby create a drop in voltage. Because voltage or electromotive pressure is the signal being measured, any drop will distort the signal markedly.

Biologic signals frequently involve looking at alternating voltages and currents. This tendency means that the EMG circuit must deal with Ohm's law, where current is equal to voltage divided by impedance. The formula would be stated as

$$I = E/Z$$

where Z is impedance. Because the frequency also changes, the factor of inductance must be accounted for. The ideal preamplifier should have high-input impedance to have the least amount of distortion and loss of amplitude, which would be the voltage of the signal. High impedance is defined as high resistance and small capacitance.

Differential amplification is the capacity of the preamplifier to amplify selectively the signals that are confined to the input exploring and reference electrodes as they relate to the ground plate. Because differential amplification concerns the response to minute voltage differences between the two points, the resistance, size, and interface of the exploring and reference electrodes should be as similar as possible to the tissue being explored. Because voltage can be likened to pressure and current can be likened to the flow of water, it is analogous to say that restricting the flow of water increases the pressure. Conversely, opening the restriction reduces the pressure quickly. The latter is referred to as a **voltage drop** and results in large distortions of the biologic signal being measured.

Another aspect of differential amplification is that the small voltages within tissue can be identified even in the midst of much higher voltages (eg, wall outlets, lights, diathermy units, and other electrical devices). The reason that the small voltages can still be detected rather than being drowned out by the larger wall currents is that the differential amplifier compares both the active electrode and the dispersive electrode to ground and thus can ignore the larger voltages that are common to both poles or electrodes as well as the ground. Therefore, voltages common to all three are rejected; this process is called **common-mode rejection ratio (CMRR)**. A good EMG should have a CMRR of 1000:1. This will allow detecting small voltages even in the field of extremely high voltages.

A **calibration signal** is usually available that will display a known signal, which can be used as a reference to measure the biologic signals against. This is crucial for reliable and consistent measurements of these tiny biologic signals.

The amplifier receives the preamplified signal, which the examiner can increase or decrease according to the needs of the particular study being conducted. The control on the face of the ENMG usually is termed sensitivity, voltage, or gain control. The EMG signals are measured in microvolts; therefore, the therapist selects a gain or sensitivity setting for EMG at 100 µV. In a motor nerve conduction study, the therapist might set the gain at 5000 µV. In conducting a sensory evoked test, a typical gain or sensitivity setting would be 10 µV.

In an effort to reduce distortion, the **frequency bandwidth** or cycles per second (Hz) over which the amplifier must operate varies for particular studies. In conducting sensory studies of conduction, it is not necessary to extend the frequency band far in the high range, whereas EMG requires a low-frequency as well as a high-frequency range to detect the wide range of signals being generated in normal and pathologic states. Electronic filters are often used to remove some characteristically annoying signals such as 60-cycle or 60-Hz wall currents.

The amplified display on the cathode ray oscilloscope is then filtered sufficiently to avoid distorting the display or reducing its amplitude, so that it is possible to measure critical components of the waveforms displayed. The displayed signal can then be transferred to a printer for a paper display that can be stored as a permanent record.

In an effort to eliminate 60-cycle interference, which is found commonly from house current, inexpensive EMG feedback devices limit the low frequencies to no lower than 100 Hz. Consequently, this process results in cutting out all of the MUPs less than 100 Hz, which includes the small motor units that fire from 5 to 15 Hz.

Amplification of the signal will decrease for alternating-current (AC) test signals at frequencies above and below the frequency bandwidth of the instrument. The bandwidth limit consists of the frequencies that reduce or attenuate the amplitude 30% or more from that encountered in the midband region. Similarly, the amplifier should have a sufficiently rapid rise time of 20 microseconds and a much slower decay time of at least 8 milliseconds.

Amplifier noise can become extremely troublesome when conducting a sensory study, which requires high amplification. The **electronic noise** usually present in newer models of EMG, when shorting out the input terminals, is between 4 µV and 7 µV. This amplifier noise will increase geometrically with the frequency bandwidth. Thus, restricting the frequency bandwidth will reduce the amplifier noise, permitting better identification of the evoked sensory response. Another factor that increases noise is the electrical resistance in the electrode circuit connecting the patient to the preamplifier. This underscores the need to reduce skin resistance and to use relatively short wire leads to connect the active biologic signal source to the preamplifier. Because this biologic signal is an alternating one, the conducting leads must not offer excessive impedance—that is, the combined effect of capacitance and inductance plus the electrical resistance of the patient circuit. It is essential to have low-impedance conducting signals from the patient through the leads to the amplifier, after which the amplifier circuit should offer high-input impedance so that the voltage will not drop asymmetrically and thereby distort the biologic signal. If electrode paste accidentally enters one terminal but not the other, the terminals would not be matched for impedance. Therefore, the difference between the terminals would be amplified, resulting in an error signal on the oscilloscope. This distortion, known as a voltage drop, attenuates (reduces) the rapid parts of the waveform and leaves the slower components unchanged. The result is a major waveform distortion.

When conducting an EMG, the size and duration of the waveforms or action potentials will be important items. The horizontal axis provides a time base that can be modified by the control on the EMG called the **sweep speed** or the **time base.** When the sweep speed is on 5, each centimeter on the horizontal axis represents 5 milliseconds (or 5/1000 of a second). If the sweep is changed to 10, each centimeter is equal to 10 milliseconds.

The vertical axis is used to determine amplitude and is also called the *gain* on the EMG. The gain or voltage can be changed. If the gain is set at 5 mV, that setting means that each vertical centimeter attained by the action potential will be 5000 μV in amplitude. Similarly, if the gain setting is changed to 100, that setting implies that each vertical centimeter is equivalent to 100 μV. When the gain has a higher number, it is less sensitive, and when the gain has a lower number it is more sensitive. If a gain setting of 2000 is used and a CAP attains a height of 2 cm, it is evident that the amplitude is 4000 μV or 4 mV.

The nerve conduction mode uses a stimulation circuit that is electronically isolated from the differential amplifier. In addition, the nerve conduction velocity mode is synchronized so that the sweep is initiated at the lefthand margin of the screen. This arrangement provides for a consistent location of the stimulus and

the evoked responses. Without this synchronization, it would be necessary to measure each distance and also to anticipate it at different locations.

Modern ENMG devices have **storage oscilloscopes** that can "freeze" the waveform on the screen for detailed study. Generally, both EMG and nerve conduction velocity tracings can be stored and, in turn, printed on paper for permanent records.

Another technological advance that is incorporated in the ENMG is the **averager.** This device amplifies only signals that arrive within a given time period, which the examiner selects to approximate the time frame in which the signal is expected to arrive. Only signals that appear regularly in that window (time frame) are amplified, thereby making it possible to identify extremely small potentials even though much larger potentials are present but fall outside this time window.

The following are common sources of distortion of electrical signals from the patient to the apparatus:

- Lead wire of an electrode is partially broken.
- Lead wire moves during recordings.
- Wrong electrodes are connected to the amplifier input.
- Stimulator electrodes are near or on the recording electrodes.
- The ground electrode is loose.
- Dried electrode paste is on the surface electrode.
- Too much electrode paste is creating a bridge between poles.
- Power cords are plugged into a receptacle near the patient.
- Fluorescent lighting is in the testing area.
- Electronic dimmers are nearby or on same circuit.
- Audio that is too high is causing feedback.
- Citizen-band radio or taxi broadcaster is nearby.
- Radio or television transmitter is nearby.
- Diathermy or other electronic equipment is nearby.
- Wall receptacle is poorly grounded.
- Examining table is metal, or a wheelchair is ungrounded.

It is important that patients not come into contact with the casing of the ENMG because there may be small **leakage currents** coming from the case. The ENMG has the power cord attached at the rear of the unit, thereby considerably reducing the possibility of contact with the patient. The shock from this source, although small, could be serious if the patient's cardiac status is unstable or if the patient has an implanted pacemaker.

Stimulators should always have the intensity control returned to zero so that a large stimulus will not be delivered to the patient inadvertently. When stimulating, the intensity should be gradually advanced to avoid an excessive amount of stimulation. Care should be exercised so that the limb to be stimulated is not on a metal or conductive surface because this contact may lead to unpredictable effects on the patient.

If short-duration pulses (0.1–0.2 milliseconds) of direct current (DC) are delivered to a nerve trunk, more and more axons are activated, beginning with the larger-diameter fibers, as the intensity of the stimulus becomes stronger. When the nerve fibers are fired simultaneously, an action potential that is an amalgamation is formed of all active units within the muscle, and it becomes a **compound action potential (CAP).** As noted earlier, a greater-than-maximal, or *supramaximal*, stimulus is used to assure that all nerve fibers are activated, thereby providing a basis for later comparison of the active fibers within a given nerve trunk.

NERVE CONDUCTION STUDIES

Motor Nerve Conduction

To study the conduction of nerve fibers that supply muscle fibers, it is necessary to place surface electrodes over the muscle to pick up the response. The cathode (black) pickup electrode is placed over the center of the belly (motor point) of the muscle selected for study, and the anode (red) is placed distally on top of the muscle tendon junction. It is important to cleanse the skin of any oils or dirt to reduce skin impedance to an acceptable level (usually 5000 µW or less) under each electrode. A moderate amount of electrode paste is placed on each cathode and anode as well as on the ground plate. Then the electrodes are secured with enough tape to assure that they will not slip or move during the stimulation (**Fig. 23–5**). It is best to have patients recline for the test because some may become lightheaded or feel faint if upright. This posture also facilitates relaxation of muscles.

With the pickup electrodes in place and with the ground plate fixed between them and the stimulating

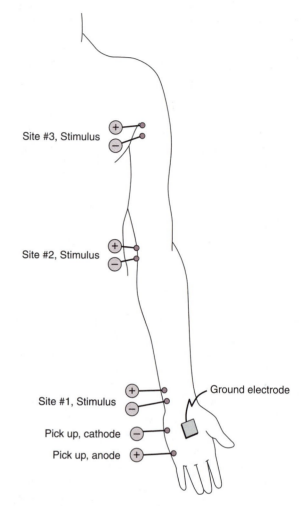

FIGURE 23–5 Placement of pickup and stimulating electrodes over the ulnar nerve on the left arm (anterior view) at three sites.

electrodes, the nerve conduction mode of the ENMG instrument is chosen. This mode typically provides a gain setting of 2–5 mV per centimeter division and a sweep speed of 5 milliseconds per centimeter division. The stimulus frequency most commonly is 1 per second; however, the therapist can activate the stimulus by pressing on a foot switch. The duration of the stimulus will depend to some extent on the state of conductivity of the nerve: that is, a diseased nerve will require a longer duration than does a healthy nerve. The therapist typically begins with a duration of 0.1 millisecond; if no response is obtained, the duration is increased to 0.2 millisecond.

A distal point is selected on the nerve to be tested next, and the cathode (black) is placed distal to the anode (red). The stimulator handle contains an intensity control that advances the stimulus gradually while pressing the electrodes firmly into the skin over the nerve. Once a response is obtained, the stimulus intensity is advanced gradually until no further increase in the amplitude of the response wave is noted. When the intensity is then advanced 10% more, the stimulus is termed a supramaximal one. This procedure is done to assure that all conducting fibers are included in the study of that nerve. Once an optimal response is obtained, the response is stored on the screen. Then a cursor is moved from the left side of the screen to the beginning of the takeoff of the negative (up-going) phase of the response wave. This duration is called the **distal latency** and is measured in milliseconds; it is the time required for the stimulus to be conducted along the motor nerves to the muscle fibers, from which the impulses are picked up and displayed as the response wave. The amplitude of that response is measured from the baseline to the peak of the negative phase and is recorded as millivolts (see **Fig. 23–1**).

Then a second site is chosen on the same peripheral nerve, and, again, a supramaximal stimulation is conducted and the response wave is stored on the oscilloscope screen. The second, proximal latency is recorded by moving the cursor to the second response wave when it first departs from the baseline in an upward sweep. Similarly, the amplitude is again measured from baseline to the peak of the negative phase (see **Fig. 23–1**).

A tape measure is used to determine the distance from the distal cathode stimulus site to the proximal cathode site, which is determined in millimeters. The skin temperature is then recorded at a distal site on the limb being tested.

The steps required to test motor nerve conduction can be summarized as follows:

1. Select the instrument component—the nerve conduction mode.
2. Use a sensitivity setting of 2–5 mV.
3. Use a sweep speed of 5 ms/division.
4. Use a stimulus rate of 1/s and a duration of 0.1 ms.
5. Position the patient in the supine position with the limb supported.
6. Prepare the skin for recording electrodes over the muscle.
7. Place the cathode (negative) recording electrode over the center of the belly of the muscle.
8. Place the anode (positive) recording electrode over the tendon of the same muscle.
9. Place the ground electrode between the stimulating and recording electrodes.
10. Tape all recording electrodes securely in place.
11. Apply the stimulating electrodes with the cathode (negative) directed distally toward the muscle.
12. Increase the intensity of the stimulus progressively.
13. Continue to increase 10% more once the impulse is maximal to assure that no axons are left out.
14. Record three responses from the distal point.
15. Record three responses from the proximal point.
16. Measure the distance from the proximal to the distal points.
17. Record the proximal and the distal latencies and the measurements from the proximal to distal stimulation sites of the cathode.
18. Determine the skin temperature over the distal limb, and record it.
19. Calculate the conduction velocity of that segment of the nerve.
20. Repeat the previous steps for the next proximal segment of the nerve.

To calculate the conduction velocity of motor components, the distal latency is subtracted from the proximal latency to obtain the time of conduction through that segment of the nerve. This conduction time is then divided into the distance measured (in millimeters) to determine the conduction velocity of that segment of the nerve. That is,

$$\text{conduction velocity} = \frac{\text{distance (millimeters)}}{\substack{\text{conduction time} \\ \text{(milliseconds)}}}$$

More than two points can be studied in the same manner if they are accessible to the electrode through the skin. By studying each segment, the therapist can compare different segments with each other to determine whether there is relative slowing in one portion versus the other or whether there is a drop in amplitude in one area versus another. Each laboratory should conduct tests on a series of normal subjects to determine the normal values for each segment. It is helpful to print these values on the reporting form. A sample reporting form for nerve conduction is shown in **Figure 23–16** on page 355).

Environmental temperature has a significant influence on nerve conduction values. These temperatures have an even greater influence when circulatory disturbance or paralysis of musculature is present.

The relationship between temperature and conduction velocity is linear for the range between 29° and 38°C. When beyond this range in temperature, the conduction velocity increases 5% per degree increase or decreases the same percentage per degree decrease. For example, in nerve conducting between 40 and 60 meters per second, if the environmental temperature decreases 1°C, the conduction velocity will decrease 2–3 meters per second. The distal latency from wrist to hand muscle will increase by 0.3 millisecond per degree of cooling for both median and ulnar nerves.

The skin temperature is often taken if these changes in conduction velocity would prove to be critical when interpreting the results on a particular patient. If testing is performed in an environment with a variable temperature, the skin temperature, the conduction velocity, and the latency values should be recorded at the same time.

Sensory Nerve Conduction

Because all fibers in a nerve trunk are stimulated simultaneously when electrical pulses of more than threshold are applied, differentiation of motor and sensory components of the peripheral nerve is achieved by placement of the pickup electrodes. To determine the sensory components of a peripheral nerve, it is customary to place ring electrodes around the fingers for the specific upper-extremity nerves to be tested and over skin areas of the feet or toes for selected lower-extremity nerves. Obviously, the motor components are also stimulated when the entire nerve trunk is stimulated; however, removing the skin pickup area from the area of discharge from the muscle provides a distinct signal that represents the sensory or skin innervation for that nerve.

Orthodromic Procedure.   Sensory axons normally, or orthodromically, conduct impulses from the periphery to the center of the body. Therefore, the therapist can stimulate on the digits and place pickup electrodes over the nerve trunk at one or more sites to permit determination of sensory conduction velocity (as in motor nerve conduction testing). This orthodromic **sensory nerve action potential (SNAP)** response will be of much lower amplitude than the motor response; therefore, the sensory conduction mode will use 10–20 µV gain settings and a sweep speed of 2 milliseconds. Because electronic noise will

be close to the signal response, it is helpful to reduce the upper part of the frequency band and compress it between 30 and 200 Hz. This narrow frequency band provides an optimal amplification of the signal.

Antidromic Procedure.   Sensory studies can also be conducted in an antidromic fashion, that is, against the normal flow of the sensory signal. In this situation, the pickup electrode is the ring around the finger (cathode proximal and anode distal). The stimulating electrode is the same one used in motor component studies. In both orthodromic and antidromic studies, the amplitude is measured from the takeoff from baseline to the peak of the negative spike. Typical upper-extremity amplitudes are 20–50 µV, whereas lower-extremity values range from 5 to 15 µV.

The distal latency is determined in the same way as motor latency, measuring the time required for the stimulus to be conducted along the sensory fibers to the first recording electrode. The sensory nerve conduction velocity is determined in the same way as motor conduction, subtracting the distal latency from the proximal latency of the sensory response, and then dividing into the distance measured between the cathode stimulation sources when performed antidromically. If orthodromic, the two times of conduction would be compared with the distance in millimeters from one pickup site to the other. The amplitudes will be much lower in orthodromic than in antidromic sensory studies; for this reason, sensory studies are subject to more interference and technical errors than are the larger amplitude motor studies.

The steps required to test sensory nerve conduction can be summarized as follows:

1. Place the patient in a comfortable supine position.
2. Prepare the skin by cleaning it with alcohol.
3. Place the recording rings or disc electrodes over the cleaned recording and stimulating electrode sites.
4. Place the ground plate between the stimulating and the recording electrodes.
5. Follow the orthodromic technique of sensory testing by (a) placing stimulating rings or clips on digits with the cathode (negative) proximal, and (b) placing the recording electrodes over the nerve that is being stimulated with the cathode

distal, and placing the ground plate between the stimulating and recording electrodes.

6. Follow the antidromic technique of sensory testing by (a) placing the recording electrodes on digits or the distal portion of the nerve being tested with the cathode proximal and the anode distal, (b) placing stimulating electrodes on the distal segment of the nerve with the cathode distal and the anode proximal, and (c) placing the ground between the stimulating and recording electrodes.

7. Select the sensory nerve conduction mode with a 10 µV gain setting and a 2 millisecond sweep speed setting.

8. Stimulate distally and pickup at the nerve at the two sites on the nerve in the orthodromic technique or stimulate on the nerve and pickup from the distal site in the antidromic technique.

9. Record three tracings from each site.

10. Record the skin temperature over the distal limb.

11. Measure the distance between the stimulating and the proximal recording electrode and the distal recording site (orthodromic technique).

12. The antidromic technique is the same as in motor nerve conduction.

13. Calculate the conduction velocity from the recorded proximal and distal latencies.

14. Record the latencies and the conduction velocity values on a chart for the particular nerve in question.

Proximal Conduction Procedure.   Selected peripheral nerves can be stimulated with the cathode directed proximally, the sweep speed reduced to 20 msec/division, and the gain increased to 200 µV. This arrangement evokes responses in the nerve that stimulate axons from distal to proximal. As stimulation of a nerve axon will be conducted in both the proximal and the distal directions, the latter will be detected at the distal latency time and will be of large amplitude (eg, 8–12 mV) and is known as an M wave. A proximal conduction observed is an H reflex, which is obtained through stimulation of the posterior tibial nerve (**Fig. 23–6**).

The F Wave.   The technique for eliciting the F wave response is as follows:

1. Place the patient in a supine, relaxed position.

2. Select the nerve conduction mode on instrument.

3. Use sweep settings of 20 ms/division.

4. Use a gain setting of 200 µV.

5. Use the procedures outlined for motor nerve conduction with regard to skin preparation, electrode placement, and so on.

6. Reverse the position of the stimulating electrode so that the cathode is directed proximally.

7. Advance the stimulation progressively, using the same frequency and duration as in motor nerve conduction. The M wave will appear at the motor latency on the left of the screen, and after several impulses a much smaller response of 50–150 µV will appear at a much longer latency.

8. Record eight long-latency F waves.

9. Measure the limb length from the seventh cervical vertebrae to the styloid process of the ulna.

10. Compare the proximal conduction with the conduction of the distal segment as a ratio of proximal to distal.

11. Compare the latency of one side with the latency of the other side, and if no limb length discrepancy exists, use the longer F wave latency to indicate proximal slowing.

The **F wave latency** is believed to represent a type of echo reaction via the alpha motor neurons that Magladery et al[6] first noted and labeled the F wave. The F wave is called a wave because it does not involve any synaptic transmission. The impulse is believed to travel antidromically proximally in the alpha motor neuron to the cell body, and then reflect back again to the motor axon to produce the extremely small and variable response wave in the muscle. If the dorsal roots (carrying sensory axons) are sectioned, the F wave is still readily elicited; therefore, it is assumed that the motor nerves are responsible for its conduction. However, whether the F wave is the product of some other mechanism, perhaps even conduction through other afferents or through afferents that enter the spinal cord through the ventral root, is not completely resolved. The F wave latency is variable within a narrow range in normal individuals, and its amplitude also changes in the same individual. These readings may represent variability in the placement of the stimulating electrode during the test or other technical factors, or the F wave could represent some form of multisynaptic transmission.

The F wave is readily obtained by using a supramaximal stimulus on the distal point of most peripheral

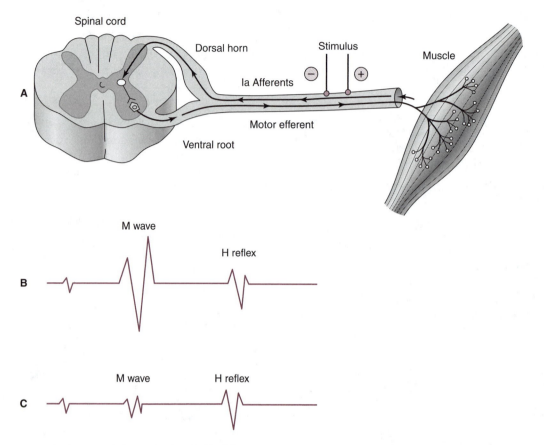

FIGURE 23–6 (**A**) An idealized H reflex under circumstances of diminishing stimulus intensity. (**B**) Both M and H responses at a threshold stimulus of 0.5 milliseconds duration and a frequency of less than 1 second. (**C**) The M wave decreases as the stimulus decreases. However, the H reflex remains constant in amplitude and duration with a stimulus of 0.5 milliseconds duration, but lower intensity at a frequency of 1 second.

nerves, and the frequency can be at 1 per second. This is not found with the H reflex testing (discussed later), which requires submaximal stimulation at irregular and widely spaced intervals.

Because the F wave is believed to reflect the adequacy of conduction of the axons proximally, it is helpful for the determination of lesions that affect the proximal portion of the axons, such as the Guillain-Barré syndrome and thoracic outlet and nerve root compression lesions. It is helpful to compare the conduction of the distal segment with the proximal segment so that a peripheral (distal) neuropathy does not provide a false positive impression of proximal slowing if the therapist looks only at the F wave conduction.

The H Reflex. The **H reflex** has been studied extensively in clinical and physiologic investigations since it was first identified by Hoffman in 1918,[7] but it was not so designated until the studies of Magladery et al.[6] The H reflex has been the subject of numerous articles over the past forty years, and Crone et al[8] and Leonard and Moritani[9] have advocated its use dynamically to determine the neural basis of movement disorders in neurologically impaired individuals. In the typical application in the clinical setting, the H reflex is used to determine the adequacy of the dorsal root containing the Ia afferents from the muscle spindle and to determine the excitability of the alpha motor neuron pool.[10] Crone and Nielsen[11] found that H-eliciting stimulations that were less than 1 second apart did not allow for the complete recovery of the H reflex to baseline levels. Similarly, the H reflex is stimulated by submaximal stimuli of longer duration (0.5 milliseconds), so that a response is elicited in the thicker afferent (spindle afferents) fibers first and not primarily to elicit motor axons (see **Fig. 23–6**).

The technique for eliciting the H reflex is as follows:

1. Position the patient prone with the head in the midline.
2. Place the recording electrode (the cathode) over the midpoint between the length of the tibial nerve from the popliteal fossa and medial malleolus, on the medial gastrocnemius, and the anode over the Achilles tendon.
3. Tape the cathode and anode stimulating electrode over the posterior tibial nerve in the popliteal fossa with the cathode directed proximally.
4. Place the ground electrode between the recording and stimulating electrodes.
5. Set the oscilloscope screen to a gain of 500 µV and a sweep speed of 20 milliseconds.
6. Set the stimulus duration for 0.5 milliseconds and the frequency for less than 1 per second or for the best elicitation by the foot switch.
7. Advance the stimuli slowly and to less than maximal so that an M response is evoked. At a latency of nearly 27–32 milliseconds, an H response should be detected.
8. Decrease the intensity after the H response is obtained to the point where the amplitude of the M response declines by 30–40% and the H response remains unchanged.
9. Record the H wave latency and its amplitude from each side.
10. Compare the latencies with each other and with normal values.

Braddom and Johnson[12] found that submaximal stimulation of the posterior tibial nerve in the popliteal fossa in 100 normal subjects with a wide age range had an H reflex latency of 29.8 milliseconds, with a standard deviation (SD) of 2.74 milliseconds. The latency is correlated with leg length and with age, so it can be said that H latency is equal to 9.14 + 0.46 leg length in centimeters + 0.1 age in years. When Braddom and Johnson measured the H latencies in 25 subjects of all ages, they noted that there was a mean difference of only 0.3 milliseconds. The standard error of the means from one leg to the other was 0.40 milliseconds. Using three standard errors from the mean, this finding would imply that 1.20 milliseconds becomes a significant difference from one limb to the other. It is useful to use this test when compromise of the lumbosacral nerve root is suspected, because it reveals S1 nerve root lesion

deficits. Obviously, an absence of the response on one side but not on the other also would be indicative of an S1 compromise on that side. Schuchmann[13] conducted H reflex testing of unilateral L5 radiculopathy and found no significant differences in the latencies (see **Fig. 23–6**).

The H response can be readily obtained from other nerves in addition to the posterior tibial when there is a lesion in the CNS, presumably because the inhibition is removed from the spinal cord circuit.

The Blink Reflex. Kugelberg[14] described the response of the orbicularis oculi to an electrode stimulus over the brow on the opthalmic branch. He noted an early ipsilateral blink reflex response with a latency of 12 milliseconds and a late response bilaterally in the orbicularis oculi muscles of 21–40 milliseconds in healthy people. The blink reflex is currently elicited with an electrical pulse to the opthalmic branch of the trigeminal nerve at the supraorbital foramen; the impulse is then conducted to the anterior hind brain and synaptically transfers the stimulus to the facial nerve, where it is then conducted to the orbicularis oculi muscles for pickup by the electrodes. Kimura et al[15] described a technique in which two channels are used to determine the simultaneous response in both eyes to stimulation on each side independently.

The procedure for eliciting the blink reflex is as follows:

1. Place the patient in the supine position on the examining table.
2. Tape the cathode disk electrode to the outer border of each eye.
3. Tape the reference (anode) electrode to the outer wall of the nostril on each side.
4. Tape the ground electrode to the chin.
5. Select the nerve conduction mode for the oscilloscope.
6. Bring up two channels with the same settings of 200 µV gain and 20 millisecond sweep speed.
7. Stimulate the opthalmic branch at the supraorbital foramen with the cathode while the anode is on the brow.
8. Use a stimulus intensity of 50 V and a duration of 0.1 milliseconds. The ipsilateral response (R1) will be 10.6 milliseconds (SD, 0.82 milliseconds) in normal subjects. The bilateral second response (R2) will be found ipsilaterally at 31.3 milliseconds (SD, 3.3 milliseconds), and the contralateral

R2 will be found at 31.6 milliseconds (SD, 3.78 milliseconds).

9. Repeat the stimulation from the opposite supraorbital site to obtain R1 and R2 responses ipsilaterally and contralaterally from that side.

10. Compare both sides for symmetry; a difference of three standard deviations from one side to the other is considered significant.

The **blink reflex test** is useful for testing individuals with facial palsy. This test can activate the proximal portion of the facial nerve, where it is frequently impaired through the facial canal in the temporal bone. A complete loss of conduction leads to an absence of ipsilateral responses but not of the contralateral responses because the trigeminal nerve is unimpaired. If conduction slows, the ipsilateral response will be prolonged, but the latency of the contralateral one will be normal.

The blink reflex also has potential value for testing individuals with blepharospasm or hemifacial spasm. It has been used to document facial and trigeminal involvement in individuals with acoustic neuromas.[16] Other applications being investigated include trigeminal neuralgia and migraine headaches.

Repetitive Stimulation of the Neuromuscular Junction.

Myasthenia gravis is the disease process most often associated with dymfunction of the neuromuscular junction. The affected area is the postsynaptic acetylcholine receptor site, with weakness and early-onset fatigue common complaints.[17] An older method of testing the neuromuscular junction used high-frequency stimulation of more than 50 Hz, which was extremely uncomfortable. The technique has been supplanted by one described by Desmedt,[18] a series of pulses applied at two pulses per second, which results in a significant decrement after the fourth pulse and a return to initial values from the fourth through the tenth pulse. Intercurrent exercise is applied after the first train of 10 pulses. Immediately after the exercise of the muscle being tested, another train of 10 pulses is applied at two per second.[18]

Summary of Nerve Conduction Studies

Nerve conduction studies must be based on sound clinical judgments, and they are actually an extension of the physical examination of the patient. As Brooke[19] suggested, therapists need to listen to patients because they are trying to say what is wrong. The selection of the test is determined by the review of the patient's history and physical findings. Nerve conduction studies depend on exacting technique and careful recording of data. The quality of the instrumentation is crucial, and staff in each laboratory should establish their own normal values.

The interpretation of the results of nerve conduction studies depends on the examiner's knowledge of neurophysiology and neuropathology. For example, a diabetic neuropathy leads to demyelination that results in slowing of conduction, whereas an alcoholic toxic neuropathy leads to degenerative changes in the axon, resulting in a reduction in the amplitude of the evoked responses. Some disorders of the peripheral nerve may not exhibit changes in the periphery if they are found initially in the proximal region of the nerve, such as in the Guillain-Barré syndrome. However, the F wave, the H reflex, or both may be delayed or absent in the same subjects because the ventral roots are implicated in this disease.

Common anatomic variations—such as the Martin-Gruber anastomosis between the median and ulnar nerves in the forearm—must be considered. Another variation may occur in the peroneal nerve in the lower leg. Sensory symptoms are often inconsistent with textbook configurations; and because there is much variation in this area, the examiner should not reach the hasty conclusion that the patient is not telling the truth. Also, reported symptoms such as numbness and hyperesthesia are frequently confusing to the examiner who is depending on the words that a patient uses to describe symptoms.

A *neuropractic lesion* (one that results in loss of conduction at one location on the nerve) at the elbow will not reveal any loss of conduction unless there is a stimulus through that segment. One major deficit in nerve conduction testing is the problem of whether the available segments of a given nerve have been studied sufficiently. Although a nerve may be transected completely, it can still conduct impulses for 72 hours after the lesion, but it will not conduct across the site of the transection. Use of statistical comparisons should not replace sound clinical judgment as well as a comparison from one limb to the other and between one nerve and another. Differences in amplitude are unreliable to a degree, but a difference of more than 10% would be of consequence if the study were performed in a standardized manner for each limb. A reduction in amplitude will be found when axons have been eliminated or have stopped conducting, because this results in a loss of many more muscle fibers from the motor unit. In an acute lesion, the loss of one axon would result in 6–700 muscle fibers (motor unit ratio); therefore, 10 axons would result in a loss of 60–7000 muscle fibers. When a lesion has been present for several months, some sprouting of neurons from other healthy ones begins to take over the denervated territory by collateral sprouting, thus reducing the impact on the amplitude to some extent and increasing the numbers of phases, producing a short-duration, low-amplitude, polyphasic motor unit action potential.

The duration of the CMAP will be prolonged if the conduction velocity within the nerve trunk is variable. This finding may be the first sign of axonal degeneration in peripheral nerves affected by Guillain-Barré syndrome or another progressive demyelinating disease of the peripheral nerves. These **demyelinating diseases** also may produce focal slowing in conduction of peripheral nerves; thus, it is important to test more than one segment in nerves that are suspected victims of this type of disorder (see **Fig. 23–7**).

Prolongation of the distal latency of a nerve may occur with localized compression of that nerve. A common site of compression is the median nerve through the carpal tunnel or the posterior tibial nerve through the tarsal tunnel. Other disorders will cause the distal portion of the nerve to die back. Sumner[20] implicated distal motor latencies as the most common early sign of toxic dying back of a nerve. They noted the wide variety of toxic agents that are encountered

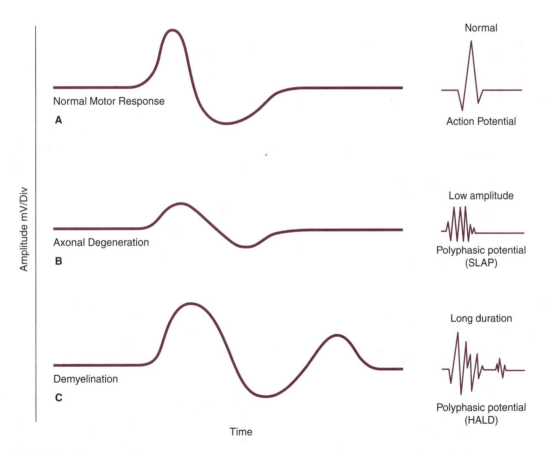

FIGURE 23–7   Effects of demyelination and axonal degeneration on the evoked motor response and the electromyogram. Axonal degeneration results in reduced amplitude of the evoked response and low amplitude EMG potentials (SLAP), whereas the response from demyelination produces a prolonged duration and a complex EMG potential that also is of longer duration. (**A**) Normal action potential. (**B**) Low short duration amplitude polyphasic potential (SLAP). (**C**) Long high amplitude duration polyphasic potential (HALD).

today, ranging from heavy metal poisoning to volatile industrial toxins; and the list steadily grows longer. These agents should be part of any screening for the etiology of a disturbance that is not readily explained by trauma or other means.

Electrophysiologic studies may uncover changes in conductivity that are not clinically apparent. Thus, it is important to distinguish between a **carpal tunnel syndrome** and a **dying-back neuropathy** caused by an industrial toxin. Clearly, if a nerve is dying back, surgical release of the transverse ligament will not improve nerve function (see **Fig. 23–7**).

Trauma to a peripheral nerve can result in a loss of conduction called *neuropraxia* or axonal degeneration; a loss of nerve continuity called *axonotmesis*; or discon-

tinuity called *neurotmesis*. In a neuropraxia, the part of the nerve distal to the lesion responds to stimulation normally but will not produce a response distal to the site of neuropraxia when stimulating above it. With axonotmesis and neurotmesis, response distal to the lesion will be good until Wallerian degeneration takes place in the distal segment; then, the response will be nonexistent if the nerve is completely degenerated or partial if the degeneration is incomplete. During regeneration, some rudimentary conduction will take place, but it will lag behind changes in the EMG. The EMG will be discussed in a later section (**Fig. 23–8**).

Failure at the neuromuscular junction results in a progressive declination of the amplitude with repetitive stimulation. When studying patients with an ab-

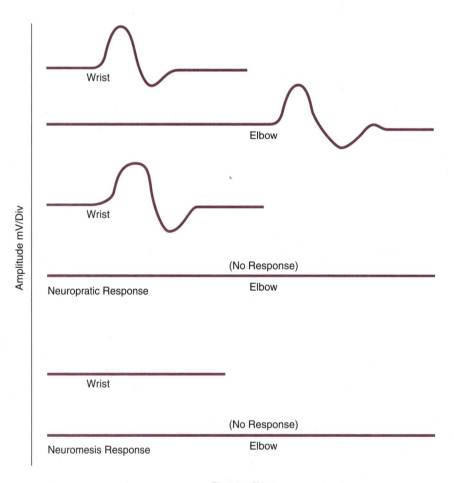

FIGURE 23–8   Comparison of neuropractic versus neurotmesis in evoked responses of the ulnar nerve at the level of the elbow. (See the normal values on the top tracing.)

normally low amplitude with a single shock, a train of pulses at 2 Hz should be applied, along with intercurrent exercise, to rule out the **Eaton-Lambert phenomenon** or the myesthenic reaction.[21] In addition, other disorders of the neuromuscular junction result in variable amplitudes if the rate is faster than 1 per second. Whenever variable amplitudes are detected, repetitive stimulation testing should be instituted.

Good technique is the most important factor in avoiding errors in nerve conduction studies. One common source of error is the placement of electrodes and their fixation to the skin. The cathode or negative recording electrode is usually black and should be fixed securely with tape after the skin is cleansed with alcohol to remove any dirt or oils. This electrode should be placed over the center of the belly of the muscle that is customarily the motor point of that muscle. If the active recording electrode is not over the motor point, it may result in an initial positive deflection followed by the negative one. This result makes it extremely difficult to determine the precise point of takeoff of the evoked CMAP. The reference electrode is then placed on the musculotendinous junction of that same muscle. Placement of the reference electrode on the tendon junction will provide the best circumstance for reliable amplitude readings. If the patient should perspire during the test, the tape may loosen, and the amplitude of the recording will become decreased or fragmentary and may even prolong the duration of the CMAP. Similarly, if the electrode paste is bridged from one stimulating electrode to the other, a partial short may occur and cause incomplete stimulation of the nerve under the electrodes.

The use of too much electrode paste, permitting paste to bridge from the active to the reference or recording electrode, will result in a distorted signal that is difficult to distinguish from a pathologic entity. Loosening of a ground electrode also will increase electronic noise (**interference**) with a greater distortion of baseline. Before calling the manufacturer's representative, check the electrodes for continuity and good fixation to the body.

Improperly placed stimulating electrodes lead to the need to increase the intensity until the stimulus is extremely painful for the patient. Adequate pressure over the nerve helps to place the electrode as close to the nerve as possible; however, if the pressure displaces the nerve from the vicinity of the stimulus, it decreases the effectiveness of the stimu-

lus. Most studies begin with stimulation of a distal point on the nerve to avoid cross stimulation from one nerve to another when close together (eg, in the median nerve at the wrist versus in the upper arm). If the therapist is careful to duplicate the response wave at each site along the nerve, you are likely to be stimulating the same nerve throughout. This duplication process also may help when confronted by anomalous innervation such as Martin-Gruber anastomosis of median and ulnar nerves in the forearm or the accessory peroneal nerve, which is found posterior to the lateral malleolus.

Patients with a considerable amount of subcutaneous fat or with a bulky musculature may require longer-duration pulses to stimulate the nerve adequately. In a large individual, this possibility may become more evident in the proximal region of the nerve, and an increased pulse width should be used if the response wave changes substantially from the distal one, which involves less tissue. Conversely, if too much stimulation is applied, it may splash to other adjacent nerves, resulting in a confusing pattern of response. When stimulating with high-intensity stimuli, the stimulus might be conducted by volume conduction to the recording electrode, which may produce a false signal that would produce a false result. This outcome is most commonly encountered in sensory conduction studies in which the motor nerves are responding and the sensory are not, thereby resulting in motor responses that are volume conducted from the muscle to the fingertips, where the recording electrode is located, when recording antidromically.

Measurement is another source of error and should always be taken from pen marks on the skin to avoid errors. The measurements are taken from stimulating cathode to cathode or from stimulating cathode to the recording cathode. The use of calipers have been recommended; however, if metal tape is used carefully, it will result in reproducible results. The measurement should be over the anatomical course of the nerve, but this position may be difficult to follow in some areas—for example, through the axilla or around the elbow for the ulnar nerve. In the latter, it is highly recommended[17,22] that the elbow be flexed approximately 90° when testing the ulnar nerve across the elbow. This position allows better approximation of the true anatomical length of the nerve when measuring across the elbow. Whichever position is used, it should be consistent from one test to the next. The shorter the distances between stimulation sites, the greater the possibility of error. This possibility is most evident in the ulnar nerve at the elbow, where the short distance from above the elbow to below the elbow can be avoided by measuring from above the elbow to the wrist and from below the elbow to the wrist. This procedure will not only produce a less dramatic drop in conduction but also avoid an error of 1 cm resulting in a major error in the determination of conduction velocity. For instance, an error of 1 cm over 10 cm is a 10% error, but a 1 cm error over 25 cm is a 4% error.

Distal latencies can be standardized to a greater extent through the process of having consistent distances from stimulating cathode to recording cathode. This distance is usually 8 cm for the hand and 14 cm for the foot.

When testing in cold climates, the examiner must allow for warming of limbs and must ensure that the environmental temperature is adequate to avoid a chill. If necessary, a heating pad or blanket can be applied for 10 to 15 minutes before testing begins. The recording of skin temperatures is essential in these circumstances to interpret the results in a reasonable fashion.

The patient's age also must be considered because the very young and the very old will have decreased conduction velocity. Other factors that affect conduction, such as peripheral vascular disease, which results in greater cooling of the part, also need attention. Determining whether a patient needs vascular surgery when vascular insufficiency and reduced conduction velocity are present is a difficult clinical task. Paralysis from a cardiovascular accident also may decrease the limb temperature and thereby reduce the conduction velocity of the peripheral nerves within that limb.

During **repetitive stimulation** of a given muscle, unless both the stimulating electrodes and the recording electrodes are taped securely to the patient, any slight movement of either set of electrodes will cause a change in amplitude. Because a change in amplitude of 10% is considered pathologic in the repetitive stimulation technique described earlier, it is crucial to avoid movement of the electrodes during the recording. In addition, the limb should be strapped to a board to ensure additional reliability of the measurements.

Studies of Specific Nerves

This section outlines the application of conduction techniques to specific peripheral nerves (boxed text pages 337–345). It outlines the instrument settings for each nerve, describes the position of the patient and the placement of electrodes, and indicates the stimulation sites used in most clinical situations (see **Box 23–1**). The sites of stimulation are labeled S1, S2, S3, and so forth. A more complete description of the conduction velocity procedure will be found elsewhere.

The following comments apply as readers review the procedures for testing specific nerves. When responses are evoked in the facial nerve, the patient may experience a flash of light with each pulse and should be counseled that this effect is natural, not harmful. The patient may experience a transient taste of metal in the mouth from slight ionization of metal fillings in the teeth; again, the patient should be told about this effect in advance. Only one site is available in the facial nerve; thus, the response to stimuli is recorded as a latency and compared with the opposite side regarding time as well as the amplitude of the CMAP.

Other peripheral nerves are recorded by the nerve and side, and each site of stimulation is labeled with the latencies from each one. As many sites as practical should be used to ensure that the lesion is not proximal to the segment studied. The amplitude is recorded for each site, and some examiners also record the temporal dispersion of the CMAP. In addition, the distance between electrodes is recorded for each site, and the difference between sites is divided by the time difference to arrive at the conduction velocity, which is also recorded for that segment.

The proximal latencies are recorded on the nerve conduction record for each nerve studied in this way. The H reflex and the amplitudes of the proximal response or reflex also are recorded. Some laboratories conduct an M conduction versus an F conduction to report a ratio of F to M by measuring the length of the limb and calculating a conduction velocity of the proximal latency versus the conduction velocity of the distal segment of the nerve. In this way, the therapist can determine whether the distal segment is faster than the proximal segment, which would pervade in a disorder of the proximal components and would be the reverse in the normal situation. All modern ENMG instruments have a variety of printing capabilities, and all the recordings can be displayed on paper with the calculated conduction velocity values, amplitudes, and CMAP waveforms.

Repetitive stimulation studies are reported as amplitude changes as compared with the initial single shock to the muscle being examined. Each series of 2-Hz pulses is calculated and displayed on a paper trace of the responses. The amplitudes that were obtained should also be noted after the brief exercise.

Box 23–1 *Nerve Conduction Velocity Study Procedures*

MEDIAN NERVE (MOTOR)

Electromyograph Instrument Parameters

Filter settings/frequency response: 10,000–10 Hz
Sweep speed: 2–5 ms/division
Sensitivity/gain: 1,000–5,000 µV/division

Patient Position

The patient is positioned supine with the arm abducted approximately 45°. The forearm is fully supinated, and the wrist is in a neutral position.

Electrode Placement

The active recording electrode is positioned directly over the anatomic center of the abductor pollicis brevis muscle. The electrode is placed half the distance between the metacarpophalangeal joint of the thumb and the midpoint of the distal wrist crease.

The reference electrode is positioned **off** the abductor pollicis brevis muscle on the distal phalanx of the thumb over bone or tendon.

The ground electrode is firmly positioned on the dorsum of the hand between the active and stimulating electrodes.

Electrostimulation

Percutaneous electrostimulation is performed at the appropriate anatomic sites in the following order:

1. Distal stimulation is performed at the wrist between the palmaris longus and flexor carpi radialis tendons. The cathode (negative) pole of the stimulator is placed proximal to the center of the active recording electrode on the abductor pollicis brevis muscle.

2. Stimulation above the elbow is performed proximal and medial to the antecubital space and proximal to the elbow crease between the belly of the biceps muscle and the medial head of the triceps muscle. The stimulator is positioned just lateral to the brachial artery to minimize the possibility of inadvertent electrostimulation of the ulnar nerve.

3. Proximal stimulation is performed in the axilla at least 10 cm proximal to the above elbow site and immediately lateral and anterior to the brachial artery.

Technical Comments

Evoked muscle action potential responses from all three sites should be similar in waveform, amplitude, and duration of response.

Wrist-site stimulation voltage, stimulus pulse duration, or both should be increased gradually and monitored carefully because a high-voltage/long pulse-width stimulation at the wrist may volume conduct to the adjacent ulnar response.

The clinical response should be observed carefully to avoid mistaking an ulnar for a median response. At the wrist, median stimulation elicits thumb palmar abduction and opposition, whereas ulnar stimulation elicits thumb adduction and metacarpal phalangeal flexion. At stimulation sites above the elbow and axilla, median-nerve stimulation elicits wrist flexion and radial deviation involving the flexor carpi radialis muscle, whereas ulnar nerve stimulation involves wrist flexion and ulnar deviation by contraction of the flexor carpi ulnaris muscle.

The wrist should be maintained in a neutral position while one measures forearm distance. Wrist flexion decreases and wrist extension increases the distance. All distance measurements should be taken with a metal tape measure. The measurement of distance should approximate the anatomic course of the nerve being tested.

ULNAR NERVE (MOTOR)

Electromyograph Instrument Parameters

Filter settings/frequency response: 10,000–10 Hz
Sweep Speed: 2–5 Ms/division
Sensitivity/Gain: 1,000–5,000 µV/division

(continued)

Patient Position

The patient is positioned supine with the arm abducted to 90° and externally rotated with the elbow in midflexion at 60°–90° palm up, and the wrist in a neutral position. When the patient is positioned supine, the palm of the hand faces the ceiling.

Electrode Placement

The active recording electrode is positioned on the ulnar border of the hand directly over the anatomic center of the abductor digiti minimi muscle at the point midway between the distal wrist crease and the crease at the base of the fifth digit at the level of the web space.

The reference electrode is positioned **off** the abductor digiti minimi muscle on the ulnar aspect of the fifth finger at the level of the web space.

The ground electrode is positioned on the dorsum of the hand between the active and stimulation electrodes.

Electrostimulation

Percutaneous electrostimulation is performed at the appropriate anatomic sites in the following order:

1. Distal stimulation is applied at the wrist, medial **or** lateral to the flexor carpi ulnaris tendon. The cathode (negative) pole of the stimulator is placed proximal to the center of the active recording electrode on the abductor digiti minimi muscle (see **Fig. 23–5**).
2. The below-elbow stimulation site is situated just distal to the medial humeral epicondyle in line with the cubital tunnel (a point midway between the medial epicondyle and the olecranon process) of the elbow and the distal wrist stimulation site.
3. The above-elbow stimulation site is located at least 10 cm proximal to the below-elbow stimulation site in line with the ulnar groove of the elbow and the midportion of the shaft of the humerus in the axilla.
4. The axilla stimulation site is located at least 10 cm proximal to the above-elbow site at the midpoint of the humerus in the axilla.

Technical Comments

Evoked muscle action potential responses from all four sites should be similar in waveform, amplitude, and duration of response.

Wrist stimulation voltage, stimulus pulse duration, or both should be increased gradually and monitored carefully because high-voltage/long pulse-width stimulation at the wrist may volume conduct to the adjacent median nerve at the wrist, eliciting a volume-conducted median nerve response.

The upper extremity should be maintained in the same standard position while the test and measurements of segmental distances are performed.

A major source of error in performing segmental studies is stimulation below the elbow and across the elbow. The below-elbow stimulation site must allow access to the ulnar nerve **before** it enters the flexor carpi ulnaris muscle in the forearm. It is important to select an above-elbow stimulation site at least 10 cm proximal to the below-elbow stimulation site.

The above-elbow stimulation can be accomplished best by positioning the stimulation electrodes at the midhumeral area just posterior to the medial intermuscular septum. Care should be taken not to stimulate too anteriorly (causing contraction of the biceps muscle by direct stimulation or stimulation of the median nerve) or posteriorly (causing contraction of the triceps or failure to stimulate the ulnar nerve).

RADIAL NERVE (MOTOR)

Electromyograph Instrument Parameters

Filter settings/frequency response: 10,000–10 Hz
Sweep speed: 2–5 ms/division
Sensitivity/gain: 1,000–5,000 μV

(*continued*)

Patient Position

The patient is positioned supine with the arm abducted approximately 45°. The elbow is slightly flexed, and the forearm is fully pronated.

Electrode Placement

The active recording electrode is positioned over the extensor indicis proprius muscle of the dorsal forearm.

The reference surface electrode is positioned away from the extensor indicis proprius muscle on the dorsum of the hand.

The ground electrode is placed between the active and stimulating electrodes on the dorsal surface of the forearm.

Electrostimulation

Percutaneous electrostimulation is performed at the appropriate anatomic sites in the following order:

1. Distal stimulation is applied at the forearm proximal to the active and ground electrodes. This site is approximately 8–10 cm proximal to the active electrode and just lateral to the extensor carpi ulnaris muscle.

2. The elbow stimulation site is situated at or about the groove between the brachioradialis muscle and the biceps tendon approximately 6–10 cm proximal to the lateral epicondyle of the humerus.

3. The axilla stimulation site is situated in the groove between the coracobrachialis muscle and the medial edge of the triceps muscle. (**Note:** The third stimulation is accomplished after the arm is externally rotated and the forearm is supinated.)

Technical Comments

This is a technically difficult test to perform. Surface or needle active (recording) electrodes can be used, but it is crucial in either case to obtain similar evoked responses from all stimulation sites. When using surface electrodes, the response commonly has an initial positive deflection. If so, this should be obtained at all sites for valid calculations. Then,

the latency is measured at the same place for all three waveforms.

Any distal extensor muscle of the upper extremity innervated by the radial nerve can be used as a recording site. The extensor indicis proprius is the most distal. To localize this muscle, the examiner should palpate it and evaluate the function during extension of the index finger.

DEEP PERONEAL NERVE (MOTOR)

Electromyograph Instrument Parameters

Filter settings/frequency response: 10,000–10 Hz
Sweep speed: 2–5 ms/division
Sensitivity/gain: 500–2,000 μV/division

Patient Position

The patient is positioned in a comfortable, relaxed side-lying position facing away from the examiner. The hip and knee are slightly flexed, with the ankle positioned in neutral. A single pillow is placed between the patient's knees for comfort and to support the limb being examined.

Electrode Placement

The active recording electrode is positioned over the anatomic center of the extensor digitorum brevis muscle in the anterior, lateral aspect of the proximal midtarsal area of the foot.

The reference electrode is placed on the tendon of the extensor digitorum brevis muscle on the fifth toe.

The ground electrode should be positioned on the lateral or medial malleolus between the active and stimulating electrodes.

Electrostimulation

Percutaneous electrostimulation is performed at the appropriate anatomic sites in the following order:

(*continued*)

1. The nerve is stimulated initially below the head of the fibula and anterior to the neck of the fibula. The stimulator is positioned to approximate the anatomic course of the nerve around the neck of the fibula.

2. Distal stimulation is applied at the anterior ankle proximal to the center of the active electrode situated on the extensor digitorum brevis muscle. The distal site at the anterior ankle is between the extensor digitorum longus and extensor hallucis longus tendons.

3. The popliteal space stimulation site is at least 10 cm proximal to the fibular neck site. The peroneal nerve is situated in the lateral border of the popliteal space near the lateral hamstrings.

Technical Comment

Evoked muscle action potential responses from all three sites should be similar in waveform, amplitude, and duration of response.

When applying proximal stimulation in the popliteal fossa, the clinical response in the leg or calf should be monitored to avoid volume-conducted stimulation of the posterior tibial nerve. Ankle eversion ensures that the peroneal nerve is being stimulated, whereas plantar flexion of the ankle indicates stimulation of the tibial nerve.

Distal stimulation is performed approximately halfway between the malleoli, lateral to the extensor hallucis longus tendon, and just proximal to the level of the anterior tarsal tunnel. Occasionally, the response can be improved by stimulating more laterally to the extensor digitorum longus tendon. In obese patients or in patients with edema or induration, the ankle response may be difficult to elicit. Increasing the stimulus intensity, the pulse duration, or both may overcome this difficulty.

Posterior Tibial Nerve (Motor)

Electromyograph Instrument Parameters

Filter settings/frequency response: 10,000–10 Hz
Sweep speed: 2–5 ms/division
Sensitivity/gain: 1,000–5,000 µV/division

Patient Position

The patient is positioned prone with a single pillow placed under the ankles to allow slight flexion of the knees.

Electrode Placement

The active recording electrode is positioned over the abductor hallucis muscle, 1 cm inferior (toward the plantar surface) and 1 cm distal (toward the great toe) to the navicular.

The reference electrode is positioned distally on the abductor hallicus muscle tendon on the medial border of the great toe.

The ground electrode is positioned on the medial or lateral malleolus between the active and stimulating electrodes.

Electrostimulation

Percutaneous electrostimulation is performed at the appropriate anatomic sites in the following order:

1. Stimulation at the ankle is performed at a point halfway between the medial malleolus and the Achilles tendon proximal to the center of the active recording electrode and proximal to the flexor retinaculum.

2. Proximal stimulation is performed at the popliteal fossa slightly lateral to the midline along the flexor crease of the knee.

Technical Comments

The prone position makes this test more convenient for the examiner. The electrical and clinical responses should be closely monitored, especially during proximal stimulation. Care must be taken to ensure that all evoked muscle action potential responses to ankle and popliteal stimulation have similar waveforms, amplitudes, and durations of response. Plantar flexion ensures that the tibial nerve is being stimulated, whereas ankle eversion indicates peroneal nerve stimulation.

The waveform often exhibits an initial positive deflection. Repositioning of the active electrode on

(continued)

the abductor hallucis muscle minimizes but may not eliminate this problem. If the active electrode is repositioned, the distance to the stimulator must be adjusted to ensure that stimulation is proximal to the flexor retinaculum. In the event that the positive deflection remains after repositioning, accept the waveform, and ensure that the waveform at each subsequent stimulation site has the same configuration and that all latencies are marked in a consistent manner.

FEMORAL NERVE (MOTOR)

Electromyograph Instrument Parameters

> Filter settings/frequency response: 10,000–10 Hz
> Sweep speed: 2–5 ms/division
> Sensitivity/gain: 1,000–5,000 µV/division

Patient Position

The patient is positioned supine in a comfortable resting position. The leg is slightly abducted and externally rotated. A pillow can be placed under the knee to maintain this position.

Electrode Placement

The active recording electrode is placed over the center of the vastus medialis oblique muscle.

The reference electrode is placed away from the muscle on the patella or medial joint line.

The ground electrode is placed on the anterior thigh between the stimulating and active electrodes.

Electrostimulation

Percutaneous electrostimulation is performed at the appropriate anatomic sites in the following order:

1. Distal stimulation is applied at Hunter's canal in the medial aspect of the thigh between the quadriceps and adductor muscles. This site is approximately 8–10 cm proximal to the active electrode.

2. Surface stimulation is performed below the inguinal ligament and just lateral to the femoral artery.

3. Surface stimulation is performed above the inguinal ligament and just lateral to the femoral artery.

Technical Comments

For recording, placement of the active electrode over the most prominent portion of the vastus medialis oblique muscle is most useful when recording the maximum motor response.

The inguinal ligament forms an arc, the convexity of which points downward, that extends between the anterior superior iliac spine and the pubic tubercle. Stimulation can be accomplished above and below this ligament approximately 4–8 cm apart.

MEDIAN (ANTIDROMIC) SENSORY NERVE

Electromyograph Instrument Parameters

> Filter settings/frequency response: 20,000–20 Hz
> Sweep speed: 1–2 ms/division
> Sensitivity/gain: 5–20 µV/division

Patient Position

The patient is positioned supine with the arm abducted approximately 45°. The forearm is fully supinated; the wrist is in a neutral position. The fingers may flex slightly when in a "resting" position.

Electrode Placement

The active recording electrode is attached to the index finger at the midpoint of the distance between the phalangeal flexion crease and the web space of the index finger so that a distance of at least 10 cm, but not more than 14 cm, is maintained between the stimulation and active electrodes.

(continued)

The reference electrode is positioned at or about the distal interphalangeal flexion crease of the index finger so that a distance of at least 3 cm is maintained between the active and reference electrodes.

The ground is positioned on the dorsum of the hand between the active and stimulating electrodes.

Electrostimulation

Percutaneous electrostimulation is performed at the wrist between the palmaris longus and the flexor carpi radialis tendons proximal to the transverse carpal ligament.

Technical Comments

Low-intensity stimulation is usually adequate to elicit the antidromic sensory response. Motor response and volume-conduction effects can be reduced by decreasing the electrostimulation intensity, decreasing the pulse width duration of the applied electrostimulation, or both. (**Note:** Motor responses from hand muscles and volume conduction are more of a technical problem when using antidromic techniques than when using orthodromic techniques.)

Special concern: Care must be taken to maintain a separation between the active and reference electrodes on the index finger. Do not allow conducting gel to bridge this interelectrode space.

MEDIAN (ORTHODROMIC) SENSORY NERVE

Electromyograph Instrument Parameters

Filter settings/frequency response: 20,000–20 Hz
Sweep speed: 1–2 ms/division
Sensitivity/gain: 5–10 μV/division

Patient Position

The patient is positioned supine with the arm abducted approximately 45°. The forearm is fully supinated; the wrist is in a neutral position. The fingers may flex slightly when in a "resting" position.

Electrode Placement

The active recording electrode is positioned directly over the cathode (distal) stimulation site used to evoke the median motor response at the wrist.

The reference electrode is positioned 2–3 cm proximal to the active electrode. This electrode is positioned so that it is directly over the anode (proximal) stimulation site used to evoke the median motor response at the wrist.

The ground electrode is positioned on the dorsum of the hand between the active and stimulation electrodes.

Electrostimulation

Percutaneous electrostimulation is applied over the digital nerve through electrodes attached to the index finger. The cathode is positioned at the midpoint of the proximal phalanx of the index finger, and the anode is positioned at or about the distal phalangeal joint line. A distance of no less than 10 cm, but no more than 14 cm, is maintained between the stimulation cathode on the index finger and the active electrode at the wrist.

Technical Comments

A low stimulation intensity is usually adequate to elicit an orthodromic sensory response. The orthodromic technique reduces the possibility of obtaining a spurious motor response.

Motor response and volume conduction effects can be lessened by decreasing the intensity of the electrostimulation, decreasing the pulse-width duration of the applied electrostimulation, or both.

(continued)

Special concern: Care must be taken to maintain a separation between the stimulation cathode and the anode on the index finger. Do not allow conduction gel to bridge this interelectrode space.

ULNAR (ORTHODROMIC) SENSORY NERVE

Electromyograph Instrument Parameters

Filter settings/frequency response: 20,000–20 Hz
Sweep speed: 1–2 ms/division
Sensitivity/gain: 5–10 µV/division

Patient Position

The patient is positioned supine with the arm abducted to 45°. The forearm is fully supinated, palm up, and the wrist is in a neutral position with the fingers slightly flexed in a "resting" position.

Electrode Placement

The active recording electrodes are positioned directly over the cathode (distal) stimulating site used to evoke the ulnar motor response at the wrist.

The reference electrode is positioned 3 cm proximal to the active electrode. This electrode is positioned directly over the anode (proximal) stimulating site used to evoke the ulnar motor response at the wrist.

The ground electrode should be positioned on the dorsum of the hand between the active and the stimulating electrodes.

Electrostimulation

Percutaneous electrostimulation is applied over the digital nerve through electrodes attached to the fifth finger. The cathode is positioned at or about the midpoint of the proximal phalanx of the fifth finger. The anode is positioned at or about the distal interphalangeal joint line of the fifth finger so that a distance of no less than 10 cm, but no more than 14 cm, is maintained between the stimulating cathode on the digit and the active electrode at the wrist.

Technical Comments

A low stimulation intensity is usually adequate to elicit an orthodromic sensory response. The orthodromic technique reduces the possibility of obtaining a spurious motor response.

Motor response and volume conduction effects can be lessened by decreasing the intensity of the electrostimulation, decreasing the pulse-width duration of the applied electrostimulation, or both.

Special concern: Care must be taken to maintain a separation between the stimulation cathode and the anode on the little finger. Do not allow conducting gel to bridge this interelectrode space.

ULNAR (ANTIDROMIC) SENSORY NERVE

Electromyograph Instrument Parameters

Filter settings/frequency response: 20,000–20 Hz
Sweep speed: 1–2 ms/division
Sensitivity/gain: 5–20 µV/division

Patient Position

The patient is positioned supine with the arm abducted approximately 45°. The forearm is supinated, palm up; the wrist is in a neutral position, and the fingers are slightly flexed in a "resting" position.

Electrode Placement

The active recording electrode is attached to the fifth finger at the midpoint of the proximal phalanx so that a distance of at least 10 cm, but no more than 14 cm, is maintained between the stimulating electrode and the active electrode. (See **Fig. 25–5**).

(continued)

The reference electrode is positioned at or about the distal interphalangeal joint line of the fifth finger so that a distance of at least 3 cm is maintained between the active and reference electrodes.

The ground electrode should be positioned on the dorsum of the hand between the active and stimulating electrodes.

Electrostimulation

Percutaneous electrostimulation is performed at the wrist, medial, **or** lateral to the flexor carpi ulnaris tendon.

Technical Comments

The intensity of sensory electrostimulation is usually adequate to elicit the antidromic sensory response. Motor response and volume conduction effects can be lessened by decreasing the intensity of the electrostimulation, decreasing the pulse-width duration of the applied electrostimulation, or both. (**Note:** Motor impulses from hand muscles and volume conduction are more of a technical problem when using antidromic techniques than when using orthodromic techniques.)

Special concern: Care must be taken to maintain a separation between the active and reference electrodes on the fifth finger. Do not allow conducting gel to bridge this interelectrode space.

SUPERFICIAL RADIAL (ANTIDROMIC) SENSORY NERVE

Electromyograph Instrument Parameters

Filter settings/frequency response: 20,000–20 Hz
Sweep speed: 1–2 ms/division
Sensitivity/gain: 5–20 μV/division

Patient Position

The active recording electrode is positioned over the portion of the nerve that can be palpated over an extended extensor pollicis longus tendon at or about the dorsal-radial aspect of the wrist.

The reference electrode is positioned distal to the active electrode in the first web space midway between the first and second metacarpophalangeal joints.

The ground electrode is placed between the active and stimulating electrodes on the dorsal surface of the forearm.

Electrostimulation

Percutaneous electrostimulation is applied along the dorsolateral border of the radius lateral to the cephalic vein at least 10 cm proximal to the active (recording) electrode.

Technical Comments

The extensor pollicis longus tendon forms the medial border of the "snuff box." By running the index fingernail along this tendon distal to the wrist, the examiner can palpate the superficial radial sensory nerve. The active (recording) electrode should be placed at the intersection of the tendon and nerve.

Stimulation of the superficial radial nerve is usually accomplished using a low-voltage, short-duration stimulus. Stronger stimulation may spread to the anterior interosseus branch of the median nerve and may produce an unwanted motor response or a volume-conducted artifact. When this problem occurs, slight flexion of the distal phalanx of the thumb is observed.

The patient may be able to help find the nerve by reporting a tingling sensation along the dorsum of the thumb, index, or second finger when a stimulus is delivered.

(continued)

SURAL (ANTIDROMIC) SENSORY NERVE

Electromyograph Instrument Parameters

Filter settings/frequency response: 20,000–20 Hz

Sweep speed: 1–2 ms/division

Sensitivity/gain: 5–10 µV/division

Patient Position

The patient is positioned in a comfortable, relaxed, side-lying position facing away from the examiner. (The patient also can be positioned supine or prone.) The hip and knee should be slightly flexed with the ankle positioned in neutral. A single pillow can be placed between the patient's knees for comfort and to support the limb being examined.

Electrode Placement

The active recording electrode is positioned inferior to and in line with the lateral malleolus and parallel with the sole of the foot.

The reference electrode is positioned distal to the active electrode along the lateral border of the foot and parallel with the sole of the foot.

The ground electrode is positioned on the medial or lateral malleolus between the active and stimulating electrodes.

Electrostimulation

Percutaneous (antidromic) electrostimulation of the sural nerve is performed 14 cm proximal to the center of the active electrode. Stimulation is performed slightly distal to the lower border of the belly of the gastrocnemius muscle at or about the junction of the gastrocnemius muscle and the Achilles tendon. Stimulation begins 14 cm proximal to the active electrode in the midline of the posterior calf and proceeds laterally (maintaining at least 10 cm but no more than 14 cm distance) until a satisfactory evoked sensory response is obtained.

Technical Comments

The major difficulty encountered when stimulating the sural sensory nerve is finding the nerve in the posterior calf. The patient may be able to help by reporting tingling along the posterior or lateral calf or the lateral foot when a stimulus is delivered.

The sensory response is often obscured by a large muscle response. This problem may be avoided by using a low-voltage stimulus intensity with a short pulse duration.

ELECTROMYOGRAPHY

The electrical characteristics of the normal motor unit are the basis for the EMG. These characteristics are detected by inserting an electrode into the muscle while the muscle is at rest, mildly contracting, and vigorously contracting. The electrical discharges within the muscle are the result of the depolarizations of the active muscle fibers connected to the particular motor unit. If the motor unit has five or six muscle fibers supplied by one axon, all of those fibers will fire at roughly the same time. This outcome results in a synthesis of the firing of each individual muscle fiber into an amalgamated MUP that represents the summation of each individually discharging muscle fiber

within the muscle (see **Fig. 23–2**). The properties of interest to the electromyographer are (1) the duration of the MUP, (2) the amplitude of the MUP, and (3) the number of phases and their configuration.

Normal Muscle

The normal MUP consists of no more than four phases; two or three phases are most typical. (See the normal motor unit tracing in **Fig. 23–3**). A phase is initiated each time that the tracing passes through baseline and is completed when the tracing returns to baseline again. The duration of the MUP is determined by the initial departure from baseline and the return of the potential to baseline again at the end of the entire potential. The amplitude is measured in one of two ways: from baseline to the peak of the negative phase or from the peak of the negative phase to the peak of the positive (down-going) phase. Obviously, the laboratory must specify how amplitude measurements are taken. The values reported in this chapter are baseline to peak of the negative phase.

Motor Unit Duration. The **MUP duration** is reported as 7 milliseconds (SD, 3.5 milliseconds).[23] The duration of the MUP is determined by the spread of the endplate zone as it relates to the total length of the muscle. For example, the abductor pollicis brevis has an endplate zone that occupies 50% of the total

length of the muscle, resulting in a duration of the MUP of 8–9 milliseconds. Conversely, the biceps brachii has an endplate zone that occupies 10% of the total length of the muscle fibers, resulting in a duration of 5–6 milliseconds for the MUP (**Fig. 23–9**).

Motor Unit Amplitude. The amplitude of the MUP is measured from baseline to peak of the negative (upward) phase, and it varies from 300 to 5000 μV in the normal individual.[23] The amplitude is representative of the size of the active membrane area with respect to the total size of the muscle. Therefore, a small muscle consisting of large individual muscle fibers

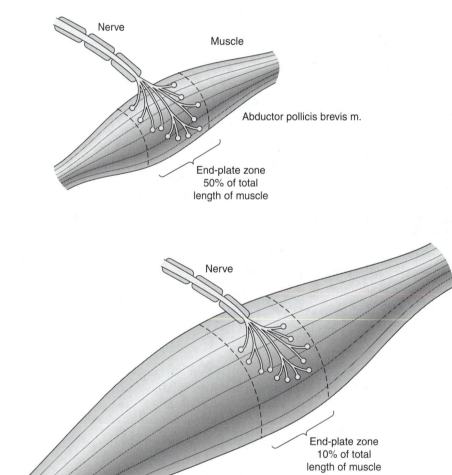

FIGURE 23–9   Relative spread of the end-plate zone versus the total length of the muscle.

such as the abductor pollicis brevis will result in a larger amplitude MUP than will the biceps brachii in a sedentary person. If the muscle fibers are hypertrophied, the amplitudes will increase slightly but will not do so in a predictable manner that is correlated with the hypertrophy. The study of MUP concerns the difference between the MUP obtained from patients and normal values (**Fig. 23–10**).

Motor Unit Phases.   The number of phases or crossing of the MUP across baseline is determined by the wave of depolarization sweeping along the muscle fibers in a synchronized fashion. If there is a wide spread to the motor endplate zone, there will be a greater tendency to have more than two or three phases because the summation of the wave of depolarization is not as well synchronized. The minimum number of phases must be two because the wave of depolarization is an alternating wave from negative to positive or vice versa, depending on the position of the recording needle electrode. When the number of phases exceeds four, the MUP is termed a **polyphasic**

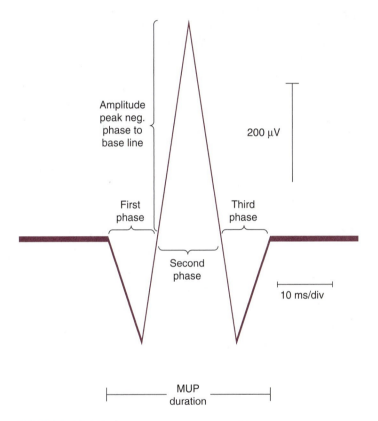

FIGURE 23–10   A normal motor unit. The motor unit consists of the anterior horn cell, its axon, the neuromuscular junction, and all muscle fibers it innervates. Motor unit potential (MUP) is the synchronous discharge of all muscle fibers innervated by the anterior horn cell. They occur during volitional activity. Initial deflection can be either positive or negative. The amplitude of the motor unit action potential depends on the number of motor unit muscle fibers in close proximity to the recording electrode. The rate of rise time of the motor unit action potential depends on the closeness of the recording electrode to the active muscle fibers. The duration of the action potential of the motor unit depends on the relative density of the muscle fibers in the recording area.

MUP. The polyphasic MUP is associated with an MUP that is in the process of reorganization, when the denervated muscle fibers are becoming innervated by collaterals from healthy motor units. This process adds many more immature muscle fibers to the original motor unit, spreading the depolarization of these additional fibers over a much larger area. The result is the addition of these multiple phases, forming the polyphasic MUP (**Fig. 23–11**).

Reorganized Motor Unit. When a motor unit is reorganizing, it causes the endplate zone to spread out because the healthy motor unit collaterals reach out to the denervated muscle fibers. Spread of the endplate zone determines the duration of the MUP, which in the reorganizing motor unit will be of longer duration. The duration may exceed 12 milliseconds; some MUPs have been recorded in excess of 20 milliseconds.

Initially, the amplitude of the reorganizing MUP is no larger than the intact MUP, and the amplitudes of some phases will be lower than normal because the previously denervated fibers are atrophic. As the newly innervated fibers increase in diameter, the amplitude of the MUP also increases. A newly organized MUP will produce a relatively short-duration, low-amplitude polyphasic action potential (**SLAP MUP**) (see **Fig. 23–7**).

A later-stage reorganized MUP will have a polyphasic action potential with a higher amplitude and a longer duration (**HALD MUP**). This type of action potential is encountered in chronic neuropathic lesions in late-stage reorganization of the motor units.

Needle-Insertion Activity. Inserting a needle into a normal muscle results in a brief burst of electrical activity known as insertional activity. When pierced, the normal muscle liberates electrical discharges that last as long as the actual insertion lasts. If the muscle is denervated (ie, the axons have degenerated after being severed), the denervated muscle fibers revert to a more primitive state that exists in the fetus before motor nerves innervate muscle fibers. When denervated, a skeletal muscle fibrillates; that is, the individual muscle fibers fire spontaneously, producing a small depolarization in all the denervated muscle fibers. Because denervated muscle is extremely sensitive to mechanical irritation, inserting the needle causes a shower of fibrillation potentials in that muscle. The fibrillation potentials are of low amplitude, less than 100 µV and of very short duration, 1–2 msec, with an initial positive deflection followed by a negative phase (**Fig. 23–12**). The **fibrillation** potential may be confused with endplate noise, which is of similar amplitude and duration but has an initial neg-

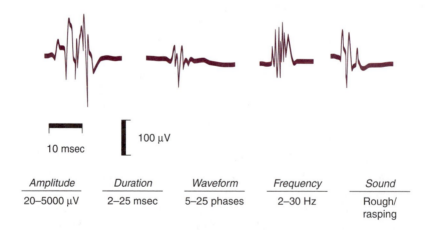

Amplitude	Duration	Waveform	Frequency	Sound
20–5000 µV	2–25 msec	5–25 phases	2–30 Hz	Rough/rasping

FIGURE 23–11 Complex (polyphasic) action potential of a motor unit with multiple phases. This probably results from asynchronous discharge of muscle fibers in the motor unit. It represents the electrical expression of a motor unit that is undergoing reorganization. Polyphasics are observed in partial compressive neuropathies and in muscular dystrophy. The initial deflection can be either positive or negative. They occur during volitional activity. High-amplitude long-duration (HALD) polyphasic potentials are usually seen in long-standing chronic neuropathies.

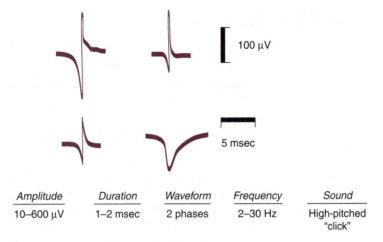

Amplitude	Duration	Waveform	Frequency	Sound
10–600 µV	1–2 msec	2 phases	2–30 Hz	High-pitched "click"

FIGURE 23–12   Fibrillation potentials representing spontaneous, repetitive discharges of a single muscle fiber. The initial deflection is positive; it indicates altered muscle membrane excitability and an unstable muscle membrane that depolarizes in a variety of circumstances and may be the result of denervation (separation of muscle from nerve), metabolic dysfunction (altered electrolytic states), inflammatory diseases (polymyositis), trauma (injection sites), or lack of trophic influence (stroke or spinal cord injury).

ative phase followed by a positive one. The endplate potential also is associated with considerable discomfort, which can be relieved readily by slight movement of the electrode that pulls the electrode away from the endplate zone of the nerve. The endplate potential is normal, not indicative of denervation (**Fig. 23–13**).

Electrical Activity at Rest.   At rest, a normally innervated muscle exhibits no electrical discharge. The baseline is isoelectric and no spontaneous discharges are noted. Conversely, denervated muscle has spontaneous discharges of fibrillation while at rest and may have trains of **positive sharp waves** that also discharge while the muscle is at rest (**Fig. 23–14**).

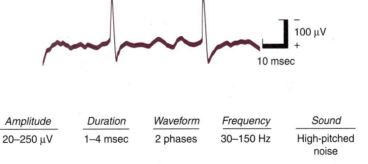

Amplitude	Duration	Waveform	Frequency	Sound
20–250 µV	1–4 msec	2 phases	30–150 Hz	High-pitched noise

FIGURE 23–13   End-plate potentials. These potentials are produced when the EMG needle electrode comes into contact with nerve fibrils within the muscle. Patients complain of increased pain when these potentials are present. Slight movements of the needle should relieve pain, eliminate the end plate "noise," and clear the screen display of these potential. The initial deflection is negative.

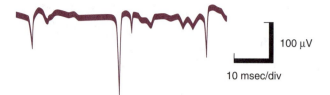

Amplitude	Duration	Waveform	Frequency	Sound
30–4000 µV	2–10 msec	2 phases	2–100 Hz	Dull "thud"

FIGURE 23–14   Positive sharp waves. These waves may represent asynchronous discharge of a number of denervated muscle fibers. They reflect an alteration in the excitability of the muscle membrane. The initial deflection is positive. Its shape is the most constant of all EMG potentials. Positive sharp waves appear spontaneously at rest and are unpredictable. They are seen in both neuropathies and myopathies.

Electrical Activity during Mild Contraction.   With mild contraction of a muscle, the smaller motor units initially discharge, followed by the large and the larger motor units as more demand is placed on the muscle for contraction force. This process is known as the Henneman size principle of motor unit recruitment. If a muscle is partially denervated, the only motor unit remaining will be the ones that the person can activate. If no further motor units can be recruited, the existing motor unit must fire at an increasing rate. If an individual is not denervated but attempts to imitate this state, only a few motor units will fire. When asked, the individual does not increase the rate of firing of those few motor units. This is a helpful method of determining how many motor units are available to a patient and whether the nerve axons are truly partially denervated.

Electrical Activity during Maximum Contraction.   When a muscle is required to contract with greater intensity, recruitment of motor units will progress through the small to large motor units and also increase the rate of firing of the motor units recruited. This process results in a complete obliteration of the oscilloscope screen with MUPs; this phenomenon is labeled a complete interference pattern and is termed good recruitment. If there are gaps in the recruitment, the recruitment is termed fair and called a partial interference pattern. If even less recruitment occurs and if there are discreet MUPs on the screen,

the phenomenon is termed a poor recruitment pattern and is called a single-unit interference pattern.

Normal muscle provides good recruitment with a complete obliteration of the baseline on the oscilloscope. This finding is recorded as good recruitment with a complete interference pattern.

Abnormal Muscle

The EMG is particularly helpful for detecting peripheral neuropathies and anterior horn cell disorders and for classfiying them regarding the degree of axonal interruption and state of recovery from the denervation.

Characteristics

Insertional Activity   Whereas insertion of an electrode into a normal muscle elicits a brief discharge of less than 100 milliseconds, a muscle that is denervated becomes highly responsive to mechanical stimuli, and inserting an electrode into it results in a shower of fibrillation potentials (see **Fig. 23–12**).

If a muscle is denervated and the muscle membrane is unstable, inserting a needle electrode may give rise to trains of positive sharp waves (see **Fig. 23–14**). The positive waves may be intermingled with fibrillation potentials. Recall that fibrillation potentials should not be confused with end-plate potentials.

The Muscle at Rest.   A denervated muscle at rest reveals spontaneous discharges without any voluntary effort on the patient's part. These spontaneous discharges may be fibrillation, positive sharp waves, or both. These fibrillation potentials should be stored on the oscilloscope screen and studied carefully to determine that they have an initial positive deflection, followed by a negative deflection, and that they are 1–2 milliseconds in duration and of 50–100 µV in amplitude. The fibrillation potentials have a sound that simulates that of fat frying in a pan or the crinkling of cellophane (see **Fig. 23–12**). Another spontaneous discharge found in denervated muscle is the positive sharp wave, which begins with an initial and a sudden positive (downward) deflection of 50–100 µV and a variable duration of 2–100 milliseconds. The sound is a popping sound and may appear in trains or a series (see **Fig. 23–14**).

When the anterior horn cells (alpha motor neurons) are undergoing degeneration or when an inflammatory state is present in that region, the muscles may reveal that fasciculation potentials are spontaneously firing. These fasciculations appear suddenly without any voluntary activation of the muscle. They are either normal bi- or triphasic MUPs, or they may be HALP or SLAP potentials (see **Fig. 23–7**). It should also be emphasized that these potentials can be found in normally innervated persons who have exercised to fatigue and the motor units are firing spontaneously as a result. These fatigue fasciculations are benign and should not, in themselves, lead to the conclusion that a neuropathy is present. The frequency of firing of benign fasciculations is regular, whereas the frequency of firing of fasciculations associated with anterior horn cell disease is irregular.

Types of Abnormalities

Neurotmesis and Axonotmesis   When a muscle is completely denervated, all the axons are completely separated from the muscle. This situation, called a **neurotmesis,** results in complete loss of voluntary recruitment of MUPs distal to the lesion. With an **axonotmesis** incomplete interruption of the axons within a nerve trunk—some surviving axons may be able to fire a few MUPs. This circumstance results in an extremely weak, tremulous contraction. The MUPs elicited will fire at a regular frequency, and when the patient is asked to contract more vigorously, the frequency of firing of those MUPs will increase. It is impossible for a person with an intact nerve trunk to duplicate this pattern of recruitment because the normally innervated muscles will recruit larger and larger MUPs while increasing the rate of firing of the previous MUPs. Partly denervated patients have no other

MUPs to recruit; thus, they fire the available MUPs at a higher frequency.

The axonotmesis lesion undergoes a reorganization known as collateral sprouting from healthy axons to supply the muscle fibers that have lost their own supply of axons. When skeletal muscle is denervated, it reverts to a more primitive embryologic state, and its surface membrane, the sarcolemma, becomes supersensitive to acetylcholine. This supersensitivy is associated with the process of attracting healthy axons to the denervated muscle fibers. The healthy motor unit sprouts additional axons, which seek out the denervated fibers, perhaps by specific RNA messengers that have neural attracting agents within them. As these sprouts attach themselves to the now-atrophic muscle fibers, the original motor unit expands to include the new muscle fibers. This activity expands the endplate zone of the motor unit and increases the duration of the MUP. The newly innervated muscle fibers are atrophic and therefore develop lower amplitude potentials that are separated from the original MUP. This process will form the SLAP units noted earlier (see **Fig. 23–7**).

As a motor unit becomes reinnervated through collateral sprouting, the previously denervated fibers begin to enlarge; therefore, the amplitude of the MUP increases. The endplate spread caused when the collaterals reach out for the denervated fibers remain spread out; therefore, the duration of the MUP increases. This process results in the HALD unit, as noted earlier (see **Fig. 23–11**).

Neuropractic Lesions.   In a **neuropractic** lesion, which represents a transient loss of conduction in a segment of the nerve, a loss of MUP recruitment will occur distal to the conduction block. Because the neuropractic lesion frequently rectifies itself within hours or several weeks, the recruitment of MUPs will reappear with the ability to conduct impulses in the nerve. It is not uncommon for the nerve to begin conduction after being stimulated electrically above and below the block. However, one cannot always predict when this will occur. The absence of spontaneous discharges at rest is another indication that this is not an axonotmesis or neurotmesis.

Myoneural Function Disorders.   In myasthenia gravis, the progressive declination of the transmission of the wave of depolarization from the nerve across the myoneural junction may eventually lead to a variable wave of depolarization of the muscle membranes. This outcome will result in a poorly synchronized firing of the MUP that is recognized as variability in the same MUP as it fires repeatedly. The amplitude of the normal MUP, or of even the neuropathic MUP, will not vary during sampling of many motor units. The duration of the MUP also may vary, depending on how many individual myoneural junctions in the motor unit fire synchronously. Because some of these junctions may be less functional than others and the junction is fired at various rates, it is apparent that more and more junctions will fail when the rate of firing increases. The high rate of firing is associated with intense contractions, which will manifest the loss of tension or weakness earliest in the course of the disease.

The Eaton-Lambert phenomenon, the myasthenic reaction, has been linked to toxicity associated with bronchogenic carcinoma of the lung.[21] This disorder is characterized by an extremely low-amplitude response with a single supramaximal stimulus. The amplitude may be only 10% of the normal expected values. When the person produces several voluntary isometric contractions, the amplitude becomes potentiated, sometimes as much as 600%.[24] This result would be recognized in EMG discharge as an initial low-amplitude response, followed by the potentiation of the response, then a progressive declination of amplitude when the neuromuscular junction becomes depleted again. A number of other neuromuscular junctional abnormalities, such as botulism intoxication, myotonia, amyotrophic lateral sclerosis, and syringomyelia, also produce EMG evidence of neuromuscular blockage.[25]

Primary Muscle Disease.   If the muscle fiber itself is diseased (eg, in muscular dystrophy), a selective process of degeneration of Type II muscle fibers may result in preservation of the Type I, or slow twitch fibers. As the Type II fibers atrophy, the EMG will reveal low amplitude MUPs in great abundance. Because the axons supplying these atrophic muscle fibers are not lost, the person can recruit them readily. A key difference between normal recruitment and myopathic recruitment is the relative ease with which the patient produces a complete interference pattern with relatively little effort.

An analysis of the MUPs reveals complex units of low amplitude and relatively short duration. The reason for the short duration is that the motor-unit territory shrinks as the total muscle shrinks; therefore, the end-plate spread will be less and will result in a decreased duration. As the muscle fibers undergo atrophy, the amplitude is reduced proportionately (see **Fig. 23–8**).

Some inflammatory muscle diseases, such as **polymyositis,** demonstrate increased irritability to the probe of the needle electrode. The insertional activity is prolonged, and scattered fibrillation may be noted when the muscle is at rest. Contraction of the muscle will result in normal motor unit discharges in the early stages; however, as the inflammatory process produces deterioration, atrophy of fast twitch fibers and a resultant drop in amplitude of the MUP occur. The inflammatory state will not result in abundant recruitment, but in its place there will be fair recruitment with partial interference patterns, albeit of lower amplitude.

Congenital or acquired **myotonia** manifests a waxing and waning discharge of MUPs when a needle electrode is inserted into affected muscles. These MUPs have a sound that resembles a dive bomber in a steep dive. The muscles are silent at rest. With moderate contraction, however, the MUPs have a variable amplitude with normal recruitment in the early stages. A distinguishing feature is an inability to terminate muscular contraction, which results in prolonged MUP discharges after a request to relax. This sustained contraction is the most debilitating feature of myotonia because it results in an inability to perform repetitive actions.

The Examination

Following a clarifying assessment of the patient's sensory, motor, and reflex statuses, the affected parts of the body to be examined are outlined. Generally, neuropathic disorders are characterized by a pattern of greater involvement in distal versus proximal muscles, whereas myopathic disease is found more commonly in proximal musculature. The purpose of the sequence of testing selected is to identify changes in muscles that will probably be affected.

If a peripheral neuropathic disorder is suspected, it is appropriate to examine the conduction velocity and distal latencies of lower extremity nerves initially. If the values are less than 40 meters per second in a middle-aged person, further consideration of a peripheral neuropathic disorder is warranted. Similarly, if the distal latencies are prolonged, they would be associated with a dying-back neuropathy.

The next part of the examination is to sample muscles from the distal extreme of the nerve distribution and another muscle at the beginning of the distribution. This procedure is repeated for each lower extremity nerve that exhibits a reduced conduction velocity and a prolonged distal latency. One common pattern would be that the more distal the nerves, the greater the manifestation of denervation. Nerves in the upper extremities would be considerably less affected in peripheral neuropathic disorders. Reduced conduction velocity values, coupled with prolonged distal latencies plus neuropathic EMG findings, would be consistent with a **peripheral neuropathy multiplex.** This designation is given when multiple nerves are involved. If only one peripheral nerve is involved, it is called a mononeuropathy.

A patient with a long history of low-back pain who was doing spring gardening that involved an excessive amount of stooping and lifting complains of pain radiating to the right leg and describes it as a streak of lightning that extends to the foot. The physical examination reveals hypoesthesia of the dorsolateral lower leg and foot on the right side. The ankle tendon jerk response is depressed on the same side. When testing the peroneal and posterior tibial nerves bilaterally, the conduction velocities are found to be symmetrical and in a range of 45–50 meters per second with distal latencies of less than 4 milliseconds. Would lumbosacral **nerve root compression** result in a decrease in nerve conduction velocity? Even if the compression compromised more than 30% of the axons within the nerve root, it would not cause any loss of conduction velocity. However, it would reduce the amplitude on the affected side versus the unaffected side. Because the lesion is found proximally in the region of the origin of the nerve, the F wave and H reflex latencies would reveal slowing in nerves supplied by the lesioned nerve root or roots. In addition, muscles would be affected in a root distribution pattern versus one that would follow a peripheral nerve distribution. For example, the therapist must select muscles that derive innervation from the same root distribution but are innervated by different peripheral nerves. In this case, the therapist may find neuropathic EMG findings in the tensor fascia latae and in the extensor hallucis longus and extensor digitorum brevis muscles, all of which derive innervation from the fifth lumbar nerve root but are innervated by two separate peripheral nerves. Further investigation of paraspinal musculature in the region of the fifth lumbar vertebrae would place the offending lesion in the nerve root—the

common source for this wide range of involvement. Normal EMG findings in the vastus medialis (L2–L4) and soleus (S1–S2) would also help to confirm a diagnosis of fifth lumbar nerve root involvement.

The Report

The reporting of EMG and nerve conduction values or electroneuromyographic findings are usually presented in a tabular form known as the ENMG or EMG report. The report is separated into two major components: the nerve conduction values and the EMG data. In addition to the data presented, the report includes the patient's history and subjective complaints, pertinent clinical findings, and the time of onset and general course of the disorder. A summary of physical findings is also included.

The nerves studied are typically presented in a tabular form, with the proximal and distal latencies of each segment and the distances of those segments of the nerve. The amplitudes for each site of stimulation are presented in millivolts for motor nerves and in microvolts for the sensory components of each nerve. In addition, the proximal latencies, F wave response, and H reflex latencies and their amplitudes are recorded for each nerve on each side (see **Fig. 23–6**).

The EMG data are presented in the manner in which the information is collected: with insertion of the electrode, with the muscle at rest, with the muscle moderately contracted, and with maximal contractile effort. The needle electrode insertion activity is recorded as brief (which is normal), prolonged, or waxing and waning (as in myotonia). When a muscle is at rest, even when the electrode is in it, the normal muscle will not have any electrical discharges. The denervated muscle will have spontaneous discharges such as fibrillation or positive sharp waves. The fibrillation potential discharge is usually recorded as few and scattered (+1), frequent and found in more than one site (+2), numerous and only a few gaps between them (+3), or abundant and continuous (+4). When positive sharp waves are identified, they are given similar ratings; however, the positive waves typically appear as trains of sharp waves and are ranked according to their duration—the shorter the duration, the lower the numerical rating.

Recording the MUPs during moderate contraction involves the process of analyzing the number of phases, the duration, and the amplitude and frequency of firing with increased demands for more contraction. Some investigators actually store 20 or 30 MUPs, determining the percentage of polyphasic

MUPs and noting which form they take, SLAP or HALP. Most normal muscles have 10% or less polyphasic MUPs. With increasing age, the percentage of polyphasic MUPs increases, possibly because of remodeling of the endplate zones. The recording of increased percentages of polyphasic MUPs in a particular nerve root, peripheral nerve, or some other anatomic distribution is helpful, along with other data, to form an impression of the site of the deficit. These percentages of polyphasicity are then listed under the column indicating waveform (**Fig. 23–15**).

Full-effort contractions are recorded when the patient contracts isometrically against the examiner's resistance. The examiner must elicit the patient's maximal effort and judge whether there is genuine input to the muscle contraction. One method of assessing this situation is to track the increase in recruitment and the frequency of firing, as noted in an earlier section. In a normal muscle, recruitment is rated as good and productive of a complete interference pattern. If the recruitment is diminished to a minor degree, it is labeled fair, and the interference pattern is labeled as partial. When the recruitment is diminished to a great extent, it is listed as poor, and the interference pattern is labeled incomplete. Poor recruitment also may be called discreet MUP recruitment.

Although the reporting forms used are varied, all of them should present complete nerve conduction values and the electromyographic data. That is, the latencies for each site of stimulation and distances between stimulus sites must be listed in a clear manner. The amplitudes of these responses and the latencies also must be juxtaposed. Then, the calculation of the conduction velocity of each segment of the nerve is entered. The EMG data should indicate the name of the muscle studied; its side; the result of needle insertion; the state during rest; the waveforms, amplitude, and duration of the motor units during contraction; and the quality of the recruitment plus the interference pattern produced. (See **Figure 23–16** for an example of a reporting form used in many laboratories.)

Application to Patient Care

Determining the pathophysiologic mechanism that underlies a clinical problem is essential to optimal patient care. A common example is an elderly patient who complains of weakness of both legs. The patient has not been diagnosed as diabetic but has not been tested specifically for diabetes in the past year. What might give rise to this weakness? The sources of weakness might include a CNS lesion; a spinal cord

Muscle	S I D E	Innervation	Insertion	At Rest	Motor Unit Configuration			Motor Unit Recruitment	Comment
					Shape	Amplitude	Duration		

DETAILED ELECTROMYOGRAPHIC FINDING

FIGURE 23–15   An example of an electromyography record, indicating the essential information needed.

Name John Doe   Age 38   Sex M   Test Date 3/25/05

Address 100 Main Street, Newark, NJ 07094   Status Priv   Case # 0018

Chief Complaint Low back pain w/ radiation to left leg   Onset Date several months

Clinical Findings Hypesthesia lateral aspect of left foot   Referring Dr.

— ELECTROMYOGRAPHIC FINDINGS —

MUSCLE AND SIDE		INSERTION	REST	MODERATE	RECRUITMENT	MAXIMUM
Ext. Dig. Brevis	(L)	prolonged	hi-frequency	25% polyphasic	fair	partial
Ext. Hallucis Longus	(L)	prolonged	hi-frequency	25% polyphasic	fair	partial
Medial Gastroc.	(L)	prolonged	hi-frequency	25% polyphasic	fair	partial
Erector Spinae L_5–S_1	(L)	prolonged	hi-frequency	25% polyphasic	fair	partial
Erector Spinae L_5–S_1	(R)	brief	silence	10/15% polyphasic	fair	partial
Erector Spinae $L_{3,4}$	(L&R)	brief	silence	10/15% polyphasic	fair	partial
Medial Gastroc.	(R)	brief	silence	10/15% polyphasic	good	complete
Anterior Tibialis	(L&R)	brief	silence	10/15% polyphasic	good	complete
Vastus Medialis	(L&R)	brief	silence	10/15% polyphasic	good	complete
Ext. Hall. Long	(R)	brief	silence	10/15% polyphasic	good	complete
Ext. Dig. Brevis	(R)	brief	silence	10/15% polyphasic	good	complete
Abductor Hall.	(L&R)	brief	silence	15% polyphasic	fair	partial

— CONDUCTION VELOCITY FINDINGS —

NERVE: Peroneal (L)	NERVE: Tibial (L)	NERVE: Peroneal (R)	NERVE: Tibial (R)
PROX: 10.4 4 mVolts	PROX: 12.2 10 mVolts	PROX: 10.8 7 mVolts	PROX: 10.5 10 mVolts
DISTAL: 4.0 4 mVolts	DISTAL: 4.0 10 mVolts	DISTAL: 4.2 7 mVolts	DISTAL: 4.0 10 mVolts
VEL: 48 M/SEC.	VEL: 45 M/SEC.	VEL: 45 M/SEC.	VEL: 59 M/SEC.
DISTANCE: 31 CM.	DISTANCE: 36 CM.	DISTANCE: 29 CM.	DISTANCE: 36 CM.
F=51.4 msecs	F=49.5 msecs	F=50.2 msecs	F=45.9 msecs
NERVE: Sural (L)	NERVE: L H-Reflex =	NERVE: R H-Reflex =	NERVE: Sural (R)
PROX:	PROX:	PROX:	PROX:
DISTAL: 3.52 104 µVolts	DISTAL: 31.2 msecs 350 µV	DISTAL: 28.9 msecs 500 µV	DISTAL: 3.51 10 µVolts
VEL: 48 M/SEC.	VEL: M/SEC.	VEL: M/SEC.	VEL: M/SEC.
DISTANCE: CM.	DISTANCE: CM.	DISTANCE: CM.	DISTANCE: CM.

IMPRESSION: The EMG findingd and prolonged proximal latencies of F waves and H reflex responses on the left side are compatible with an L_5–S_1 radiculitis on the left side.

FIGURE 23–16   An example of an electrodiagnostic report. Some typical recordings of muscle and nerve conduction values are shown.

disorder; a peripheral nerve disease; a myoneural junctional disorder; a muscular disease; or psychological factors such as depression, anxiety, or an emotional disorder. The ENMG may delineate whether the weakness derives from the motor neuron, the peripheral nerve or nerves, the myoneural junction, or the muscle itself. The testing of CNS disorders also can be evaluated with cortically evoked studies of the spinal cord, brain stem, or auditory and visual systems. The latter studies are special applications of electrophysiology that is covered in other sources.[26]

Another benefit to the physical therapist is to monitor progress or regression in specific patients. With serial ENMG studies, one can establish realistic goals and expectations. Prediction regarding when these goals can be attained are rendered more precise; therefore, attainment of function can be predicted with more certainty. The therapist must guide the patient who has sustained a foot drop or peroneal palsy regarding what intervention is required and whether orthotic support is indicated and what type. If, in the latter case of foot drop, the ENMG reveals axonotmesis at the neck of fibula in the common peroneal nerve, it is known that peripheral axons will regenerate at a rate of approximately 1 inch (2.5 cm) per month. If the peroneal nerve is 27 cm long, it is evident that this patient has a recovery period of 2 years and some months. During that 2-year wait, it is essential to avoid stretching paralyzed muscles; thus, the patient must be fitted with an orthosis. The type of orthosis should be one that distorts normal locomotion the least because the patient will be walking with this device for 2 years, and habit patterns are established in less time than that (**Table 23–1**).

Another consideration regarding the patient with a common peroneal palsy is to determine when to begin electrical stimulation, or even whether one should begin electrical stimulation confirmed by the ENMG data. For example, according to Davis,[27] the presence of fibrillation is a contraindication for electrical stimulation of denervated muscle. He suggested that once fibrillation has subsided, it may be more appropriate to stimulate the skeletal muscle. The major questions that arise are these: If this stimulation is to take place over two or more years, is it reasonable to expect a patient to comply over this period? And if the patient does so, will that compliance result in improved function of the target muscle? Pachter et al[28] explored some of these issues in animal studies and concluded that stimulation produced some benefits but only for relatively short periods. Kosman[29] cautioned that these studies on denervated animal models are not applicable to the longer durations needed for human regeneration; therefore, he opted against elec-

TABLE 23–1   *Normal Conduction Values*

Nerve	Distance (cm)	Amplitude (using 6 mm disk)	Nerve Conduction Velocity (msec)	Distal Latency (msec)
Ulnar				
Motor (forearm)	6.5	6–16 mV	49–71	≤ 3.5
Sensory (5th digit)	11.0	>10 mV		≤ 3.0
Sensory (palm)	10.0			≤ 2.4
Median				
Motor (forearm)	8.0	4–18 mV	49–70	≤ 4.4
Sensory (index)	13.0	> 15 μ V		≤ 3.5
Sensory (palm)	10.0	≥ 30 μ V		2.4
Radial sensory				
Disk electrode	10.0	> 15 μ V		≤ 2.5
Peroneal				
Motor (foreleg)	9.0	2–12 mV	43–58	≤ 6.6
Sural sensory				
Behind lateral malleolus	14	5–50 μ V		≤ 4.0
Post Tibial Nerve				
Abductor Hallucis Brevis (knee > ankle)	12.9	3–26 mV	41–53	≤ 7.0
Abdi Digiti Minimus	19.0	2–16 mV		≤ 7.3

trical stimulation for such long periods. The electromyographic findings also reveal early reinervation to determine when it is appropriate to institute muscle reeducation. Obviously, when SLAP discharges are uncovered in a previously denervated muscle, the therapist must actively exercise those muscles to the point of tiredness but not fatigue.[29] The SLAP discharges are seen only on the EMG; they are not visible contractions. Therefore, the EMG is absolutely necessary to identify these early electrophysiologic changes and to provide feedback to the patient.

REVIEW QUESTIONS

1. An elderly woman who was receiving chemotherapy for a bronchogenic carcinoma is now in remission but is complaining of dizziness. Is this patient a candidate for an ENMG? What would you look for if you knew that chemotherapy produces lesions in peripheral nerves?

2. If the elderly woman's conduction velocity of both peroneal nerves is 36 milliseconds and she is 63 years old, would that conduction velocity be viewed as abnormal?

3. If a response of the ulnar nerve is obtained at the wrist and also at the elbow but no response is obtained above the elbow, what does this result indicate?

4. If the distal latency of the median nerve is 4.75 milliseconds and the latency of the ulnar nerve is 2.75 milliseconds, what is the possible significance of these findings?

5. If the F wave latency of the right median nerve is 32 milliseconds and if the F wave latency of the left medial nerve is 29 milliseconds, what is the significance of this difference?

6. In the case described in Question 5, if abundant polyphasic MUPs were found in muscles innervated by the fifth and sixth cervical nerve roots on the right side, would this outcome be compatible with the findings in Question 5?

7. To perform an antidromic test of the sural nerve, where should the recording electrodes be placed?

8. In an individual with legs of equal length, an H reflex latency of 32 milliseconds is found on the left side and a latency of 28 milliseconds is found on the right side. Is this difference within normal variation? If not, what type of problem does it indicate?

9. What would be indicated by a 2+ shower of fibrillation potentials in muscles innervated by the ulnar nerve distal to the elbow?

10. What EMG findings might be found in muscles innervated by the fifth lumbar nerve root that was severely compressed by a herniated lumbar disk 18 days earlier?

KEY TERMS

electroneuromyography (ENMG)
nerve conduction
electromyography
dysesthesia
hypoesthesia
amplitude
proximal and distal rule
motor unit
supramaximal stimulus
resting membrane potential

depolarization
hyperpolarization
accommodation
action potential
fasciculations
motor action potential (MAP)
compound motor unit potential (cMUP)
recruitment
motor unit potential (MUP)

size principle of recruitment
graded junctional potential
endplate potential
electromyograph (EMG)
differential amplifier
impedance
voltage drop
common-mode rejection ratio (CMRR)
calibration signal

frequency bandwidth
amplifier noise
electronic noise
sweep speed
time base
storage oscilloscopes
averager
leakage currents
compound motor potential (CMP)
distal latency
sensory nerve action potential (SNAP)

F wave latency
H reflex
blink reflex test
demyelinating diseases
carpal tunnel syndrome
dying-back neuropathy
Eaton-Lambert phenomenon
interference
repetitive stimulation
MUP duration
polyphasic MUP

SLAP MUP
HALD MUP
fibrillation
positive sharp waves
neurotmesis
axonotmesis
neuropractic
polymyositis
myotonia
peripheral neuropathy multiplex
nerve root compression

REFERENCES

1. Brown MC, Ironton R: Suppression of motor nerve terminal sprouting in partially denervated mouse muscles. *J Physiol* 1977; 272:70.

2. Weddell G, Feinstein B, Pattle RE: The electrical activity of voluntary muscle in man under normal and pathological conditions. *Brain* 1944; 67:178.

3. Buchthal F, et al: Motor unit territory in different human muscles. *Acta Physiol Scand* 1959; 45:82.

4. Henneman E, Somjen G, Carpenter DO: Functional significance of cell size in spinal motorneurons. *J Neurophysiol* 1965; 28:560–80.

5. DeLuca CJ, Lefever RS, McCue MP: Behavior of human motor units in different muscles during linearly varying contractions. *J Physiol* 1982; 329:113–28.

6. Hoffmann P. Uber die Beziehungen der Sehnenreflexe zur willkurlichen bewegung and zum tonus. *Z Biol* 1918; 68:351.

7. Magladery JW, MacDougla DB Jr: Electrophysiological studies of nerve and reflex activity in normal man: Identification of certain reflexes in electromyogram and conduction velocity of peripheral nerve fibers. *Bull Johns Hopkins Hosp* 1950; 86:265.

8. Crone C, Hultborn, H, Illert, M. Reciprocal Ia inhibition ankle flexors and extensors in man. *J Physiol* 1987; 389:163–85.

9. Leonard CT, Moritani T: H reflex testing to determine the neural basis of movement disorders of neurologically impaired individuals. *Electro Clin Neurophysiol* 1992; 32:341–49.

10. Johnson EW, ed. *Practical Electromyography*. Baltimore: Williams & Wilkins; 1988.

11. Crone C, Nielsen J: Methodological implications of the post activation depression of the soleus H-reflex in man. *Exp Brain Res* 1989; 78(1):28.

12. Braddom RL, Johnson EW: Standardization of H reflex and diagnostic use in S1 radiculopathy. *Arch Phys Med Rehabil* 1974; 55:161.

13. Schuchmann JA: H reflex latency in radiculopathy. *Arch Phys Med Rehabil* 1978; 59:185.

14. Kugelberg E: Facial reflexes. *Brain* 1952; 75:385.

15. Kimura J, Powers JM, Van Allen MW: Reflex response of orbicularis occuli muscle to supraorbital nerve stimulation. *Arch Neurol* 1969; 21:193.

16. Lyon LW, VanAllen MW: Alterations of the orbicularis occuli reflex by acoustic neuroma. *Arch Otolaryngol* 1972; 95:100.

17. Kimura J: *Electrodiagnosis in Diseases of Nerve and Muscle*. 3rd ed. New York: Oxford University Press; 2001.

18. Desmedt J, ed.: *New Developments in Electromyography and Clinical Neurophysiology*. Basel, Switzerland: Karger; 1973.

19. Brooke M: *A Clinician's View of Neuromuscular Diseases*. 2nd ed. Baltimore: Williams & Wilkins; 1986.

20. Sumner AJ: Axonal Polyneuropathies. In: Sumner AJ, ed. *The Physiology of Peripheral Nerve Diseases*. Philadelphia: Saunders; 1980; 340–57.

21. Lambert EH, Eaton LM, Rooke ED: Defect of neuromuscular conduction associated with malignant neoplasm. *Am J Physiol* 1956; 187:617.

22. Nelson RM, Currier DP: *Clinical Electrotherapy*. 2nd ed. Norwalk, CT: Appleton & Lange; 1991.

23. Goodgold J, Eberstein A: *Electrodiagnosis of Neuromuscular Disease.* 3rd ed. Baltimore: Williams & Wilkins; 1983.

24. Elmqvist D, Lambert EH: Detailed analysis of neuromuscular transmission in a patient with the myasthenic syndrome sometimes associated with bronchogenic carcinoma. *Mayo Clin Proc* 1968; 443:689.

25. Kugelberg E, Taverner D: Comparison between voluntary and electrical activation of motor units in anterior horn cell diseases on central synchronization of motor units. *Electroenceph Clin Neurophysiol* 1950; 2:125.

26. Halliday AM: *Evoked Potentials in Clinical Testing.* Edinburgh: Churchill Livingstone; 1982.

27. Davis HL: Is electrostimulation beneficial to denervated muscle? A review of results from basic research. *Physiother Can* 1983; 35:306.

28. Pachter BR, Eberstein A, Goodgold J: Electrical stimulation effect on denervated skeletal myofibers in rats: A light and electron microscopic study. *Arch Phys Med Rehabil* 1982; 63:427.

29. Kosman AJ, Osborne SL, Ivy AC: The effect of electrical stimulation on denervated muscle in rat. *Am J Physiol* 1946; 145:447.

IV

Mechanical Agents

This section presents the use of mechanical forces for therapeutic interventions. Specifically, it addresses distraction forces in the form of traction, and compressive forces in the form of external compression. The physical principles, interaction of mechanical forces on physiological effects, instrumentation, procedures, and indications/contraindications of traction (Chapter 24) and external compression (Chapter 25) are included in this section. Each chapter contains updated methods for applying traction and external compression as part of therapeutic interventions.

Hydrotherapy, which is both a thermal and a mechanical agent, is also included in this section (Chapter 26). The physical properties of water that can assist with exercise and functional training are presented. Specific interventions with whirlpools, Hubbard tanks, therapeutic pools, and contrast baths are also presented in the hydrotherapy chapter.

24

Spinal Traction

JOSEPH WEISBERG, PT, PhD

THERESA A. SCHMIDT, MS, PT, OCS

Chapter Outline

Spinal traction is the application of a mechanical or manual force or a system of forces to the spine in a way that separates or attempts to separate the vertebrae and elongates the surrounding soft tissue. A more appropriate term would be **distraction.**[1-2] Traction is an ancient therapeutic tool that was described at the time of Hippocrates, circa the fourth century B.C. In the 1950s, Cyriax popularized the use of traction for lumbar disc lesions.[3] Until 1990, however, traction was used mainly to treat fractures, dislocations, and deformities of the spine. At the beginning of the twentieth century, traction was used before casting and for stretching of the soft tissue surrounding the spine of patients with scoliosis. Since then, traction has been refined to become an intervention designed to manage specific disorders. However, follow-up studies on the use of spinal traction to treat chronic and acute musculoskeletal disorders of the spine failed at that time to establish its effectiveness.[4-17] Over the past 25 years, interest in traction has grown, and new methods have been developed.[18-28] More recent studies have documented successful outcomes with the use of spinal traction. Falkenberg et al[29] demonstrated the positive effect of using traction to unload the axial spine to reduce muscle activity as measured by electromyography (EMG).[29] Abdulwahb[30] studied the effect of cervical traction on reflex activity in cases of C7 radiculopathy. In the study, cervical traction reduced radicular symptoms and improved reflex activity.[30] Mesazaros et al[31] reported improvement in **straight leg raise (SLR)** mobility of the lower extremity after application of continuous lumbar traction at 30% and 60% of body weight in patients with a positive SLR test. Additional research is needed to determine the optimal parameters for traction applications and to prove its efficacy in treating specific disorders.

The use of positional traction, in which gravity provides the distracting force, has been refined,[32] and techniques for spinal traction such as positional traction, inversion traction,[33] Goodly polyaxial traction, Goodly-Shement lumbar lift, Cottrell 90/90 Backtrac, and autotraction have been developed. These methods apply precise and gentler forces that are based on sound neurophysiologic and biomechanical principles. With these techniques, the patient is positioned in a way that promotes maximal separation between the vertebrae, and some of the units permit the patient to exercise while in traction.[34-36] The new trac-

tion techniques, combined with the clinician's improved abilities to evaluate and tailor precise intervention to specific disorders, enable today's physical therapist to treat patients with traction more effectively. This chapter covers the lumbar and cervical traction techniques that are used for many musculoskeletal and neurogenic disorders, excluding fractures and dislocations.

The literature supports the fact that spinal traction can elongate the spine.[37-40] To elongate the spine, the muscles and the ligaments must be elongated, and the space between the vertebral bodies—the articulating facets—and the **intervertebral foramen (IVF)** must be increased. These changes are claimed to promote relaxation in the paraspinal muscles,[29] reduce the bulging in a herniated disc,[41-42] reduce pressure on nerve roots in the area of the IVF,[43] and improve reflex activity in cases of radiculopathy.[30]

TYPES OF TRACTION

Many different types of traction are available.[44] This chapter details them in the following sections.

Mechanical Traction

- *Continuous traction* is applied with a constant force (weight) for several hours each day, usually for 10–14 days. Because of the long duration, only a small amount of force can be applied. The purpose of this type of traction is to reduce the pressure exerted on the spine by muscles and other soft tissues while the patient is kept on complete bed rest. It also functions to immobilize the patient. (**Figs. 24–1, 24–2**).[44-45]

- *Sustained traction* also is applied continuously, but usually for no longer than 30–45 minutes. Because of this relatively short duration, greater forces can be applied.[44-45] With this type of traction, relief of symptoms may be achieved,[34] soft tissue can be stretched, and separation of bony surfaces is possible.[36]

- *Intermittent mechanical traction* involves a mechanical device that alternately applies and releases the traction for brief intervals, usually from 15–60 seconds. This form of traction also uses relatively high forces. Its purpose is to separate bony surfaces, mobilize the joint, stretch soft tissues, and relax the muscles around the joints. The duration

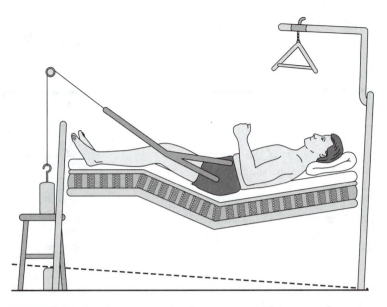

FIGURE 24–1   Continuous lumbar traction. This type of traction is applied continuously with a constant force for several hours each day, usually for 10–14 days. (*Adapted with permission from* Low Back Pain Syndrome *R Cailiet. 1978, FA Davis.*)

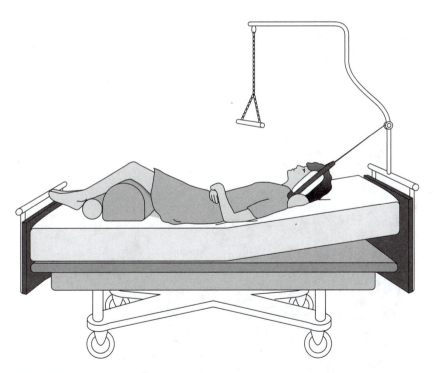

FIGURE 24–2   Continuous cervical traction. This type of traction is applied continuously with a constant force for several hours each day, usually for 10–14 days.

of intervention is usually 10–30 minutes (**Figs. 24–3, 24–4**).[44]

- *Positional traction* is applied by positioning the patient in a way that will affect the relationship of the bony surfaces in the area treated. The purpose is to alleviate pressure on an entrapped nerve and to relax the muscle in spasm. This can be done unilaterally or bilaterally. The advantages of positional traction are that the patient may perform the technique at home, the position may be modified, the force is low, and no equipment is needed.[46] The duration of intervention is usually 5–30 minutes. **Figure 24–5** shows unilateral lumbar positional traction. **Figure 24–6** shows bilateral cervical positional traction.

- *Gravity-assisted traction* can be applied in most situations. With this type of traction, the patient is placed in a position that favors distraction. Intervention duration is usually 10–30 minutes. In addition, the traction device is applied in a way that permits gravity to help the overall distraction of the targeted tissue. Some of these units permit the patient to regulate the amount of pull, thus preventing the possibility of exceeding the tolerance of the tissue. **Figure 24–7** shows gravity-assisted cervical traction, and **Figure 24–8** shows gravity-assisted lumbar traction.

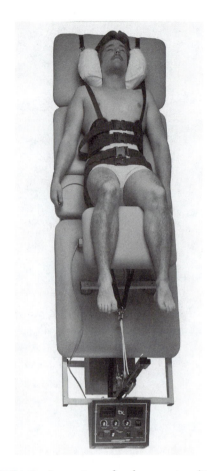

FIGURE 24–3   Intermittent lumbar traction (*Reproduced with permission from Chattanooga Group, Hixson, TN.*)

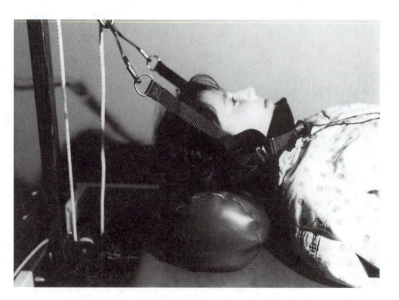

FIGURE 24–4   Intermittent cervical traction

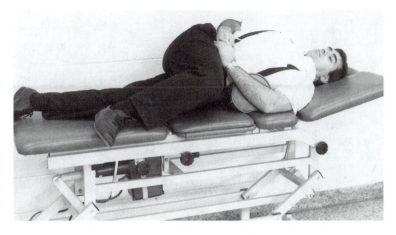

FIGURE 24–5   Unilateral positional lumbar traction.

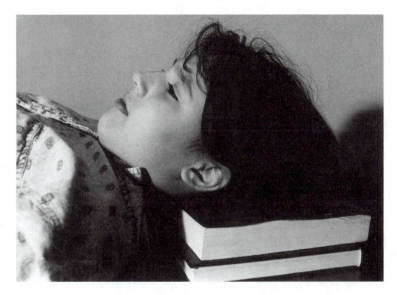

FIGURE 24–6   Bilateral positional cervical traction.

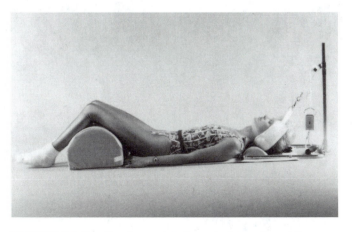

FIGURE 24–7   Gravity-assisted cervical traction. (*Courtesy of VMG Medical, Staunton, VA.*)

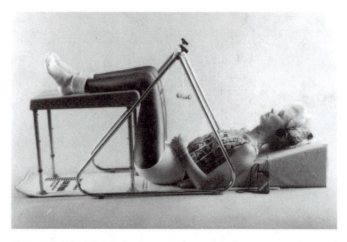

FIGURE 24–8   Gravity-assisted lumbar traction. (*Courtesy of VMG Medical, Staunton, VA.*)

- *Traction by inversion* requires the patient to be held in an inverted position. The traction force is gravity. Traction by inversion may be performed by suspending the patient by the ankles or by applying pressure through the thighs (**Figure 24–9**). During an inversion traction intervention, the patient can exercise the trunk muscles while in the inverted position.[33] The

duration of this intervention is usually 5–15 minutes. Any type of inversion traction has been shown to stress the cardiovascular system and to cause a temporary rise in systolic and diastolic blood pressure, headache, visual disturbance, nasal congestion, and petechiae on the eyes and pharynx.[47] **Figure 24–9** shows lumbar traction by inversion. Because of the documented poten-

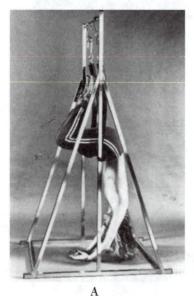

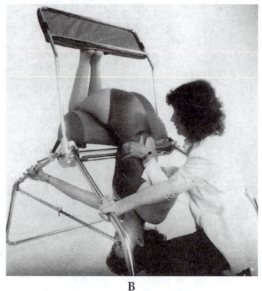

A   B

FIGURE 24–9   Examples of traction by inversion: (A) without exercise and (B) with exercise. (*Courtesy of VMG Medical, Staunton, VA.*)

tially deleterious effects of gravity inversion traction, **it is not recommended.**[47]

- *Traction in water* requires the patient to be suspended vertically in the water with a floating ring around the chest while weights are attached to the ankles. The duration of intervention is usually 6–30 minutes. The warm water may help relax the muscles (see **Fig. 24–10**).

- *Autotraction* may be of two types. One uses a multiplane automatic traction table with a force determined by the patient.[5] An autotraction table has two sections that can be set at different angles in different planes. In addition, the table can be manipulated from the horizontal to the vertical position, and the patient can lie on it in a prone, supine, or side-lying position. These characteristics of the autotraction table permit the therapist to position the patient passively in a position that is most comfortable and that utilizes the principles of positional traction and gravity-assisted traction. The intervention duration is usually 20–60 minutes. This type of traction also permits the use of exercise techniques to rehabilitate the patient. **Figure 24–11** shows the autotraction table.

- A patient may also apply self-traction using positioning against gravity combined with the force of the patient's arms to pull the body into a position of relief. In sitting self-traction, the patient presses up on the hands, using the arms of a chair to relieve weight from the spine.[46] In another method of self-traction, the patient suspends the body from an overhead bar, to relieve weight from the lower extremities, using their weight to exert a pulling force on the lumbar spine.[46]

Manual Traction

Manual traction is applied by the therapist, usually for 15–60 seconds or as a sudden thrust. Unlike mechanical traction, the therapist may immediately monitor the patient's response and may alter the direction and amount of traction force to achieve intervention goals. This type of traction can also be used as an examination tool to determine whether mechanical traction is indicated.[43] Various positions are tried to find the most comfortable one (**Figs. 24–12, 24–13, 24–14**).

Results of Intervention

The result of traction depends on the diagnostic category, strength and direction of the applied force, type of traction, technique, and length of time the force is applied. The amount, duration, and direction of the applied force for any given intervention depends on the following:

- The preferred practice pattern established or diagnostic category (eg, disc herniation, osteoarthritis, muscle spasm).
- The spinal level at which pathology is present.
- The weight and the position of the part being treated, the inertial state of the body (at rest or in motion), the contour and texture of the body surfaces, and the surface on which the patient rests.
- The nature of the surface on which the body part is resting and the size of the area in contact with the table. (The force of friction that opposes the movement differs from surface to surface; it is equal to the product of the body weight and the coefficient of friction of the surfaces: skin, cloth, and the material on the surface of the intervention table. Use of a split table for lumbar traction corrects this problem.)[48–49]
- The type of traction (continuous, intermittent).
- The strength and direction of the applied force.
- The duration of intervention.
- The technique.
- The patient's condition (general health, age, sex).
- The patient's tolerance.

Table 24–1 summarizes the different therapeutic traction techniques and their effects.

APPLICATIONS

In general, when applying traction, the therapist should aim for maximum results with the minimum amount of force. This technique will reduce some of the complications, such as skin irritation from tight harnesses, pressure on blood vessels, and pain arising from the use of high forces, thus permitting more patients to benefit from this type of intervention. To accomplish this goal, it is necessary to do the following:

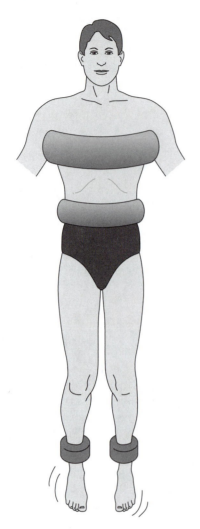

FIGURE 24–10 Lumbar traction in water. Weight can be placed on either the waist or the ankles.

- Minimize the amount and duration of force needed to overcome friction and to achieve separation. The magnitude of the force will be directly proportional to the frictional resistance of the surfaces and to the resistance of the soft tissue. Surface resistance to traction depends on the weight of the body segment undergoing traction and on the frictional coefficient of the surfaces. Usually half the body weight is required to overcome friction.[50]

- Ensure that the direction of the applied force is in line with the desired direction of distraction. The rope angle of a split table should be close to zero to eliminate most frictional resistance. On a continuous table, the traction rope should be more than a 15° angle, but there remains a significant frictional force to resist the traction, according to Goldish.[48]

- Ensure that the joint is placed in a position that will achieve maximal elongation of the spine while allowing the muscles to relax[46] so that the ligaments of the joint will be relaxed. Reilly et al[51] reported that the supine position produced statistically significant increases in posterior separation of upper lumbar vertebrae with the hips at 90° flexion. Weatherell[2] studied the effects of prone or supine positioning on **surface electromyography (SEMG)** activity of lumbar sacrospinalis muscles during traction at 50% body weight. They found that the optimal level of relaxation was achieved by the sixth minute in prone and the eighth minute in supine.[2]

The application of these principles is explained in the section on techniques.

TABLE 24–1   *The Effects of Using Different Traction Techniques*

	Technique							
Effects	**Continuous Sustained**	**Sustained**	**Intermittent**	**Manual**	**Positional**	**Gravity Assisted**	**Inversion**	**Traction in Water**
Distraction		X	X	X	X	X	X	X
Stretching soft tissue	X	X	X	X	X	X	X	X
Relaxing muscles	X	X	X	X	X	X	X	X
Mobilizing joints			X	X				
Immobilization	X							
Temporary relief of compression		X	X	X	X	X	X	X

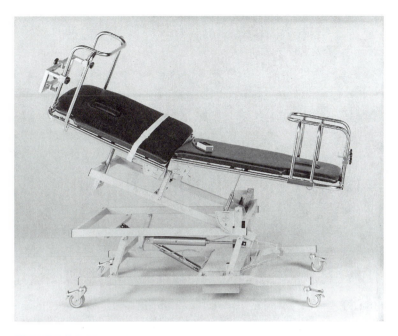

FIGURE 24–11   Table for autotraction.

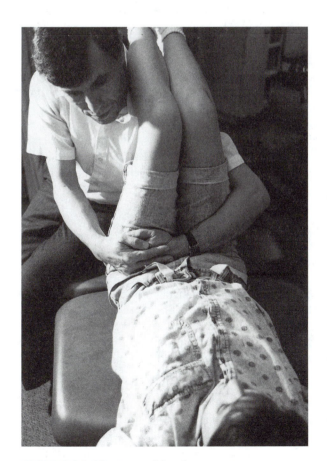

FIGURE 24–12   Manual lumbar traction.

INDICATIONS AND CONTRAINDICATIONS

Indications

The indications and rationale for spinal traction are contained in **Box 24–1.**

Contraindications

Like any other intervention modality, traction should not be used indiscriminately and is contraindicated in some disease processes and in some conditions for which spinal motion may be harmful. **Box 24–2** contains the contraindications and rationale for not using spinal traction.

Several of the newest cervical traction devices are designed to avoid exerting pressure on the TMJ. A cervical strap without the chin strap may be used for this purpose (**Fig. 24–15**). The Saunders cervical traction unit provides for cervical traction in the supine position. The Saunders unit uses a halter that applies a frictionless force through the occiput only, holding the cervical spine and occiput with padded foam wedges to achieve a purchase on the neck and occiput posteriorly.[25–26] The unit is available in both clinical and home models (**Figs. 24–16**). The Pronex 7 (**Figure 24–17**) traction unit by EMPI, Inc.,

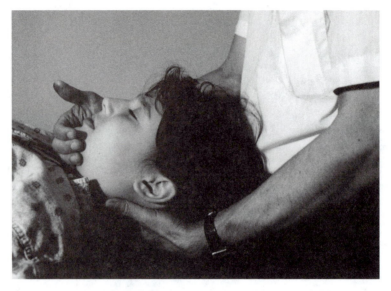

FIGURE 24–13   Manual cervical traction while the patient is in the supine position.

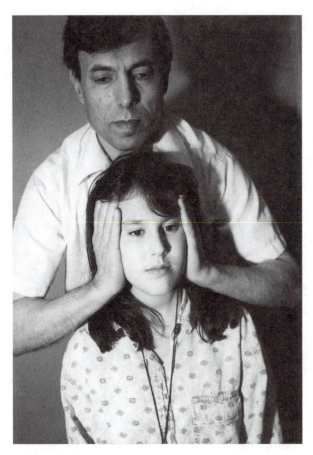

FIGURE 24–14   Manual cervical traction while the patient is in the sitting position.

consists of two inflatable foam moldings: one holds the occiput, and the other presses on the trapezius to stabilize the unit. There is a bladder-inflated bellows between the upper and lower moldings, which is inflated to allow for distraction. This arrangement avoids pressure on the TMJ.[28] **Figure 24–18** shows another example of a cervical home traction unit using a cervical strap.

The remainder of this chapter discusses the procedures for mechanical traction to the lumbar and cervical areas. The discussion includes the rationale for the intervention and specific instructions concerning its application.

Lumbar Traction

Position

To apply traction effectively, the technique must be tailored to the disorder. The therapist must consider the desired outcome for the intervention (eg, spasm reduction, intervertebral joint opening, joint capsule stretch). The mode of traction, continuous (sustained) or intermittent, must be considered. Saunders recommends sustained traction for disc protrusions, and intermittent mode for joint hypomobility and degenerative disc disease (DDD).[22] However, a review of the literature failed to demonstrate a significant difference between sustained and intermittent trac-

Box 24–1 *Indications for Spinal Traction*

Indication	Rationale
Spinal nerve root impingement from: • disc herniation • narrowing of intervertebral foramen • spinal stenosis • degenerative disc disease • osteophyte encroachment • spondylolisthesis	Reduce intervertebral pressures to decrease symptoms associated with nerve root impingement or irritation.
Subacute joint pain	Stimulate mechanoreceptors to block painful input associated with apophyseal facet joint dysfunction.
Chronic degenerative joint disease	Maintain apophyseal facet joint mobility and preserve spinal ROM when used with active and passive exercise.
Spinal hypomobility	Increase extensibility of soft tissues associated with the spine when used with active and passive exercise.
Paraspinal muscle spasm	Alter muscle spindle firing by elongation of the muscles in spasm.

tion. No difference in normal sacrospinalis muscle activity was found on SEMG by Hood et al,[52] in a study comparing sustained and intermittent traction of 80 lbs. Letchuman and Deusinger[53] confirmed their findings in their comparisons of sustained and intermittent traction at 50% body weight in patients with low back pain.

Lumbar traction can be administered in the supine or prone position. The patient's comfort and response will determine the choice of position. Traction can be applied unilaterally or bilaterally. With unilateral dysfunctions such as hypomobility of a facet joint or muscle spasm, unilateral traction is more effective.[54] The position of the patient's spine (flexion, extension, or neutral) depends on the dysfunction. When positioning the patient for intervention, the therapist must consider these principles:

1. The patient's position should provide optimal separation between the articulation surfaces. Onel et al[35] evaluated sustained supine traction effects on lumbar disc herniations using CT scans. A 45 kg (99 lb) load produced separation of the disc spaces and apophyseal facet joints, increase of neural foramina, and reduction of herniated nucleus pulposus (HNP) in median and posterolateral protrusions. They theorized that posterior longitudinal ligament (PLL) tension and creation of negative pressure in the intervertebral space assists in the reduction of disc herniations. Little effect was noted for lateral or large fragmented median protrusions, which are not adjacent to the PLL.[35]

2. The joint position should be as close to midrange or neutral as possible because the more relaxed the joint capsule and the ligaments, the less force is required to achieve the desired amount of distraction.

3. The sacrospinal muscles must be relaxed to allow for vertebral separation. In a comparison of SEMG of paraspinal muscles in normals during sustained pelvic traction at 50% body weight, Weatherell reported significantly less sacrospinalis muscle activity in prone compared with in supine.[2] Deets[55] attributed the narrowing of cervical intervertebral spaces during seated cervical traction to the inability of the patients to relax their muscles when seated. Andersson[12] found increased disc pressures in subjects who performed active autotraction, whereas passive manual lumbar traction had an insignificant effect on disc pressure.

Box 24–2 *Contraindications for Spinal Traction*

Contraindication	Rationale
Local and systemic diseases affecting spinal structures: • spinal tumors and cancer • infections • rheumatoid arthritis • advanced osteoporosis	Decreased integrity of spinal structures (ie, joints, ligaments muscle, bone) may create spinal instability that should not be exposed to excessive traction forces
Acute sprains, strains, and inflammation	Excessive traction forces may create further stress on areas of acute sprain, strain, and inflammation (inflammatory conditions, such as rheumatoid arthritis, cause joint laxity or instability, and excessive traction may therefore cause joint subluxation).
When spinal movement is contraindicated	Continuous traction (low loads for immobilization) to prevent movement may be indicated, whereas excessive traction forces may be harmful.
Spinal hypermobility	Hypermobility may be an indication of decreased spinal structural integrity that should not be exposed to excessive traction forces.
Peripheral vascular disease	Areas with compromised circulation may be further occluded with the pressure exerted by traction corsets, halters, or straps.
An increase in signs or symptoms associated with spinal dysfunction	Increased pain radiation, sensory loss, or numbness may be an indication that traction is aggravating the present dysfunction.
Over areas where harness or corset pressures may be harmful	Lumbar and thoracic harness pressures could have a harmful effect in such cases as pregnancy, hiatal hernia, abdominal aneurysm, uncontrolled cardiac or pulmonary disorders, and patients with skin sensitivity (ie, diabetes).
Poor patient tolerance	If the patient is anxious or claustrophobic, the inability to relax may offset the benefits of traction (may use manual and positional traction techniques).
Temporomandibular joint (TMJ) dysfunction	Compressive forces from a mandibular harness may aggravate TMJ dysfunction[50–51] (may use manual traction or devices that do not use a mandibular harness).

There are no standard intervention approaches to traction; individual patient response will vary. Each intervention must be tailored to the individual and to the specific pathology involved. For example, Onel[35] reported that patient response to 90 lb sustained traction was related to the type, direction, and degree of disc herniation. The position of patients will also depend on their tolerance. According to the McKenzie theory, the prone position is used because the spine can be extended. In extension, the forces are theoretically directed on the disc anteriorly (**Fig. 24–19**).[56] However, this will be the position of choice only if the patient can tolerate the position well and benefit from it; only then can the therapist assume that the herniation may be reduced by the intervention.

For patients who cannot tolerate the extended position, the neutral position is attempted. The neutral position is a midrange position between flexion and

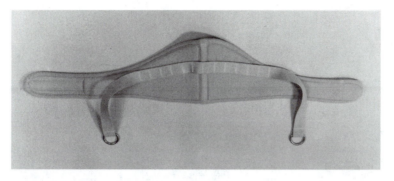

FIGURE 24–15   Cervical strap without the chin strap.

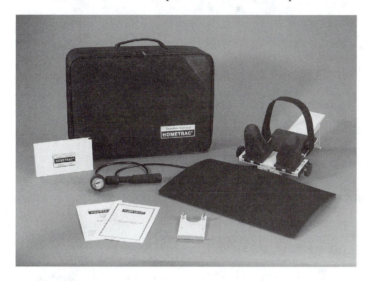

FIGURE 24–16   Home unit for cervical traction. (*Courtesy of Empi, Inc. St. Paul, MN.*)

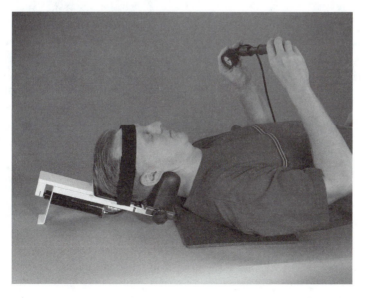

FIGURE 24–17   Application of pneumatic cervical traction. (*Courtesy of AliMed, Inc., Dedham, MA.*)

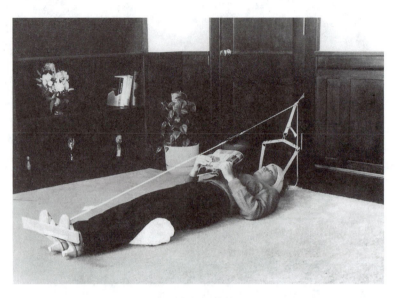

FIGURE 24–18   The patient applies intermittent traction.

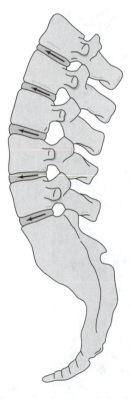

FIGURE 24–19   Lateral view of the lumbar spine in extension.

extension and can be assumed while in either the prone or supine position. If the patient cannot tolerate the neutral position, the flexed position is attempted *with caution.* Recall that most herniations are in a posterolateral direction; therefore, a force on the disc that is applied anteromedially may help to reduce the herniation. During extension of the spine, the forces on the disc are directed anteriorly. Adding lateral bending toward the affected side by applying unilateral positional traction might further direct the herniation medially (ie, toward the center of the disc) and thus be more effective. A patient may not tolerate a particular position because the forces applied are not moving the nucleus pulposus in the intended direction but instead are exerting even more pressure and thus producing more pain. In such a situation, the therapist explores another position.

An optimal position for treating patients with encroachment on the IVF with traction is one that will permit maximal opening of this foramen. In unilateral dysfunction, side bending toward the unaffected side and rotation of the upper part toward the affected side will increase the amount of opening of the foramen at the affected side (see **Fig. 24–5**). Saunders[54] recommends use of unilateral traction for facet joint restrictions, positioning in lateral flexion to the unaffected side.

The author has found clinically that dysfunction of the facet joint is best treated in flexion. The amount of flexion is determined by the level of the facet being treated. This procedure is done by positioning the patient on the table and flexing the hip slowly with one hand while the other hand is on the spine at the appropriate segmental level. As the hip is flexed, the spine will begin to flex at some point. The movement will begin from below L5-S1 and move upward. Once the movement reaches the involved segmental levels, it can be felt by the palpating hand. The segment then will continue to move to the extent that the structure permits. At the midpoint between the beginning and the end of the range of segmental movement is the neutral position of a segmental level—the point at which the ligaments around the joints are lax. It has been observed clinically that the L5-S1 segmental level requires about 45° to 60° of hip flexion to achieve laxity in the joints involved. To achieve laxity at the L4-L5 segmental level, 60° to 75° of hip flexion is required. To achieve laxity at the L3-L4 segmental level, 75° to 90° of hip flexion is required. With the respective degree of hip flexion, the therapist can assume that each respective facet is in the mid (neutral) position. In this position, the ligaments of the facets and the joint capsule are lax, thus permitting separation of joint surfaces.

Equipment

The following equipment is needed for lumbar traction:

- a pelvic corset that fits snugly over the iliac crests
- a thoracic harness that fits around the lower thoracic ribs below the xiphoid process
- a spreader bar with a rope attached at each end
- a machine that continuously or intermittently applies the pulling force
- a split traction table
- a mechanical traction unit

Both the pelvic and the thoracic harnesses are placed next to the patient's skin to eliminate slippage. These harnesses should be strapped in such a way as to overlap slightly (**Fig. 24–20**).

The most effective traction table is one that splits in the middle, thus minimizing the resistance of the friction force to the traction (**Fig. 24–21**). Because the coefficient of friction between a human body and a mattress is approximately 0.5, traction on a similar surface will require a force of one-half the patient's body weight to move that part of the body horizontally.[48] During lumbar traction only about half of the body weight is pulled; in other words, a traction force of about one-fourth of the total body weight is required just to overcome the frictional force.[49] Applying

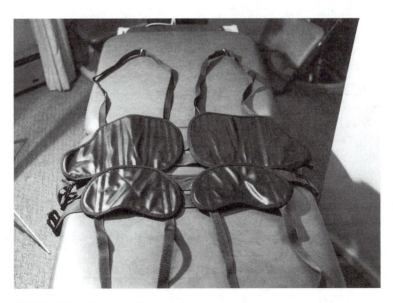

FIGURE 24–20   Overlapping harnesses.

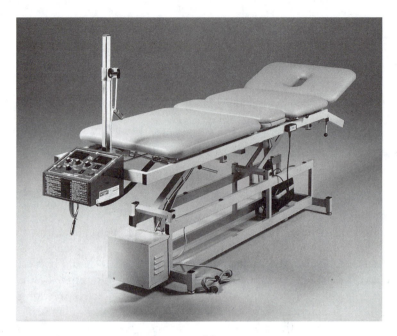

FIGURE 24–21   A split traction table.

lumbar traction on a table that is split virtually eliminates this force; thus, almost all of the traction force applied is used to distract the tissue.

At the beginning of the intervention, the table should be closed in order to ensure that the slack from the harnesses has been removed during the first few pulls. Release the catch to allow the table to open. Once the table is opened, the intervention begins.

Force and Frequency

A large amount of force is required to effect structural changes in the lumbar spine. Most authors agree that to separate segmental levels effectively, the force must be greater than 50% of body weight. Some authors indicate that a force as high as 200 pounds may be required.[14,36] On the initial visits, low force should be used (25–50 lb), gradually increasing at the tolerance of the patient.[46] This technique prevents muscle guarding and allows for accommodation and for assessment of the patient's reaction. Once the therapist has established that the patient is tolerating the low forces (25–50 lb) well, higher forces can be administered to achieve a therapeutic effect.

The setting of the on-and-off cycle is determined by the patient's condition and tolerance. Disk involvement requires longer on-times (60 seconds) and shorter off-times (20 seconds). Joint involvement requires a shorter on-time (15 seconds) and the same amount of off-time (15 seconds).[15]

The frequency of intervention can vary greatly, from twice daily to once weekly. There is no conclusive evidence of an optimal frequency of intervention or exact duty cycle (on-time/off-time ratio) for traction.

Procedure

The therapist must determine the optimal parameters of traction intervention for the given practice pattern. Before initiating the intervention, the therapist should carry out the following steps:

1. Arrange the pelvic corset and the thoracic harness on the table in the position that they will be placed on the patient.

2. Place the patient on the table in the desired position (flexion, neutral, or extension), and put a pillow under the patient's head. The split should be at the level of the affected spinal segment.

3. The pelvic corsets are applied to the skin to avoid any slippage. Attach the lumbar corset first, just over the iliac crest. Next, apply the thoracic harness with the upper limit just below the xiphoid process. Let it overlap slightly to allow for the minor slippage that will occur. Both appliances must fit snugly.

4. Attach the rope to the corset with the hook or the spreader bar.

5. Turn on the power. Select the amount of force, the mode, the on-off cycle, and the duration of intervention. The parameters chosen must be within the patient's tolerance and comfort.

6. Turn on the machine, and let it pull for a few seconds to remove the slack from the straps.

7. Release the catch of the table to allow the lower part to move.

8. Start the timer.

9. Some units have a patient alarm with a cutoff switch. Be sure to instruct the patient to turn off the unit if discomfort or peripheralization of symptoms is experienced.

When the intervention is completed, slowly reduce the tension on the rope. If the rope is released too suddenly, it may rebound and cause discomfort as the disc pressure changes abruptly. Once the rope is slack, undo the corset and the harness and encourage the patient to rest for a few minutes before getting up.

Precaution: In some cases of disc protrusion, the patient may experience discomfort after traction; this is known as the rebound effect. Saunders[44] recommends keeping the intervention short, under 8–10 min. Theoretically, as the intradiscal pressure decreases during traction, pain is alleviated. Disc pressure increases again as the traction is removed, as the osmotic pressure changes, resulting in greater pressures and pain.[44] The author has found clinically that the rebound effect may be relieved by gentle stabilization exercises prior to return to the upright position and by allowing the patient to rest for a few minutes before standing up.

CERVICAL TRACTION

Cervical traction is used to treat facet, disc, and soft-tissue dysfunctions. Intervention is guided by the same principles discussed in the section on lumbar traction. In addition, it is advisable to perform the vertebral artery test (**Fig. 24–22**), which determines whether the vertebral artery might be compromised in certain head positions (especially extension and rotation).

A comparison of the patient's pain before and after intervention can be made using the visual analogue scale to measure the patient's response to cervical traction. Assessments such as changes in range of motion, SEMG, SLR angle, or functional abilities are more objective. Measurements are taken and recorded before and after traction. Usually the response to intervention is immediate, but it does not always last; repetitive interventions may bring lasting relief. It is

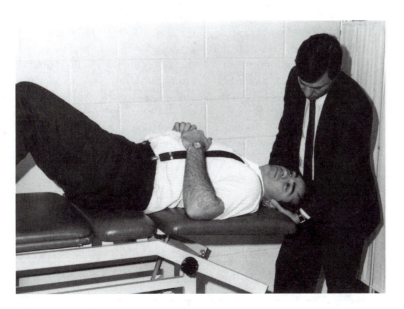

FIGURE 24–22   The vertebral artery test.

best to combine traction with patient reeducation in body mechanics and proper posture, therapeutic exercise, manual therapy, and other modalities as part of a complete plan of care.

Although the effects of cervical traction have been studied for many years, more research is needed to determine its effects on specific dysfunctions. Studies currently under way not only may increase our understanding about the effects of traction but also help us to be more precise in its application.

Position

When the intervention is administered, the patient is positioned both for comfort and security in order to promote relaxation. If the patient's paraspinal muscles are not relaxed, other modalities (eg, manual therapy, massage, thermal agents, ultrasound) can be used before the traction to help achieve relaxation. Relaxing the muscles before traction is preferable because it permits better distraction from the onset of the intervention.

Cervical traction can be administered to patients in the sitting or the supine position; however, the supine position is clearly preferred.[36,54] In the sitting position, the weight of the head (approximately 12–14 lb) must be overcome before any distractive forces of the traction can affect the tissues. In the supine position, if the head rests on the traction table, more of the traction force is directed toward distraction of the tissues. To open the posterior intervertebral spaces and minimize the effects of the friction forces, it is recommended that the rope angle be 35° to 45°,[32,54] whereas the head-neck angle is slightly flexed to a position that should not exceed 20° to 30° (**Fig. 24–23**). To select an optimal angle of pull, it is necessary to decide whether the goal is to open the posterior or anterior aspect of the cervical intervertebral spaces. Saunders[25] states that an angle of pull of 15° flexion is best to decrease a forward head posture, to straighten the cervical curve, and to open up the IVF. Saunders developed a supine cervical traction unit that provides a frictionless surface, which has an angle of pull adjustable from 15° to 25° flexion.[25] This device it uses a foam wedge to contact the occiput for distraction, thereby avoiding undue pressure on the TMJ. Maitland recommends using a pad between the molar teeth to transfer forces from the chin halter to the cranium to avoid irritating the TMJ.[45]

Wong et al[32] studied the effect of 3.5 kg (7.7 lb) traction force at 0°, 15°, and 30° traction angles on the separation of cervical vertebrae. Using X-ray, they found that the facet joint space at C5-6 and C4-5 actually increased in slight extension and that it increased in neutral for C2-C5. They cautioned against the use of extension because of possible discomfort and for cases of instability or vertebrobasilar artery insufficiency. Most anterior separation occurred in 30° of flexion, and less so in neutral. Anterior separation decreased in extension. Posterior separation was best achieved in neutral horizontal position, and less so in 30° flexion.[32]

Equipment

The apparatus available to provide mechanical cervical traction consists of a halter that fits the patient's head and a machine that intermittently or continuously applies the pulling force to the halter by means of a rope and a spreader bar (**Fig. 24–24**).

To apply traction correctly, an appropriate head halter must be used. The most appropriate halter seems to be one that allows for adjustment of the angle of pull, from neutral to 25° flexion. The device should enable the traction pull to be exerted from the occiput, not the chin. In most cases, the halter concentrates the traction force posteriorly, where it is most beneficial in flattening the cervical lordosis, stretching the cervical paraspinals and opening the IVFs posteriorly. According to Saunders, the rope should be at 15° from the horizontal for optimal results.[26] The unit should be capable of exerting 0–40 lb of force (see **Fig. 24–23**).

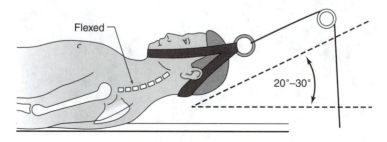

FIGURE 24–23   Using the angle of pull to achieve cervical flexion.

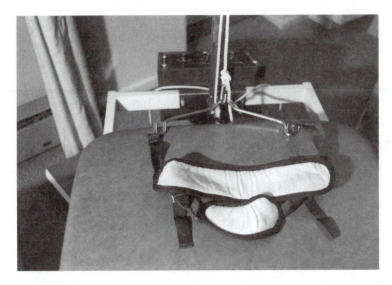

FIGURE 24–24 Mechanical cervical traction apparatus.

Force and Frequency

The amount of force necessary to demonstrate a change in the upper cervical area is 10–15 lb. In the middle and lower cervical region, it is 25–50 lb.[26]

The intervention time is relatively brief, usually 5–10 min for disc dysfunction and 10–15 min for other conditions. The patient's comfort is the determining factor when establishing the duration of intervention. There is no substantial evidence in the literature regarding optimal intervention duration for cervical traction. Weatherell[2] reported that it took 6–8 min to relax the sacrospinalis muscles during lumbar traction, as shown by SEMG. Longer durations have been used to treat disc herniations, up to 40 minutes.[46]

Unilateral traction can be incorporated in the intervention of unilateral dysfunctions. With this technique, the therapist is able to direct a stronger force to one side of the cervical spine, to open the IVF on that side. With this technique, a stabilizing strap must be used over the patient's chest so that the patient will not align the body with the angle of the rope (**Fig. 24–25**).

Procedures

Before initiating the intervention, the therapist must carry out the following steps:

1. Prepare the table, adjusting the angle of the rope or unit for the specific dysfunction (usually about 15° flexion). Place a pillow or bolster under the

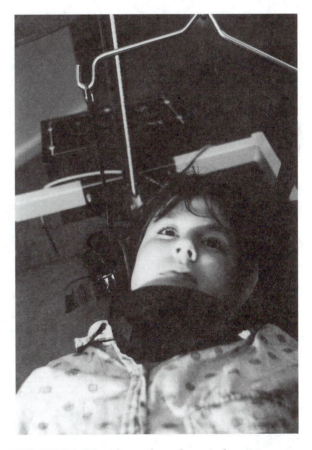

FIGURE 24–25 The unilateral cervical position.

patient's head when flexion is desired, if using a soft harness. Another pillow under the knees can be used to promote relaxation.

2. Position the patient and adjust the halter on or under the occiput, according to the instructions of the manufacturer.

3. Attach the halter to the spreader bar or rope. The rope must be slack to attach the spreader bar. The slack should be removed before the intervention.

4. Select the force, the mode (continuous or intermittent), the duration of the duty cycle (on-off cycle), and the duration of the intervention. The suggested amount of force to use initially is 10–15 lb. Then gradually increase the force to achieve the desired amount of pull that the patient can tolerate, usually up to 30–40 lb.

5. Turn on the machine and make certain that the pull that the patient experiences comes from the occiput. Monitor the patient's response, and adjust the harness accordingly.

6. Stay with the patient for the first few minutes of traction to assess the response and make adjustments in force or time according to tolerance. Establish a call system prior to leaving the patient alone. Some units have a patient cutoff switch in the event that the patient becomes uncomfortable. Instruct the patient in its operation, and advise to relax during the intervention for best results.

7. At the conclusion of the intervention, release the rope gradually, then remove the bar and halter from the patient, and instruct the patient to rest for a few minutes before arising.

The frequency of intervention will depend on the patient's response. Many clinicians administer traction from twice daily to once a week. There is no substantial evidence in the literature to support a given frequency of traction intervention.

If necessary, cervical traction may be given while the patient is in a sitting position. If the sitting position is elected, it must be done with the proper angulation of the rope. The instructions for cervical traction in a sitting position are the same as those for the supine position except for the amount of flexion, which is determined by the position of the chair in relation to the line of pull. Care must be taken to ensure that the patient follows instructions, especially those regarding the specific head position. If the patient's neck is not aligned, the effectiveness of the intervention will be reduced. It has been shown that the neck muscles do not relax well in sitting, and intervertebral separation is not adequately achieved in sitting, as compared with supine.[57]

Manual Cervical Traction

Cervical traction is often applied manually as both an examination and a therapeutic intervention. This technique is a type of joint mobilization in which the therapist applies a distraction force to the occiput of the patient in either supine or sitting position. A full explanation of the use of manual traction and mobilization of the neck is beyond the scope of this chapter (see **Figs. 24–13**, **24–14**).

Precautions

It is important to take the following precautions when using cervical traction:

• The therapist should instruct the patient to report all symptoms, not just pain. Patient monitoring is crucial for a favorable outcome.

• Increased pain and increased neurologic signs or symptoms are cause to discontinue traction immediately.

• Always perform a vertebral artery test to rule out vertebrobasilar insufficiency. Nausea, visual changes, and dizziness can be triggered by traction. Positions that increase neurologic signs must be avoided.

• Peripheralization of symptoms is a sign of additional nerve irritation. Decreased pain accompanied by an increase in positive neurologic signs during traction is an indication of abnormal nerve root involvement. If these symptoms or any other neurologic symptoms occur, traction should be stopped. The therapist documents the incident and consults with the patient's physician.

• Centralization of symptoms is a normal response to traction. As nerve root pressure is reduced, symptoms tend to move from the periphery (eg, leg pain, paraesthesia) to the center (eg, back pain) at the site of the impingement.

• It is highly recommended that all patients have spinal X-rays prior to receiving spinal traction.

DOCUMENTATION

Documentation of intervention using traction must include the following:

• type of traction device applied
• area treated

- force
- mode: continuous or intermittent; if intermittent, include on/off times and reset force (the force applied during the rest period)
- duration
- position of the spine in degrees
- body position
- response to traction

PREFERRED PRACTICE PATTERNS

In 2001, the American Physical Therapy Association (APTA) published the second edition of the *Guide to Physical Therapy Practice*. The guide describes the diagnostic categories that may benefit from the application of a variety of physical therapy interventions, including traction. Mechanical and manual traction are listed as specific direct interventions under Physical Agents and Mechanical Modalities, and Manual Therapy Techniques, respectively. The types of mechanical traction include sustained (continuous), intermittent, and positional (gravity or autotraction).

The musculoskeletal preferred practice patterns for traction are as follows:

- *Pattern G:* impaired joint mobility, motor function, muscle performance, range of motion, or reflex integrity secondary to spinal disorders
- *Pattern F:* impaired joint mobility, motor function, muscle performance, and range of motion associate with localized inflammation
- *Pattern E:* impaired joint mobility, muscle performance, and range of motion associated with ligament or other connective tissue disorders
- *Pattern D:* impaired joint mobility, motor function, muscle performance, and range of motion associated with capsular restriction

Manual traction only is listed for neuromuscular patterns:

- *Neuromuscular Pattern A:* impaired motor function and sensory integrity associated with congenital or acquired disorders of the central nervous system in infancy, childhood, and adolescence
- *Neuromuscular Pattern C:* impaired motor function and sensory integrity associated with progressive disorders of the central nervous system in adulthood
- *Neuromuscular Pattern E:* impaired motor function and sensory integrity associated with acute or chronic polyneuropathies

REVIEW QUESTIONS

1. Identify the different types of spinal traction.
2. Identify the ways in which external forces can be produced for therapeutic spinal traction.
3. Identify the indications for spinal traction.
4. Identify the precautions and contraindications for spinal traction.
5. Provide the rationale for using traction to (a) increase spinal ROM, (b) reduce disc herniation, and (c) decrease neck pain and muscle spasm.
6. When using a cervical halter, where should the traction forces be applied? In which area should traction forces be avoided?
7. Identify the positioning of the thoracic harness and lumbar corset when performing lumbar traction.
8. Identify the principles that influence the position choice when performing lumbar traction.
9. Identify the appropriate poundage that should be used when performing cervical and lumbar traction.
10. Identify the "preferred practice patterns" for which traction is indicated.

KEY TERMS

spinal traction
distraction

straight leg raise (SLR)
intervertebral foramen

surface electromyograpyhy
(SEMG)

REFERENCES

1. Saunders HD: Lumbar traction. *J Orthoped Sports Phys Ther* 1979; 1(1):36.

2. Weatherell VF: Comparison of electromyographic activity in normal lumbar sacrospinalis musculature during static pelvic traction in two different positions. *J Orthoped Sports Phys Ther* 1987; 8(8):382–90.

3. Cyriax J: The treatment of lumbar disc lesions. *Brit Med J* 1950; 2:1434.

4. Christy B: Discussion on treatment of backache by traction. *Proc R Soc Med* 1955; 48:811.

5. Larsson V, Sholer U, Lindstrom A, et al: Auto traction for treatment of lumbago-sciatica. *Acta Orthop Scand* 1980; 51:791.

6. Lindstrom A, Zachrisson M: Physical therapy on low back pain and sciatica: An attempt at evaluation. *Scand J Rehabil Med* 1970; 2:37.

7. Mathews J, Heckling H: Lumbar traction: A double-blind control study for sciatica. *Rheumatol Rehabil* 1975; 14:222.

8. Weber H: Traction therapy in sciatica due to disc prolapse. *J Oslo City Hosp* 1973; 23(10):167.

9. Ljunggren AE, Walker L, Weber H, et al: Manual traction versus isometric exercises in patients with herniated intervertebral lumbar discs. *Physiother Theory Pract* 1992; 8:207.

10. Pal B, Magnion P, Hossian MA, et al: A controlled trial of continuous lumbar traction in the treatment of back pain and sciatica. *Br J Rheumatol* 1986; 25:181.

11. Crisp EJ: Discussion of the treatment of backache by traction. *Proc R Soc Med* 1955; 43:805.

12. Andersson BJG, Schulz AB, Nachemson A: Intervertebral disc pressures during traction. *J Rehabil Med* 1988; 9(suppl):88.

13. Goldie I, Landquist A: Evaluation of the effect of different forms of physiotherapy in cervical pain. *Scand J Rehabil Med* 1970; 2C3:117.

14. Van Der Heijden GJ, Beurskens AJ, Koes BW, Assendelft WJJ, DeVet HC, Bouter LM: The efficacy of traction for back and neck pain: A systematic, blinded review of randomized clinical trial methods. *Phys Ther* Vol, 1995; 75(2):18–29.

15. Pellecchia GL: Lumbar traction: A review of the literature, journal of orthopedic and sports physical therapy. 1994; 20(5):262–67.

16. Beurskens AJ, DeVet HC, Koke AJ, Lindeman E, Regtop W, Van Der Heijden GJ, Knipschild PG: Efficacy of traction for non-specific low back pain: A randomized clinical trial. *Lancet* 1995; 346:1596–1600.

17. Beurskens AJ, Van Der Heijden GJ, DeVet, HC, Koke AJ, Lindeman E, Regtop W, Knipschild PG: The efficacy of traction for lumbar back pain: Design of a randomized clinical trial. *J Manip Physiol Therapeutics* 1995; 18(3):141–47.

18. Lind G: *Auto-Traction Treatment of Low Back Pain and Sciatica.* University of Linkoping; Linkoping, Sweden; 1974. Thesis.

19. Larsson U, Choler U, Lindstrom A: Auto-traction for treatment of lumbago-sciatica. *Acta Orthop Scand* 1980; 51:791.

20. Nossi L: Inverted spinal traction. *Arch Phys Med Rehabil* 1978; 59:367.

21. Kaltenborn F: In Kent B, ed. *Proceedings of the International Federation of Orthopedic Manipulative Therapists.* Vail, Colorado; 1977.

22. Saunders H: Evaluation, treatment and prevention of musculoskeletal disorders. In: *Educational Opportunities.* Minnesota; 1985.

23. Saunders HD: Unilateral lumbar traction. *Phys Ther* 1981; 61(2):221–25.

24. Oudenhoven RC: Gravitational lumbar traction. *Arch Phys Med Rehabil* 1978; 59:510.

25. Saunders HD: Cervical traction: Effective treatment for disc herniation and headache pain. *A Literature Review,* 1–4. 1995. The Saunders Group, Inc.

26. Saunders HD: *Frequently Asked Questions about Cervical Traction,* 1–4. 1995. The Saunders Group, Inc.

27. Saunders HD: Lumbar traction: Effective treatment for disc herniation and radicular symptoms. *A Literature Review,* 1–4. 1995. The Saunders Group, Inc.

28. Nitz A: *Case Study: Pronex Cervical Traction.* EMPI Inc., October 1995.

29. Falkenberg J, Podein RJ, Pardo X, Iaizzo PA: Surface EMG activity of the back musculature

during axial spinal unloading using an LTX 3000 lumber rehabilitation system. *Elecrtromyography Clin Neurophys* 2001; Oct–Nov;41(7):419–27.

30. Abdulwahb S: The effect of reading and traction on patients with cervical radiculopathy based on electrodiagnostic testing. *J Neuromusculoskeletal System* 1999; 7(3):91–96.

31. Meszaros TF, Olson R, Kulig K, Creighton D, Czarnecki E: Effect of 10%, 30%, and 60% body weight traction on the straight leg raise test of symptomatic patients with low back pain, journal of orthopedic and sports. *Phys Ther* 2001; 31(9):525–27.

32. Wong AMK, Leong CP, Chen C-M: The traction angle and cervical intervertebral separation. *Spine* 1992; 17(2):136–38.

33. Gianakopoulos G, Waylonis GW, Grant PA, Tottle DO, Blazek JV: Inversion devices: Their role in producing lumbar distraction. *Archives of Physical Medicine and Rehabilitation*. 1985, February; 66:100–02.

34. Gupta RC, Ramarao SV: Epidurography in reduction of lumbar disc prolapse by traction. *Arch Phys Med Rehab* 1978; 59:322–27.

35. Onel D, Tuzlaci M, Sari H, Demir K: Computed tomographic investigation of the effect of traction on lumbar disc herniations. *Spine* 1989; 14(1):82–90.

36. Colachis SC, Strohm BR: Effects of intermittent traction on separation of lumbar vertebrae. *Arch Phys Med Rehab* 1969; 50(5):251–58.

37. Basmajian JV: *Manipulation, Traction and Massage*, 3rd ed. Baltimore: Williams & Wilkins; 1985:174.

38. Colachis SC Jr, Strohm BR: Cervical traction relationship of time to varied tractive force with constant angle of pull. *Arch Phys Med Rehabil* 1965; 46:815.

39. Colachis SC Jr, Strohm BR: Effects of intermittent traction on separation of lumbar vertebrae. *Arch Phys Med Rehabil* 1969; 50:251.

40. Twomey LT: Sustained lumbar traction: An experimental study of long spinal segments. *Spine* 1985;10(2):146–49.

41. Judovich B: Herniated cervical disc: A new form of traction therapy. *Am J Surg* 1952; 84:646.

42. Mathews JA: The effects of spinal traction. *Physiotherapy* 1972; 58:64.

43. Christie BGB: Discussion on the treatment of backache by traction. *Proc R Soc Med (Physical Med)* 1972; 58:64.

44. Saunders HD: Use of spinal traction in the treatment of neck and back conditions. *Clin Orthoped Related Research* 1983; 179:31–38.

45. Maitland GD: *Vertebral Manipulation*. London: Butterworth;1986.

46. Cameron M: *Physical Agents in Rehabilitation: From Research to Practice*. Philadelphia: Saunders; 1999.

47. Zito M: Effect of two gravity inversion methods of heart rate, systolic brachial pressure, and opthalmic artery pressure. *Phys Ther* 1988; 68:20–25.

48. Goldish GD: A study of the mechanical efficiency of split-table traction. *Spine* 1989; 15:218–19.

49. Judovitch BD: Lumbar traction therapy: Elimination of physical factors that prevent lumbar stretch. *JAMA* 1955; 159,459.

50. Judovich BD: Lumbar traction therapy and dissipated force factor. *Lancet* 1954; 74:411.

51. Reilley JP, Gersten JW, Clinkingbeard JR: Effect of pelvic-femoral position on vertebral separation produced by lumbar traction. *Phys Ther* 1979; 59:282–86.

52. Hood CJ, Hart DL, Smith HG, Davis H: Comparison of electromyographic activity in normal lumbar sacrospinalis musculature during continuous and intermittent pelvic traction. *J Orthoped Sports PhysTher* 1981; 2(3):137–41.

53. Letchuman R, Deusinger RH: Comparison of sacrospinalis myoelectric activity and pain levels in patients undergoing static and intermittent lumbar traction. *Spine* 1993; 18(10):1361–65.

54. Saunders H: Unilateral lumbar traction. *Phys Ther* 1981; 61:221.

55. Deets D, Hands K, Hopp S: Cervical traction: A comparison of sitting and supine positions. *Phys Ther* 1977; 57:255.

56. Paris S: Anatomy as related to function and pain. *Orthoped Clin N Amer* 1983; 14(3):475–89.

25

External Compression

BERNADETTE HECOX, PT, MA

LAURA F. JACOBS, MD, PhD

Chapter Outline

Physical therapists have been using the concept of compression for years. External compression has been used to treat extremity edema in individuals with such diseases as chronic venous insufficiency and lymphedema. In addition, external compression has been used to help shape the residual limb following amputation in preparation for prosthetic fitting. After long periods of bed rest, patients who are placed in an upright position for the first few times, either on a tilt table or in the parallel bars, may have external compression applied to their lower extremities to prevent orthostatic hypotension. When a patient sustains a traumatic injury such as ligamentous tear in the ankle, RICE—Rest, Ice, Compression, and Elevation—is used to prevent swelling and the resulting pain that would follow.

Chapter 5 discussed the pathophysiologic basis for edema and mentioned various agents for the control of swelling. Traditional intervention with patients who have peripheral edema relies on the use of simple mechanical forces. They include elevation of the affected limb, ace wrapping, gradient compression stockings and sleeves, and massage. A commonly used mechanical modality for treating extremity edema, **intermittent pneumatic compression (IPC),** is presented in this chapter. The use of IPC has increased since the early 1970s. In addition to being used to control or reduce edema, IPC pumps are used to treat many other peripheral problems, including traumatic edema (subacute and chronic), venous insufficiency, lymphedema, leg ulcers, amputated limbs, wound healing, arterial insufficiency, and contractures—as well as to prevent possible thrombophlebitis. Intermittent pneumatic compression is also used for dialysis patients.

EQUIPMENT

Intermittent pneumatic compression (IPC) units, as the name implies, are basically air pumps. They intermittently force air into inflatable sleeves or boots into which an upper or lower extremity has been inserted. Thus, the air pressure surrounding the extremity increases. In turn, this applied pressure increases the pressure of the fluids in the interstitial spaces to a level higher than that of the lymph and blood vessels. The resulting pressure gradient encourages the fluids in the interstitial spaces to return to the venous and lymphatic vessels. Because the air pressure is applied intermittently, it acts somewhat like a pump, moving fluids back toward the heart.

The following items are required for IPC:

- An IPC unit containing (1) an on-off switch, (2) a dial to control pressure, (3) a dial to control inflation time, or time on, (4) a dial to control deflation time, or time off, and (5) a pressure or air outlet to which rubber hosing is attached (**Figs. 25–1, 25–2, 25–3,** and **25–4**).
- Inflatable sleeves and boots.
- A sphygmomanometer and stethoscope to measure the patient's blood pressure before intervention.
- Marking pencils for marking the skin, and a tape measure for measuring the part being treated before and after intervention.
- Standardized charts or paper for recording the measurements (**Fig. 25–5**).
- A stockinette to be placed on the part being treated for absorption of perspiration and for hygiene.
- Pillows, an incline board, or another device for elevating the part being treated.

TECHNIQUE OF APPLICATION
Preintervention

The extremity to be treated should be examined and compared with the contralateral limb in cases of unilateral involvement prior to IPC. Note the contours and definitions of joints. If they are not visible, edema or poor circulation may be present. On the dorsum of the foot, for example, tendons and veins are normally

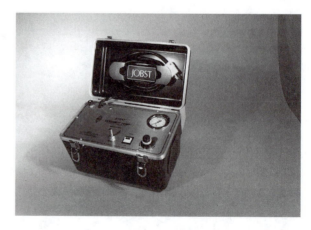

FIGURE 25–1   Portable intermittent compression extremity unit. (*Reproduced with permission from the Jobst Institute, Inc., Toledo, OH.*)

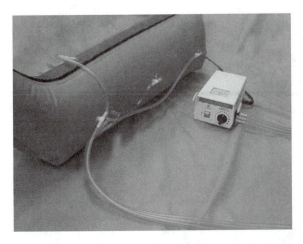

FIGURE 25–2 Portable sequential intermittent compression unit with lower extremity sleeve.

seen, but they may not be evident if there is edema. Absence of normal hair growth on the toes and lower leg may reflect poor circulation. Consider the color and quality of the skin in the affected area. Increased erythema, caused by capillary congestion, may reflect the presence of infection or cellulitis. The therapist should evaluate the integrity of the skin, particularly areas that may be fragile and ready to break down. Wounds and pressure sores are always of concern, and open areas and wound drainage should be noted. Additionally, taut or shiny skin may indicate edema. Hemsoderin deposits—dark-brown skin coloration, particularly in the calf area—may be a sign of chronic

venous engorgement. Again, compare the skin to the same area on the contralateral limb if possible.

Sensitivity and pain may be associated with presence of edema. Evaluation should include the patient's complaints of pain quality and frequency. Primary lymphatic disease tends not to be painful, whereas conditions such as cellilitis may be very painful.

The visual evaluation of the extremities for peripheral vascular disorders is followed by physical examination. Among the considerations are limb/skin temperature; status of the peripheral pulses; presence of pain/induration/pitting; and limb strength, endurance, and joint range of motion (ROM). Using the back of the hand, note any unusual warmth in areas of concern, especially compared to the contralateral limb. It is important to determine both distal (indurated) and soft (pitted) areas, and to assess the degree of induration or pitting. Chronic venous disease may start as pitting edema, but fibrosis may cause the area to become nonpitting and indurated.

Before initiating the intervention, the therapist carries out the following steps:

1. Explain to the patient the procedure and the sensations of pressure likely to be experienced, and advise the patient about the duration of intervention. Instruct the patient to call out if at any time if the compression causes pain, numbness, or paresthesia. Some therapists suggest that patients move their fingers or toes occasionally during the "inflation off" periods.

2. Place the patient in a comfortable position, because the intervention may last a relatively long time.

3. Take the patient's pulse and blood pressure. It is recommended that the pressure from the unit not exceed the diastolic pressure because it could occlude return of blood. However, the Jobst Corporation, which produces one of the compression units that will be discussed, claims that the diastolic pressure can be exceeded because the pressure is on for a relatively short time when in the intermittent compression mode.

4. Remove jewelry, and perform skin inspection as noted before.

5. Test the limb for pressure sensation. If the limb is extremely pressure sensitive, the patient will have to be monitored closely. If a "deep thrombus" is

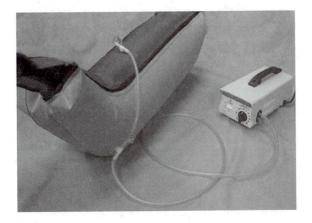

FIGURE 25–3 Non-sequential compression pump with lower extremity sleeve.

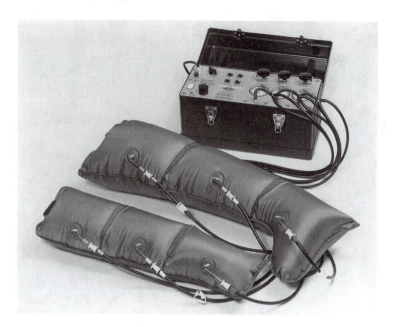

FIGURE 25–4   Intermittent compression pump with sequential air filling. Note that the compression garment has divided sections (cells). The pressure varies in each cell; it is highest in the distal cell and is lower in each more proximal cell. (*Reproduced with permission from Wright Linear Pump, Imperial, PA.*)

CHART INFORMATION

Patient Name _____ Diagnosis _____

ID# _____

(other pertinent information) _____

Extremity being treated: Right Lower Extremity _____

<table>
<tr><td rowspan="3">Locations to be marked for measuring on lateral aspects of the extremity</td><td></td><td>**Treatment Dates**</td><td colspan="2">**9/12/93**</td><td colspan="2">**9/13/93**</td><td colspan="2">**9/15/93**</td><td colspan="2">**9/18/93**</td><td colspan="2">**9/22/93**</td></tr>
<tr><td></td><td></td><td>**Pre-tx**</td><td>**Post-tx**</td><td>**Pre-tx**</td><td>**Post-tx**</td><td>**Pre-tx**</td><td>**Post-tx**</td><td>**Pre-tx**</td><td>**Post-tx**</td><td>**Pre-tx**</td><td>**Post-tx**</td></tr>
<tr><td>Example</td><td>9" prox to LE</td><td>35"</td><td>34 1/2"</td><td>35"</td><td>34Æ</td><td>35"</td><td>34"</td><td>34"</td><td>33 1/2"</td><td>33 1/2"</td><td>32 1/2"</td></tr>
<tr><td></td><td>6" prox to LE</td><td></td><td></td><td></td><td></td><td></td><td></td><td></td><td></td><td></td><td></td></tr>
<tr><td></td><td>3" prox to LE</td><td></td><td></td><td></td><td></td><td></td><td></td><td></td><td></td><td></td><td></td></tr>
<tr><td></td><td>At LE</td><td></td><td></td><td></td><td></td><td></td><td></td><td></td><td></td><td></td><td></td></tr>
<tr><td></td><td>9" prox to LM</td><td></td><td></td><td></td><td></td><td></td><td></td><td></td><td></td><td></td><td></td></tr>
<tr><td></td><td>6" prox to LM</td><td></td><td></td><td></td><td></td><td></td><td></td><td></td><td></td><td></td><td></td></tr>
<tr><td></td><td>3" prox to LM</td><td></td><td></td><td></td><td></td><td></td><td></td><td></td><td></td><td></td><td></td></tr>
<tr><td></td><td>1" prox to LM</td><td></td><td></td><td></td><td></td><td></td><td></td><td></td><td></td><td></td><td></td></tr>
<tr><td></td><td>4" prox to MH</td><td></td><td></td><td></td><td></td><td></td><td></td><td></td><td></td><td></td><td></td></tr>
<tr><td></td><td>2' prox to MH</td><td></td><td></td><td></td><td></td><td></td><td></td><td></td><td></td><td></td><td></td></tr>
<tr><td></td><td>At MH</td><td></td><td></td><td></td><td></td><td></td><td></td><td></td><td></td><td></td><td></td></tr>
</table>

FIGURE 25–5   A sample chart for recording pre- and posttreatment measurements of the girth of a lower extremity. The patient information at the top of the chart may vary, depending on the clinic. The points to be measured will vary according to the patient's size, LE = lateral epicondyle, LM = lateral malleolus, MH = head of the fifth metatarsal, PRE TX = pretreatment, POST TX = post treatment, PROX = proximal.

suspected, do not treat without consulting a physician.

6. Use bony prominences for reference points, and mark the skin approximately every 2 or 3 inches. Measure and record the girth at each marking (see **Fig. 25–5**).

7. Connect the unit to the wall outlet.

8. Place the stockinette on the part being treated, and smooth out all wrinkles. When an amputated limb is treated, the stockinette is often placed over the elastic bandage used to shape the stump.

9. Apply the boot or sleeve. Some slide on, whereas others have zippers.

10. Elevate the treated limb to a horizontal position or higher to allow gravity to help drain the fluids.

11. Attach the rubber hose to the garment and to the air outlet on the IPC unit.

12. Set the on-off dials to the desired inflation-deflation times. (Home units may have the inflation and deflation times preset in a ratio of 3:1–90 seconds on, 30 seconds off.)

13. Turn the power on.

14. Turn the pressure dial to the desired pressure. It will register *only* when the machine is in the inflation cycle.

15. Stay with the patient for the first few inflations and deflations to make certain that the patient is not uncomfortable or experiencing tingling or pain and that the pressure output is stabilized at the desired level.

Postintervention

All of the following procedures should be completed while the limb is still elevated: in other words, before the patient assumes a dependent position that might allow fluids to flow distally again.

1. At the end of intervention, turn the pressure off when the machine is in the deflation cycle.

2. Turn the power off.

3. Disconnect the tubing from the machine.

4. Remove the garment and stockinette.

5. Check the skin for pressure areas or creases from the stockinette.

6. Remeasure and record the girth of the limb at distances previously marked to determine whether the intervention made progress in decreasing swelling.

7. Apply a compression garment or ace bandage. (Before applying compression garments, many therapists have patients perform range of motion or resistive exercises or both with the treated part in the elevated position.)

The usual intervention time for massive edema is at least 2–4 hours; however, the intervention time will depend on the problem addressed. Continue the interventions, always comparing the before-and-after measurements to determine progress and the point at which a plateau is reached in the circumference of the limb. At that point, the patient should be ready to be fitted with a custom-made compression garment.

DOSAGE

Pressure on the upper extremity usually should not exceed 40–60 mm Hg; pressure on the lower extremity usually should not exceed 40–70 mm Hg. The dosages shown on **Tables 25–1** and **25–2** are based on those suggested by the Jobst Institute and Huntleigh Technology Inc. All companies that produce IPC units provide their own guidelines for each model, and they will provide more detailed intervention guides on request. Therapists should follow the guidelines for the specific model being used.

INDICATIONS AND CONTRAINDICATIONS FOR EXTERNAL COMPRESSION

Box 25–1 contains the common clinical uses and rationale for the use of external compression.

Contraindications and reasons for not using external compression are presented in Box 25–2.

MODIFIED UNITS

In addition to the standard models of IPC, some units have extra features: for example, the Wright linear pump, the Huntleigh sequential system, the NormaTec pneumatic compression pump, and the Jobst Cryo/Temp® unit (**Fig. 25–6**). The Wright linear pump (see **Fig. 25–4**) may increase the elimination of edema because it offers compression through different "cells" in the garment that give more pressure

TABLE 25–1   *Treatment Guidelines Recommended by the Jobst Institute, Inc.*[*]

Indications	Pressure (mm Hg)	Recommended Treatment Periods	Inflation Time (on)	Deflation Time (off)
Postmastectomy lymphedema	30–50	Two treatment periods a day for 3 hrs	80–100 s	25–35 s
Edema of lower extremities	30–60	Two treatment periods a day for 3 hrs	80–100 s	25–35 s
Peripheral edema and venous stasis ulceration	85	One treatment period for 2½ hrs three times a week	80–100 s	30 s
Stump reduction	30–60	Three treatment periods a day for 4 hrs	40–60 s	10–15 s
Hand edema	30–50	Two treatment periods a day of 30 min to 1 hr each	Extension position: 5–10 minutes	Flexion position: 5–10 min

Note: In general, pressures for the upper extremity should not exceed 40–60 mm Hg, and pressures for the lower extremity should not exceed 40–70 mm Hg. Pressures lower than 30 mm Hg are usually not recommended.

TABLE 25–2   *Treatment Guidelines Recommended by Huntleigh Technology Inc.*[*]

Indications	Pressure (mmHg)	Treatment	
		Minimum/Day	Total
Venous ulcers	50	Two 2 hr periods	As necessary (not less than 6 wks)
Edema (venous)	40–80	Two 2 hr periods	4–8 wks
Lymphatic edema	70–90	2 hrs	As necessary (not less than 6–8 wks)
Traumatic edema	50	2 hrs	As necessary
Stump forming	20–50	1 hr	4–6 wks

[*]These lists should be used only as a guide. Pressure and treatment periods can be varied to suit the individual requirements. The system should be used intensively initially, then reduced as improvements are obtained. The use of elasticized stockings to maintain control between treatments is recommended for certain conditions. In traumatic edema the use of ice packs may greatly aid in the reduction of pain and swelling.

Note: In general, pressures for the upper extremity should not exceed 40–60 mm Hg, and pressures for the lower extremity should not exceed 40–70 mm Hg. Pressures lower than 30 mm Hg are usually not recommended.

distally than proximally: eg, 90 mm Hg at the ankle, 70 mm Hg at the knee, and 50 mm Hg at the proximal thigh. The most distal cell has the highest pressure, which is the mean of the systolic and diastolic blood pressures.[8] Theoretically, this gradient pressure promotes the flow of fluid (edema) from the distal to the proximal part of a limb. This type of unit can be useful in the intervention with lymphedema because it prevents the backflow or reverse flow "to the areas of relatively decreased resistance."[9] Klein et al[9] reported

that the Wright linear pump was effective in treating lower extremity lymphedema in adults.

The Huntleigh sequential system has three chambers; each is filled sequentially, starting with the distal and moving to the proximal chamber. Theoretically, this arrangement should enhance the movement of fluid in a limb in a proximal direction.

The NormaTec pneumatic compression pump provides a dynamic pulsing compression within a segmental sleeve. Each segment within the sleeve can be

Box 25–1 *Indications for Therapeutic External Compression*

Indication	Rationale
Traumatic edema	Mild compression to control the leakage of vascular fluid into the interstitial tissue
Chronic edema in individuals with decreased mobility	Compression to create a pumping effect for individuals with a decreased muscle pump due to paralysis and/or weakness
Lymphedema	Compression for individuals with stasis within the lymphatic system (ie, individuals with congenital or acquired lymphatic dysfunction) to prevent pain, infection, decreased function, and skin breakdown[1,2]
Venous stasis wounds	Compression removes edema and prevents venous pooling so that the wound is able to heal (an absorptive dressing with an unna boot or compression wraps would be indicated)
Residual limb shrinkage	Compression following amputation helps to shrink and shape the residual limb in preparation for prosthetic fitting[3]
Prevention of thrombophlebitis	Compression post-operatively to maintain venous return when the calf and lower extremity muscle pump is decreased[4,5]
Tissue healing and scar management for wounds and burns	Mild compression for postoperative wounds[6] Stronger compression after suture line healing to help model the laying down of new scar tissue Control of hypertrophic scarring for individuals with burns
Arterial insufficiency	Mild compression to increase venous return to provide more blood flow into the arterial circulation[7]
Hand contractures and edema	Compression with pneumatic pump, finger wrap, and glove to manage edema and maintain ROM following surgery, trauma, and stroke
Renal insufficiency	Mild compression if not contraindicated to minimize extremity edema due to kidney dysfunction

individually controlled so that areas with compromised skin integrity, sensitivity, and other conditions in which less compression is indicated can still be treated.

The Jobst Cryo/Temp® therapy system combines two components of the RICE intervention described in **Chapter 14**: cooling of a limb with either intermittent or continuous controlled compression (see **Fig. 25–6**).[10] Two types of Cryo/Temp units are available. The large "professional" or hospital unit stands 32 inches high, has its own refrigeration mechanism that does not require ice or water, and comes with different-sized sleeves that remain completely dry and fit on different limbs. The temperature is adjustable and thermostatically controlled, and ranges from 32°F (0°C) to room temperature. A compression on-off time cycle allows compression to be on for as long as 180 seconds and off for as long as 60 seconds. Gauges indicate the temperature and pressure. Two separate controls allow two different limbs to be treated simultaneously.

A smaller portable "home" Cryo/Temp unit is available for foot, ankle, knee, hand, wrist, and elbow injury intervention. With this unit, only one injured part can be treated at a time. Like the hospital unit, the temperature and pressure of this unit are adjustable. However, it offers only intermittent compression at a preset time of 90 seconds on and 30 seconds off. The unit has a gauge to indicate pressure. The temperature selected is determined by the injury. If a deep muscle or joint is involved, a low temperature is selected.

Box 25–2 *Contraindications for External Compression*

Contraindication	Rationale
Edema from acute pulmonary edema and congestive heat failure	Compression will bring more fluid to a system that is already overburdened and will increase stress on the heart and lungs.
Completely obstructed lymphatic vessels	Compression will be effective only after clearing the area of obstruction.
Presence of deep vein thrombosis and obstructed venous vessels	Compression could dislodge the thrombus and create an embolism to the heart, lungs, or brain.
Unstable acute fractures	Compression could cause movement at an unhealed fracture site.
Acute local infections	Compression and resultant perspiration could spread infection.
Severe peripheral arterial occlusive disease	Compression could contribute to further arterial occlusion.

If continuous pressure is used, the pressure dial is lowered to zero once the intervention is completed so that the sleeve or garment can be removed easily. The temperature dial should be turned down.

The combination of cold and compression may help to reduce the bleeding and edema, and, in turn, to reduce the pain caused by the pressure of the edema on structures in and around the injured area. The home unit can be useful for patients who cannot come to the clinic often.

The combination does have a few disadvantages. Some patients cannot tolerate cold; however, as men-

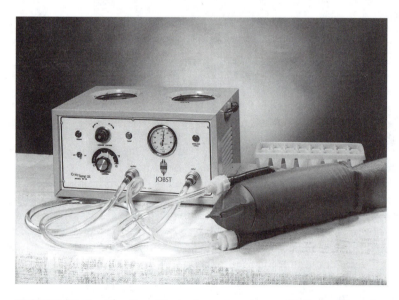

FIGURE 25–6   The Cryo/Temp therapy system, which combines intermittent pressure with cooling. (*Reproduced with permission from the Jobst Institute, Inc., Toledo, OH.*)

tioned earlier, the temperature can be controlled. The amount of pressure must be low and carefully selected if there is any danger that bleeding can be exacerbated. If intervention is applied over a fracture site, the therapist must be certain that the fracture is well aligned. (Physical therapists usually do not treat such cases.)

DOCUMENTATION

As in other areas of physical therapy, ample clinical documentation demonstrates positive results with using IPC. The manufacturers have supported research to substantiate these benefits. In 1990 an independent study comparing the effects of IPC and electrical stimulation on posttraumatic hand edema showed significant reduction of edema with IPC.[11]

This study supports the findings of previous studies and clinical observations; however, further investigations must still be conducted. At present, the comparison of girth measurements before and after intervention and from intervention to intervention is a good clinical indication of the effectiveness of IPC.

In physical rehabilitation, IPC is an accepted treatment whenever the danger of excessive or prolonged swelling warrants its use: for example, after a mastectomy or surgery on a shoulder or an ankle. As was mentioned in **Chapter 5,** tissues stretch accordingly when edema is prolonged, thus encouraging more edema. Aggressive physical therapy, including IPC interventions, active exercise, proper positioning, and compressive garments can do much to prevent the development of chronic swelling.

REVIEW QUESTIONS

1. Why is intermittent pneumatic compression (IPC) contraindicated for patients with a congestive heart problem?

2. Why is IPC contraindicated for patients with thrombosis?

3. When using IPC on a patient who has arterial insufficiency, what precautions must be taken?

4. When using IPC to treat a patient who has stasis ulcers in the leg, what pressure and intervention periods are recommended? For how long should the intervention continue?

5. A 40-year-old woman is being treated with IPC after a radical mastectomy. How can IPC help reduce the postoperative lymphedema? How much pressure should be applied, and for how long?

6. Why is a stockinette placed on the part to be treated with IPC?

7. For what cases would the combination of cold and compression, as with the Cryo/Temp®, be useful?

8. Before treating chronic edema in a 45-year-old man's leg, his blood pressure proves to be 140/120. What effect, if any, would these pressures have on the amount of pressure selected for the IPC intervention?

9. What is the optimal positioning for an individual receiving IPC for lower leg, ankle, and foot edema?

10. What additional interventions should be employed after and between IPC interventions to maintain edema reduction?

KEY TERMS

Intermittent Pneumatic
   Compression
Lymphedema
Residual Limb Shrinkage

Thrombophlebitis
Pulmonary Edema
Peripheral Arterial Occlusive
   Disease

Sequential Pneumatic
   Compression

REFERENCES

1. Sanderson R, Fletcher W: Conservative management of primary lymphedema. *Northwest Med* 1965; 64:584–88.

2. McNair TJ, Martin IJ, Orr JD: Intermittent compression for lymphedema of arm. *Clin Oncol* 1976; 2:339–42.

3. Redford JB: Experiences in use of a pneumatic stump shrinker. *Inter-clin Inform Bull Prosth Orthot* July 1973; 12(1).

4. Allenby E, Pflug J, Boardman G, et al: Effects of external pneumatic intermittent compression on fibrinolysis in man. *Lancet* 1973; 2:1412–14.

5. Clark WB, et al: Pneumatic compression of the calf and postoperative deep vein thrombosis. *Lancet* July 6, 1974; 2:5.

6. Pflug J: Intermittent compression: A new principle in the treatment of wounds? *Lancet* August 10, 1974.

7. Henry JP, Windos T: Compensation of arterial insufficiency by augmenting the circulation with intermittent compression of the limbs. *Am Heart J* 1965; 70(1):77–88.

8. Klein M, Alexander M, Wright J, et al: Treatment of lower extremity lymphedema with the Wright linear pump: Statistical analysis of a chronic trial. *Arch Phys Med Rehabil* 1988; 69:203–06.

9. Alexander M, Wright E, Wright J, et al: Lymphedema treated with linear pump: Pediatric case report. *Arch Phys Med Rehabil* 1983; 64:132–33.

10. Cryo/Temp® Therapy Systems. Product News. Toledo, OH: Jobst Institute.

11. Griffin J, Newsome L, Stralka S, et al: Reduction of posttraumatic hand edema: A comparison of high-voltage pulsed current, intermittent pneumatic compression, and placebo treatments. *Phys Ther* 1990; 70:279–86.

26

Hydrotherapy

BERNADETTE HECOX, PT, MA

PETER M. LEINANGER MS, PT, OCS, CSCS

Chapter Outline

When water is used as a treatment for physical or psychological problems, it is termed **hydrotherapy.** Medical hydrotherapy can be defined as the internal or external use of water in any of its three forms—solid, liquid, or vapor—to treat disease or traumas. "Internal use" refers to treatments such as drinking mineral waters, administering enemas, or douching. In the United States, the word *internal* can be omitted from a physical therapy definition because physical therapists do not treat internally. According to this definition, hot and cold packs, ice modalities, and moist air cabinets are all considered hydrotherapy modalities. Many people also include melted paraffin because it is fluid. In essence, however, the medium for hydrotherapy is water.

Water has unique physical properties, including buoyancy, hydrostatic pressure, surface tension, cohesion, adhesion, and fluidity, in addition to its well-recognized thermal properties. By immersing the patient's body or part of the body in water, therapists use these properties when performing many therapeutic procedures. **Table 26–1** outlines the primary treatment procedures for which immersion in water is useful and the specific properties of water that warrant its use. Because all the properties listed are inherent in water, all act on an individual simultaneously. However, this chapter discusses each individually.

Immersion Hydrotherapy
Thermal Effects

Hydrotherapy modalities are considered to be superficial thermal modalities because only the body surface contacts the water and the skin is virtually waterproof. However, when the body is immersed in water, physiologic changes may occur that are different from those arising from other superficial thermal modalities.

Immersion Factors. When the body or body part is immersed in water, the entire circumference of the immersed part is treated simultaneously. Nonfluid superficial modalities may be applied to only one surface of the body. The melted paraffin-mineral oil bath and Fluidotherapy® also are immersion modalities, but their thermal properties differ from those of water.

Thermal Properties of Water. In comparison with the thermal properties of the paraffin mixture, water has higher specific heat and thermal conductivity values; thus, it contains more heat per temperature and conducts heat more rapidly (see Table 9–3). Because of these thermal properties, water is a good means of heating or cooling the body rapidly.

Heat Transfer with Immersion. The primary means of heat transfer between skin and water is convection. However, assuming that the immersed body part remains completely still, a limited amount of heat gain or loss may occur via conduction between the skin and the water molecules immediately adjacent to the skin. This adjacent water layer may act as a "sealer," deferring further conduction. Everyone has experienced this sealer effect. If an individual sits still in a tub of very warm water, the water next to the skin soon begins to feel cooler, but when the individual swishes the water a little or moves about in it, the cooler water is pushed aside and the warmer water

TABLE 26–1   *Purposes of Immersion Hydrotherapy and the Properties of Water that Warrant Its Use*

Purpose	Property of Water
Hot or cold treatment modality	Thermal properties
Environment for performing therapeutic exercise procedures (muscle strengthening, balance, ambulation, and range of motion)	Buoyancy, hydrostatic pressure, surface tension, cohesion, and turbulence used for resistance/assistance.
Environment in which to improve circulation, reduce edema, or both	Thermal properties and hydrostatic pressure
Treatment of skin problems and open wounds; debridement; removal of dressings; application of topical medications in solution; skin lubricant	All pressure factors and fluidity and turbulence
Psychological	Any and all properties

comes close to the skin. The water then feels warmer again. The diver's wet suit exemplifies the use of this sealer effect as a means of insulation. In therapy, agitators are placed in whirlpools primarily to move the water and prevent this sealer effect.

Actually, even if an individual could remain completely still, some convection would occur. The heat transfer by conduction between the skin and adjacent water molecules results in a temperature of the adjacent water that differs from that of the rest of the water in the tub. This temperature gradient sets up convection currents, and heat transfer by convection begins (see **Chapter 9**). The convection power of water is 25 times greater than that of air.[1] Swimming increases the convection as the body moves through the water; agitators do the same because the water is forced to move across the body.

Physiologic Effects of Immersion. The physiologic and therapeutic effects resulting from the thermal properties of water are similar to those attributed to any heat or cold modality discussed in **Part 2.** However, the tissues affected may be different from those affected by other superficial modalities. Because the body part is surrounded by water, both agonist and antagonist muscle groups are affected simultaneously. When the entire body segment is surrounded by a substance containing much heat, there is less opportunity for normal local heat-loss mechanisms to be effective; therefore, heat may conduct to deeper tissues than is the case with other superficial modalities.[2,3] If so, it may be possible to effect the healing of slightly deeper tissues more than is possible with other superficial heat modalities and to elongate (stretch) deeper tissues such as tendons and capsules more effectively. It has been shown that nonelastic tissues can best be lengthened while heated, but with many heat modalities, the stretching procedures must wait until the heat has been removed. The precise mechanisms for heat transfer from water to the body core are not clearly understood. Nadel points out that the thickness of the subcutaneous fat layer is inversely proportional to changes in internal temperature. Whether this is the case simply because fat, a thermal insulator, influences the conduction of heat, or whether other thermal regulatory mechanisms are involved is unclear.[4]

Systemic physiologic changes in water, including changes in all vital signs (core temperature, blood pressure, pulse rate, and respiration), may be much greater than with other superficial heat modalities because the body's means of heat loss are much less. For example, if the total body is immersed, as with a Hubbard tank treatment, and the water temperature is greater than the skin temperature, there is virtually no way for sweat to evaporate or for surface heat to radiate to a cooler environment. The ambient temperature in which the patient is existing while in the water is the water temperature, not the room temperature that the therapist is experiencing, and the humidity of the patient's environment is 100%.

The room temperature and humidity also must be considered. If the air in the room is extremely humid—as it may be because there is so much water in the area—some heat loss may occur through radiation, but there is little chance for heat loss through the evaporation of sweat. This fact is significant not only for patients but also for everyone else in the hydrotherapy area. Changes in vital signs, fainting, or both may be experienced by anyone in the area. Thus, it is important to keep the room as well ventilated as possible. The temperature of the room should be cool enough to allow some heat to escape but warm enough to avoid chilling the patient when leaving the water. A room temperature of 78°F (25.5°C) with a relative humidity of 50% is suggested.[5] Although Campion[6,8] suggested an air temperature of at least 86°F (30°C) for pediatric hydrotherapy areas, she stated that it must be lower than the water temperature. To avoid chilling, the patient is always wrapped in dry towels or cotton blankets after coming out of the water.

Aquatic Therapeutic Exercise

Exercising in water has great value. Patients with limited standing balance can stand with reduced fear of falling, patients with limited ability to bear weight on joints in the lower extremities can walk, patients with weak muscles can move body parts, and peripheral and cardiac muscles can be strengthened. Since exercising in water is often useful, this chapter discusses the properties of water and the ways that they apply in therapeutic exercise. Extensive hydrotherapeutic exercise programs are beyond the scope of this book but can be found in the literature.[6–12,69–71]

Buoyancy. **Buoyancy** is defined as the upward thrust of water acting on a body that creates an apparent decrease in the weight of the body while immersed. Archimedes' Principle tells us that the upward thrust experienced by a fully or partly immersed body is equal to the weight of the water it displaces. The amount of water displaced depends on the density (mass/unit volume) of the immersed body relative to the density of water (see **Chapter 9**).

Water density does not remain constant; it varies with temperature and atmospheric pressure. The density of salt water is greater than that of fresh water; thus, an individual floats more easily in the ocean than in a fresh-water lake. The density of any volume of water is proportional to its depth. Because deeper water supports the water above, its density is greater.

The densities of various substances, measured in g/cm,^{3} are described by a pure number value called **specific gravity (SG)** that is given to each substance. The SG value for pure water at 4°C is 1.0. Whether another substance will float or sink in water can be determined by comparing its SG value to that of pure water. Specific gravity values for substances relevant to this discussion are given in **Table 26–2**.[7,9,13–16]

An object whose SG, thus its density, is equal to pure water (1.0) will float submerged just below the surface of the water. If the SG of the object is *greater* than 1.0, the object will sink at a rate that depends on the difference in SGs. For example, aluminum (SG = 2.7) will sink, but it will do so more slowly than iron

(SG = 7.8). If the SG of the object is *less* than 1.0, the object will displace a proportional amount of water. For example, the SG of ice is approximately 0.92; thus, 92% is in the water and 8% is floating above. What can be seen floating in Arctic waters is indeed just the tip of the iceberg.

Air is far less dense than water (SG = 1.21 × 10^{-3}), so air-filled pillows, toys, and even surgical gloves blown up like balloons can be used to support body parts and to increase a patient's ability to float. Because the SGs of oak and pine woods are less than 0.1, they can be useful as floats if dry. Even wooden seats or crutches can be used to help support a body part or prevent a patient from sinking. Floats also can be used for resistance exercises to increase the resistance encountered when pushing down into the water against the effects of buoyancy.

The SG of the average human body with air in the lungs is approximately 0.974, slightly less than water; thus, the body floats nearly submerged but 2.6% is fortunately above water. If the floating is prolonged, it is hoped that this part above water will be the face. Because air is considerably less dense than water, if an individual inhales deeply, more of the body will be above water; but on exhaling completely, the body

TABLE 26–2   *Specific Gravity of Different Substances**

Substance	Specific Gravity Value
Pure water	1.0
Salt water	1.024
Ice	0.917
Air	1.21 × 10^{-3}
Average human body with air in lungs	0.97
Average human body without air in lungs	1.1
Fat (subcutaneous)	0.85
Bone (varies with density)	
Femur	1.85 (approx)
Vertebral body	0.47 (approx)
Substances used for hydrotherapy equipment	
Wood	
Oak	0.72
Pine	0.42
Aluminum	2.7
Iron	7.8

*From Skinner A, Thomson A,[7] Lehmann J,[15] and McCordle W, Katch F, Katch V.[16]

may sink because the SG of a body without air is approximately 1.1.

The differences in people's sizes and shapes and the differences in the SG values of various tissues can explain why some people float more easily than others. On average, approximately 60% of an adult's body is water, which tends to equalize the body's SG with that of the surrounding water. The SG of fat is lower than water, which tends to let the body float, but the SG of some bone may be greater than water, which tends to let the body sink. Therefore, a person with dense bones and little fat will have more difficulty floating than one who has more fat and less dense bones. Conversely, if two people's arms are of equal length and bone structure, but one person is obese and the other is thin, and both are standing neck high in water, the obese person will have more difficulty adducting the arms down under the water.

Because buoyancy counteracts weight, when ambulation is desired to maintain a patient's muscle strength, function, or both, but weight bearing is contraindicated—for example, after surgery or an injury to a lower extremity—the patient can walk safely in water that is up to the neck. As the patient improves, the water level can be lowered gradually, decreasing the apparent weightlessness. Dancers, runners, and other athletes commonly use this technique to keep in shape while recovering from injuries that necessitate non–weight bearing.

If a body segment is relaxed, weak, or paralyzed, by allowing buoyancy to lift the part, the segment can move upward toward the water surface. Resistive exercises can be performed by downward movements against this upward thrust. By positioning the body correctly, all joint movements can be performed either with or against buoyancy. Just as gravity assists with downward movements out of the water, buoyancy assists with upward movements in the water. Therefore, positions for resistance or assistance exercises are always the opposite when in water than when out of water.

Kinesiological rules for torque (the moment of a force) are as useful when planning hydrotherapy exercises as when planning exercises out of water. The torque (τ) is equal to the rotary force (F) times the lever arm distance (L); thus

$$\tau = F \times L$$

The rotary component of a force is at a right angle to the moving segment. (For more complete informa-

tion regarding torque, the reader is referred to kinesiology or biomechanics texts.[17,18,19]

When performing movements out of water, the effect of gravity (a vertical downward force) on the rotary movement of a body segment is greatest when the segment is horizontal (ie, at a 90° angle from the vertical) and the rotational component of this gravitational force decreases as the segment moves toward the vertical (ie, the angle changes from 90°). Similarly, when movements are performed in water, the effect of buoyancy (a vertical upward force) is greatest when the segment is horizontal and diminishes as the segment approaches the vertical **(Fig. 26–1)**.

Just as the **center of gravity (COG)** is used as a reference point when analyzing the effect of gravity at a given angle as a movement is performed out of water, the **center of buoyancy (CB)** of a body segment is the reference point used to analyze the effect of buoyancy on movements at a given angle when performed in water. The CB pertains only to the center of the part of the body that is immersed in the water.

Both the COG and the CB can be used to measure the lever arm distance of a rotating segment. The farther that either the COG or the CB is located from the axis of rotation, the longer the lever arm distance, thus the greater its effect on the torque produced. The COG or CB can be changed by adding external objects. Adding weights to the distal end of an extremity places the COG more distally; similarly, holding a balloon or float at the hand or foot places the CB more distally, increasing the lever arm distance for the torque produced upward by buoyancy **(Fig. 26–2A and B)**. Thus, a balloon placed in a hand in water adds resistance to an arm pushing down into the water, but it assists an arm positioned nearly vertical in the water to rise **(Fig. 26–2C and D)**. Bending a knee or an elbow moves the COG or CB proximally, thus shortening the lever arm and reducing the torque resulting from either gravity or buoyancy **(Fig. 26–2E, F, and G)**.

When horizontal movements are performed out of water, the effect of gravity is neutralized. Similarly, the influence of buoyancy is neutralized when performing horizontal movements in water. However, buoyancy will give an upward support to a body segment performing such movements. Because gravity and buoyancy are counteracting forces, the body is stable when the COG and CB are aligned vertically. If they are not, rotation occurs **(Fig. 26–3A and B)**. Knowledge of the COG and CB can be helpful when

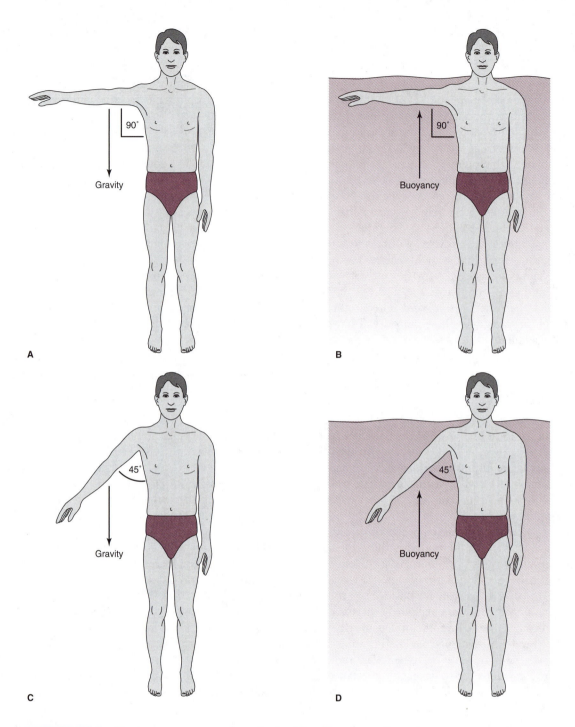

FIGURE 26–1 Rotary components of gravitational and buoyancy forces on an arm at various angles. F_t = total force, and F_r = rotary component of the total force. In the horizontal position, ie, at a 90° angle between the arm and the vertical (the trunk), the total forces of both gravity and buoyancy are rotary forces ($F_t = F_r$). At a 45° angle, the F_t of both gravity and buoyancy must be resolved into rotary components and either a compression or a distraction component; thus, the F_r is less than the F_t. (**A**) When the arm is held at a 90° angle, gravity is a downward vertical force. (**B**) When the arm is held at a 90° angle in water, buoyancy is an upward vertical force. (**C**) With the arm at a 45° angle, the F_t of gravity is resolved into rotary and distraction components, and the F_r is less than the F_t. (**D**) With the arm at a 45° angle in water, the F_t of buoyancy is resolved into rotary and compression components, and the F_r is less than the F_t.

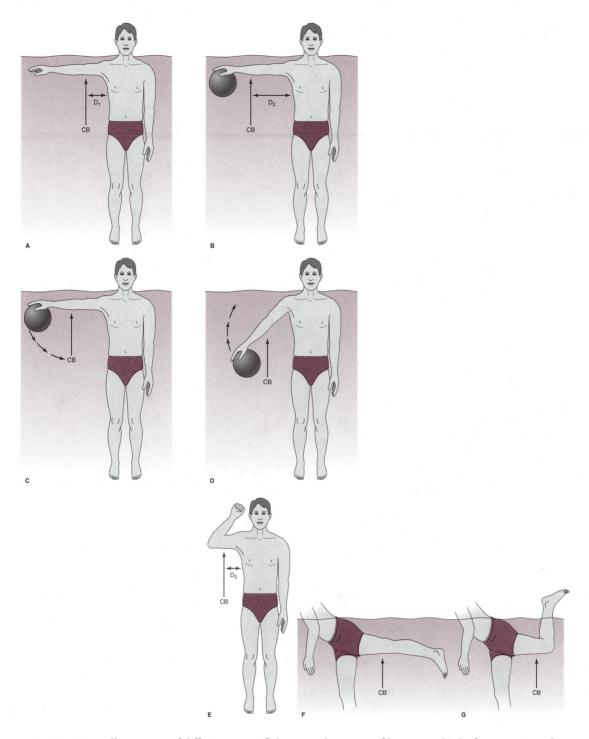

FIGURE 26–2 Illustrations of different ways of changing the center of buoyancy (CB) of an extremity, thus changing the lever arm distance and the resulting torque. This can increase the resistance or assistance that buoyancy produces to movements in water. (**A**) The lever arm distance (D_1) to the CB of an arm in water is shown. (**B**) An inflated balloon is held in the hand. This moves the CB distally, lengthening the lever arm distance (D_2), thus increasing the torque resulting from buoyancy. (**C**) The balloon adds resistance to downward movements, thus opposing buoyancy. (**D**) The balloon assists buoyancy with upward movements. (**E**) Bending an elbow moves the CB proximally, thus shortening the lever arm distance and decreasing the torque. Consequently, a downward movement meets less resistance, and upward movements receive less assistance. (**F** and **G**) Similarly, bending the knee alters the effect of buoyancy.

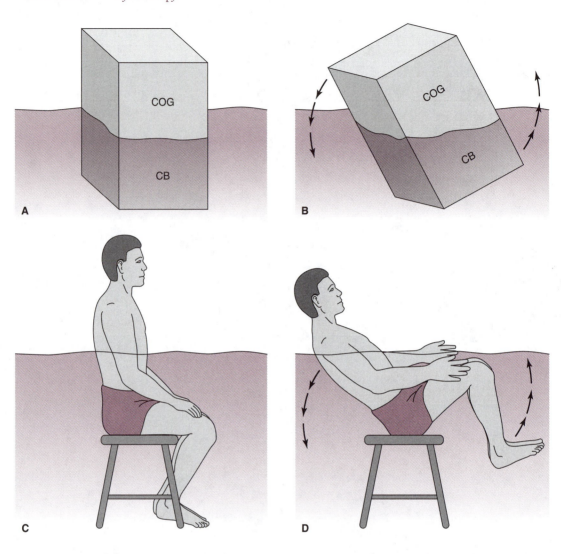

FIGURE 26–3   When the center of gravity (COG) of a portion of an object that is out of water is in vertical alignment with the center of buoyancy (CB), the object is stable. When it is not in vertical alignment, the object rotates. (**A**) Because the COG and the CB are vertically aligned, the box is stable. (**B**) Because the COG and the CB are not vertically aligned, the box rotates. (**C**) A person sitting partially immersed in water with the COG and the CB in vertical alignment is in a stable position. (**D**) If the COG of the portion of the sitting person that is out of the water is not vertically aligned with the CB of the portion in the water, the person tips over.

planning exercises to improve balance or the ability to recover to the vertical after being tipped off balance. Weak patients must be guarded carefully, however, because they can easily be tipped over by the rotation **(Fig. 26–3C and D).**

Hydrostatic Pressure.   **Hydrostatic pressure** is the pressure exerted by the water on the immersed body.

Water surrounds the immersed part, conforming to and enclosing any shape. According to Pascal's law, when a body part immersed in fluid is at rest, the fluid will exert equal pressure on all surface areas at a given depth **(Fig. 26–4).** The effect of this pressure is significant when treating patients with respiratory problems. The pressure can be used as a resistance when doing exercises to improve lung expansion; however,

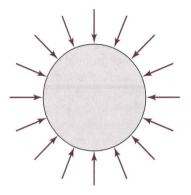

FIGURE 26–4 Equal hydrostatic pressure at any given depth.

patients with serious respiratory problems may have difficulty breathing if their lungs cannot expand adequately against so much external pressure.

Because pressure increases with the density of the fluid and the density of water increases with its depth, a pressure gradient is established between surface water and deeper water (22.4 mm Hg for each 30.5 cm).[20]

Thus, standing and walking in water can be helpful to patients who have circulatory problems of edema in the legs or feet if the edematous body part is positioned correctly in the water. The distal part, if deeper in the water, will be subject to more pressure. This pressure gradient encourages return flow of fluids in a proximal direction from the extremity **(Fig. 26–5)**.

The combined effects of buoyancy and hydrostatic pressure can be helpful when a patient is practicing standing balance. The pressure provides support equally around the body, and if the patient should fall a little off the vertical when immersed while standing, buoyancy can help in regaining the vertical position **(Fig. 26–6)**.

When explaining differences in the effect of water on a stationary body versus a moving one, Kolb's differentiation of hydrostatic and hydrodynamic pressure is useful. Kolb categorizes both buoyancy and the equal pressure that still water exerts on a static object as **hydrostatic pressures** and categorizes the pressures caused by movement of either the object or the water as **hydrodynamic pressures**.[21]

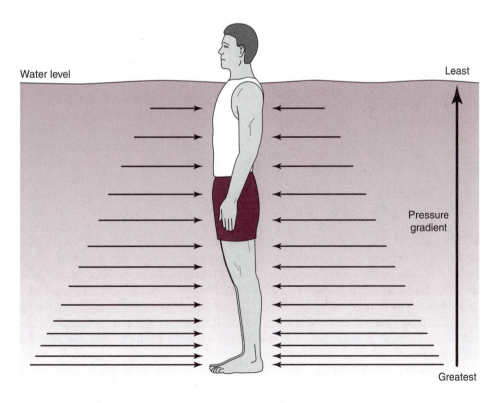

FIGURE 26–5 The effects of hydrostatic pressure when a patient is standing in water. Density increases with depth increasing the pressure

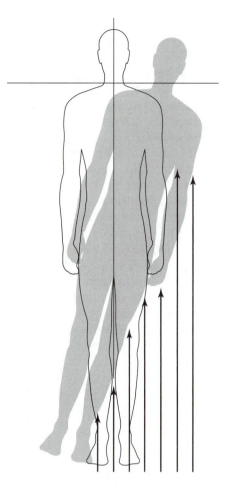

FIGURE 26–6   Temporary displacement of a vertical body. Buoyancy assists recovery.

When walking in water, an individual will encounter the pressures inherent in the fluid. To move the water in the path as the body moves forward requires pushing against the pressure that the water is exerting. The faster the individual walks, the more resistance is encountered and the more demands are made on the walking muscles. Conversely, in the "wake" of a body moving in water (ie, immediately behind), there is much less pressure. If a patient is extremely weak, the therapist might walk in front of the patient. The patient who is close behind, in the therapist's wake, will not encounter as much pressure. Baby ducks swimming in line behind their mother exemplify this phenomenon.

Other Properties.   Other properties of water to be considered in relation to hydrotherapy exercises are

(1) surface tension, (2) cohesion, (3) adhesion, and (4) turbulence.

Surface tension: Water molecules on the surface have a greater tendency to hold together; thus, resistance is slightly greater on the surface. Any driver who does a belly flop experiences that tension. Therapeutically, this increased resistance is usually insignificant, but if someone is extremely weak, horizontal movements may be performed more easily in the water just beneath the surface rather than at the surface.

Cohesion: This is the tendency of water molecules to adhere to each other. The greater the cohesion, the greater the viscosity. This cohesion contributes to the resistance encountered while moving through water because some force is required to separate the water molecules.

Adhesion: This is the tendency of water molecules to adhere to molecules of other substances. This property is observed daily. Water drops cling to the body or to the sides of a glass. A damp sponge cleans dirt off a surface better than a dry sponge. It is this adhesion to the sides of therapeutic tanks that requires that they be wiped dry after cleaning. This property of water has no significant influence on movements in water. However, it is a factor when doing volumetric measuring because water drops adhering to the sides of a container are not measured in overflow volume.[22]

Turbulence: Webster's defines a turbulent fluid flow as one in which "the velocity at a given point varies erratically in magnitude and direction." This movement is in contrast to a smooth "streamline" flow, in which the direction is unchanged.

The movement of objects in water can cause the water to move in circular patterns, creating small whirlpools or eddy currents—turbulence. Moving a body segment through water creates some turbulence. Obviously, a body encounters greater resistance moving through turbulent water or against the current than through calm water or with the current. The faster the movement, the greater the turbulence, which puts more demand on muscles. Skinner and Thomson[7] stated that "the quicker the movement, the greater the turbulence and therefore an exercise may be progressed by increasing the speed at which it is taken."

Many studies have been carried out to determine the effects of static immersion or exercise in water. Johnson et al[11] compared identical upper- and lower-extremity exercises performed by healthy young adults on land and in water, and found that both heart rate and oxygen consumption were greater when exercises were performed in water. These investigators suggested that "the metabolic requirement of exercise performed in water is greater than when the same exercise is done on land," and they note that the cardiac recovery cost was reduced.[11] More recently, Kirby et al[23] studied the oxygen consumption of healthy young adults who were exercising while immersed in a pool heated to 96.8°F (36°C), with a pool area temperature of 77°F (25°C) and a relative humidity of 53%. It is interesting that they found no significant difference in oxygen consumption when a subject sat quietly in the pool, neck high in water, than when resting on land. Exercise ranging from light (walking in the pool) to heavy (running in place) produced proportional increases in oxygen consumption and a gradual increase in aerobic demands. Kirby et al concluded that the higher-intensity exercise appeared to "be within range that is likely to induce aerobic training"—that such exercises might be beneficial for some patients. However, they warned that the exercises should be used with caution because they could "represent a risk to patients with unstable cardiac disease."

It should be noted that few published studies can be found that compare the benefits of aquatic and land therapeutic exercise. A 1990 unpublished study[24] did compare the effects of an exercise program on land versus water on subjects with arthritic knees. The results showed a *significantly greater increase* in knee joint range of motion (ROM) and *decrease* in perception of pain for the aquatic group vis-à-vis the land group. Although the study was well executed, the population was small; a duplication of the study with more subjects would be useful. A study in 1997[66] demonstrated improved isometric strength and ROM in the joints of individuals with osteoarthritis. This study was based on intervention included with the Arthritis Foundation Aquatic Program.

More recent studies[67,68] have compared the physiologic effects of exercise in the water versus on land. In the study by Cassady and Neilsen,[67] cardiovascular responses to similar exercises in water and on land were analyzed. A subsequent study by Butler[68] compared the response of the vastus medialis muscle during a single leg squat on land and in water at various depths. This information may prove helpful when rehabilitating patients with various orthopedic conditions, including osteoarthritis (OA), rheumatoid arthritis (RA), and postsurgery.

Peripheral Circulation and Edema

Heat is indicated to hasten healing through increased metabolism and increased blood flow to an area. However, heat applications may cause edema or venous pooling (see **Chapters 3 and 5, Table 5–1**). The rationale for the use of compression to reduce edema and to increase venous return is cited in **Chapters 5 and 25.** When a body part is immersed, the tissues are compressed by the hydrostatic pressure of the surrounding water.

If the distal part of an extremity is lowest in the water, the pressure gradient between the surface and deeper water favors reduced accumulation of fluid in distal parts. Although fluid accumulation is common in distal parts while "dangling" extremities out of water, in water the effect of gravity is counteracted by the effect of buoyancy.[20,25] On the basis of the effects of water pressure, full body (head out) immersion is recommended as a treatment for "diuretic-resistant" edema in patients with cirrhosis and nephrosis.[26,27] It might also be assumed that, in water relative to out of water, the probability of edema or venous pooling at any given temperature is also diminished. Studies of head-out immersion in thermoneutral water at 95°F (35°C) indicate that there is an increase in venous return from the periphery to the central body and a shift of fluid from the interstitial space to the capillaries. These changes have been attributed to the hydrostatic pressure.[28,29]

Traditionally in physical therapy, whirlpool treatments are used for problems involving the extremities, both for their thermal effects and for hydro exercise. However, the effect of whirlpool treatments on edema is debatable. Magness et al,[30] using as subjects both healthy adults and patients with rheumatoid arthritis, lymphedema, and hemiplegia, showed that when an upper extremity was passively immersed in water at various temperatures 92–112°F (33.3–44.4°C), edema in both the healthy and the patient populations did increase; the increase was proportional to the increase in water temperature. The authors suggest that the heat produced the edema and that if the extremity had been active while immersed, the effect might have been ameliorated.

Walsh's[31] reports of studies yet unpublished indicate that swelling occurs with or without exercise in water. The temperatures of the water used in these studies were about 98.6°F (37.6°C) and 104°F (40°C).

The meager evidence available suggests that the effect of heat may be confused with that of immersion. Yet one should not necessarily throw out the bathwater with the baby (the heat). Exercise in thermoneutral water and utilization of hydrostatic pressure may be inoilated in conditions in which edema is of great concern. Research is needed to determine the effect on edema of water at such temperatures. In other conditions, the use of hydrotherapy for heat as well as other benefits should be continued until more conclusive evidence is available.

Skin Problems and Open Wounds

The fluidity properties of water make it a useful substance for treating skin problems and open wounds. *Fluidity* means the rate of flow of a substance. For example, catsup is not as fluid as water. Every liquid has a certain viscosity (ie, a certain amount of friction between the molecules of that substance that causes resistance). The amount of resistance determines the rate of flow of that liquid, its fluidity. The fluidity of water enables it to get into all crevices quickly and thus reach all skin and surface openings regardless of position or shape. The cleansing effect of water, sometimes referred to as the **lavage effect,** is the result of this fluidity. Water is useful in therapy for lubricating dry areas, for removing dressings painlessly, and for debridement of dead tissues from ulcers or burns or after cast removal. Pulsed lavage is increasingly being employed for wound debridement as described in a study by Luedtke-Hoffmann and Shafer[72] (see later section of this chapter on pulsed lavage).

Because many chemicals can dissolve in water, a topical medication in solution with water or lubricating oils can be transported to any or all surface areas. Oils, of course, float on top of the water.

When an external force causes water to move more rapidly, the water can exert greater pressure on the body. The massage showerhead currently sold commercially exemplifies this tendency. In therapy, whirlpool agitators with the force directed toward the body are used to create a massage effect, enhance the lavage cleansing effect, or assist in removing dressings and dead tissues. In cases in which only a slight increase in pressure is required and the amount of pressure must be well controlled, a dental water irrigating device may be used. A study of normal adults comparing 20–30 min soaks, agitation, and brief sprays showed that agitation followed by spraying was "significantly better than any single technique in removing bacteria."[32]

Psychological Effects

Most healthy people feel invigorated after taking a bath or shower and enjoy some relief from daily anxieties. Changes in patients' attitudes, the improvements observed during treatments, and patients' reports of feeling good after a tank or pool treatment may be the result of the psychological effects of immersion in water as much as or more than the physiologic effects.

Psychology offers various reasons for these emotional and behavioral changes. People often identify bathing with a leisure-time activity. This identification encourages relaxation. In water, a person can be surrounded by a neutral-to-warm environment that is also physically supportive because of the buoyancy and pressure properties of water. Receiving this external comfort and support can be emotionally supportive and can help relieve anxiety.

In psychiatric settings, with the increased use of pharmacotherapies and psychotherapies, the use of physical therapies has declined considerably.[33] However, hydrotherapy treatments are still being used in selected cases to alleviate the symptoms of neurotic and psychotic patients.[34] It is natural for a patient with a physical problem to have accompanying psychological problems. Although the hydrotherapy treatment is given for physically beneficial reasons, psychological problems may be relieved as well.[35]

In this section we have attempted to acquaint the reader with various factors that make hydrotherapy an important physical therapy modality. However, despite the popularity of this modality and the belief in its usefulness, reports of its effects in a disabled population are meager. Most hydrotherapy study populations are made up of healthy young adults. Few studies that compared the effectiveness of water immersion with that of other modalities could be found in the recent literature. Whether physiologic effects of hydrotherapy are the result of the thermal or the other properties of water needs more investigation.

Hydrotherapy does have certain advantages over other modalities; for example, water is readily available and easy to use. Although hydrotherapy treatment may appear to be relatively inexpensive, this is not necessarily true. The cost of buying, maintaining, and cleaning hydrotherapy equipment such as whirlpools and Hubbard tanks, not to mention the municipal charges for water and the energy to heat it, may make these treatments expensive. This cost is ultimately absorbed by patients. For cost reasons, such treatments should not be given capriciously, but neither should they be avoided when they are the treatment of choice. If the therapist prefers holistic interventions, tank or pool treatments are frequently the optimal ones available because both the mind and the body may benefit.

WATER IMMERSION MODALITIES
Whirlpool and Hubbard Tanks

The two most common modalities used in clinics for immersion in water are whirlpool tanks and **Hubbard tanks;** the two share much in common. Their common features are discussed first, and then specific information pertaining to each is provided.

Both types of tank can be used in hot or cold thermal modalities, and both transfer heat primarily by convection. Both utilize the properties of water for the therapeutic purposes shown in **Table 26–1.**

Equipment. Both whirlpool tanks and Hubbard tanks are made of stainless steel or plastic, which can be easily cleaned. If cared for properly, these tanks will last for decades. The water is supplied by plumbing similar to that for a bathtub. The tanks include the following:

- Hot water and cold water mixing valves
- A temperature gauge that indicates the temperature of the water flowing into the tank
- A water thermometer attached to the inside of the tank to indicate tank water temperature
- An agitator (a turbine ejector aerator)
- A seat (or stretcher in a Hubbard tank)
- A gravity drain

The agitator in the tank mixes the water so that all water in the tank has approximately the same temperature. Agitators are designed so that they can be raised, lowered, and pivoted to direct their force at various levels and angles. Some agitators are movable; they are attached to a rail on the outside of the tank and the top edge, and can slide to any position along the tank. The agitator forces air through openings that *must be immersed* in the water; this force increases the rate of water flow. The amount of force produced by the agitator can be varied manually by ejector controls located out of the water. If the force is trained directly toward one part of the body, it can have a stimulating effect, which is sometimes called a micromassage effect. Patients with low-back pain, for example, often enjoy the agitation force directed toward the painful area. This added force and the increased water flow can also assist in both removal of dressings and debridement.

Precautions Regarding Agitators. Although the agitator has no exposed moving parts that might injure the patient, care must be taken not to allow a finger, toe, or loose bandage to plug agitator openings. Because the agitator is motorized, attached to an electric source, and used in water, great care must be taken that there are no breaks in the wiring or insulation. Even a minor problem in any part of the electrical mechanism can cause serious electric shock, or even electrocution.[36] The motor must be securely fastened outside of the tanks. **All personnel must be aware that if a live motor of any sort falls into water, anyone in that water can be electrocuted.**[31] This equipment must contain hospital-grade plugs, and the receptacles must be fail-safe hospital grade. All equipment must be provided with ground fault interrupters, (GFI). All hydro equipment must be checked for current leakage at least every 6 months. **Never allow the person in the water to switch the agitator off or on.**

Additives. Opinions vary concerning the need for solutions added to the water. Although solutions were commonly used in the past, current literature recommends no additives unless they are absolutely required for bactericidal properties.[37] Chemical additives are known to be cytotoxic, which cause delay in the formation of granulation tissue and epithelialization. Clinical decision making on the use of chemical additives must balance the importance of bactericidal properties with the delay in healing time. If solutions are used, recommended concentrations are included in the manufacturer's label on the container. Providone-iodine,[38] saline solutions, or bactericidal agents—including sodium hypochlorite (household bleach)—can be added for the treatment of open wounds, but toxic levels must be avoided. Richard[39] provides much information to guide the therapist when using these additives. McGuckin et al[40] reported an outbreak of wound infections caused by *Pseudomonas aeruginosa* that coincided with the discontinuance of the use of sodium hypochlorite (Clorox®) in Hubbard tank treatments and ceased when the use of the disinfectant resumed. Steve et al[41] studied the effects of chloramine-t with burn patients and showed that this additive was effective relative to its concentration: 200 ppm was far more effective than 100 ppm. For patients with dry skin (eg, after cast removal) or for those receiving many water treatments, bath oil can be added. A 4% solution of lidocaine has been suggested to reduce pain during debridement.[42] Adding a scented, colored water softener or foaming solution can be a pleasant bonus for the patient. Care must be taken to ensure that patients have no allergic reactions to any solutions used.

General Considerations

The common clinical applications and rationale for hydrotherapy are listed in Box 26–1.

The contraindications for hydrotherapy are similar to the contraindications associated with the use of other superficial thermal modalities presented in Chapters 13 and 14. Box 26–2 summarizes the contraindications for localized and full immersion hydrotherapy interventions.

Preparation of Tanks.   Tanks must be thoroughly clean before water is added. Cleaning procedures are discussed later in this section. Tanks should be filled and ready for patients just before the time of treatment. Although there is much heat in the volume of water contained in these tanks, the water will cool down. Thus, the temperature should be checked at the time of treatment to ensure that it is correct. Allow 10–15 min for complete filling of the tanks.

Indications and Contraindications.   The effects of the properties of water on an immersed body or body part have been discussed earlier in this section. **Tables 26–3 and 26–4** list common indications and relative contraindications for hydrotherapy as related to the effects of the properties of water. Physical therapists must always be alert to factors that contraindicate hydrotherapy for patients who otherwise might benefit from this modality (eg, in cases in which there is a danger of cross-contamination or cases in which hydration might exacerbate a skin condition.[43]

Precautions.   Any part of the body that is immersed in water loses its means of heat escape; the heat cannot radiate from that part of the body, and the sweat cannot evaporate. When a substantial part of the body is in very warm water, the body temperature may increase, and systemic mechanisms that increase heat loss, heart rate, blood pressure, and respiration may change greatly in an effort to maintain thermal homeostasis. **Vital signs must be monitored.** The patient's oral temperature should be monitored whenever the water temperature is higher than 100°F (37.8°C). Patients may faint or experience heat distress. Therefore, **the patient must never be left alone during or after a hydrotherapy treatment.**

Box 26–1 *Indications and Rationale for Hydrotherapy*

Indication	Rationale
Wound debridement	Mechanical agitation of water to assist in removing necrotic tissue
Pain and associated muscle spasm	Increased thermal and mechanical sensory input
	Increased blood flow to wash out inflammatory chemicals associated with pain and muscle spasm
	Cold immersion to decrease nerve conduction velocity and muscle spindle afferent activity
Individuals with generalized weakness	Buoyancy to eliminate the effects of gravity and to allow individuals with weakness in their antigravity muscles to ambulate and perform therapeutic exercise during a full body immersion
Subacute and chronic inflammation	Increased blood flow and cellular activity to assist in the inflammatory and healing process following injury or overuse (use low temperatures directly after trauma and increased temperatures following the acute inflammatory response)
Individuals with inability to bear weight through lower extremity joints and spine (ie, arthritis, postoperative restrictions)	Buoyancy to eliminate the effects of gravity and to allow individuals to ambulate and exercise with less trauma and compression through the spine and lower extremities during a full body immersion

Box 26–2 *Contraindications for Hydrotherapy*

Contraindication	Rationale
Severe hypertension or hypotension	Hot or cold full body immersions may exacerbate blood pressure problems.
Fever	Hot full body immersions may further increase core temperature.
Patients with significant cardiac and pulmonary dysfunction	Tolerance for full body immersion or extreme temperatures may be poor.
Patients with hypersensitivity to thermal stimuli	If not using neutral temperatures, may cause an adverse reaction to thermal stimuli (ie, cold uticaria).
Bowel and bladder incontinence	Prevent contamination in a therapeutic pool being used by others.
Poor peripheral circulation	If not using neutral temperatures, may cause tissue damage due to inability to shunt blood to the intervention area.
Impaired mentation and/or fear of water	Tolerance and feedback from the patient may be limited.
Thrombophlebitis	Thermal and mechanical stimuli may cause a thrombus to be dislodged.
Skin and lymphatic cancer (safety in the presence of cancer has not been determined)	Thermal and mechanical stimuli may increase tissue metabolism.

Opinions vary concerning the amount of activity and the temperature of water that will maintain normal core temperature. Houdas and Ring[1] reported that if a healthy adult is resting immersed in water at a temperature of approximately 91°F (33°C), thermal neutrality is maintained; that is, the vasomotor activity will maintain stable core temperature. If the person is exercising strenuously, at three times the resting metabolic rate, a water temperature as low as 79°F (26°C) will maintain thermal neutrality. McArdle et al,[15] also referring to healthy adults, reported that the optimal water temperature for swimming is 82–86°F (27.8–30°C). This temperature-activity information may serve as a guideline for treating orthopedic patients who are otherwise healthy. However, temperature ranges must be modified for more seriously debilitated people.

Bierman and Licht[44] reported 3°F (1.7°C) core temperature elevation when subjects stood in 104°F (40°C) water for 10 min. It is interesting that the study reported by Kirby et al[23] found no significant change in oral temperature while the subjects were immersed in 96.8°F (36°C) water, regardless of the intensity of their activity. However, the duration of immersion was not reported.

Frequently, patients are apprehensive about hydrotherapy tank treatments and the difficulty of getting into the tanks, especially if lifts are required for safe transfers. Being transported on the lifts can be frightening. Therapists must realize this possibility,

reassure the patient, and handle all aspects of the treatment with skill to gain the patient's confidence.

Before the treatment, the therapist must check patients' records for any problems that would contraindicate an immersion hydrotherapy and use the records as a guide regarding how closely the patients' vital signs must be monitored. When patients come out of the water, they may be chilled. Therefore, they should be dried immediately and covered with cotton blankets or towels to keep warm until they become adjusted to the air temperature.

Whirlpool Interventions

Whirlpool tanks are available in various sizes, from a size just large enough for a hand or foot to a size large enough for an adult to be seated comfortably (**Fig. 26–7**). Lo-Boy®, which is similar to a bathtub, allow the legs to be extended in a horizontal position. A common size found in clinics is large enough to immerse an entire extremity and allow free movements of the joints of arms or ankles and feet. However, it is difficult to immerse a shoulder joint comfortably. Larger tanks can be equipped with a seat so that an adult can sit with much of the body immersed in the water. A seat, usually made of stainless steel or plastic, can be adjusted to various depths in the water and can easily be removed when not needed (**Fig. 26–8A**).

A high chair is often placed outside the tank. This placement enables patients to sit outside the tank and

TABLE 26–3   *General Indications for Warm and Hot Immersion Therapy*

Indication	Therapeutic Effect	Property of Water
Subacute and chronic soft tissue injuries such as joint strains, sprains, or low-back problems	Decreases swelling (edema)	Pressure
	Hastens healing	Thermal
	Decreases pain/spasms	Thermal
	Increases range of motion	Buoyancy and thermal
	Increases strength	Buoyancy and pressures as resistance
Shortened tissues contractures, scars	Causes relaxation	Thermal and psychological
	Increases extensibility of nonelastic tissues	Thermal
	Softens scar tissue	Fluidity and thermal
	Assists active motion	Buoyancy
Arthritis: osteo and subacute, chronic rheumatoid	Increases joint mobility	
	Decreases pain	Thermal and buoyancy
	Increases range of motion	
Postfractures	Removes dry scaly skin	Fluidity and pressure
	Increases range of motion	Thermal and buoyancy
	Increases strength	Antibuoyancy pressure
Open wounds, burns, decubitii	Cleanses debrides, Increases circulation	Fluidity and pressure
Partially healed wounds or burns	Softens scar tissue Prevents contractures	Thermal and buoyancy
Muscle spasms	Increases circulation	Fluidily (turbulence forced pressure)
	Decreases pain	Thermal
Muscle weakness caused by central or peripheral nervous system involvement or by disuse	Increases range of motion Increases strength	Buoyancy and antibuoyancy pressure
Tension, anxiety, or other emotional or psychological problems	Relieves symptoms	Thermal and hydrostatic pressure

immerse much of their lower extremity in the water. The chair also can be used to facilitate lowering patients into a sitting tank. They first sit on the locked chair outside the tank, place their legs in the tank, and then lower themselves onto the tank seat. Many patients need one or two people to help them with this transfer **(Fig. 26–8B).**

Hard rubber handgrips, similar to those used on crutches, are usually placed on either side of the tank rim. These can be used to improve the patients' grip while they lower themselves into the tank, or they can be positioned to reduce pressure on vessels and nerves in popliteal or axillary areas if these areas are pressing on the rim of the tank. Motorized lifts are available

and are especially useful for transferring patients into a Lo-Boy® **(Fig. 26–8C).**

Dosage.

Water Temperature.   Depending on the size of the body area immersed and the patient's physical status, an effective hot or very hot whirlpool may range from 103° to 105°F (40–42°C).[43,44] If the patient is sitting waist or chest high in water, the temperature should be at the lower end of the range to avoid great increases in core temperature. If only one extremity is immersed, the upper range can be used, provided that the patient is otherwise healthy. The temperature should never be so high that the patient is uncomfort-

TABLE 26–4   *General Contraindications for Immersion Hydrotherapy**

Contraindication	Rationale
Cardiac dysfunctions	Heart cannot adapt to changes needed for thermal homeostasis adjustment.
Respiratory dysfunctions	Inability to resist hydrostatic pressure, tolerate heat, or both.
Decreased thermal sensation	Inability to report overheating or overcooling. Avoid hot or cold water; recommend cool through warm range (approx. 80°F–98°F) (26.7°–36.7°C)
Severe peripheral vascular disease (diabetes, arterial sclerosis)[†]	Contraindication for heat.
Danger of bleeding or hemorrhage*	Contraindication for heat.
Acute rheumatoid arthritis[‡]	Contraindication for heat.
Surface infections (including all fungus infections)[†]	Infection may spread to other areas or cross-contaminate via water.
Uncontrolled bowels (if pelvic area is in water)	Contamination is avoided.
Some dermatological conditions (atopic eczema; Senile or winterpruritus and ichthyosis)	Skin hydration may exacerbate some dermatologic conditions. Water removes natural skin moisture.

*These contraindications are relative to the intensity of the heat and the amount of body immersed.
[†]Avoid water temperatures higher than about 95°F.
[‡]Always and a bactericidal agent to the water.

able, and the therapist must be alert to changes in vital signs and observable signs of distress.

Duration of Intervention.   The usual duration of an effective intervention is approximately 20 min. If ROM or therapeutic exercises are also done in the tank, the time may be extended.[45]

Intervention Procedures.

1. Remove the patient's clothes from the area to be treated.
2. Inspect the skin for conditions that may invite cross-contamination or may be exacerbated by moisture.
3. Test for thermal sensitivity.
4. Drape the patient properly. Use towels to protect clothes on other areas of the body from getting wet.
5. Help the patient immerse his or her body or body parts, having a second person help if necessary.
6. Place a towel roll over the hand grip under the axilla or knee to avoid pressure on nerves or blood vessels if only the extremity is immersed and the patient leans against the edge of the tank.
7. Advise the patient against getting fingers or toes near the opening in the agitators and against turning agitators off or on.
8. Loosen the bolts, and rotate and adjust the height of the agitator to the desired position. Tighten the bolts securely. Be careful that the agitator does not rise quickly (buoyancy) and hit you in the face while adjusting. Do *not* adjust the agitator while the motor is on.
9. Turn on the agitator.
10. Reassure and remind the patient that someone will always be in the area.
11. Monitor vital signs as necessary.

Note: If the patient is to sit in the water, advise the patient to urinate before beginning the intervention.

Postintervention Procedures.

1. Remove the body part from water.
2. Dry thoroughly.

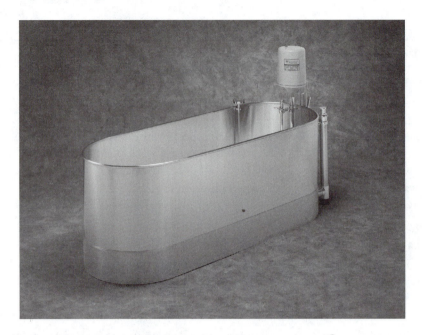

FIGURE 26–7   A "sit in" sized whirlpool tank or Lo-Boy®. (*Reproduced with permission from Whitehall Electro Medical Co., Inc. Hackensack, NJ.*)

3. Check skin condition, and check for unusual changes in vital signs.
4. Avoid chilling by keeping the body covered or wrapped.
5. Assist the patient in dressing if necessary.

Frequently, the whirlpool intervention is followed immediately by ultrasound (underwater method) while the patient is still in the tank. Berger[46] stressed the importance of therapists' wearing rubber gloves during these interventions. He advised **that all equipment should be plugged in to ground fault interrupters.** Obviously, the agitator should be off not only for safety but also for preventing ultrasound from diverging flow.

Hubbard Tank Interventions

The Hubbard tank, named after the engineer who designed it, is a large tank with a shape that resembles a keyhole. These tanks are available in various sizes. Generally, the tank is approximately 8 feet long. The width is approximately 6 feet near one end, which enables a supine person to fully abduct the arms, and is approximately 4 feet wide near the other end, which allow the legs to abduct. At midside, the width narrows to 36 inches, enabling the therapist to get closer to the patient than is possible with a rectangular-shaped tank. The tank is deep enough to allow full-body immersion while sitting or lying on a stretcher **(Fig. 26–9).**

Indications and Contraindications.   Hubbard tanks are usually used for wound care, ROM, and therapeutic exercise, for people who need full-body interventions for conditions also including arthritis or multiple burns. The tanks are also useful for those who should remain in a lying position (eg, patients who have spinal cord injuries; patients who have had hip surgery or fractures; or patients with back, shoulder, or neck problems that warrant hydrotherapy.

The contraindications to Hubbard tank interventions are listed in **Table 26–4.** Special considerations should be given regarding patients with severe cardiac or respiratory problems because they may be unable to adjust to any excessive external pressure caused by the water or to temperatures that may strain the cardiorespiratory systems, patients with loose bowels, and pregnant women in the first trimester if the heat is sufficient to raise the core temperature greater than 102°F (38.9°C) for 20 min because this temperature may be harmful to the fetus.[47] Exposure in the first trimester of pregnancy to heat in the form of hot tub, sauna, or fever has been shown to be associated with an increased risk of neural tube defects such as spina

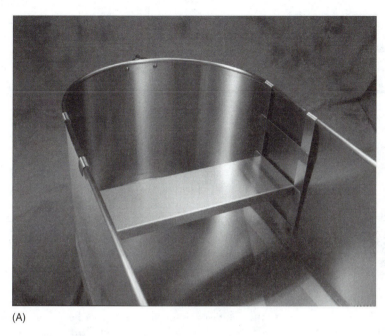

(A)

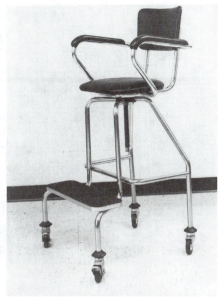

(B)

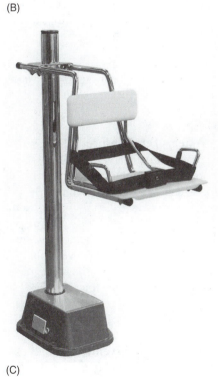

(C)

FIGURE 26–8   Accessories for a hydrotherapy tank. (**A**) An adjustable seat. (**B**) A mobile adjustable-height hydrochair. (**C**) A motorized chair lift. (A *Reproduced with permission from Whitehall Electro Medical Co., Inc. Hackensack, NJ.*) (B and C *Reproduced with permission from Ferno ILLE, Williamsport, PA, a division of Ferno-Washington, Inc., Wilmington, OH.*)

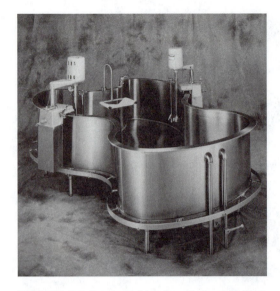

FIGURE 26–9   A Hubbard tank for full body immersions. (*Reproduced with permission from Whitehall Electro Medical Co., Inc. Hackensack, NJ.*)

bifida. The hot tub appeared to have the strongest effect of any single heat exposure.[48]

Dosage.

Water Temperature. The water temperature range is 90°–102°F (32.2°–38.8°C). Frequently, the temperature of water used in clinics is about 97–100°F (36.1–38.8°C). This temperature may be pleasurable and have a sedative effect, but realize that most of the body is immersed in this heat. Whenever ambient temperature is in this range, vital signs, including the core temperature, will change over time. Thus, temperatures in the lower part of the range may be required for patients who cannot tolerate these changes—those with cardiac or respiratory problems or preexisting fevers, or those who will be exercising in the water.

Duration of Intervention. The usual duration is 20 min.[45] If other interventions will be done while in the tank, the time can be extended to 30 min.

Procedures. Patients should wear a bathing suit or light-textured clothing that will not feel uncomfortable when wet and that can be removed easily. Hospital gowns or proper draping are acceptable. Disposable paper swim clothes manufactured especially for these interventions are available commercially. Some patients like to wear a cap to keep their hair dry. Patients should be advised to urinate before beginning intervention.

The following steps should be carried out during the intervention:

1. Position the patient, usually supine, on a stretcher designed specifically for use in water.
2. Secure the patient to the stretcher with straps to keep any body parts from floating off the stretcher **(Fig. 26–10).**
3. Secure an air-filled pillow or towel roll to the stretcher, and place it under the patient's head.
4. Position extremely weak or debilitated patients on the stretcher outside the tank, and use a motorized or hydraulic lift to suspend the stretcher, which then rotates or slides on a track to transport the patient over the tank. Then lower the stretcher into the tank. To ensure safety with these transfers, two people should assist the patient. The stretcher must be steadied, and the head must not be allowed to drop during transfer.
5. Lower the stretcher just to the water line so that the patient can become accustomed to the feeling of the water before being completely immersed.
6. Secure the head of the stretcher to the hooks in the tank so that the patient's head is elevated appropriately.
7. Immerse the patient to the depth necessary, keeping the head elevated.
8. Fasten the stretcher securely.
9. Place agitators in the appropriate positions, and turn them on.
10. **During intervention, monitor the patient's vital signs, and do not leave the patient unattended.**

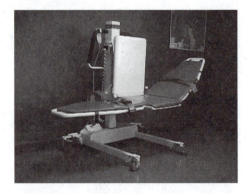

FIGURE 26–10 An electric lift and stretcher for Hubbard tank intervention. (*Reproduced with permission from Whitehall Electro Medical Co., Inc. Hackensack, NJ.*)

As a responsible physical therapist, ensure that motorized equipment (agitators and lifts) are maintained in good working order and are checked periodically for both electrical and mechanical safety.

Postintervention Procedures.   As soon as the intervention is completed, proceed as follows:

1. Lift the patient and stretcher to just above the water line, and cover the patient immediately with cotton blankets or dry towels. Let the stretcher drip water into the tank before moving it over dry floor.

2. Remove the patient's wet clothes, and dry the patient thoroughly, always keeping the patient covered for modesty and warmth.

3. Return the stretcher to an adjacent area, and lower it onto a table or plinth.

4. Help the patient dress, always making certain that the patient is not chilled.

Pulsed Lavage.   Pulsed lavage is an intervention that uses an electrical device to administer saline or water under low pressure to irrigate and debride a wound.[37] An early example of this intervention was the use of Water Pik® (Teledyne Water Pik, Fort Collins, Colorado). The handheld unit can be used in any clinical setting or even in the patient's home. The pressure setting is typically between 4 and 15 pounds per square inch, and the saline is connected to the unit via standard IV tubing. Most pulsed lavage units have negative pressure that facilitates removal of the saline and pathogens from the irrigation site.[49,50] The size of the single-use application head is interchangeable depending upon the area designated for intervention.

Pulsed lavage is indicated for most cases of venous or arterial insufficiency and many other wounds.[37] The pressure component allows debridement of shallow tunneled areas or other invaginations that are difficult to cleanse. Its mechanical properties coupled with mild negative pressure can enhance debridement and wound healing, and therefore pulsed lavage is indicated for all stages of wound healing.[50–52] Clinical research, minimal with this modality, has supported its use as an appropriate wound care intervention.[49,52]

Contraindications and precautions include close proximity to healthy structures that could be damaged by pressure application of saline and/or negative pressure.[37] This includes patients with recent skin grafts, exposed nerve or blood vessels, or surgical repairs, or those who should not receive any intervention in which water pressure (agitation) is potentially injurious.

Application of this intervention follows standard precautions used in wound care. Proper sterile technique, draping, and therapist and patient protection from splashing fluids are essential. Setup includes collection of fluid if negative pressure is not being used. Facility policy and procedures must be followed throughout the intervention and wound dressing afterward. Manufacturer instructions for each lavage unit must be reviewed by all staff members before using the equipment.

In comparison with whirlpool, pulsed lavage is easily transportable, can treat small wounds on almost any body part, is more cost-effective, and has a lower chance of cross-contamination.[37] However, it cannot be used with large wounds, many components are single-use items, and it can be messy to administer.

Walking Tanks.   Hubbard tanks may have an additional "walking trough," which is approximately 32 inches deep, below the floor of the regular tank. (It may be countersunk into the floor.) In some models, the center floor of the basic tank acts as a cover for the trough that can be lifted out when the trough is needed. When the trough is not needed, the cover keeps the trough area dry **(Fig. 26–11).**

Walking tank interventions are indicated for any patients who require non-weight-bearing standing or ambulation activities (eg, during early recovery from some injuries of the lower extremity or surgical procedures) and for neurologic patients who require practice in sitting or standing balance or ambulation.

The trough is equipped with parallel bars and a chair or stool at each end. Patients can practice walking and all forms of hydrotherapeutic exercises in the water. The water level can be altered to meet each patient's needs; for example, it can be shoulder high for non-weight-bearing standing or ambulation and can be lowered gradually as the patient is able to bear more weight.

Some patients need to be transferred into the water by a sling halter or a chair lift. As with stretcher transfers, two people are needed for this transfer. For safety and for reducing the patient's anxiety, the therapist should be in the water before the patient and be ready to assist as the patient is lowered into the water.

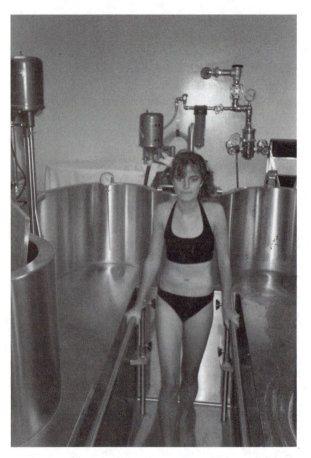

FIGURE 26–11 A Hubbard tank with a walking trough.

Cleaning and Maintenance of Tanks

It is important to keep all hydrotherapy equipment clean and in good condition. In each clinical setting, the procedures used are recorded and must always be followed. In hospital facilities, any laxity in the care and cleaning of equipment may lead to the department's failure to pass the periodic inspections of the American Hospital Association and the American Medical Association, as well as endangering the patient or damaging equipment.

All physical therapists, physical therapy assistants, and aides should be capable of cleaning tanks thoroughly and efficiently. Although hydrotherapy aides usually clean the tanks, the therapist is responsible for the proper instruction of the aides and for strict adherence to the cleaning protocol.

Cleaning procedures may vary to some extent in each setting, but they are basically the same. The procedures presented here were taken from those used in three large rehabilitation centers, although each center's protocol had slight variations.

Equipment. The equipment required includes disinfectant solutions, protective gloves, brushes with handles that enable all crevices to be scrubbed, buckets, many clean dry towels, and a water hose. Special hoses are available that can select and spray either the disinfectant or clean water, making this task much easier. In some clinics, disposable plastic liners are used for all patients. Cleaning is still required, but it takes less time.

At present, there is no conclusive evidence to recommend any one disinfectant.[43] Studies and reported observations suggest that sodium hypochlorite (5.25%) as contained in household laundry bleach is an effective and inexpensive disinfectant.[40,43] However, Turner et al[53] pointed out that, over time, chlorine corrodes the surface of stainless steel tanks. Their investigation showed that manual scrubbing with a standard germicidal detergent was effective in reducing bacterial contamination except for drains and bottoms of tanks, which could not be adequately scrubbed.

Procedures. Tanks must be cleaned before and after each patient. They also must be cleaned before water cultures are taken. **Everyone must be careful not to splash the disinfectant solution on anyone's skin. Should this problem occur, rinse the area immediately and thoroughly with cool water.**

The procedure for cleaning the tanks is as follows:

1. Put on protective gloves.
2. Drain all the used water completely.
3. Rinse the entire tank and all equipment used for interventions, being sure that all openings in agitators and all drains are included.
4. Wipe out thoroughly all surfaces that touched the water, using a clean towel. (Some clinics put alcohol on the towel.)
5. Spray and wash the entire inside of the tank, including the drains, and the outside of the agitators with lukewarm (not hot) water and the disinfectant delivered through the special hose attached to the tank. The disinfectant is delivered through the hose by depressing the small lever under the nozzle head. Release it to stop the flow of the disinfectant. If this hose is not available, mix the disinfectant with water in a bucket, and pour it on all surfaces, and then rinse with water

using a regular hose. Follow each manufacturer's directions regarding the percentage of disinfectant and water in the bucket. Be sure that the solution reaches all parts of any equipment, agitators, and water thermometers that were in the water during the intervention. Usually, disinfectant is left on approximately 1 min.

6. Lower the agitators into the disinfectant solution in the bucket, being sure that all openings are in the solution. Turn on the motors for approximately 20 seconds. Turn off the motors. Remove the agitator from the bucket.

7. Rinse the entire tank with water delivered through the hose until all residue is drained. Include all equipment in this rinse.

8. Rinse a final time with water at approximately 115°F to hasten drying.

9. Post a READY sign on the tank.

10. Wipe both the inside and the outside dry after the final use for the day. Be sure that clean towels are used for the inside.

11. Clean the outside of the tank once a week with a stainless steel cleanser, usually a cream or powder. Remove any mineral deposits or discoloration from the inside of the tank with chlorine cleanser.

Some tanks are designed to reduce contamination by eliminating the crevices at the intersection between the floor and the walls. The interior surface is curved and seamless, resembling the design of most bathtubs.

Procedures for isolation patients   Isolation patients include those with burns or other acute infectious lesions, surface ulcers, pressure ulcers, and AIDS-related eruptions. For these patients, tank interventions are useful for cleansing the wounds, changing dressings, applying medication in solution, and debriding dead tissues. Therapists should not intervene with such patients unless they are well trained in all techniques to avoid cross-contamination or endangerment of the patient in any way. The specialized intervention procedures are beyond the scope of this book. Currently, tank interventions for isolation patients are being replaced by sprays, showers, and topical medications.

Note that when a patient's burns have healed sufficiently, a tank is useful for preventing contractures in scarred areas and for increasing ROM. At this stage, when the patient is no longer considered an isolation patient, only normal precautions need be taken.

Tanks cannot be completely sterile because the drain must ultimately be connected to a sewer system.[54] However, every effort should be made to treat patients in as sterile an environment as possible. Sterilized plastic tank liners are used in an attempt to decrease contamination. Additional cleaning procedures may be required when preparing tanks for, and after treating, isolation patients. These procedures are as follows:

1. Follow the usual cleaning procedures up to and including Step 7.

2. Refill the tank with a solution of hot water (approximately 115°F, 46°C) and disinfectant.

3. Allow the solution to stand for approximately 5 min. (Some clinics use the agitator during this period.)

4. Drain thoroughly.

5. Rinse thoroughly.

6. Proceed with Step 8 of the usual cleaning procedures.

Tanks must be cleaned immediately after each isolation patient and, in some clinics, again before the next patient uses the tank.

Therapeutic Pools

Although pools are an expensive addition to a physical therapy department, they are extremely valuable for patients in the rehabilitation stage of disability. With some adaptation and creativity, the expense of aquatic therapy can be minimized. The number of home hydrotherapy systems has steadily increased in recent years.[55] Home hydrotherapy rehabilitation has proven to be an effective adjunct to more structured hospital and clinic programs. The primary purpose of pools is therapeutic exercise.

Pools ideally should be equipped with ramps, stairs, and lifts to help patients get in and out, and with parallel bars and attachments for stretchers or chairs that are immersed. The floor of the tank typically is graded to vary the depth of the water, allowing for increased safety and an array of interventions. For rehabilitation purposes, in addition to the properties of water that can facilitate rehabilitation, creative therapists can devise methods of doing exercises that can be fun. All pools should have an assortment of floats, beach balls, and inflatable toys to be used during the exercises **(Figs. 26–12, 26–13).** Pools in pediatric rehabilitation centers

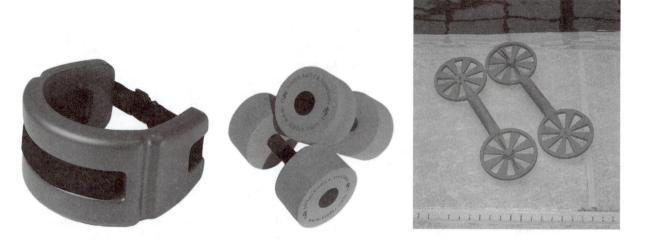

FIGURE 26–12   Floatation devices including belt, hand floats, and resistive paddles.

are extremely popular because swimming, water games, and enjoyable exercises motivate the children to carry out the necessary therapy. Campion's text presents many creative hydrotherapy ideas.[6] Pools are recommended for athletes and dancers who are recovering from injuries to maintain their general strength, flexibility, and function while remaining non-weight-bearing. A modified pool that is approximately 4 feet deep and 12 feet wide (Swimex®) is available for hydrotherapy. It is designed so that a one-directional flow of current can be activated in the water in the upper region. The rate of flow can vary, enabling patients to exercise against a current "set" for an appropriate amount of resistance.

Generally, the temperature of the water in therapeutic pools is warmer than in a regular indoor pool. Temperatures of approximately 90°–100°F (32–38°C), usually between 94° and 98°F (34.4–36.7°C) are rec-

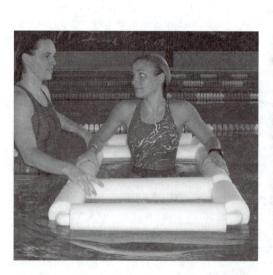

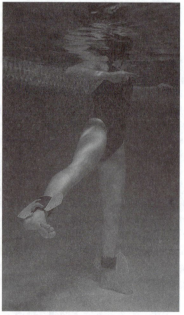

FIGURE 26–13   Clients using floatation devices and/or ankle straps while exercising in pool setting.

ommended. As mentioned earlier, Kirby et al[23] found no change in the oral temperature of healthy subjects regardless of the intensity of activity at 96.8°F (36°C), but Houdas[1] believed that the temperature at which thermal neutrality is maintained at rest in water is slightly lower than 94°F. Houdas also stated that healthy people who are exercising at three times their resting metabolic rate can maintain thermal neutrality in a water temperature as low as 79°F (26°C); in the rehabilitation setting, however, such a low temperature is not advised. A study by Peterson[56] determined that exercising in water at 94°F was appropriate for a patient with multiple sclerosis without producing unwanted heat sensitivity or excessive fatigue. Past studies[57,58] have recommended reduced temperatures between 83° and 85°F.

Broach and Dattilo[59] demonstrated the benefits of aquatic therapy with four adults with relapsing-remitting multiple sclerosis. The participants displayed improved gross motor behavior, stair walking, and bicycling.

Be aware that the amount of exercise may determine the optimal temperature. Sagawas et al[60] showed that, in cool water, exercise rather than resting is more advantageous for maintaining core temperature, but if the water temperature is approximately 77°F (25°C), an ordinary man cannot generate enough heat through exercise to maintain his core temperature. Conversely, if the pool temperature is in the higher range, 98°F (36.7°C), exercise must be limited.

Konlian[61] presented support for aquatic therapy in the intervention of low-back injuries. The author concluded that aquatic therapy, by itself or in conjunction with land-based intervention, is effective in the intervention of low-back injuries. The author recommends temperatures of 83°F for acute pain and 91°–94°F for subacute or chronic pain when rehabilitating patients with low-back injuries. Aquatic therapy allows the therapist to implement exercises earlier in the rehabilitation process and is effective in improving the patient's functional outcome.

A study by Mobily and Verburg[62] showed promising results of the application of aquatic therapy in the intervention of fibromyalgia. Intervention resulted in decrease of acute pain and subsequent improvement in functional activities. It should be noted that the study was conducted on a 59-year-old female, limiting generalization to a larger group.

The advantages of initially practicing walking, standing, and therapeutic exercise in water were discussed earlier in this chapter. However, there may be no direct carryover to standing and walking out of water. Both patient and therapist must be prepared for a transition period when progressing to functions out of water. Contraindications and cross-contamination precautions are similar to those given for Hubbard tank interventions.

Contrast Baths

Intervention with **contrast baths** involves placing one or more extremities alternately in very hot and very cold water. Clinically, whirlpool tanks are usually used; for home interventions, patients can use pails or tubs.

Because superficial blood vessels constrict while in the cold water and dilate while in the hot water, contrast baths are considered to be a vascular exercise limited to peripheral blood vessels.[43] This procedure can increase superficial blood flow in the extremities to a remarkable degree, and it is believed to hasten healing.

An early study, Moor et al[63] reported that a 30-min contrast bath produced a 95% increase in local blood flow when one lower extremity alone was immersed. When all four extremities were immersed, there was a 100% increase in blood flow in the upper extremities and a 70% increase in the lower extremities. The literature contains few studies about the effects attained with contrast baths—for example, changes in muscle strength and in recovery time from fatigue. The reported studies are not in agreement and are inconclusive.

Dosage.   The recommended water temperatures for the cold bath range from 59° to 68°F (15°–20°C). Those for the hot bath should range from 105° to 110°F (40.6° to 43.3°C).[64] There are several variations in the timing used. One example is 3–4 min in the hot water, followed by 30–60 seconds in the cold water.

Procedures.   It is usual to begin with the hot bath and to continue alternating for approximately 30 min, with the final immersion in the cold. Keep in mind, however, that for vascular exercise, the contrast in temperature is more important than the sequence in which it is applied. It may be advisable, especially for the first intervention, to begin both hot and cold at the more moderate ends of the temperature range, then gradually to move toward the extreme ends of the ranges, within the patient's tolerance.

Indications and Contraindications. Contrast baths are most commonly used for athletic injuries. This modality is also used for leg ulcers or for orthopedic problems (ie, arm or leg joint strains or sprains). However, these indications are valid only if the patient is otherwise in good health, because patients experience extreme thermal shocks with each change in temperature.

The contraindications are similar to those for other thermal modalities (see **Chapters 13 and 14**): cardiovascular problems, peripheral vascular diseases (especially arterial sclerosis), a tendency toward hemorrhage, loss of sensation, pregnancy, and hypersensitivity to temperature.

Precautions. Autonomic fight-or-flight reactions should be expected because substantial alteration and fluctuation in pulse and blood pressure will occur during the intervention. Consequently, therapists must be alert for any signs of distress. The patient's pulse should be monitored frequently throughout the intervention.

If the volume of water is not great, the water temperatures may change markedly during an intervention. Thus, water thermometers should be monitored to ensure that the contrast in temperature remains consistent throughout the intervention. If necessary, more ice can be added to the cold water, or more hot water can be added to the hot bath. Be careful when adding the hot water if the body part is already immersed.

Other Modalities

Although currently not used extensively in the United States, many other forms of hydrotherapy exist. Because they are popular in other countries and are occasionally used in the United States, this chapter discusses them briefly. More complete descriptions for their intervention procedures can be found in other texts.[9,45,63,64]

Moist Air Cabinets. Approximately one-half of the patient's body can be placed in a **moist air cabinet.** The patient is usually supine but can be prone or side-lying. Water is heated to 103°–113°F (40°–45°C), and air is forced past the water, absorbing much of the moisture; thus, the humidity in the air is extremely high. The air then circulates throughout the cabinet. During a 15–20 min intervention, the patient's core temperature usually increases 3°F. The high humidity prevents evaporation of sweat in the areas of the body that are in the cabinet. The patient will sweat profusely after intervention to cool down. Patients with chronic low back and arthritis pain report relief, are able to move with greater ease, and exhibit increased range of motion after these interventions.

Sitz Baths. In a **sitz bath,** the water covers the pelvic region. There are tubs specially constructed so that just the pelvic and peroneal areas are in the water. Portable units designed to fit over toilets and maintain the desired temperature are available for home use. However, as a home intervention, patients often sit in bathtubs with water covering that area.

Hot sitz baths require a temperature of 105°–115°F (40.5°–46°C). The duration can range from 2 to 10 min. This intervention is intended to reduce pain, increase circulation in the pelvic area, and enhance tissue healing. Dodi and Bogoni[65] showed that at a water temperature of 104°F (40°C), internal anal pressure decreased significantly, whereas this outcome did not occur with water temperature at either 41°F (5°C) or 73.4°F (23°C). They suggested that the pressure change reduces pain. The indications for hot sitz baths are for women after a birth or a hysterectomy; for patients after a hemorrhoidectomy; and for patients with prostatitis, cystitis, or chronic pelvic inflammatory diseases.

Cold sitz baths require a temperature of 35–75°F (1.7–24°C). The duration can range from 2 to 10 min. This intervention is intended to increase the tone of smooth muscles (atonic constipation) and to reduce uterine bleeding. Although urologists and gynecologists prescribe sitz baths, more investigation is needed to determine the benefits.

Scotch Douche. In the **Scotch douche,** a shower spray of alternating hot (100–110°F, 37.8–43.3°C) and cold (80–60°F, 26.7–15.5°C) water is passed over the body. First the hot, then the cold, spray is passed up and down the back of the person standing in a shower stall. This procedure, alternating hot and cold, continues for several min. The same procedure is carried out on the front of the body. This intervention is invigorating and is also used with patients who have emotional or psychiatric problems.

Peloids and Fango. **Peloids** (mineral mud) and **fango** (moor peat) are heated and applied to the body in a manner similar to the way that hot packs are applied. Many people believe that the mineral content of these muds enhances the benefits received from a heat modality.

Wet Sheets. Wet sheets are used in some psychiatric settings. The patient is completely wrapped in wet sheets at 60–70°F (15–21°C). While wrapped in the sheets, the patient experiences three changes in sensation of temperature: cool, neutral, and then very hot, during which profuse sweating occurs. This intervention is said to reduce anxiety states to a great degree.

Sauna Baths. Sauna baths are popular in the general population in both the United States and Europe. First, the individual rests in a room that has walls, floor, and benches made entirely of wood. The air is extremely dry (low humidity). Stones or bricks are heated so that the air in the room is 140–176°F (60–80°C) or higher.[10] The person sweats profusely, and because the air is dry, the sweat easily evaporates, cooling the body. Thus, the high temperature can be tolerated—but only for brief periods. The next procedure is to take a brief cold shower (or roll in snow) and then return to the sauna. The two procedures can be repeated. Note that although some people enjoy this activity and the feeling of well-being that it pro-vides, sauna baths place a great strain on all the heat-loss mechanisms and may lead to cardiac or heat accidents. Sauna baths are contraindicated for cardiac patients, the elderly, and women in the first trimester of pregnancy. Members of many ethnic groups do take sauna baths throughout life and claim no ill effects; perhaps they become conditioned and therefore don't experience or notice greater reactions with increasing age.

Spas. Areas of effervescent, sparkling water (ie, carbon dioxide springs) can be found throughout the world. Many people strongly believe that these springs have great healing power and report some rejuvenation of health and spirits after spending time at these spas, which are often considered to be resorts. Saratoga Springs in New York state and Nauheim and Mannheim in Germany are examples of these spas. At these resorts, massage and other hydro facilities such as saunas, steam baths, and mud baths are usually available.

REVIEW QUESTIONS

1. What are some of the advantages of hydrotherapy when compared with other superficial thermal agents?

2. How is heat transferred during hydrotherapy interventions?

3. What type of patients would benefit from the effects of buoyancy during a full body immersion?

4. What are the physical properties of water that will influence active exercise during a full body immersion?

5. What water temperature range should be used when using hydrotherapy to treat open wounds?

6. What is the relationship between an object's specific gravity and its ability to float?

7. What are the contraindications for placing an individual in a therapeutic pool?

8. What are the indications for using contrast baths?

9. What is pulsed lavage, and what is it indicated for?

10. Why is vigorous exercise contraindicated in a therapeutic pool with a high temperature?

KEY TERMS

hydrotherapy
buoyancy
specific gravity (SG)
center of gravity (COG)
center of buoyancy (CB)
hydrostatic pressure
hydrodynamic pressure

surface tension
cohesion
adhesion
turbulence
lavage effect
Hubbard tanks
walking tank

contrast baths
moist air cabinet
sitz bath
Scotch douche
peloids
fango

REFERENCES

1. Houdas Y, Ring F: Human *Body Temperature*. New York: Plenum Press; 1982; 69, 192.

2. Clarke R, Hellon F, Lind A: The duration of sustained contractions of the human forearm at different muscle temperatures. *J Physiol* 1958; 143:454–73.

3. Abramson D, Mitchell R, Tuck S: Changes in blood flow, oxygen uptake, and tissue temperature produced by the topical application of wet heat. *Arch Phys Med Rehabil* 1961; 42:305.

4. Nadel E: *Problems with Temperature Regulation During Exercise*. New York: Academic Press; 1977; 91–120.

5. Atkinson G, Harrison A: Implications of the Health and Safety at Work Act in relation to hydrotherapy departments. *Physiotherapy* 1981; 67:263–65.

6. Campion M: *Hydrotherapy in Pediatrics*. Rockville, CO: Aspen; 1985.

7. Skinner A, Thomson A, eds: *Duffield's Exercise in Water*, 3rd ed. London: Bailliére-Tindall; 1983; 20.

8. Forster A, Palastanga N: *Clayton's Electrotherapy: Theory and Practice*, 8th ed. Philadelphia: Saunders; 1981.

9. Licht S, ed: *Medical Hydrology*. New Haven, CT: Elizabeth Licht; 1963; 181, 196, 207, 247, 291–99.

10. Golland A: Basic hydrotherapy. *Physiotherapy* 1981; 67:258.

11. Johnson B, Stromme S, Adamczykj J, et al: Comparison of oxygen uptake and heart rate during exercise on land and in water. *Phys Ther* 1977; 57:273–78.

12. Davis B, Harris R: *Hydrotherapy in Practice*. London: Churchill Livingstone; 1988.

13. Lehmann J: *Therapeutic Heat and Cold*, 4th ed. Baltimore: Williams & Wilkins; 1990.

14. Halliday D, Resnick R: *Fundamentals of Physics*, Extended 3rd ed. New York: Wiley; 1988.

15. McArdle W, Katch F, Katch V: *Exercise Physiology*. Philadelphia: Lea & Febiger; 1986; 162, 491–94.

16. Evans F: *Mechanical Properties of Bone*. Springfield, IL: Charles C Thomas; 1973; 166.

17. Smith L, Weiss EL, Lehmkuhl D: *Brunnstrom's Clinical Kinesiology*, 5th ed. Philadelphia: Davis; 1983.

18. Levangie P, Norkin C: *Joint Structure and Function*, 3rd ed. Philadelphia: Davis; 2001.

19. Enoka R.: *Neuromechanical Basis of Kinesiology*. Champaign, IL: Human Kinetics Books; 1988.

20. Greenleaf J: Physiological responses to prolonged bed rest and fluid immersion in humans. *J App Physiol Environ Exer Physiol* 1984; 57:619.

21. Kolb M: Principles of underwater exercise. *Phys Ther Rev* 1957; 37:361–65.

22. Beach R: Measurement of extremity volume by water displacement. *Phys Ther* 1977; 57:286–87.

23. Kirby RL, Sacamno JT, Balch DE, et al: Oxygen consumption during exercise in a heated pool. *Arch Phys Med Rehabil* 1984; 65:275–78.

24. Douros M: *Comparison of the Effects of Aquatic Therapy vs. Therapeutic (Land) Exercise on the Increase of the Range of Motion of the Osteoarthritic Knee*. New York: Program in Physical Therapy, Columbia University; 1990. Master's thesis.

25. National Aeronautics and Space Administration: *Physiologic response to water immersion in man—a compendium of research*. Washington, DC: NASA Technical Memo X–3308.

26. Bank N: Letter to the editor. *N Engl J Med* 1980; 302:969.

27. Brown CD, et al: Water immersion–induced diuresis in the nephrotic syndrome—secondary ref. Presented at American Society of Nephrology, November, 1979.

28. Epstein M: Renal effects of head-out water immersion in man: Implications for an understanding of volume homeostasis. *Physiol Rev* 1978; 58:529–81.

29. O'Hare J, Heywood A, Dodds P: Water immersion in rheumatoid arthritis. *Bri J Rheumatol* 1984; 23:117–18.

30. Magness J: Swelling of the upper extremity during whirlpool baths. *Arch Phys Med Rehabil* 1970; 51:297.

31. Walsh M: Hydrotherapy. In: Michlovitz S, ed. *Thermal Agents in Rehabilitation*, 3rd ed. Philadelphia: Davis; 1996; 76, 139–67.

32. Niederhuber S, Stribley R, Koepke G: Reduction of skin bacterial load with use of the therapeutic whirlpool. *Phys Ther* 1975; 55:482–86.

33. Kolb LC, Brodie HK: *Modern Clinical Psychiatry*. Philadelphia: Saunders; 1982.

34. Singh H: Treating a severely disturbed self-destructive adolescent with cold wet sheet packs. *Hosp Commun Psychiat* 1986; 37:287–88.

35. Tarnowski KJ, Rasnake KL, Drabman RS: Behavioral assessment and treatment of pediatric burn injuries: A review. *Behavior-Ther* 1987; 18:417–41.

36. Arledge R: Prevention of electric shock hazards. *Phys Ther* 1978; 58:1216.

37. Myers B: *Wound Management: Principles and Practice*. Upper Saddle River, NJ: Prentice Hall; 2004.

38. Smith P, ed: *Infection Control in Long-Term Care Facilities*. New York: Wiley; 1984; 133.

39. Richard R: The use of chlorine bleach as a disinfectant and antiseptic in whirlpools. *Phys Ther Forum* August 29, 1988; 7–8.

40. McGuckin M, Thorpe R, Abrutyn E. Hydrotherapy: An outbreak of *Pseudomonas aeruginosa* wound infections related to Hubbard tank treatments. *Arch Phys Med Rehabil* 1981; 62:283–85.

41. Steve L, Goodhart P, Alexander J: Hydrotherapy burn treatment: Use of chloramine-t against resistant microorganisms. *Arch Phys Med Rehabil* 1984; 65:301–03.

42. *Every Inch & 1/2*. Suggestions from a reader. Publication of The Jobst Institute, Toledo, OH; undated.

43. Belanger A: *Evidence-Based Guide to Therapeutic Physical Agents*. Baltimore: Lippincott Williams & Wilkins; 2002.

44. Bierman W, Licht S: *Physical Medicine in General Practice*. New York: Paul Holber; 1952: Ch. 2.

45. Hayes K: *Manual for Physical Agents*, 5th ed. Upper Saddle River, NJ: Prentice Hall; 2000.

46. Berger W: Electrical shock hazards in the physical therapy department. *Clin Management* 1985; 5:30.

47. Smith D, Clarran S, Harvey M: Hyperthermia as a possible teratogenic agent. *J Pediatr* 1978; 92:878–83.

48. Milunsky A, Ulcickas M, Rothman K, et al: Maternal heat exposure and neural tube defects. *JAMA* 1992; 268:882–85.

49. Luedtke-Hoffman K, Shafer DS: Pulsed lavage in wound cleansing. *Phys Ther* 2000; 80(3):292–300.

50. Scott RG, Loehne HB: Treatment options: Five questions and answers about pulsed lavage. Adv. *Wound Care* 2000; 13(3):133–34.

51. Hess CL, Howard MA, Attinger CE: A review of mechanical adjuncts in wound healing: Hydrotherapy, ultrasound, negative pressure therapy, hyperbaric oxygen, and electrostimulation. *Ann Plast Surg* 2003; 51(2):210–18.

52. Haynes L, Brown M, Handley B, et al: Comparison of Pulsavac and sterile whirlpool regarding the promotion of granulation tissue. *Phys Ther* 1994; 64(5):S4.

53. Turner A, Higgins M, Craddock JC: Disinfection of immersion tanks (Hubbard) in a hospital burn unit. *Arch Environ Health* 1974; 28:101–04.

54. McMillan J, Hargiss G, Nourse A, et al: Procedure for decontamination of hydrotherapy equipment. *Phys Ther* 1976; 56:567–70.

55. Hope J: HydroWorx to launch rehab pools for home. *Central Penn Business Journal* 1999; 15:3–11.

56. Peterson C: Exercise in 94°F water for a patient with multiple sclerosis. *Phys Ther* 2001; 81:1049–58.

57. Peterson JL, Bell GW: Aquatic exercises for individuals with multiple sclerosis. *Clinical Kinesiology* 1995; 49:69–71.

58. Woods DA: Aquatic exercise for patients with multiple sclerosis. *Phys Ther* 1992; 46:14–20.

59. Broach E, Dattilo J: Effects of aquatic therapy on adults with multiple sclerosis. *Therapeutic Recreation Journal* 2001; 35:141–54.

60. Sagawas S, Shiraku, Yousef M, et al: Water temperature and intensity of exercise in maintenance of thermal equilibrium. *J App Physiol* 1988; 65:2413–19.

61. Konlian C: Aquatic therapy: Making a wave in the treatment of low-back injuries. *Orthopaedic Nursing* 1999; Jan/Feb:11–20.

62. Mobily KE, Verburg MD: Aquatic therapy in community-based therapeutic recreation: Pain management in a case of fibromyalgia. *Therapeutic Recreation Journal* 2001; 35:57–69.

63. Moor F, et al: *Manual of Hydrotherapy and Massage*. Mountain View, CA: Pacific Press; 1964.

64. Kottke F, Lehmann J, ed: *Krusen's Handbook of Physical Medicine and Rehabilitation*, 4th ed. Philadelphia: Saunders; 1990.

65. Dodi G, Bogoni F, Infantino A, et al: Hot and cold in anal pain. *Dis Colon & Rectum* 1986; 29:248–51.

66. Suomi R, Lindauer, S: Effectiveness of Arthritis Foundation Aquatic Program on strength and range of motion in women with arthritis. *Journal of Aging and Physical Activity* 1997; 5:341–51.

67. Cassady SL, Neilsen DH: Cardiorespiratory responses to calisthenics performed with upper and lower extremities on land and in water at given cadences. *Phys Ther* 1992; 72:532–40.

68. Fuller RA, Dye KK, Cook NR, Awbrey BJ: The activity levels of the vastus medialis oblique muscle during a single-leg squat on the land and at varied water depths. *J Aquatic Phys Ther* 1999; 7:13.

69. Sova R: *Essential Principles of Aquatic Therapy and Rehabilitation: A Study Guide for the Aquatic Therapy and Rehabilitation Industry Certification.* Chassell, MI: Challenge Publications; 1999.

70. Ruoti RG, Morris DM, Cole AJ: *Hydrotherapy: Principles and Practice.* Boston: Butterworth-Heinemann; 1997.

71. Reid, Campion M: *Aquatic Rehabilitation.* Philadelphia: Lippincott; 1997.

72. Baird CL: First-line treatment for osteoarthritis: Nonpharmacologic intervention and evaluation. *Orthopaedic Nursing* 2001; Nov/Dec(20):13–20.

PART V

Photochemical Agents

This section presents radiant energies with specific frequencies, wavelengths, and photochemical effects. Based on their physiological effects, ultraviolet radiation and low-level laser can be used for therapeutic purposes. The physical principles, physiological effects, instrumentation, procedures, and indications/contraindications for ultraviolet radiation (Chapter 27) and low-level laser (Chapter 28) are included. Each chapter contains research literature to support the use of these modalities and stresses the importance of continued research to advance the development of intervention efficacy.

27

Ultraviolet Radiation

JOSEPH WEISBERG, PT, PhD

JOSEPH A. BALOGUN, PT, PhD, FACSM

Chapter Outline

The use of sunlight for healing purposes is ancient. References to sun gods are found in the writings of ancient Egypt and Greece. In 525 B.C., Herodotus concluded that the energy of the sun affected bone growth. Throughout the centuries that followed, sunbathing was prescribed for conditions such as arthritis, sciatica, weight loss, ulcers, scurvy, rickets, and general weakness. In 1877, Downes and Blunt proved that sun rays could kill bacteria.[1]

Artificial **ultraviolet (UV)** light was developed during the nineteenth century. In 1859, the relationship between artificial ultraviolet irradiation and erythema was discovered. In 1893, Niels Finsen introduced the use of artificial ultraviolet light from a carbon arc to treat skin disorders such as lupus vulgaris, for which he received the Nobel Prize. The mercury vapor lamp was developed early in the twentieth century.[2] Today, ultraviolet light is readily available to the general public, mostly for tanning purposes, and to the medical profession for specific therapeutic purposes, primarily tissue repair, exfoliation, and wound healing. However, the reasons for administering UV therapy are decreasing because more efficient methods of achieving the same intervention goals have been developed.

Physical Principles

The term *ultraviolet* (*ultra* = beyond) was first used by J. Ritter in 1801. This term is misleading because the wavelengths referred to are actually below the wavelength of visible light (less than 400 nm); thus, a more accurate term would be "infraviolet." Angström (1868) was the first to map out the wavelengths of this part of the spectrum. The unit of measurement used to describe the wavelength was the angstrom unit (Å(1 Å = 10 nm). At present, a nanometer is the unit of measure used (1 nm = 0.1 Å).

Ultraviolet radiation (UVR) is produced when the electrons in stable atoms are activated to move to higher orbits, thus creating an unstable state. As these electrons move back to their original orbit, energy is given up as electromagnetic radiation. This energy has the property of both discrete particles (photons) and continuous waves. The emission and transmission of this energy has been explained by the quantum and electromagnetic wave theories (see **Chapter 7**).

The range of radiant energy designated as ultraviolet (UV) extends from approximately 180 nm to approximately 400 nm. The frequencies range from approximately 1.65×10^{15} cycles per second (cps) to approximately 7.5×10^{14} cps[3] (cps has now been replaced by Hz). The ultraviolet rays are in the range immediately below violet of the visible spectrum (**Fig. 27–1**). Within the ultraviolet range, the longer wavelengths are referred to as **near ultraviolet rays** because they are nearer to the visible light and are considered to be beneficial to life in general (between 290 nm and 400 nm). For example, UV at this range helps with the production of vitamin D, and photosynthesis in general. The shorter wavelengths are referred to as the **far ultraviolet rays** because they are farther away from the visible light (between 180 nm and 290 nm) and are generally considered to be harmful to life. For example, UV light at this range is used

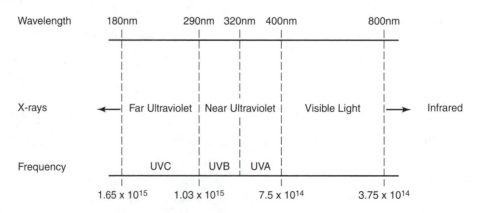

FIGURE 27–1   Portion of the electromagnetic spectrum containing ultraviolet and visible light.

to sterilize instruments. Some authors separate the ultraviolet radiation into three bands: UV-A (320–400), UV-B (290–320), and UV-C (200–290).[4,5] This classification, although well accepted, may vary slightly (± 5 nm) in the literature.

The sun is the natural source of UVR. Five to 10% of the sun's energy is in the UV range (180–400 nm).[6] The ozone layer of the earth's atmosphere filters most of the harmful UV rays. Most, but not all, of the sun's UV rays that reach the earth's surface after filtration range from 290 to 400 nm. The actual UV rays from the sun reaching the earth will depend on (1) variation in the amount of energy radiated from the sun, (2) variation in the earth's distance from the sun (season of the year), (3) time of day, (4) condition of the atmosphere (the ozone layer, dust, moisture), (5) latitude, and (6) altitude.

Ultraviolet-A (320–400 nm) accounts for 6.3% of the sunlight during the summer, and it has long been considered innocuous, but recent studies have shown that it is carcinogenic.[1] Ultraviolet-A is responsible for 80% of the cytotoxic effects of solar-radiation ultraviolet.[1] Some bands of UV-A easily penetrate through the atmosphere and through most sunscreens.[1] In fair-skinned individuals, up to 50% of the UV-A radiation will reach the dermis! Artificially produced UV-A are used by dermatologists for **psoralen phototherapy (PUVA),** and it is the primary wavelength emitted in newer tanning salon generators.[1]

Ultraviolet-B (290–320 nm) accounts for only 0.5% of the sunlight during the summer, and it is often called "sunburn spectrum" because it damages the skin and causes skin cancer. Ultraviolet-B generated by the sun is almost completely absorbed by the atmosphere, but a sufficient amount passes through to affect human skin. Irradiation of the skin with UV-B can precipitate marked endothelial swelling, focal eosinophilic infiltration in the areas exposed, decline in epidermal growth factor receptor sites, and systemic immunological changes. Repeated exposure to moderate doses of UV-B alters skin structure and adversely affects subsequent wound tensile strength.[1]

Ultraviolet-C (200–290 nm) is the shortest wavelength in the ultraviolet spectrum emitted from germicidal lamps, and it constitutes a major component of extraterrestrial lights.[1] Ultraviolet-C is completely filtered by the ozone layer, and little actually reaches the earth's surface.[2] It is toxic to one-cell organisms.[1]

PHYSIOLOGIC AND PSYCHOLOGICAL EFFECTS

In biological tissue, UV rays are absorbed within 0.22 mm of the surface. Therefore, when normal skin is exposed to UV radiation, 80–90% reaches the dermis. In addition, it is important to realize that skin reflects the shorter wavelength rays more than it reflects the longer wavelength rays. Therefore, the amount of UV rays with shorter wavelengths affecting the skin is proportionally less.[7] The UV rays absorbed by the tissue are capable of breaking chemical bonds, which leads to the formation of new chemical bonds, thus producing photochemical effects. This process is caused by a chain of reactions; therefore, the net effect of UV intervention is delayed, appearing over a period of time after the intervention is given. The specific photochemical effect produced by UV rays differs at various wavelengths. For example, rays of 254 nm or 299 nm are the most effective wavelengths for producing tanning (**Fig. 27–2**). Rays of 254 nm or 297 nm are the most effective in producing erythema (**Fig. 27–3**). Rays of wavelength between 250 and 270 nm have a predominantly bactericidal effect. Some bands obviously have a multiple effect (**Fig. 27–4**).[8]

The specific effect of UV light depends on the wavelength. For example, a relatively long wavelength (297 nm) will produce erythema that will develop slowly (within 24 hours) and will disappear slowly (in more than 10 days). A shorter wavelength (254 nm) will produce peak erythema in 6 hours, which will disappear within 4 days.[8,9]

The beneficial effects of ultraviolet can be summarized as follows:

- **Erythema.** Erythema is defined as redness of the skin produced by congestion of the capillaries. Erythema promotes wound healing by increasing the blood supply to the treated area. If the dosage is sufficiently high, the UV rays will initiate an inflammatory response.[10] It is believed that the vasodilation is caused by the liberation of histaminelike substances in concert with other vasodilators.[11] This, in turn, stimulates the formulation of granular tissue, leading to tissue repair. Note that erythema occurs as a result of enlargement and engorgement of minute blood vessels in the corium (the superficial layer of the dermis), not as a thermal reaction. Erythema is

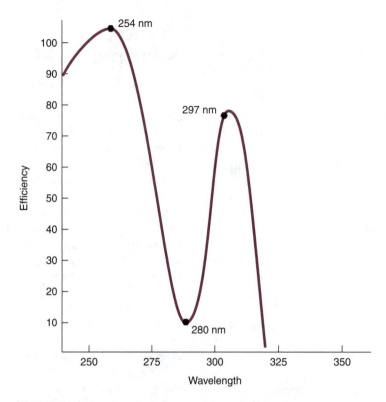

FIGURE 27–2   Production of pigmentation in relationship to the wavelength. Wavelengths of 254 nm or 299 nm are the most effective tanning rays. (*Adapted from S Licht.*)

best achieved with wavelengths of 254 nm and 297 nm (see **Fig. 27–3**).

- **Pigmentation.** Pigmentation is the production of melanin in the deeper strata of the epidermis. The melanin ascends into the more superficial zones, causing a darkening of the skin (tanning) and thickening of the corneum. In turn, this partially blocks penetration of UV rays, thus providing protection from sunburn. Tanning is best achieved with wavelengths of 254 nm and 299 nm (see **Fig. 27–2**).

- **Destruction of bacteria.** The destructive effect of UV rays on bacteria was demonstrated as early as 1877 by Downes and Blunt.[1] The bactericidal effect is best achieved with wavelengths ranging from 250 nm to 270 nm (**Fig. 27–4**). These rays exterminate bacteria by suppressing their synthesis of DNA and RNA.[8] Ultraviolet rays in these ranges can be used to sterilize air and water. Clinically, UV is used to destroy bacteria in ulcers and other types of wounds. Furthermore, it increases the resistance to airborne infection by stimulating reticuloendothelial cells, which increases the production of

circulatory antibodies.[11,12] In addition, the destruction of bacteria enhances the tissue repair process.

- **Thickening of the epidermis.** Ultraviolet radiation causes thickening of the epidermis in all layers, with the exception of the basal layer.[13,14] This may have a protective function, but its usefulness is questionable.

- **Exfoliation of epidermal cells.** Ultraviolet radiation causes the exfoliation (sloughing off) of dead epithelial cells at the stratum corneum, the most superficial layer of the epidermis. Thus, it is used to treat acne vulgaris.[7]

- **Formation of vitamin D.** Historically, UV was useful in treating patients with a deficiency of vitamin D. Currently, however, this vitamin is readily available in the diet and in supplements.

- **Increased production of red blood cells.** Even though this effect has been demonstrated, ultraviolet is not currently used for this purpose.[9]

- **Stimulation of steroid metabolism.** Ultraviolet radiation promotes vasomotor responses causing an antirachitic effect.[15]

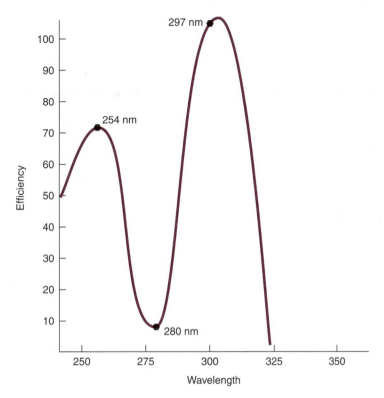

FIGURE 27–3   Production of erythema in relationship to the wavelength. Wavelengths of 254 nm and 297 nm are the most effective in producing erythema. (*Adapted from S Licht.*)

- **Psychological effects.** Sunshine in general promotes the feeling of well-being. Many people equate tanning with health; thus, we can say that UV promotes the feeling of well-being.[7]

The photochemical effect of excessive doses of UV irradiation can lead to shock.[10] This condition reduces the pulse rate, respiration, and blood pressure, and can be life-threatening. The early, clinically observable sign is that the patient suddenly becomes pale. Even doses within the clinical range can at times cause an extreme reaction in patients who have preexisting conditions that make them photosensitive. The student is reminded of the inverse squares law and the cosine law, both of which apply to UV radiation. The distance of the application from the surface of the body and the angulation of the rays will affect the dose that the body receives.

In the event that the patient is overexposed, some authors suggest that the patient be treated within 1 hour by luminous infrared lamp or fluorescent light for at least 10 min. This treatment has been claimed to cause photoreactivation, which will thus diminish the effect of UV irradiation.[16,17]

CONTRAINDICATIONS AND PRECAUTIONS

Contraindications

Box 27–1 summarizes the contraindications associated with the use of UVR. Further details related to these and other precautions are presented in the following section.

Because the cornea absorbs UV wavelengths over 295 nm, the eyes of the patient and operator must be well protected with goggles at all times. Ultraviolet irradiation is contraindicated for only a few conditions:

- Photosensitivity (photosensitive patient, such as one with albinism, might not tolerate even a minimum dosage)
- Porphyrias (a rare metabolic disorder)
- Pellagra (dermatitis due to severe niacin deficiency)
- Discoidlupus erythematosus (inflammatory dermatitis due to lupus)

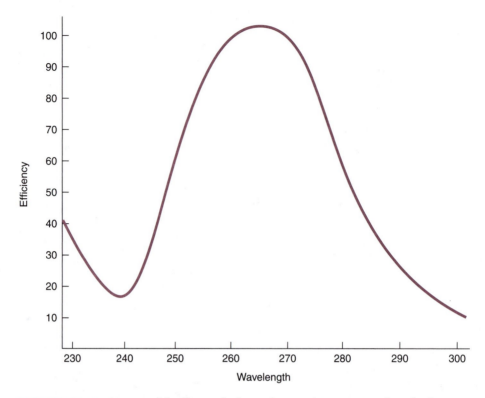

FIGURE 27–4   Bactericidal effects of ultraviolet irradiation. Wavelengths between 250 nm and 270 nm are most effective.

- Sarcoidosis or xeroderma pigmentosum (chronic progressive granulomatous reticulosis involving organs including the skin)

- Fever, active pulmonary tuberculosis, severe cardiac involvement, acute diabetes, and acute skin pathologies

Precautions

Caution should be taken with patients who have any of the preexisting conditions in the following list, because each condition increases their sensitivity to UV rays. When it is necessary to treat such patients with UV rays, the overall dosage should be lowered.

Box 27–1 *Contraindications and Precautions for UVR Interventions*

Contraindication/Precaution	Rationale
Active pulmonary tuberculosis	Exacerbation of infection
Significant cardiac, kidney, and liver disease	Decreased tolerance to UVR
Hyperthyroidism, diabetes mellitus	Severe itching from interaction of UVR with thyroid medications and insulin
Acute eczema or dermatitis	Exacerbation of acute skin conditions
Systemic lupus erythematosus	Exacerbation of associated symptoms
Recent exposure to other radiation therapies	Increased risk for skin carcinoma
Fever	Elevation of core temperature
Photosensitivity (acquired or drug related)	Poor tolerance and exaggerated physiological resposnses

- Patients with little pigmentation, often seen in blonds and redheads. (A patient with albinism may not tolerate even a minimum dosage.)
- Patients with conditions such as syphilis or alcoholism because of photochemical hypersensitivity; cardiac or renal diseases because their tolerance is lower; initial acute onset of psoriasis; acute eczema, herpes simplex, systemic lupus erythematosus; active pulmonary tuberculosis because UV may exacerbate it; hyperthyroidism and diabetes because UV causes itching; cancer because UV may increase anemia; and infants, the elderly, or patients receiving chemotherapy because of low tolerance.
- Patients who have ingested certain foods such as strawberries, eggs, or shellfish before the intervention.
- Patients who are taking any of the following medications: birth control pills (because of hormonal changes, UV can produce undesirable blotching), sulfonamides, sulfonylurea, griseofulvin, tetracycline, quinine, endocrines, gold or other heavy metals, diuretics, insulin, phenothiazines, psoralens, or tar. Exposure to UV while taking these medications heightens the effect of the medication. (When in doubt, consult the physician, pharmacologist, or the *Physicians' Desk Reference*.)
- Patients who received superficial heat (hot pack infrared) before the UV intervention.[18]
- Patients with a history of skin cancer.

PUBLIC HEALTH CONCERNS

In the general population, tanning is often associated with beauty. Recent scientific studies demonstrating the carcinogenic effects of artificial ultraviolet light, used in tanning salons, have prompted increased interest in this public health issue. Over 1 million Americans visit tanning salons daily with possible risks of developing skin and eye burns, cataracts, wrinkles (photo aging), and nonmelanoma skin cancer.[19] A greater concern relates to the projection by the American Cancer Society that over 7,000,000 cases of basal cell and squamous cell skin cancer and 32,000 cases of malignant melanoma will be diagnosed annually.[20]

The incidence of skin cancer still continues to rise, despite the step-up in public health education cam-

paigns in the mass media urging people to wear large sunglasses, sun screens, hats with 3-inch brims, and protective clothing made from tightly woven fabrics during recreational activities in the sun.[4] As part of the public education efforts to convey the risks of overexposure to UV, the National Weather Service now reports the **experimental ultraviolet index (EUI)** daily.[20] The EUI is a prediction of the peak UV radiation level (noon standard time). It is classified into the following categories:

0–2	minimal EUI level
4	low EUI level
6	moderate EUI level
8	high EUI level
10–15	very high EUI level[20]

At 0–2 EUI level, it is expected that individuals most sensitive to sun (ie, a person who tans easily) will burn in 30 min, whereas the less sensitive individuals (persons who do not tan easily) can stay in the sun for about 2 hours. At 15 EUI level, individuals most sensitive to sun can burn in under 5 min, and those least sensitive can burn in 20 min.[20]

Sunscreen is a popular staple recommended for individuals who have to stay in the sun for any period of time, because it provides a physical barrier against the sun. Sunscreens manufactured before 1970 primarily contained zinc oxide and titanium oxide. They were not cosmetically well accepted because they resembled white greasepaint when applied to the skin. The first invisible chemical sunscreen, para-aminobenzoic acid (PABA), was developed in early 1970; when applied to the skin, it is capable of absorbing UV-B radiation.[21]

Many chemical sunscreens—which fall into the categories of benzophenones, cinnamates, and salicylates—have been manufactured and are capable of absorbing a limited spectrum of UV rays. The ingredient in the chemical sunscreens is usually combined to provide broader spectrum protection. Information on the product **sun protection factor (SPF)** is not provided on most sunscreens.[21] The SPF is calculated by determining the time required to produce an erythema reaction when sunscreen is applied over the skin divided by the time it takes to produce the same shade of erythema reaction without sunscreen application.[21] A sunscreen with SPF 10 would theoretically allow the individual wearing it to stay in the sun ten times longer than when the same individual is unprotected.

Sunscreens are now available in PSFs up to 50, and some are able to provide both UV-A and UV-B protection. Sunscreens with an SPF value of 15 and above are recommended because they provide wider spectrum protection than those with lower SPFs. For effective protection against skin cancer, the right amount of sunscreen (a minimum of 1 ounce) should be applied at least 10 to 20 min before going into the sun. Furthermore, irrespective of the sunscreen's SPF label, it should be reapplied every 1 to 2 hours while in the sun.

Allergic reactions to sunscreens are common; there, it is important to pretest them before applying to the entire body or face. Apply a small amount of the sunscreen to the extensor surface of the hand. Continue to observe for up to 6 hours the skin reaction or any untoward effect produced as a result of the application of the sunscreen.

A common myth is that people of color are not as susceptible as light-skinned individuals to the risks and dangers associated with overexposure to sunlight.[20] Although it is true that, in general, the **minimal erythermal dose (MED)** for people of color is higher than for fair-skinned people, appropriate intervention precautions and public health education recommendations should be observed for all patients irrespective of the texture and color of their skin.

Although sunscreens, when used appropriately, offer some protection against skin cancer, a false sense of security may have been created in the general population, because sunscreen users tend to stay longer in the sun to get a "good tan." Paradoxically, several epidemiological studies have revealed that people who normally use sunscreen had a higher incidence of skin melanoma.[2] This finding initially suggested that the ingredients in sunscreens themselves may be carcinogenic. Fortunately, laboratory analysis of the ingredients in sunscreens did not reveal any carcinogen. On the basis of these findings, scientists now attribute the higher rate of melanoma in individuals who use sunscreen to their longer exposure to sunlight. Prolonged exposure to sunlight increases the risk for UV-A absorption, which may suppress the body's capacity to combat skin-cell damage.[20]

There is encouraging news for individuals whose summer is not complete without a good tan. Artificial tanning products (skin bronzers) are now available, and they have been found to be harmless.[2] They are particularly needed for individuals with a family history of skin cancer and for those with pale skin and blue eyes, keratoses, and freckles.[21]

EQUIPMENT

Most UV generators that are used clinically in physical therapy consist of a quartz tube filled with argon gas and some liquid mercury. The quality of the quartz tube is such that it permits the UV rays to go through to affect the target tissue. When the lamp is turned on, the argon gas is heated by the passing current. The heat produced vaporizes the mercury, causing the emission of the UV and visible violet rays.

Three common UV generators are in clinical use; they are referred to as hot-quartz and cold-quartz generators. The *hot-quartz generator* (**Fig. 27–5**) is an air-cooled, high-pressure mercury vapor lamp. This type of generator uses low voltages (30–110 V) and high currents (5 A). The UV rays emitted under these conditions are in both the near and the far bands.

The other common type of generator, the cold-quartz generator, operates in a manner similar to the hot-quartz generator but at a lower temperature. It uses a high voltage (as high as 3000 V), low current (15 mA), low temperature, and low pressure. More than

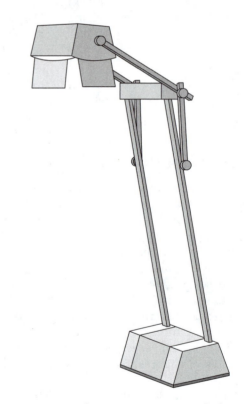

FIGURE 27–5   A hot quartz generator. (*Adapted from GE Miller, Inc.*)

90% of its emission after filtration is 253.7 nm, which is bactericidal.[16] These generators are smaller than hot-quartz generators, they are portable, and they can be used in close proximity to the body (**Fig. 27–6**).

Another cold-quartz generator, which is more common in Europe, is the Kromayer® lamp, with wavelengths between 200 and 400 nm. It operates in the same way as the hot-quartz generator. The beam of the lamp is about 4 cm in diameter, and it is commonly placed 1 inch from the skin surface when treating an open wound. Because it is water-cooled, it has a low heat output (**Fig. 27–7**).

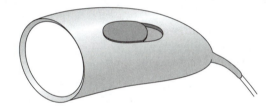

FIGURE 27–6 A cold quartz generator. (*Adapted from GE Miller, Inc.*)

DOSAGE
Minimal Erythemal Dose

To determine the therapeutic dosage for each patient, the following procedure should be performed:

1. Prepare an erythrometer, which can be made from a piece of paper, cardboard, exposed X-ray film, or fabric measuring 4 inches by 8 inches. Cut small holes approximately 3/4 of an inch wide in six different shapes about 3/4 of an inch apart (**Fig. 27–8**).

2. Clean and dry the surface to be tested. Make certain that the skin of the area selected for the test has not been previously exposed to UV radiation. Tape the erythrometer to the flexor aspect of the forearm or to the lower abdomen. Use the lower abdomen if the forearm is too small or if it is unavailable for another reason. These are the areas of choice because they are flat, are rarely exposed to the sun, and are more photosensitive.

3. Cover all the holes in the erythrometer.

4. Drape the patient completely.

5. Put on goggles, and give a pair to the patient.

6. Position the UV lamp directly over the area (so that the UV beam is perpendicular) and 30 inches (76 cm) away.

7. Turn on the generator to preheat for 5 min, being sure that the shutters are closed.

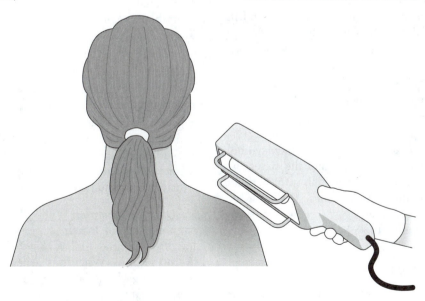

FIGURE 27–7   Application of a portable UVC lamp for treating an infected wound.

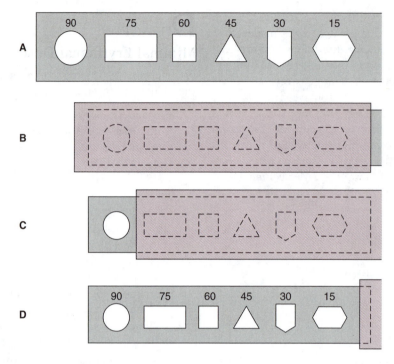

FIGURE 27–8 An erythrometer. (**A**) The cardboard with the cut holes. (**B**) The cardboard with the cover. (**C**) The cardboard with one hole exposed. (**D**) The cardboard with all holes exposed and the time exposures lableled in seconds.

8. Open the shutters and expose the first hole, keeping the remaining holes covered. After 15 seconds, uncover the second hole. Continue uncovering each subsequent hole at 15-second intervals until all the holes are uncovered.

9. When 90 seconds have elapsed since the first hole was uncovered, cover the patient, and close the shutters. In this way, the first hole will have received 90 seconds of exposure, the last hole only 15 seconds.

10. Instruct the patient to check the area every 2 hours while awake and to record which symbols appeared, which ones faded, and the times that each one appeared and faded. This information is used to determine the patient's MED, or the amount of infrared exposure required to show erythema lasting up to 48 hours.

Ultraviolet Doses

Hot Quartz Generator. The parameters for the various doses are as follows:

- Suberythemal dose (SED), no evidence of erythema
- Minimal erythemal doses (MED), evidence of erythema lasting 24 hours
- First-degree erythemal dose (E1) (2.5 × MED), evidence of erythema lasting as long as 48 hours.
- Second-degree erythemal doses (E2) (5 × MED), evidence of intense erythema with edema, peeling, and pigmentation that will last as long as 72 hours.
- Third-degree erythemal doses (E3) (10 × MED), produces erythema with severe blistering and exudation and should be limited to an area no larger than 25 sq cm. **Note:** Change in pigmentation may occur simultaneously.

Cold Quartz Generator. The MED for cold quartz from a distance of 1 inch (2.5 cm) is 12–15 seconds, E1 = 36–45 seconds, E2 = 72–90 seconds, and E3 = 135–180 seconds. When this generator is used in direct contact with the body, 55% of the dosage should be used. This may be appropriate when deeper penetration is desired.

The dose with the cold quartz method depends on the condition. Healing wounds can be treated with a MED of E3. Exposure of the intact skin to UV radiation may require more exposure to get the same effect. Generally, mucosal surfaces can tolerate a dose that is twice as high as the epidermal surfaces can tolerate. However, because there is no epidermal covering that might thicken, the dosage remains the same.

PROCEDURES

General Instructions

1. The intervention room should be well ventilated to eliminate the accumulation of poisonous ozone gas[3] from the warm-up. (Short UV wavelengths, 184.9 nm, are readily absorbed by the oxygen in the air to form ozone and nitrogen oxides.)

2. Wipe off the envelope (bulb) and the reflectors at least once a day (if in use), preferably with 95% ethyl alcohol. Use nap- or lint-free toweling to avoid leaving any fibers behind. Any dust, oil, or water film on the envelope or the reflector will diminish the amount of UV energy reaching the patient.

3. Position the lamp so that the rays are perpendicular to the area to be treated. Measure the distance from the lamp to the highest surface of the area. (A distance of 30 inches, 76 cm, is commonly used at the start.)

4. Cleanse the skin to be treated.

5. Completely cover all skin area (including hair) until intervention time, when the involved area will be exposed for a timed dose.

6. Protect the patient's and your own eyes with special goggles designed for this purpose. Other glasses and sunglasses do not protect from reflection from the side. Eyes need this protection because of poor circulation in the superficial structure of the eye. Thus, the energy absorbed from the UV rays concentrates in a small volume of tissue and damages that tissue.

7. The hot quartz generators should be warmed up 5 to 10 minutes (or as indicated by the manufacturer's manual) before the intervention, with the shutters closed to protect the patient and yourself.

8. Begin timing as soon as the shutters are open and intervention time is on.

9. Carefully monitor the exposure time. The dose is determined according to the MED. (Remember that the dose can be intensified by increasing the exposure time or shortening the distance between the lamp and the patient.)

10. Immediately cover the exposed area after the intervention, and then close the shutter.

11. Record the exposure time and lamp distance. If the facility has more than one lamp, specify the lamp used.

During the intervention, the therapist should avoid exposing his or her own body. In addition, the therapist must remember that hot quartz lamps must cool sufficiently to reestablish the original gaseous state before they are turned on again. The lamps should be restandardized by the company representative after every 100 intervention hours.

Generalized Intervention with Hot Quartz

When intervention is sought for conditions such as generalized dermatitis or localized psoriasis, the following procedures must be followed:

1. Position the patient in the supine position with the face turned to one side and with the palms up. Cover the patient, providing an extra protective covering over the nipples, umbilicus, genitalia, hair, and eyes.

2. Center the lamp over the superior half of the patient's body 30 inches (76 cm) away from the sternum.

3. Expose the upper part of the body for the dosage indicated, using the anterior superior iliac spine and the borderline between the upper and lower part of the body.

4. Close the shutters, and cover the patient.

5. Position the generator over the lower part of the patient's body.

6. Expose the lower area for intervention.

7. Close the shutters, and cover the patient.

8. Do the same for the back, using the posterior superior iliac spine as the dividing landmark, and expose the upper and lower parts in the same manner as before while the patient is prone. Make certain that the arm is now positioned with the palm down and that the other side of the face is now exposed. (To avoid double exposure,

record the original position.) Be extra careful with obese patients because landmarks are not clearly visible. Furthermore, fat rolls and the umbilicus area should be exposed with care.

9. Subsequent interventions should be conducted in the same manner, but the duration per area usually can be increased by 5 seconds each time. The increment by which the dosage is increased will depend on the patient's sensitivity to UV radiation. When the total exposure for each area reaches 3 min, the distance can then be reduced to avoid increasing the exposure time further.

Local Intervention with Hot Quartz

The procedures for treating local conditions are the same as for generalized exposure, but the UV rays are applied to a local area. Closer distances can be used for this type of intervention, and the exposure time should be recalculated according to the formula

$$T2 = \frac{(T1\ d2^2)}{(d1^2)}$$

where T2 = new exposure time, T1 = initial exposure time, d1 = initial distance, and d2 = new distance.

Never use a hot quartz generator closer than 15 inches (about 38 cm) to the patient because the intensity of the UV will be extremely high and regulating the dosage will be difficult. No dose should be repeated until the erythemal effect of the previous dose has disappeared.

The therapist is responsible for positioning the patient carefully for intervention to avoid over- or underexposure. Duplication of exposure can easily occur if one is not careful, especially if whole-body irradiation is used. One-half of the face, either the anterior or the posterior surfaces of the upper extremities, and the lateral aspect of the lower extremity are especially vulnerable.

When treating local areas, it is important to keep a precise record of the area treated to avoid overexposure in subsequent interventions. Charting the area by means of bony landmarks is helpful.

Underexposure can occur if the lamp or body part is not clean or is not optimally positioned. For example, in treating the ventral surface of the arm, the neutral position of the arm (that is, with the lateral aspect perpendicular to the lamp) is not optimal. The UV rays will be parallel to the volar surface of the arm, leading to underexposure.

Local Intervention with Cold Quartz

Cold quartz is used most commonly to treat decubitus (pressure) ulcers for the bactericidal healing effects. Because the UV is applied to an open wound, the skin is not a mediating factor. There is no need to determine the MED for this intervention. Exposure time for the different doses is predetermined.

When operating the cold quartz generator, the therapist should carry out the following steps:

1. Wash the area with soap and water and clean the wound of any debris.
2. Dry the area thoroughly.
3. Cover the area with a sterile drape when treating open wounds.
4. Put on the goggles, and give the patient a pair.
5. Drape the bulb end of the unit.
6. Turn on the unit for 1–3 min to warm it up.
7. Position the lamp perpendicular to the skin surface at a distance of 1 inch (2.5 cm). You can ensure the correct distance either by placing the lamp on doughnut gauze that is 1 inch thick or by taping to it tongue depressors that protrude 1 inch (2.5 cm)
8. Expose the wound for the required time.
9. Turn off the lamp.

The effectiveness of the UV intervention depends on the output of the lamps—their output diminishes as they age. The effectiveness of the lamp is reduced long before the bulb is completely burned out. For that reason, the lamp must be checked after every 100 hours of use or at least once a year.

Many large facilities have their own meters to calibrate UV lamps.[22] Commercial calibration facilities serve those users without in-house facilities.

Intervention Frequency and Progression

Ultraviolet radiation intervention should not be applied on an intact skin until the previous erythema reaction has completely disappeared. A MED can be applied daily because the erythema reaction produced would have disappeared within 24 hours. An E1 dose can be repeated on alternate days, whereas E2 doses can be repeated every 3–4 days.

Ultraviolet radiation therapy can be administered daily for open wounds and decubitus ulcers without increasing the dose applied. To maintain the same response, the intervention dose required for an intact skin must be increased, because of the anticipated thickening of the epidermis and the melanin formation. For MED and E1 interventions, the dose must be increased by 25% and 50%, respectively, with each ensuing intervention. An E2 dose should be increased by 75% with each ensuing intervention. When sessions are missed, the dose should be decreased by 25% of the previous dose. Following prolonged discontinuation of intervention or after peeling of the skin, the initial dose is used.

COMMON INDICATIONS

Psoriasis

One common use of UV radiation is in the intervention for psoriasis (but not in the acute stage of the first manifestation).[23] Ultraviolet radiation (E2 dose) can be used alone to achieve exfoliation or in conjunction with medication, tar paste, or ointment.[24–27] The two types of UV interventions for psoriasis that are considered to be safest and most effective are the TUVAB and the PUVA. **TUVAB** is an acronym for tar and ultraviolet A and B, three antipsoriatic agents also known as the **Goeckerman regimen**. The intervention involves the application of tar ointment, followed by exposure to ultraviolet radiation. With this type of intervention, it is theorized that UV rays damage the DNA, thus inhibiting the cells from proliferating as rapidly. **PUVA** is an acronym for psoralen and UV-A. The patient ingests psoralen and is then exposed to UV-A. It is theorized that the psoralen binds to the DNA and damages it when it is irradiated with UV. Patients must be warned that for 24 hours after ingesting psoralen, they must wear UV-opaque goggles to protect the lens of the eyes.[28] It is important to note that PUVA has recently been associated with an increased incidence of skin cancer, liver disease, and some tumors. It is still an acceptable intervention, but only for selected severe cases.[29]

Acne Vulgaris

Ultraviolet radiation is used to achieve exfoliation.[30] The intervention for this condition involves local or general body irradiation three times a week, beginning with an MED and progressively increasing the dosage with subsequent intervention (up to 16–20 MED). It has been suggested that patients who show spontaneous remission of the acne during the summer are better candidates for this intervention. Obviously, the interventions are given during the winter.

Uremic Pruritus

Ultraviolet irradiation has proved to be helpful to patients who have uremic pruritis.[30] The intervention for this type of itching involves general body irradiation with a suberythemal dose every 3 or 4 days.

Jaundice

Ultraviolet irradiation also is used to help prevent jaundice in newborns.

Wounds

Ultraviolet radiation has been used to treat poorly healing wounds. A more detailed duscission of UVR for wound healing follows this section.

Box 27–2 *Common Clinical Uses and Rationale for Ultraviolet Radiation*

Indication	Rationale
Psoriasis	Promote exfoliation of superfical skin layers.
Acne Vulgaris	Promote exfoliation of superfical skin layers.
Uremic Pruritis	Relieve skin itching associated with chronic renal failure.
Jaundice	Assist in the elimination of billirubin.
Wounds	Increase circulation in the skin.
	Promote new cell production from the basal cell layer.
	Boost responses of the immune system.
	Kill bacteria.

Overview of UVR in Wound Management

Physical therapists are frequently consulted in the management of recalcitrant (indolent) ulcers and infected wounds, particularly pressure sores. To promote healing, physical agents are used in conjunction with antibiotic therapy (a course of antibiotic medications and/or topical gel). Relevant studies on the effects of UVR on wound healing are presented next.

Evidence from the Literature

Several case studies[31–34] have documented the effectiveness of UVR in the intervention with ulcers. In a recent case study, Thai et al[35] investigated the effects of UVR on indolent ulcers. Three patients with chronic ulcers infected with methicillin-resistant *Staphylococci aureus* were treated with UVR. Two of the three ulcers had complete closure within 1 week of intervention with UVR. The authors concluded that UVR is a "promising adjunctive therapy for chronic wounds containing antibiotic-resistant bacteria." Despite the preceding finding, there is still skepticism about the clinical value of UVR, in part because of a lack of well-controlled clinical studies documenting its effectiveness in the various conditions for which it is recommended.

Willis et al[36] in 1983 evaluated the effectiveness of UVR in the intervention with pressure ulcers. Eighteen patients with pressure ulcers were randomly assigned to active UVR or placebo intervention groups. Intervention was administered in direct contact with the ulcer using the Kromayer® lamp with wavelengths between 200 and 400 nm. The surrounding skin was screened to within 1 mm of the edge of the ulcer. Wound healing was significantly less ($p<0.02$) in the UVR-treated group (6.3 plus/minus 0.6 weeks) as compared with the placebo group (8.4 plus/minus 0.5 weeks). Analysis of the data, controlling for patient's age and initial size of the ulcer, did not change the outcome of the findings. The authors concluded that "in spite of growing skepticism about its effectiveness, it appears that ultraviolet radiation may play a useful role in the intervention with pressure sores."

In 1988, Ohali[37] compared the efficacy of UVR and Eusol® (wet dressing) in promoting wound healing. Ten patients, each with multiple skin ulcers, were recruited. With each patient as his or her own control, one of the ulcers was randomly assigned to UVR, and the other ulcer received Eusol® dressing (dosage was not specified). Using the Kromayer® lamp, the ulcers treated with UVR received E2 dose to the periphery of the ulcer and E4 dose to the crater of the ulcer. Ultraviolet radiation was administered three times per week. Measurement of surface area of each ulcer was obtained weekly, and photographs of the ulcers were taken at regular intervals. The results revealed that both Eusol® dressing and UVR were effective ($p<0.001$) in promoting the healing of the ulcers. At the end of the fifth week of intervention, the surface areas of the UVR-treated ulcers (32.8 plus/minus 49.6 cm^2) were smaller than those treated with Eusol® dressing (110.6 plus/minus 101.6 cm^2). On the basis of the findings in this study, the author concluded that UVR is an effective physical agent in promoting wound healing and wondered why "patients are denied a very effective method of intervention."

In 1986, Basford et al,[38] in a randomized, controlled-design study, compared the effectiveness of low-energy HeNe laser irradiation, cold-quartz UVR, and saline "damp-to-dry" dressing (occlusive membrane) in the intervention of wounds. Six pigs were randomly assigned into three two-pig groups. Wounds assigned to laser intervention received two minimal erythemal dose (MED) interventions (15-second exposure), twice daily, for 6 days per week. The dressing of the occluded wounds (Tegoderm®) was checked and replaced as needed twice daily, 6 days per week. All intervention groups appeared to heal faster than the occluded wounds. With the dosages used, the amount of bacteria colonization and wound strength in all intervention groups were similar. The lack of a statistically significant difference observed in the UVR-treated wounds may be attributed to the low dose of UVR used in this study.

To date, there are only two well-controlled studies in humans,[36,37] and both studies showed positive results from UVR in wound healing. On the basis of the available literature, we conclude that UVR may be an underrated but effective physical agent beneficial for well-selected patients. However, further studies are warranted to ensure the optimal dosage and intervention parameters necessary to obtain satisfactory responses.

The therapeutic effect of UVR in promoting wound healing is generally attributed to its erythematous effect, which causes stimulation of the repair process and the thickening of the epidermis.[39–42] There is some evidence to show that UVR (predominantly UV-B wavelength) has bactericidal effect.[43,44]

In 1976, Atun[43] investigated the effect of exposure to different dosages (1 MED to 20 MED) of UVR on bacterial flora obtained from the pressure ulcers of 21 patients. The samples (n = 974) were cultured on blood agar plates and incubated for 24 hours. The bacterial flora decreased gradually from 1 MED (1 min exposure time) to 6 MED of UVR exposure. The rate of decrease in bacterial flora remained about the same at 6 MED as that observed at 20 MED exposure. The findings of this study buttressed the widely known "bactericidal" effect of UVR.

A follow-up study by High and High[44] in 1983 revealed that, with exposure times equivalent to E2 (5 MED) and E3 (10 MED) doses, UV-B rays can successfully attenuate the growth of bacteria and fungi. At E4 (20 MED) dose, bacteria and fungi are completely destroyed.[44] Exposure time greater than E4 dose is therefore not justified in the management of ulcers. Although not supported by research, many clinicians recommend an MED-E1 (2.5 MED) dose for the periphery of an infected or indolent ulcer to increase blood supply and an E3 (MED) dose at the crater of the ulcer for its bactericidal effect.

Protocol

Wound management by a physical therapist must be part of an intervention plan that addresses both the skin breakdown (ulcer) and the overall functional activity of the patient. The therapist must evaluate and institute interventions that restore normal body function (blood flow, pain, edema, immobility, etc.) and provide care that promotes healing (eg, dressing and the use of physical agents).[45]

Before the initial intervention, the MED for the patient must be determined as discussed earlier. The MED is needed to calculate the appropriate dose required for intervention. The area selected for testing the MED must be as close as possible to the site of the wound. Both for hot quartz and cold quartz generators, the burner of the UVR lamp should be switched on for 5 min before intervention to allow the lamp to stabilize and work at its full capacity. Appropriate routine precautions described in **Chapter 4** should be followed. The following protocol is recommended in the management of ulcers by UVR:[37]

1. Obtain sterilized transparent cellophane papers.

2. Clean two layers of the sterilized cellophane paper with isopropyl rubbing alcohol, and place them directly on the surface of the wound.

3. With a pair of scissors, cut the outer layer of the cellophane paper and retain. Discard the inner layer of the cellophane paper that was directly in contact with the wound surface.

4. Place the tracings on the cellophane paper under a plain white sheet of paper, and trace the outline of the wound surface area on the white paper.

5. Cut the outline of the wound from the white paper, and transpose the paper on a piece of sterilized gauze. Use scissors to make an aperture of the size of the wound on the sterilized gauze.

6. Cleanse the surface of the wound with saline solution and/or topical cleansing agent.

7. Irradiate the skin surrounding the wound with MED/E1 dose to stimulate peripheral circulation.

8. Affix the gauze around the wound to expose only the crater of the wound. Care must be taken **not** to expose the newly healed tissue and surrounding skin to E3 dose.

9. Administer an E3 dose to the crater of the wound. For cold-quartz generators, E3 dose is obtained when the ulcer is irradiated for about 135–180 seconds at a distance of 1 inch (2.5 cm) from the skin. For hot quartz generators, E3 dose is calculated as 10 times the MED dose determined for the skin surrounding the ulcer.

10. Apply topical antibiotic solution/gel, and cover the wound with sterilized gauze, securing it with zinc oxide plaster or bandage.

11. For the water-cooled quartz (eg, the Kromayer®) generator, allow the water pump to continue running for 5 min after the burner is switched off in order to cool the burner.

12. Observe and document patient response to the intervention. Record the lamp used and dosage of intervention—that is, the distance of the lamp (cm) from the skin and duration (seconds) of exposure to UVR.

13. For follow-up interventions, the dosage for the crater of the ulcer remains the same because of the absence of epidermal covering.

14. For the skin surrounding the ulcer, the MED dose should be increased by 25% and the E1 dose by 50% of the preceding dose to maintain the same level of response.

15. Decrease the exposure time by 25% of the previous dose for every intervention missed.

Evaluation of Wound Healing

In a managed-care health system where third-party providers require objective documentation of intervention outcomes for reimbursement purposes, clinicians must be familiar with available and convenient methods of evaluating the effectiveness of the intervention. There are various methods of measuring wound surface area.[46,47] Techniques including photography and manual tracing of the wound perimeter can also be used to evaluate the effectiveness of interventions.

REVIEW QUESTIONS

1. Identify the position of ultraviolet radiation (UVR) in the electromagnetic spectrum and the individual ultraviolet bands with their respective wavelengths.

2. Identify and describe the physiological effects of UVR.

3. Identify the precautions and contraindications for the use of UVR.

4. What factors influence an individual's sensitivity to UVR?

5. Identify the indications for the use of UVR.

6. Provide the rationale for using UVR for wound healing.

7. Describe how to perform a minimal erythemal dosage (MED) test.

8. Describe what constitutes a (a) suberythemal dosage, (b) minimal erythemal dosage, (e) first-degree erythemal dosage, and (d) second-degree erythemal dosage.

9. Describe the technique for applying UVR to a poorly healing wound.

10. How can UVR efficacy for wound healing be evaluated?

KEY TERMS

ultraviolet (UV)
ultraviolet radiation (UVR)
near ultraviolet rays
far ultraviolet rays

psoralen phototherapy (PUVA)
experimental ultraviolet index
  (EUI)
sun protection factor (SPF)

minimal erythemal dose (MED)
TUVAB
Goeckerman regimen
PUVA

REFERENCES

1. Licht S. History of Ultraviolet Therapy. In: Licht S, ed. *Therapeutic Electricity and Ultraviolet Radiation*, 2nd ed. New Haven, CT: Elizabeth Licht; 1967; 200.

2. Harber LC, Bickers DR: Introduction to Photobiology. In: *Photosensitivity Diseases: Principles of Diagnosis and Intervention*. Philadelphia: Saunders; 1981; 3–9.

3. Anderson WT: Instrumentations for Ultraviolet Therapy. In: Licht S, ed. *Therapeutic Electricity and Ultraviolet Radiation*, 2nd ed. New Haven, CT: Elizabeth Licht; 1967; 214–15.

4. Anderson TG, Wadinger TP, Voorhees JJ: UV-B phototherapy: An overview. *Arch Dermatol* 1948; 120:1502–07.

5. Schafer V: Artificial Production of Ultraviolet Radiation: Introduction and Historical Review. In: Urback F, ed. *The Biological Effects of Ultraviolet Radiation, with Emphasis on the Skin*. New York: Pergamon; 1969; 93.

6. Brown I, Meng MJ: *Fundamentals of Electrotherapy: Course Guide*. Madison, WI: American Printing & Publishing; 1972; 10.

7. Scott BO: Clinical Uses of Ultraviolet Radiation. In: Stillwell KG, ed. *Therapeutic Electricity and Ultraviolet Radiation*, 3rd ed. Baltimore: Williams & Wilkins, 1983; 234.

8. Fischer E, Solomon S: *Physiological Effects of Ultraviolet Radiation*, 2nd ed. New Haven, CT: Elizabeth Licht; 1967; 258–73.

9. Hausser KW, Vahle W: Sunburn and Suntanning. In: Urback F, ed. *The Biologic Effects of Ultraviolet Radiation, with Emphasis on the Skin*. New York: Pergamon Press; 1969; 7.

10. Scriber WJ: *A Manual of Electrotherapy.* Philadelphia: Lea & Febiger; 1975; 49.

11. Holti G: Measurements of the vascular responses in skin at various time intervals after damage with histamine and ultraviolet radiations. *Chem Sci* 1955; 14:143–55.

12. Kahn J: Physical Agents: Electrical, Sonic and Radiant Modalities. In: Scully RM, Barnes MR, eds. *Physical Therapy.* Philadelphia: Lippincott; 1989; 894–97.

13. Nutini LG: Tissue Repair. In: Glasser O, ed. *Medical Physics II.* Chicago: Yearbook; 1950; 1124.

14. Daniels F Jr, Brophy D, Lobitz WC: Histochemical responses of human skin following ultraviolet irradiation. *J Invest Dermatol* 1961; 37:351.

15. Wadsworth H, Channugam A: *Electrophysical Agents in Physiotherapy.* New South Wales, Australia: Science Press; 1980.

16. Griffin JE, Karselis TC: *Physical Agents for Physical Therapists,* 3rd ed. Springfield, IL: Charles C Thomas; 1982; 269.

17. Weisberg, J: *Monthly Skin News.* 1988: 1(4).

18. Montgomery PC: The compounding effects of infrared and ultraviolet irradiation upon normal human skin. *Phys Ther* 1973; 53:489–496.

19. Tanning salons may cause cancer, other diseases. *PT Bulletin* March 22, 1996.

20. Protect skin from sun's ultraviolet radiation. *PT Bulletin* August 17, 1994.

21. Sunscreen. *Harvard Women's Health Watch.* 1999 (April); 6.

22. *Safety Bulletin.* New York: Columbia University, Department of Environmental Health and Safety. June 1985. Health Sciences Revision #6.

23. Bryant BG: Intervention of psoriasis. *Am J Hosp Pharm* 1980; 37:814–20.

24. Solomon WM, Netherton EW, Nelson PA, et al: Intervention of psoriasis with the Goeckerman technique. *Arch Phys Med Rehabil* 1955; 36:74–77.

25. Fusco RU, Jordan PA, Kelly A, et al: PUVA intervention for psoriasis. *Physiotherapy* 1980; 66(2):39–40.

26. Klaber MR: Ultraviolet light for psoriasis. *Physiotherapy.* 1980; 66(2):36–38.

27. Shurr DG, Zuehlke RI: Photochemotherapy intervention of psoriasis. *Phy Ther* 1981; 62(1):33–36.

28. Psoriasis update. *J Coll Phys Surg Columbia Univ* 1986; 6(1).

29. Psoriasis therapy linked to cancer. *PT Bull* October 5, 1988.

30. Gilchrest BA, Rowe JW, Brown RS: Relief of the uremic pruritis with ultraviolet phototherapy. *N Engl J Med* 1977; 297(3):136–38.

31. Freytes HA, Fernandez B, Fleming WC: Ultraviolet light in the intervention of indolent ulcers. *Southern Medical Journal* 1965; 58:223–26.

32. King R, Paver K, Poyzer: Photochemotherapy in psoriasis. *Medical Journal of Australia* 1979; 2:57.

33. Rich WG: Intervention of ulcers with ultraviolet radiation. *Medical Journal of Australia* 1979; 2:58.

34. Llewellyn DJ, Lahive KM: The intervention of smallpox vaccination ulcers with ultraviolet light. *Physiotherapy* 1965; 51:86–88.

35. Thai TP, Houghton PE, Campbell KE, Woodbury MG: Ultraviolet light C in the intervention of chronic wounds with MRSA: A case study. *Ostomy Wound Management* 2002; 48(1):52–60.

36. Willis EE, Anderson TW, Deattie BL, Scott A: A randomized placebo-controlled trial of ultraviolet light in the treatment of superficial pressure sores. *Journal American Geriatric Society* 1983; 31:131–33.

37. Ohali AB: The efficacy of ultraviolet radiation in the healing process of skin ulcers. Thesis submitted for the MS degree in physiotherapy, Faculty of Health Sciences, Obafemi Awolowo University, Ile-Ife, Nigeria. 1988. Supervisors: Nwuga VCB, Balogun JA.

38. Basford JR, Hallman HO, Sheffield CG, Mackey GL: Comparison of cold-quartz ultraviolet, low-energy laser, and occlusion in wound healing in a swine model. *Arch Phys Med Rehabil* 1986; 67:151–54.

39. Davidson SF, Brantley SK, Das SK: The reversibility of UV-altered wound tensile strength in the hairless guinea pig following a 90-day recovery period. *Brit J Plastic Surg* 1992; 45:109–12.

40. Davidson SF, Brantley SK, Das SK: The effects of ultraviolet radiation on wound healing. *Brit J Plastic Surg* 1991; 44:210–14.

41. Das SK, Brantley SK, Davidson SF: Wound tensile strength in the hairless guinea pig following

irradiation with pure ultraviolet-A light. *Brit J Plastic Surg* 1991; 44:509–13.

42. Rader M, Fluke DJ, Pollard EC: Induced repair in *Escherichia coli:* Induction by ultraviolet light at −79°C. *Biochemistry and Photobiology* 1980; 32:701–02.

43. Atun IH: The bacterial flora of decubitus ulcers and the effects of ultraviolet light on this flora. *Mikrobiyol Bull* 1976; 10(1):3–15.

44. High AS, High JP: Intervention of infected skin wounds using ultraviolet radiation: An in vitro study. *Physiotherapy* 1983; 69:359–60.

45. Prost MA: Treating people with wounds and getting paid for it. *Advance for Physical Therapists* January 19, 1998; 33–34.

46. Balogun JA, Abidoye AB, Akala EO: Zinc iontophoresis in the management of bacterial colonized wounds: A case report. *Physiotherapy Canada* 1990: 42:147–51.

47. Bohannon RW, Pfaller BA: Documentation of wound surface area from tracings of wound perimeters: Clinical report on three techniques. *Phys Ther* 1983; 63:1622–24.

28

Low-Level Laser Therapy

JOSEPH WEISBERG PT, PhD

DONNA ADAMS PT, MA

Chapter Outline

The word *laser* is an acronym for **L**ight **A**mplification by **S**timulated **E**mission of **R**adiation. Its application for medicinal purposes is extensive, and laser technology continues to advance rapidly. **Low-level laser,** which is also referred to as **low-energy laser irradiation (LELI),** has been used in Europe for more than a decade, yet its effectiveness has not been scientifically established. Clinical observation is the basis for therapeutic claims such as reducing pain and spasm, promoting healing, and decreasing inflammation. Recent research both supports and rejects these claims. Presently, the Food and Drug Administration (FDA) has classified the low-power laser as a class III medical device. Therefore, practitioners interested in utilizing this device must obtain an investigational device exemption, as stated in FDA regulation 812.2 (b).[1] However, low-level laser therapy was approved by the FDA for use as an intervention for carpal tunnel syndrome in February 2002.

Physical Principles

Light is a form of radiant energy with wavelengths that can vary between 100 and 10,000 nanometers within the electromagnetic spectrum. This capacity places laser light in the visible light band of the electromagnetic spectrum (see **Chapter 7**). Three lasers that are gaining interest in physical therapy are the HeNe (helium neon) laser, the GaAs (gallium arsenide) laser, and the gallium-aluminum-arsenide (GaAlAs) laser. In this chapter, both of the gallium lasers will be discussed as one type of laser; the difference between the two is the amount of aluminum in the semiconductor material. All units have the laser characteristic of single wavelength. Laser beams are produced by electrical or mechanical stimulus to various forms of matter (for this chapter, HeNe, GaAs, and GaAlAs). The stimulus brings about a change in the position of the electrons of an atom (**Fig. 28–1**) causing photons to be released. Photons, being the energy component of light, are absorbed as energy when they collide with other HeNe atoms, rendering the atom "unstable." Stimulated emission of photons will occur to return the atom to a stable or ground state. Emitted photons collide with other atoms, causing the release of additional photons. This process rapidly continues, resulting in a chain reaction that cumulatively causes the emission of radiation.

In a laser, the molecules are stimulated in a closed chamber with reflective and semireflective surfaces. As photons rapidly reflect off these surfaces, they align in identical phase, direction, and frequency. This rapid process continues, and the emission of radiation is amplified. Amplification continues until the chamber can no longer contain the energy produced. The laser beam is then ejected out of the reflective chamber, through a semipermeable mirror to a

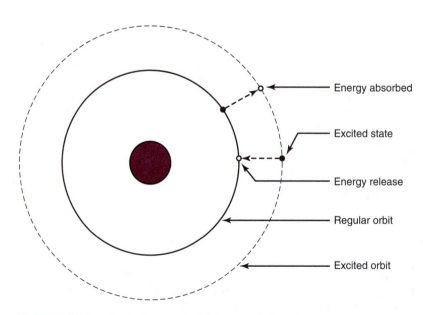

FIGURE 28–1   Excited state of electrons and the release of energy.

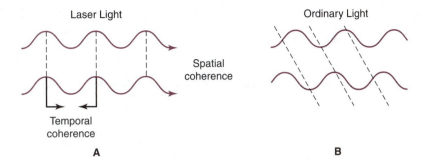

FIGURE 28–2   (A) Phase characteristics of laser light. The wavelengths have temporal coherence—all the waves emitted by individual gas molecules have the same wavelength. The wavelengths also have spatial coherence: that is, all the waves travel in the same direction. (B) Phase characteristics of ordinary light.

fiberoptic monofilament in an HeNe laser or to a diode in a GaAs laser, which directs the beam to the target tissue.

Laser light is emitted in a parallel-organized fashion, unlike the light emitted from incandescent or fluorescent light sources. Laser has three properties that are unique to it as compared with ordinary light. These properties are coherence, monochromaticity, and collimation.

Coherence

Coherence light, unlike ordinary light, consists of identical parallel waves that propagate with close approximation—that is, in the same phase (temporal coherence) and in the same direction (spatial coherence) (**Fig. 28–2**). The properties of temporal and spatial coherence minimize divergence of the laser beam. The coherent properties will result in the energy being concentrated in one area (**Fig. 28–2A**). **Figure 28–2** and **28–3** show the difference between laser and ordinary light.

Monochromaticity

Ordinary light is a mixture of many different wavelengths, whereas each laser unit emits energy of a single wavelength. For example, the HeNe laser produces a red laser beam with a wavelength of 632.8 nm (see **Fig. 7–2**). This falls within the visible red light band of the electromagnetic spectrum. The (GaAs) laser produces a laser beam within the infrared band at 910.0 nm. The literature suggests that the clinical significance of this monochromatic characteristic is that certain wavelengths have characteristics that affect biologic tissue in a particular way. Wolbarsht[2] indicated that a wavelength of 632.8 nm (red laser from HeNe) is "in tune with the resonance of the biological tissue," thereby affecting it in a positive way and possibly enhancing healing. The recommended term to describe the use of lasers for photobiomodulation is low-level laser therapy (LLLT). Monochromaticity is the most significant characteristic of LLLT that results in a cellular response through producing heating effects.[3]

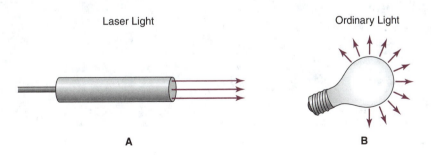

FIGURE 28–3   Wave direction of (A) laser light and (B) ordinary light.

Collimated Beam

Collimation refers to the minimal divergence, or moving apart, of the photons in a laser beam. This capacity maintains the photons moving in a parallel fashion, concentrating the beam of light on the target area—as contrasted to the illumination characteristics of ordinary light (see **Fig. 28–2**).

TYPES USED IN PHYSICAL THERAPY

Lasers are available in high or low power. High-power lasers are those with power of more than 60 mW (CO_2, Argon, and YAG lasers). These lasers can cause thermal damage to the tissues and are primarily used in surgical procedures. Low-power lasers (HeNe and GaAs) commonly referred as **cold lasers** or LLLT, use less than 60 mW of power and cause minimal to no thermal responses. The use of LLLT for pain management and wound healing is a relatively new application in the medical field. Power output used in physical therapy protocol is generally less than 1 mW on continuous mode and about 0.5 mW on pulsed mode. Most commonly utilized by the physical therapist is the HeNe laser (**Fig. 28–4**). The red laser light that this device produces is due to electric stimulation of a tube filled with helium and neon gases (atoms). Electric stimulation of these gases causes the emission of radiation at a wavelength of 632.8 nm, which is in the red band of visible light. The effects produced by laser on biologic tissue penetrate the tissue to a depth of about 0.8–15.0 mm via photochemical reactions.[4,5] Note that although the GaAs laser produces a beam in the infrared band, it is not a thermal modality. The low power and the pulsed beam negate any heating effect.

PROPOSED MECHANISM OF ACTION

Biostimulation refers to the application of electromagnetic energy by low-level laser therapy to biologic tissues. Theoretically, on the basis of the dosage, the application of this energy can **stimulate or inhibit** the biochemical, physiologic, and proliferative activities of cells.[6] There are few controlled studies in the literature substantiating any proposed mechanism of action for laser effects. Documented case studies and empiri-

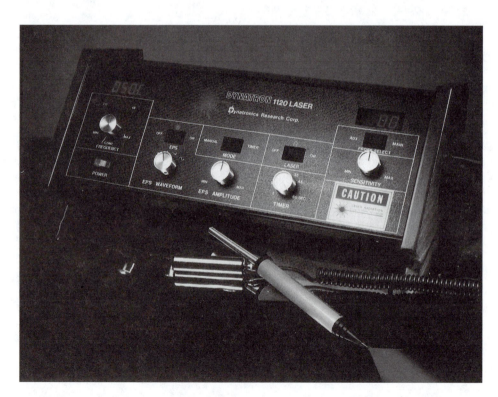

FIGURE 28–4   Helium-Neon (HeNe) laser. (*Reproduced with permission from Dynatron Research Co.*)

cal evidence indicate that the application of laser is effective in wound care and pain management.[3]

Success using laser therapy appears to depend greatly on dosage delivered. The effects of laser conform to the Arndt-Shultz principle by which weak stimuli augment physiologic activity, moderately strong stimuli impede physiologic activity, and very strong stimuli seize physiologic activity.[6] The therapeutic window of effective doses has been shown to exist between 0.5 J/cm^2 and 4 J/cm^2. Doses above this therapeutic window may be used in cases in which the bioinhibitory properties of laser are desired, for example, to dampen the rheumatoid process.[7]

DOSING

Energy density (the dosage) for laser irradiation is measured in J/cm,[2,8] where 1 Joule is equal to 1 W/sec. Dosing is therefore dependent on the power output of the laser unit in mW, time of exposure in seconds, and laser beam area in cm^2. The HeNe laser delivers a continuous waveform and has an average power of 1.0 mW. The GaAs laser delivers a pulsed waveform and has an average power of 0.04–0.4 mW. The objective of laser therapy is to deliver a specific quantity of Joules/cm^2; therefore, once the average power is determined, the intervention time per cm^2 can be calculated. For example, to deliver 1 J/cm^2, using an HeNe laser with average power of 1.0 mW,

$$T = (E/P) \times A$$
$$T = (1 \text{ J/cm}^2/0.001 \text{ W}) \times 0.01 \text{ cm}^2$$
$$T = 10 \text{ seconds}$$

where

T = intervention time for given area

E = energy in J per given cm^2

P = average power of laser unit

A = area of laser beam (0.01 cm HeNe laser)

There are charts available to assist in calculating intervention times for a variety of pulses.

CLINICAL APPLICATIONS

The use of laser irradiation for therapeutic purposes is relatively new; therefore, the physiologic and biologic effects of this application are still being explored. **Box 28–1 lists the two main clinical applications and corresponding rationale for the use of the low-level laser.** The effects of low-level laser are subtle, appearing to occur primarily at the cellular level. The strongest clinical support for LLLT is in pain management, especially rheumatic disorders, and for cutaneous wounds and ulcers.[3] Laser beams, like all other forms of radiant energy, can be absorbed by, reflected from, or transmitted through the media in which they travel. The effects of laser beams on biologic tissue are directly related to wavelength, depth of penetration, and dose. Wavelength, angle of incidence, and skin color affect the depth of penetration of the laser beam. Shorter wavelengths scatter more and therefore do not penetrate as deeply as longer wavelengths do. Laser beams applied at an angle of 90° incur less reflection of the laser beam from the tissue. Since there is less reflection of the applied energy, more energy is absorbed by the tissue. Up to 99% of laser energy is absorbed in superficial dermis. Darker skin color absorbs more energy than lighter skin color.[8] In addition, the condition of tissue plays an important role in the intervention outcome; dehydrated tissue and poor blood supply, for example, will absorb less energy than tissue that is well hydrated with good blood supply.

RECENT RESEARCH

Support—however, not confirmation—for the use of laser for therapeutic purposes has been strengthened through recent scientific investigation. The proposed physiologic and clinical effects attributed to LLLT include pain reduction, accelerated tissue healing, and possible retarding of biochemical changes during immobilization. Rood et al[9] found that laser had no effect on proliferation of normal keratinocytes in vitro; however, laser significantly affected migration of keratinocytes into wounds. This process of migration is critical to re-epithelialization and therefore is critical to wound healing. HeNe irradiation has been shown to alter the synthesis of differentiation-specific proteins of fibroblasts (collagen);[8] however, it appears that it does not alter the keratinocyte differentiation. Lucas et al[10] reported the results of using LLLT as an adjunct to standard decubitus care in 86 patients. LLLT had no significant effect on healing time in Stage III decubitus ulcers.

A meta-analysis completed by Beckerman et al[11] in 1992 assessed the efficacy of laser therapy on musculoskeletal disorders and skin disorders. They concluded, "Laser therapy appears to have specific

Box 28–1   *Indications and Rationale for Therapeutic Low-Level Laser Radiation*

Indication	Rationale
Tissue healing	Stimulate collagen formation by activation of fibroblasts and other cells involved in the proliferative phase of wound healing.
	Promote vasodilation.
Pain modulation	Decrease nerve conduction velocity.
	Alter the action of inflammatory chemicals involved in acute inflammation.
	Promote vasodilation.

therapeutic effect, especially for posttraumatic joint disorders, myofacial pain, and rheumatoid arthritis."[11] This supports earlier research suggesting LLLT reduces most of the symptoms found secondary to rheumatoid arthritis.[10] Carati et al[12] reported a favorable effect on lymphedema. As an intervention for postmastectomy lymphedema, participants received placebo or one cycle or two cycles of LLLT to the axillary region of their affected arm. Results revealed that two cycles of LLLT were effective in reducing the volume of the affected arm, extracellular fluid, and tissue hardness in one-third of patients after three months of intervention. No improvement occurred in a control group. King et al[13] have demonstrated the effectiveness of low-power laser auriculotherapy in significantly increasing the experimental pain threshold. Kleinkort and Foley[14] found similar effects of HeNe laser intervention on pain threshold. Walker[15] attributes laser analgesia to the release of serotonin and endogenous opiates. Enwenka[16,17] has shown laser to promote collagen synthesis and fibroblast proliferation along with augmenting the "tensile strength, tensile stress, and energy absorption capacity of healing tendons." Their research in 1990 showed that a daily application of low density (1J/cm^2) for 14 days was sufficient to increase density of collagen fibrils and load-bearing capacity in healing rabbit Achilles tendons.[18] Eckerdal et al[19] suggest that laser therapy, given as they describe, is an effective supplement to the traditional therapies used in the intervention of trigeminal neuralgia. Intervention protocol in their study consisted of 2J/trigger point, once a week for 5 weeks with a total cumulative energy density being 9.2 J/cm^2. Weintraub[20] demonstrates exceptional results with low-level laser therapy on patients with carpal tunnel syndrome. Electrophysiologic studies were performed on the median nerve pre and post each laser intervention. Significant improvement with elimination of clinical symptoms was identified in 77% of cases studied.[20] Flaws in the study design were apparent; however, the clinical observation is consistent with the proposal that laser interventions are a beneficial supplement in pain management. Use of LLLT as an intervention for carpal tunnel syndrome has good scientific support and FDA approval. As an example, Branco and Naeser[21] reported significant improvement in patients with chronic postsurgical failure (39 when using two types of LLLT, TENS, and secondary alternative therapies). More than 90% of subjects either had no pain or their pain was reduced by more than 50%. All subjects with prior failed surgical outcomes responded well. One- to two-year follow-up supported long-term positive effects in over 90%. Akai et al[22] conclude from their study that low-level laser has a "possibility for prevention of biochemical changes to bone and cartilage brought on by immobilization." Effective dosage used in this study was 3.9–5.8 W/cm^2. This dosage is much higher than others report using. Kana et al[23] claims intervention intensities should range from 40 to 50 mW/cm^2, achieving an energy density of 1–4 J/intervention. In 1999, DeSimone et al[24] demonstrated in vitro inhibition of the bacterial species *Staphylococcus aureus* and *Pseudomonas aeruginosa*. These findings may play a significant role in the use of laser therapy for wound care. Among all the supportive research, there are also those who conclude that "there is no difference between laser and the placebo"; the importance of this "placebo effect" is individually based.[25] Vasseljen[26,27] shows laser to have positive effects on the symptoms of "tennis elbow"; however, these effects were no better than "traditional intervention."[26,27] Vecchio,[28] in his study, concludes that laser therapy is no better than placebo intervention of rotator cuff tear. It is obvious that continued, well-controlled studies are necessary to prove the efficacy of laser therapy.

PROCEDURES

The operation of most laser units is simple. Here are the procedures for operating the Dynatron 1120 HeNe laser unit (see **Fig. 28–4**):

1. Expose and cleanse the skin, and explain the procedure to the patient.
2. Turn on the power switch.
3. Set the timer to the selected duration (for pain, 16–20 seconds; for wounds, 20–30 seconds per area).
4. Select the frequency (5–20 pulses per second (pps) for tissue healing and 20–80 pps for pain).
5. Find the low-impedance spots on the skin when the intervention requires this step.
6. Activate the laser by pressing the button on the wand (point finder). A light will stay on for the duration selected.
7. Turn off the power, and place the wand back in its holder.

Measuring Skin Impedance

The Dynatron 1120 has within it an electrical circuit that can measure skin impedance (see **Fig. 28–4**). To find the low-impedance spots, the therapist must have the patient hold an inactive electrode in one hand while the therapist completes the circuit by holding the wand used to find the spot. As the therapist moves the tip of the point finder along the skin in the suspected area, the low impedance values of the trigger points and acupuncture points are displayed relative to the impedance values of the surrounding tissue.

Determining the Dosage

The accepted dosage appears to lie between 0.5 J/cm^2 and 4 J/cm^2. Higher doses have been shown to have detrimental thermal and inhibitory effects on cellular physiology. The time and frequency of intervention is selected accordingly. Some suggested intervention dosages are as follows:[27]

Wound healing: 0.5–1.0 J / cm^2
Trigger point intervention: 1–3 J / cm^2

INDICATIONS AND CONTRAINDICATIONS

Many claims have been made regarding the effectiveness of LLLT in promoting tissue healing and pain management, including pain associated with trigger points.[3]

Since the low-power laser is a class III device, it poses an insignificant risk to humans unless the laser beam is directed toward the cornea of the eye. However, because little is known about the long-term effects, the therapist should avoid using lasers on pregnant women, the fontanels of infants, cancerous tissue, hemorrhagic areas, and photosensitive skin areas.[3] **Box 28–2 summarizes the contraindications and reasons for not using the low-power laser.**

The use of low-power laser as a therapeutic modality in physical therapy is gaining interest. More research is needed, however, to substantiate claims of its

Box 28–2 *Low-Level Laser Contraindications*

Contraindication	Rationale
Into the eyes	Potential damage to the retina or cornea may occur.
Over areas with active bleeding or suspected hemorrhage	Stimulation may promote vasodilation that contributes to further bleeding.
Over cancerous tissue	May increase tissue metabolism.
During pregnancy	Possible stimulation of the endocrine system may occur (effects yet to be determined).

usefulness. Because of the FDA regulations, data from investigative clinicians have been accumulating and will soon be analyzed. In addition, many research studies are in progress. If the data from these reports support the earlier and more-recent claims of LLLT effectiveness, the use of these devices by physical therapists will become unrestricted.

REVIEW QUESTIONS

1. What does the acronym LASER mean?
2. What does the acronym LLLT connote?
3. What are the properties of lasers that are different from ordinary light?
4. How does the Arndt-Shultz principle relate to the use of laser as an intervention?
5. What are the clinical indications for using laser?
6. What are the contraindications for LLLT?
7. Describe the method of clinical application of laser as an intervention.
8. What could physical therapists be doing to support or expand the use of this intervention?

KEY TERMS

low-level laser therapy (LLLT)
low-energy laser irradiation (LELI)

coherent light
collimation

cold lasers

REFERENCES

1. FDA Office of Training and Assistance, Center for Devices and Radiological Health: Fact Sheet. *Laser Biostimulation.* August 1985.
2. Wolbarsht ML, ed: *Laser Application in Medicine and Biology.* Vol 33. New York: Plenum; 1977.
3. Belanger AY: *Evidenced-Based Guide to Therapeutic Physical Agents.* Baltimore: Lippincott Williams & Wilkins; 2002.
4. Kleinkort JA, Foley RA: Laser acupuncture: Its use in physical therapy. *American Journal of Acupuncture* 1984; 12:51–56.
5. Kroetlinger M: On the use of laser in acupuncture. *Acupunct Electrother Res* 1980; 5:297–311.
6. Griffen, JE, Karselis, TC: Introduction to the Electromagnetic and Acoustic Spectra. In: Griffen, JE and Karselis, TC, eds: *Physical Agents of Physical Therapists,* 2nd ed. Springfield, IL: Charles C Thomas; 1982; 34–35.
7. Laakso L, Richardson C, Cramond T: Factors affecting low level laser therapy. *Australian Physiotherapy* 1993; 39(2).
8. Goldman L, Rockwell J: *Lasers in Medicine.* New York: Gordon & Breach; 1971.
9. Rood P, Haas A, Graves P, et al: Low-energy helium neon laser irradiation does not alter human keratinocyte differentiation. *J Invest Dermatol* 1992; 99:445–48.
10. Lucas C, van Gemert MJ, de Haan RJ: Efficacy of low-level laser therapy in the management of stage III decubitus ulcers: A prospective, observer-blinded multicentre randomized clinical trial. *Lasers Med Sci* 2003; 18(2):72–77.
11. Beckerman H, Bouter L, Cuyper H, et al: The efficacy of laser therapy for musculoskeletal and skin disorders: A criteria-based meta-analysis of randomized clinical trials. *Phys Ther* 1992; 72(7).

12. Carati CJ, Anderson SN, Gannon BJ, Piller NB: Treatment of postmastectomy lymphedema with low-level laser therapy: A double-blind, placebo-controlled trial. *Cancer* 2003; 98(12):2742.

13. King C, Clelland J, Knowles C, Jackson J: Effect of helium-neon laser auriculotherapy on experimental pain threshold. *Phys Ther* 1990; 70(1).

14. Kleinkort JA, Foley RA: Laser acupuncture: Its use in physical therapy. *American Journal of Acupuncture* 1984; 12:51–56.

15. Walker JB: Relief from chronic pain by low-power irradiation. *Neurosci Lett* 1983; 43:339–44.

16. Enwemeka C, Cohen E, Weber DM, Duswalt EP: The biomechanical effects of GaAs laser photostimulation on tendon healing. *Phys Ther* 1992; 72(6).

17. Enwemeka C, Gum S, Reddy K, et al: Combined ultrasound, electric stimulation, and laser promote collagen synthesis with moderate changes in tendon biomechanics. *Am J Phys Med Rehabil* 1997; 76(4).

18. Enwemeka CS, Rodriguez O, Gall NG, et al: Morphometric of collagen fibril populations in HeNe laser photostimulated tendons. *J Clin Laser Med Surg* 1990; 8:151–56.

19. Eckerdal A, Bastian HL: Can low-reactive-level laser therapy be used in the treatment of neurogenic facial pain? A double blind, placebo-controlled investigation of patients with trigeminal neuralgia. *Laser Therapy* 1996; 247–52.

20. Weintraub M.: Noninvasive laser neurolysis in carpal tunnel syndrome. *Muscle and Nerve* 1997; 20:1029–31.

21. Branco K, Naeser M: Carpal tunnel syndrome: Clinical outcome after low-level laser acupuncture, microamps transcutaneous electrical nerve stimulation, and other alternative therapies—an open protocol study. *J Altern Complement Med* 1999; 5(1):5–26.

22. Akai M, Mariko U, Maeshima T, et al: Laser's effect on bone and cartilage change by joint immobilization. *Laser Surg Med* 1997; 21:480–84.

23. Kana JS, Hutschenreiter G, Haina D, et al: Effect of low-power density laser radiation on healing open skin wounds in rats. *Arch Surg* 1981; 116:293–96.

24. DeSimone N, Christianson C, Dore D: Bactericidal effect of 0.95 mW helium-neon and 5 mW indium-gallium-aluminum-phosphate laser irradiation at exposure times of 30, 60, and 120 seconds on photosensitized *Staphlococcus*. *Phys Ther* 1999; 79(9): 839–46.

25. Malm M, Lundeberg T: Effect of low-power gallium arsenide laser on healing of venous ulcers. *Scand J Plast Recontr Hand Surg* 1991; 25:249–51.

26. Vasseljen O, Hoegn N, Larsen S: Low-level laser versus traditional physiotherapy in the treatment of tennis elbow. *Physiotherapy* 1992; 78(5):329–34.

27. Vasseljen O, Kjeldstad B, Johnsson A, et al: Low-level laser versus placebo in the treatment of tennis elbow. *Scand J Rehab Med* 1992; 24:37–42.

28. Vecchio P, Cave M, King V, et al: A Double-blind study of the effectiveness of low-level laser treatment of rotator cuff tendonitis. *Br J Rheumatol* 1993; 32:740–42.

VI

Additional Clinical Applications

This section addresses the use of electromyographic (EMG) feedback (Chapter 29) for rehabilitation of individuals with neuromuscular and musculoskeletal dysfunction. It presents biofeedback training principles and discusses biofeedback instrumentation. Chapter 30 introduces the reader to pelvic floor rehabilitation and the underlying pathologies encountered in these interventions, which include such agents as neuromuscular electrical stimulation (NMES) and biofeedback.

29

Biofeedback

GARY KRASILOVSKY, PT, PhD

Chapter Outline

Biofeedback (BF) refers to procedures used to assist a person in learning, through auditory or visual means, to gain some voluntary control over physiologic responses. These may be responses not ordinarily under voluntary control or ones that the individual generally has the ability to control but presently cannot for some reason. Using some external means of monitoring, BF enables a person to receive information about a physiological event as it is occurring. By receiving this information instantaneously, the individual may correct and/or gain better control of the event being monitored.

The simplest and most common forms of BF are commonplace visual and auditory cues. For example, a clinician may give verbal cues to guide the patient as an activity is being performed (auditory), or the patient can observe the activity in a mirror while performing it (visual). However, audio or visual information revealed through electronic BF devices or other equipment has the advantage of being objective. For example, by standing on two sets of scales, an individual can see whether the weight is equally distributed over each side of the body, or by observing the display of an EMG can determine whether a muscle is increasing or decreasing its intensity of contraction.

The feedback that an individual receives when performing an activity can be used for either positive or negative reinforcement. When BF indicates that an activity is being done incorrectly or has not achieved the desired goal, the patient can make adjustments to alter the audio/visual information being received and thus improve performance.[1] This immediate display of an event as it occurs can be useful for clinicians when documenting performance and monitoring progress.

This chapter discusses (1) EMG feedback, (2) the clinical uses of BF, (3) galvanic skin response, and (4) thermal feedback. The primary focus of the chapter will be on electromyographic (EMG) feedback as it is used to improve motor control in patients with impairments due to cerebral vascular accident (CVA), impaired selective recruitment of specific prime movers (eg, biceps for elbow flexion), inability to activate a muscle after trauma or surgery (including myoelectric prosthesis training), dystonia, and other neuromuscular/orthopedic conditions. An introduction to kinesiological EMG is also included to facilitate further utilization of this research methodology.

PROCEDURES

When using biofeedback for such activities as altering electrical activity in skeletal muscle, altering cutaneous skin temperature, or redistributing weight bearing, there are several procedures that are followed. These procedures include (1) detection and amplification of the presenting physiologic response, (2) conversion of the response to some easy-to-process form of information, and (3) immediate feedback of this information to the patient.

These stages of BF training are designed to help the patient to do the following:

- attain awareness of both present and desired physiologic activities and movement patterns;
- gain control of specific bodily activity; and
- transfer self-control to functional use.

As the first step in regaining control over a bodily function like muscle activation, the patient must obtain information about performance. For example, a patient who sustained a stroke 6 weeks ago may be unaware of excess ankle plantar flexion during stance due to a sensory deficit. The first step in retraining ankle control is making the patient aware of the difference between the present movement pattern and the desired normal movement. Once this awareness is achieved, the patient is ready for the second stage of retraining.

The second stage in gaining control over an activity requires concentration, repetition, and knowledge of performance. Through repetition of a corrected muscle activation, performance will improve and become easier. Eccentric ankle plantar flexion control for the stroke patient is not an easy task. The activity must be performed as correctly as possible, with immediate feedback. *The key is repetitive performance, with the patient receiving immediate knowledge of performance indicating when the task was performed correctly or incorrectly.* Eventually, performance is demanded of the patient without immediate feedback, but simply with monitoring by the therapist. Correct performance demonstrated repeatedly indicates that the subject has gained control over the desired activity. Training does not stop here.

In the third stage, the patient learns to transfer this self-control to functional use. Functional gains demonstrate that training in the clinical setting has carryover to all settings. After the patient has gained control of ankle movements, the training becomes more diversified. For example, ankle dorsiflexion without inversion may first be controlled by the patient in a chair or supine with the knee extended, but training must be expanded to include all functional activities that require this muscular control. Training in standing, during an isolated swing phase, and eventually a stance phase (on the involved side), must be continued until the patient has the same level of isolated control. Until this last training stage is accomplished, there will not be functional carryover.

In order to achieve the desired goals of training, the therapist should adhere to the following:

- Focus on a specific task that results in short-term functional gains.
- Train in a calm, nondistracting environment.
- Give brief, clear verbal commands. These commands should assist the patient in interpreting the biofeedback information and test the patient's understanding.
- Avoid patient fatigue, which will occur quickly during the early training sessions. Frequent rest periods are essential.
- Encourage correct performance, and correct errors as they occur. The therapist must motivate the patient.
- Include repetition until functional carryover occurs without BF.
- Gradually increase the difficulty of exercises. This increase helps the patient achieve steady improvement without undue frustration.
- For optimal carryover, incorporate training into functional use in daily living.
- Provide a home program to enhance the effectiveness of the training sessions.
- Begin rehab with limb supported, and advance to unsupported.
- Provide a distal contact with appropriate resistance.
- Use facilitation techniques such as quick stretch, tapping, vibration, quick icing, and/or neuromuscular electrical stimulation. These should be withdrawn as soon as the patient is capable of achieving activation without these external techniques.

Electromyographic (EMG) Feedback

The **electromyographic (EMG) feedback** signal is a display of action potentials generated by one or more motor units. The motor unit is the functional unit and is composed of one anterior horn cell (AHC), the axon, and all the muscle fibers innervated by that AHC. A motor unit fires in an all-or-none fashion, producing a motor unit action potential (MUAP) that can be picked up with surface or needle electrodes. This action potential is analogous to the recordings taken when performing an electrocardiogram. Each MUAP is produced as a summation of the discharge of all muscle fibers in that motor unit. In EMG BF, the raw EMG signal of each motor unit is not displayed. Instead, a simplified format called *integrated EMG* is shown. The integrated EMG displays the activity of the muscle being monitored. This display is proportional to the extent of the muscle contraction.[2] The integrated EMG signal will become larger as more motor units are recruited. It is important to realize that the EMG signal is greatly affected by the muscle length and corresponding electrode spacing on the muscle being monitored.[3] A more detailed description is included in the kinesiological EMG section at the end of the chapter. Specific techniques for recording will also be discussed later in this chapter.

Motor Unit (MU) Recruitment

Motor unit recruitment is the primary factor in determining the quantity of EMG feedback. As more motor units (MUs) are recruited, the signal displayed on an EMG feedback device becomes larger. *Recruitment* refers to the number of MUs and the frequency of firing of each MU. Recruitment begins with the small, Type I (slow-twitch and fatigue resistant) MUs.[4] Tension generated by these motor units is very small. As slightly more tension is required, the frequency of firing of these Type I MUs will increase to about 15 per second. If additional tension is needed, a second Type I MU is recruited at a lower frequency of firing. The frequency of firing will increase as more tension is required. This sequence of increased rate of firing and recruitment of additional MUs continues as greater force is required. Throughout this process, Type I MUs are recruited first for slower-speed, low-effort activities. As speed and/or effort increases, type IIa MUs are recruited. These MUs are fast-twitch but fatigue-resistant. The last type of MUs recruited are Type IIb, which are fast-twitch, generate high tension, and are rapidly fatiguing. For further description of various aspects of MUAPs, refer to **Chapter 22**.

EMG Feedback Devices

A variety of devices is available for performing **EMG feedback (Fig. 29–1).** Most small portable units have one or two channels. Desktop units have 2 to 6 or more channels. All have audio and visual modes. Some units are capable of interfacing with computers for expanded data acquisition and menus of data display.[a–f] (See Notes for Biofeedback Systems at the end of this chapter for referenced manufacturers from which such information can be obtained.)

Modes of Feedback.   The most common displays of EMG feedback are visual and auditory. Visual feedback may consist of a light bar, a series of lights that illuminate proportional to the amount of activity; a meter with the indicator needle moving from left to right to indicate increased activity; a computer monitor that presents a rising or lowering bar graph, with each bar representing one channel (some isokinetic equipment has this available); and a sinosoidal wave sweeping slowly across a screen, increasing in slope proportional to the physiologic event being monitored (two channels can be represented by two colors) (**Fig. 29–2**).

Auditory feedback will typically consist of a clicking sound increasing with a frequency proportional to muscular activity. Most units provide this feedback

continuously while in operation, and some have feedback available in an all-or-none fashion, using a threshold or goal for turning the auditory feedback on or off. Most devices provide a visual goal to serve as a target for performance. This visual goal may trigger auditory feedback when the threshold is achieved. The therapist sets the threshold or goal to a specific level of activity, and the auditory feedback begins only if that level is achieved.

To enhance training, the threshold may be set at a level that the patient can achieve on the basis of previous performance and then can raise during the training session. **Tables 29–1** and **29–2** provide examples of an EMG feedback intervention data form that is used to document the setup and patient performance.

For inhibition of an overactive muscle, the threshold is set so that the device will either turn on or off when the level of activity falls below the threshold. Here is a clinical example. On attempted elbow extension, a patient's triceps are activated, but coactivation of the biceps restricts movement. To inhibit bicep activity, the auditory feedback can be set to click proportional to biceps activity, resulting in auditory feedback proportional to the biceps response. The triceps activity could be displayed visually, or not at all.

The modes of feedback are related to the selection of a one- or two-channel unit. Two-channel units have training advantages over one-channel (eg, two channels allow comparision from side to side in evaluating gait). The first channel can be used to monitor the prime mover, or the problematic, muscle but a second channel offers flexibility in training and additional feedback to the patient and therapist. For example, with spasticity or rigidity, the antagonist

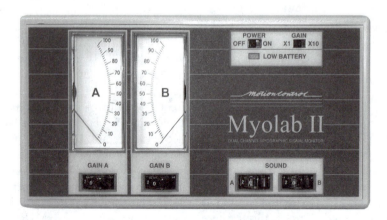

FIGURE 29–1   EMG unit. (*Reproduced with permission from Motion Control, Inc., Salt Lake City, UT.*)

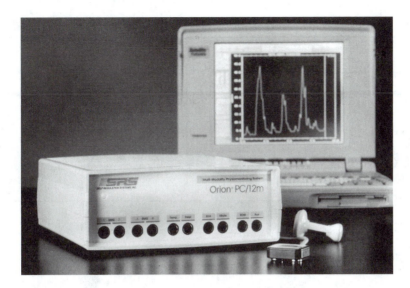

FIGURE 29–2 Computer monitor EMG display. The Orion® PC office system shows a typical biofeedback display during pelvic floor contractions. Note that multiple biofeedback modalities are possible with this unit, including monitoring temperature and respiration as well as multiple simultaneous muscle groups. The Perry Vaginal™ sensor is also shown. (*Courtesy of SRS Medical Systems, Inc., Burlington, MA.*)

muscle can be monitored along with the prime mover. A stabilizer muscle can be monitored while monitoring the primary mover. Both muscles being trained are displayed on the visual channel, and the muscle being inhibited (the secondary muscle) uses the auditory feedback channel. When working on inhibition as a goal, the auditory channel is the channel of choice because it allows patients to close their eyes and relax while focusing on gaining control of the overactive muscle. This feature obviates the need for the patient to watch the feedback device while trying to inhibit a muscle.

Amplifier and Specifications. All EMG feedback devices sold today meet or exceed minimum requirements. They address an amplification range between 0.1 and 1000 μV. The frequency spectrum for most EMG signals recorded with surface electrodes is in the range of 20 to 500 Hz.[2]

Types of Electrodes. Surface electrodes are the most common recording electrodes used in therapeutic EMG. There are many types of surface electrodes (**Fig. 29–3**). They include round discs 1–2 cm in diameter with a wire lead soldered to the back; block

electrodes with two or three round silver-silver chloride–coated metal discs embedded in a plastic housing; and singular round silver-silver chloride electrodes encased in a plastic cup that surrounds the electrode.[g] Electrodes are also available that have a built-in preamplifier. Smaller-diameter (4 mm) electrodes record from a smaller area of the muscle than do larger ones. In general, smaller-diameter electrodes are better for training. Electrodes may be reusable or disposable. Even the disposable electrodes can be reused if cleaned and dried immediately after each use. Needle electrodes are highly specific. They record only from a very small area within the individual muscle in which they are inserted. Needle electrodes (ie, intramuscular electrodes) are primarily used for diagnostic and kinesiological EMG studies. More details on the electromyographic signal display and instrumentation are discussed in the section on kinesiological EMG.

Surface electrodes are commonly employed because they are noninvasive and easy to apply and use. They are clean and are easy to obtain and to apply to the patient. However, they may pick up electrical activity from adjacent muscles (**volume conduction**) and therefore are nonspecific for one small muscle.

TABLE 29–1   *EMG Feedback Intervention Data: Facilitation*

PATIENT: _____ AGE: _____ DIAGNOSIS: _____

ONSET OF DISABILITY: _____ DISABILITY: _____

THERAPEUTIC GOAL: _____

ELECTRODE PLACEMENT: _____

POSITION OF PATIENT & LIMB: _____

ASSISTIVE DEVICES: _____ SENSATION: _____

FEEDBACK: AUDIO _____ VISUAL _____ APHASIA? _____

THERAPIST: _____

EMG Output

Date	Settings	AROM	Initial	Final	Velocity of motion	Comments

Notes: _____

_____

_____

_____

_____

_____

TABLE 29–2   *EMG Feedback Intervention Data: Inhibition*

PATIENT: _____ AGE: _____ DIAGNOSIS: _____

ONSET OF DISABILITY: _____ DISABILITY: _____

THERAPEUTIC GOAL: _____

ELECTRODE PLACEMENT: _____

POSITION OF PATIENT & LIMB: _____

ASSISTIVE DEVICES: _____ SENSATION: _____

FEEDBACK: AUDIO _____ VISUAL _____ APHASIA? _____

THERAPIST: _____

Resting EMG Readings

Date	Settings	Spasticity	Velocity of Motion	Initial	Final	Threshold	Comments

Notes: _____

_____

_____

_____

_____

_____

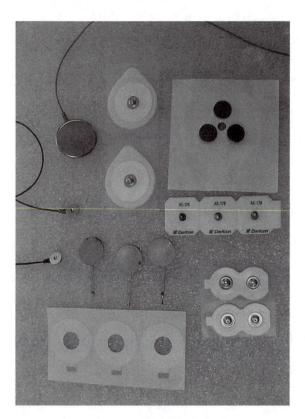

FIGURE 29–3   Recording electrodes.

Surface electrodes can be used only to record from superficial muscles, and they are susceptible to movement artifact (electrical noise) (**Table 29–3**).

Electrodes with built-in preamplifiers have many advantages. Although these are more expensive, they do eliminate changes in resistance that may occur between the electrode and the skin, and they are less sensitive to movement artifact. Deep muscles can be monitored only using needle electrodes. If these are not disposable needles, they require sterilization. These do, however, eliminate the disadvantages of surface electrodes.

When using surface electrodes, only superficial muscles can be monitored. It is best to determine what goals are the most important and realistic for the patient, and then to choose therapeutic techniques that will have the greatest impact on achieving these goals. Since BF units use one or two channels, the therapist must carefully select the most appropriate muscles to accomplish the goal. The larger the muscle belly, the easier to isolate its recording. Activity from smaller muscles in close proximity can be recorded, but greater care must be used to determine whether the signal is from the target muscle. An antagonist muscle can produce volume conduction[1,5] (displaying electrical activity from adjacent muscles) that will be picked up from electrodes on the opposite side of the limb. Many clinicians recommend using a two-channel unit even if only one muscle is going to be trained. The second channel can be used to monitor for volume conduction from adjacent active muscles and to determine whether the signal you are getting is from the target muscle. Many publications detail optimal electrode placement sites for specific muscles.[6–9]

EMG Biofeedback Procedures

Electrode Placement.   Proper electrode placement is essential for maximal benefit of EMG feedback. Both active electrodes should be located over the belly of the muscle, in a line that is parallel to the arrangement of muscle fibers. The distance between the two electrodes has a direct effect upon the amplitude of the action potentials. The closer the electrodes are, the lower will be the amplitude of the EMG signal (because of a smaller recording area); and the farther apart the electrodes are, the higher will be the amplitude of the EMG signal. For example, it has been shown that on the forearm extensors, electrodes placed 6 cm apart on average recorded 20% higher amplitude than those placed 3 cm apart.[10] On forearm flexors, the amplitude would vary on average 60% with electrodes placed 7 cm apart versus 3.5 cm. Recall that the farther apart the electrodes are, the greater will be the possibility of recording electrical activity from adjacent muscles caused by volume conduction. Electrodes should not be placed over bone, scar tissue, or tendon. A third electrode, or *ground* electrode, is attached on adjacent tissue near the muscle to be tested. The ground electrode must be larger in area than the recording electrodes. Low-intensity electrical stimulation can be used to localize the muscle belly by observing the clinical response of the contraction.

Recording Setup

1. Lightly abrade and cleanse the skin to reduce skin resistance. If body hair is present over the muscle to be monitored, shaving the area first will help improve adherence of the adhesive collar to the skin. This will also assist in relocating the electrode site

TABLE 29–3   *EMG Electrodes: Advantages and Disadvantages*

Advantages—Surface	Disadvantages—Needle Electrodes
Many types and sizes of electrodes are available, including disposable and reusable.	Reuseable needles must be sterilized and burrs removed.
Can include a built-in preamplifier for improved performance.	Monopolar electrodes record from large area.
Is noninvasive. Is easy to clean and apply to patient.	Is invasive. Daily use is not practical.
Is inexpensive and easy to purchase.	Needles are more expensive.
Electrodes can be embedded in plastic to control distance between each recording electrode.	Electrode placement is not easily replicable.
Advantages—Needle Electrodes	**Disadvantages—Surface Electrodes**
Is only electrode that can record from deep muscles.	Can record only from superficial fibers of superficial muscles.
Used for diagnostic testing and kinesiological evaluations.	Can be used only for general biofeedback applications.
Record primarily from the muscle they are inserted in (no volume conduction).	May pick up EMG signal from adjacent muscles (volume conduction).
Has less risk for movement artifact.	Has increased risk of movement artifact.
Has quick insertion (setup) time.	Setup time is longer than for needle electrodes.

during an ongoing training program. Cleanse the area with alcohol, and completely dry the skin.

2. Prepare the electrodes, being sure that they are clean.

3. Mark the skin where the electrodes are to be placed.

4. Apply gel evenly to the electrode to ensure good contact between the electrode and the skin. Too little gel will reduce the recording of the muscle action potential, and too much gel will allow too much movement between the electrode and the skin and will increase the recording area of the electrode. If the gel spreads out from under the electrode, it may come in contact with the adjacent electrode or gel. This contact will form an electrode gel bridge, causing the two adjacent electrodes to act as one large electrode, and the recording will be compromised.

5. Place the electrodes on the patient. Be sure that they are bonded well to the skin, allowing no electrode movement. Methods include adhesive collars, velcro bands, and adhesive tape; any

method can be used as long as the electrodes are held in place. Secure the adhesive collar or tape first, *not* pressing down on the middle of the electrode. The use of electrodes with smaller surface area, embedded in a plastic cup, with the recording surface slightly recessed within the cup, is one workable choice. This allows filling the "well" to the surface of the plastic with gel and using either double-sided adhesive collars or tape.

6. Place the two smaller (active) electrodes over the belly of the targeted muscle, and place the larger (ground) electrode on adjacent tissues equidistant from both active electrodes.

7. When removing electrodes, mark the middle of the recording sites with indelible ink to ensure consistent placement of each electrode on the next session.

8. *For outpatients:* Provide the patient with a marking pencil to remark the electrode sites when necessary. Another method to improve consistent electrode placement is to use a transparency placed over the body part being monitored.

Surface landmarks can be marked directly on the transparency, and a hole punch can be used to indicate each electrode location. Any skin blemishes or landmarks can also be used.

The most common cause of artifact while performing EMG feedback is due to poor setup. To minimize artifacts and electrode impedance, observe the following:

1. Electrodes must be clean and in good condition.
2. There must be adequate gel producing a good interface between the skin and the electrode.
3. The electrode wires between the electrode and the amplifier must be secure, with as little movement as possible to eliminate movement artifact. Shorter wires reduce the possibility of artifacts (although they make movement more difficult).
4. If a computer monitor is being used for the visual display, neither the electrode wires (leads) nor the patient should get close to the monitor. An electromagnetic field exists around any electrical component.

The wires from the recording electrodes should not cross over any other wires, especially any power cords. The electromagnetic field produced by these components will be picked up by the EMG device, producing an unwanted signal. The therapist should not touch the visual display on the monitor while touching the patient. Since the patient is grounded, the clinician will act as a conductor of static electricity from the face of the monitor to the patient. Türker[11] provides a detailed description of problems associated with the recording and interpretation of EMG signals, including equipment components and recording techniques.

Troubleshooting. If the baseline level of feedback is elevated, check the following:

1. Be sure that the patient is not contracting any nearby muscles.
2. Determine whether the artifact is rhythmical. It may be 60-Hz interference from fluorescent lights (turn them off to see whether doing this eliminates the artifact); or if you are recording near the upper chest or shoulder, you may be picking up EKG or respiratory muscle activity.
3. With the patient relaxed, check that the two electrodes and ground are well-attached to the patient. If this step does not solve the problem, there are a couple of simple solutions:

- If the wires between the electrodes and BF unit are removable, replace one wire between one electrode and one amplifier channel. If the problem still exists, replace the second wire connector. Occasionally, there is an intermittent break in one of the wires, and this can cause artifacts.

- If the wires are not removable, then check that there is adequate gel between each electrode and the skin. You can do this by pushing down on the middle of the electrode or by checking that the electrode is in good contact with the skin. If the adhesive tape used is slack across the electrode, then the electrode can easily lift off the skin. If this step does not solve the problem, redo the patient setup with new electrodes. At least one unit has built-in electrode testing capability.[h] This will assist you in determining the problem site and correcting it as efficiently as possible.

Clinical Applications of EMG Feedback

Clinical research shows that BF can effectively be used to achieve control of key components for higher functional training.[12–21] *Common clinical applications for surface EMG biofeedback are listed in Box 29–1.*

Electromyographic BF is used in the training of patients with neuromuscular deficits that have resulted in poor motor control due to hyperactivity, hypoactivity, or poor position sense and balance. Electromyographic BF is used also in myoelectric prosthetic training and in transfer and gait training. An important component of a BF program is the evaluation of the patient, with appropriate documentation.

The evaluation and documentation must include a full history with adequate details for replication; passive ROM; types of pathologic synergistic movements and isolated control present; functional usage, with emphasis on highest level of functional ability; and functional limitations and their possible etiology. Testing variables such as patient and limb position, time of day, sequence of activities preceding evaluation, and instruction for muscle activation of inhibition should be included to improve testing reliability.

Upper Motor Neuron Lesions (UMNLs). Electromyographic BF may be used to help the therapist determine the muscular activity associated with the patient's limitations. It has been used extensively and has shown excellent results in the retraining of pa-

Box 29–1 *EMG Clinical Applications and Rationale*

Clinical Application	Rationale
Paralysis in individuals with CNS lesions	Assist in improving motor control and facilitate cortical output to the paretic muscles.
During reinnervation following a PNS lesion	Enhance recruitment of the motor units that are intact during the reinnervation process.
Specific strengthening of muscles with disuse atrophy	Maximize recruitment of desired muscles during muscle strengthening interventions.
Pelvic floor muscle dysfunction (See Chapter 30)	Strengthen and increase awareness of pelvic floor musculature and/or relax overactive musculature.
Spasticity in individuals with CNS lesions	Increase awareness and gain strategies to control hypertonicity.
Prevention of muscle substitution patterns	Increase awareness and gain control over inappropriate muscle recruitment patterns.
Promotion of relaxation for syndromes that cause pain	Increase awareness and control of excessive muscle activity in the presence of pain.
Promotion of relaxation for situations that increase anxiety	Increase awareness and control of excessive muscle activity in the presence of stress.

tients who have sustained a cerebral vascular accident.[12–21] When trunk position feedback or EMG feedback was used appropriately, the patient's gait showed greater improvement than when these feedback devices were not included in the rehabilitation program.

In an evaluation of the critical factors for success in post-CVA patients receiving biofeedback, Wolf et al[22] found no significant relationships between patient outcome and side of hemiparesis, age, sex, or number of BF sessions. They also found a higher probability of recovery of function in the lower extremity compared with the upper extremity. A 1-year follow-up of these patients revealed excellent carryover of the original gains made.[23] Recovery of function in the upper extremity requires a higher degree of control compared with the lower extremity. An investigation of upper-extremity improvement using EMG feedback in patients with a chronic CVA revealed that gains could be made in patients who sustained a CVA 1–4 years prior to the onset of a training program.[13] However, improvement in functional activities was not statistically assessed, only gains in control over key upper-extremity muscles. Sunderland[24] compared recovery of function in the upper extremities of patients with acute stroke who received EMG feedback in addition to their usual physical therapy. Patients receiv-

ing the EMG feedback achieved statistically significant levels of improvement compared with the group receiving unspecified physical therapy. In a critical review of EMG biofeedback research, Wolf[25,26] points out the need for functional measures to determine intervention outcomes following EMG feedback interventions.

The training approach is based on the evaluation and a listing of goals determined by the therapist and the patient. Typically, limitations to higher function in a patient post-CVA are due to impaired ability to recruit and control MUs, which presents as weakness in the agonist or overactivity in antagonist MUs and/or overactivity in other muscle groups of the extremity. Training should be based on improving control over muscles to achieve better motor performance. The basic concept of *specificity of training* applies when using this modality. The training must progress to the point of performing the exact activity that the patient is being prepared to perform independently. Carr and Shepherd[27] advocate the use of biofeedback as an appropriate tool to be utilized in conjunction with their approach that stresses functional movements.

The term **spasticity** is sometimes used incorrectly as all-inclusive for UMNL problems including coactivation. Spasticity and coactivation may be seen concurrently in a patient, but they are two different problems with different intervention approaches. In this chapter, *spasticity* refers to an increased response to stretch; and **coactivation,** or loss of selective control, refers to the undesired simultaneous discharge of MUs in multiple muscles.

A clinical example of spasticity is the activation of an antagonistic muscle such as the biceps during passive or active elbow extension. In cases of severe biceps spasticity, slow movements into elbow extension may help reduce the effects of spasticity. Coactivation can present only during voluntary active movements. When observing a patient who has sustained a CVA attempting to reach forward, the therapist may see a synergistic pattern with shoulder elevation and abduction, elbow flexion, pronation, and finger flexion, along with an inability to eliminate any of these components.[28,29] This inability selectively to recruit the individual components is a loss of selective control. Among factors that increase this coactivation is effort. The greater the effort of the patient in performing an activity, the greater the possibility of an associated reaction producing coactivation. Therefore, it is important to reduce the patient's effort through a training sequence such as the one that follows. Eventually, all activities being trained must be performed in a functional setting, with the level of effort being appropriate for the activity.

When recruited selectively, muscles that are part of a pathologic synergy pattern may be weak and may display difficulty producing and grading force production. Difficulty moving quickly and decreased exercise tolerance may be partly due to disuse and deconditioning. Endurance may also be greatly impaired. Eccentric training in patients with spasticity is a very effective approach to improve control,[29] but it does not produce a change in the patient's level of spasticity or antagonist muscle recruitment. Some clinicians[30] believe that decreasing spasticity does not increase motor control but that an increase in control and strength will decrease spasticity. The recommendation is that exercise should be more aggressive and individualized in these patients.

Hypertonicity.   Biofeedback can be used to assist a patient to learn a desired movement. The dual focus of intervention should be (1) activating the agonist while (2) controlling the amount of activity in the antagonist muscle. The sequence of training is a progression from simple to more complex movements as

the patient gains voluntary control over the muscles and movements being trained. To receive positive feedback, electrodes are initially placed close together over the involved muscle or muscle group, requiring control of only a segment of the entire muscle. As control improves, spacing the electrodes farther apart will elicit control over a greater proportion of the entire muscle. For example, a specific wrist flexor may be monitored initially, and eventually the electrodes placed over all of the flexor muscles. The progression of difficulty starting with one degree of freedom of movement is optimal. As control is acquired, another level of difficulty is added.

Suggestions for retraining by decreasing undesired muscle activation are described as follows:

- *Inhibit muscle during passive stretch.* Slowly elongate the problematic muscle passively, with the patient receiving EMG feedback of the level of muscle activation. Follow the sequence of training (awareness, control, carryover) at slow rates of passive elongation, progressing to functional rates of elongation.

- *Inhibit muscle following stretch.* Training should include maintaining control of MUs firing while the muscle is held in an elongated, functional position.

- *Inhibit (antagonist) muscle during voluntary movement by the prime mover.* During slow, voluntary movement (example, extension), maintain activation of the extensor muscle(s) while controlling the undesired flexors.

- *Inhibit muscle following a contraction.* For example, during reciprocal movement, the patient and the therapist must concentrate on quickly inhibiting the prime mover for one direction to allow for the reciprocal movement in the opposite direction.

- *Inhibit muscle during movements at other joint.* Associated reactions[28,30] often occur when patients use excessive effort to move. Only muscles that are necessary as stabilizers or prime movers are normally activated. Following a CVA, this selective control is lost, and the focus of intervention is to inhibit the associated reactions during functional training. As an example, the patient should become aware of what is occurring at the ankle plantar flexors during sit-to-stand activities or what is occurring at the hand during movements at the shoulder or elbow.

- *Inhibit during coactivation at that joint.* For example, a patient presents with overactivity of the gastrocnemius muscle during attempted ankle dorsiflexion. At first glance, the patient may not need strengthening of the dorsiflexors but may need awareness of excess activity in the gastrocnemius. The focus is not just inhibition, but training selective activation of the dorsiflexor while eliminating coactivation of the antagonist muscle.

There can be overlap in this progression, and the goal is always to achieve a more normalized movement pattern. *After any training session, ask the patient to practice the functional activity to assess carryover.*

Hypotonicity. Patients who have sustained a CVA, an incomplete spinal cord injury, or a peripheral nerve injury may present with severe weakness or flaccidity. Their basic movement deficit is due to an inability to recruit MUs in the affected muscles. The intervention approach is to increase MUs recruitment using the BF device, which will increase awareness of what they did to get a positive response. The goal is to obtain a signal, with or without limb movement, and then to increase the amplitude of the BF signal. In the more severe deficits, an isometric or an eccentric contraction against gravity may be all that is expected. Isometrics provide unlimited time to generate a contraction, and eccentric training allows training throughout a ROM even if the person cannot move against gravity (however, eccentrics produce lower microvolt readings than concentrics or isometrics). Functional activities require the ability to integrate all three types of muscle contractions. The EMG feedback approach is similar for weakness because of lower motor neuron lesion (LMNL).

Some patients with paretic or flaccid muscles may not respond quickly to a BF training program focused on producing normal movement patterns. This possibility may occur in a flaccid patient who is post-CVA, a patient with a peripheral nerve injury, or a recently postoperative orthopedic patient. In these cases, for optimal results, EMG feedback may be complemented by other therapeutic approaches, such as facilitation techniques of quick stretch, tapping, vibration, quick icing, and neuromuscular electrical stimulation. Electromyographic feedback can be combined with neuromuscular electrical stimulation (NMES), whereby the NMES is triggered by a certain (even if very low) threshold level of EMG activity. The NMES then produces a stronger contraction in the muscle being retrained, allowing patients to feel the movement that they are initiating. Research has shown that NMES combined with EMG feedback can be a very effective training tool.[31]

Neuromuscular electrical stimulation can also be used by the therapist in problem solving why a patient is not able to recruit a muscle. For example, a patient had a CVA, but with good ankle recovery except in the evertors. Is the deficit related to the CVA, or possibly to peroneal nerve compression at the fibula head? To evaluate before intervening with an EMG, use any AC NMES unit. Try stimulating the unresponding muscle group, and look at the response. If the weakness (or absence) is due to an UMNL, then the muscle should respond to AC stimulation. If there is no response to stimulation, then the problem may be in the peripheral nerve. Test the unit on yourself first.

Dystonia. *Dystonia* refers to abnormal, involuntary movements that can occur in any muscle group, may worsen with fatigue or emotional stress and anxiety, and are absent during sleep. The sustained muscular contractions produce twisting, repetitive movements and/or sustained abnormal postures of the limbs, head, or trunk.[32] A well-known example is spasmotic torticollis (ST), which is manifested by head extension, lateral flexion, and rotational components. Medical and surgical management includes pharmacology, surgery, and botox injections.[33] The ST form of dystonia has responded well to EMG feedback.[34] A long-term follow-up[35] revealed a 58% success rate based on 8–12 weeks of BF training. Long-term functional carryover occurred in 40% of all patients participating in the BF training and in 73% of the patients who had achieved at least some gains during the initial training program.

Patients with ST are trained by monitoring the EMG activity of bilateral sternocleidomastoid (SCM) muscles. Initial training will focus on obtaining awareness and relaxation of the overactive muscle. Eventually, strengthening the opposite SCM will be included. Brudny[34] and Cleeland[36] support the use of EMG feedback for improving control and muscle relaxation in patients with movement disorders.

Myoelectric Prosthesis. A myoelectric prosthesis is a power-driven prosthesis that uses electrical activity of a muscle or muscles to control the motorized component of the device. Movements performed typically include finger opening and closure, and elbow flexion and extension. The physical therapist may work with the patient in training voluntary control over the muscles in the stump to be used for control of the prosthesis. Many techniques described for EMG feedback training apply to training the patient for using a myoelectric prosthesis.

The first step in training is the selection of optimal control sites. The more distal are these sites on the residual limb, the easier it is for the prosthetist to incorporate them into the design of the prosthesis. Systems such as the Utah Arm[1] use one pair of sites for controlling the prosthetic components. Once the site selection is made, training proceeds as follows:

1. Teach the patient to activate the same muscle group on the uninvolved extremity to optimize the ability to identify target muscle contractions.

2. Ask the patient to perform bilateral contractions of the same muscle groups with the recording electrodes over the target muscle on the involved extremity.

3. Eventually, focus on activation of the target muscle on the involved extremity with relaxation of the antagonist muscles.

As training is started on selective control of the hand or elbow component, the recording electrodes should be moved around to locate the optimal site for EMG recording. Electrode placements may vary in the distal segment of the residual limb because of muscle reattachment. Training sessions are easier when using a device with a preamplifier incorporated into the surface electrodes, as described earlier.

A signal as small as 5 µV can trigger the device to turn on, with isolated contraction of the target muscle desired for smooth control of the prosthesis. Since myoelectric prosthesis provides reciprocal movements, a contraction of a specific agonist muscle group is used for one directional movement, and the contraction of the antagonist group will control the opposite directional movement of the prosthesis. Motor control is a function of the electrical difference between the two control sites, not necessarily the strongest signal at each site. A difference of 20–30 µV is preferred for good prosthetic control.[37] Training focuses on the patient's developing the ability to activate one muscle group while simultaneously keeping other muscle groups relaxed. Agonist/antagonist muscle pairs, separated anatomically by the greatest distance, are optimal control sites.

Once control is achieved, the therapist turns to the task of strengthening the control muscles and increasing their endurance for repetitive activities. Training will continue after delivery of the prosthesis and will include all functional aspects of use. These aspects (eg, graded controlled grasp and movement, reciprocal control, switching between hand and forearm, or elbow control) include essentially all movements required to achieve full control of the prosthesis. Once basic control of the prosthesis is achieved, training will continue to achieve functional control in as normal a movement pattern as possible. Compensatory movements of the trunk or shoulder are discouraged if the prosthesis has the capability of providing a normal movement pattern.

Balance and Weight Transfer.   Providing information on the relative position of their center of mass in relation to their base of support (weight-bearing distribution) helps patients maintain or improve upright posture and ambulation. A normal degree of postural sway occurs during static stance, requiring ankle strength[38] and sensory feedback.[39] Normal ambulation requires controlled weight transfer during the gait cycle. The training sequence begins where control is deficient. If standing upright is asymmetrical, with impaired weight bearing on one side, training begins with bringing the center of mass in midline, with an upright posture and equal weight bearing. Symmetrical stance is a common problem for patients with neurologic and orthopedic conditions who have limited or impaired weight bearing. When a patient is referred for partial weight bearing, a specific amount of weight bearing is not always indicated; interpretation is left to the therapist. A variety of clinical interventions focus on improving lower-extremity weight bearing by increasing strength and sensory awareness.[28–30,40] These clinically based techniques rely on the therapist's providing verbal feedback to the patient.

Forms of BF have been documented to greatly assist patients in gaining an awareness of the amount of weight that they are transferring onto the target limb.[40–42] Weight bearing can be objectively measured and taught with a variety of devices. Bathroom scales[43] are the least expensive and most readily available to instruct a patient in a predetermined amount of weight bearing. The patient places the left foot on one scale and the right foot on another, and accurate information is provided on the amount of weight

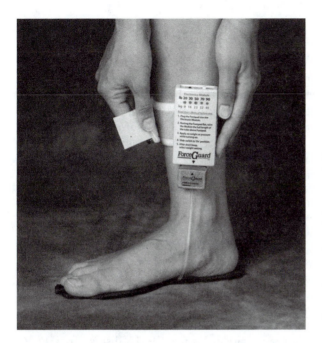

FIGURE 29–4   Force Guard weight-bearing system. The system enables the clinician and the patient to hear when the prescribed weight limit is being exceeded during therapy or at home. (*Used with permission from Impact Monitors, Inc., Longmont, CO.*)

placed on each foot. There are commercially available devices for functional training during ambulation[j,k] (**Fig. 29–4**). These devices fit inside the patient's shoe and can be calibrated to provide feedback based upon a predetermined amount of weight bearing. Utilization of an objective measurement tool to inform patients of their motor performance fits well within current relearning theories. Force plates and other highly sophisticated equipment[l] also exist for retraining and testing balance, weight shifting, finding center of pressure, and achieving vestibular rehabilitation. These devices can provide information on three aspects of balance: postural sway, postural symmetry, and limits of stability.

Using a feedback device to monitor upright trunk position has produced excellent results in improved sitting balance in patients who have sustained an acute stroke.[44] Compared with a control group receiving only standard physical therapy, 75% of patients receiving trunk angle feedback and physical therapy gained sitting balance after 10 days, compared with 15% of the control group. There was no significant difference in patients achieving sitting balance or ambulation at discharge. There was a significant differ-

ence in the overall rehabilitation period, with the BF group requiring a mean of 9.45 weeks and the control group 13.8 weeks to achieve the same goal.[44]

GALVANIC SKIN RESPONSE

Galvanic skin response (GSR) is defined as "the measurement of the change in the electrical resistance of the skin in response to emotional stimuli."[45] Sweat, which contains salt and increases conductivity, is produced as a response to an increase in the level of autonomic nervous system activation. A lie detector test, for example, depends on the GSR. Some GSR devices look like a computer mouse, with two stainless steel surfaces for two fingers to rest upon. The devices work by sending a minute electrical current through the skin, usually on the fingertips or the palm. The mode of feedback provided to the patient is typically in the form of a digital display, a light bar, or an audio feedback such as tone changes or clicks.

Skin impedence changes in response to many variables. For example, stress or pain results in overactivation of the sympathetic nervous system, which can be recorded through these changes in skin conductance.[46] Effects of this excessive stress response include increases in blood pressure, muscle tone, heart rate, and hormonal release. Training in GSR has been used to heighten awareness of an exaggerated stress response,[46] which is the first step in learning to reduce the associated symptoms. However, compared with thermal feedback training (later), there are few peer-reviewed publications on GSR.

Skin impedance varies greatly with the area of the body.[47] For example, the forearm has greater resistance than the palm. When using GSR as a measurement, a true baseline reading should be taken for comparison during training.[48] The site chosen for recording skin conductance is very important for optimal technique. It has been highly recommended that the distal phalanx be used for all measurements of skin conductance in the hand.[49]

Thermal Feedback

Thermal feedback, which is also called **temperature feedback (TFB),** is a modality that is used to help alleviate symptoms in patients with a variety of vascular-related disorders. For example, muscular (or tension) headaches respond well to EMG feedback, whereas many patients with migraines respond best to thermal feedback.[50]

Temperature feedback utilizes thermal sensors, placed on the body part, that provide immediate feedback on skin temperature. Just as stress results in increased muscle tone and increased GSR, so also it produces vasoconstriction in the extremities with resultant cooling of skin temperature. Temperature feedback is a modality that can indicate when vasodilation occurs with resultant increased skin temperature.

Migraine Headaches.   Migraines are believed to be caused by increased blood flow in cerebral blood vessels, with concurrent shunting of blood away from the extremities. One intervention approach has included skin-temperature BF with the goal of increasing peripheral blood flow and shunting blood away from the head. Results have been fairly positive.[51,52,53] When comparing temperature feedback, relaxation training, and cognitive training, children who were most successful in headache reduction were those who achieved the ability to increase finger temperature during their training sessions.[54]

Vascular Dysfunction.   Saunders et al[55] conducted a study using thermal BF of hand temperature followed by foot temperature, combined with autogenic training sessions in a patient with diabetes and peripheral vascular disease. Foot temperature rose during each TBF session, and the starting temperature was higher with successive sessions. By the twelfth session, IC symptoms had ceased, and follow-up at 1 year and 4 years revealed maintenance of these gains. In addition, with vasospastic conditions such as Raynaud's disease, TBF-induced vasodilation has been shown to be effective in reducing symptoms associated with vasoconstriction.

Hypertension.   The effectiveness of TBF in the management of hypertension has been debated extensively in the literature. Positive results have more often occurred on subjects who were not on medication,[56,57] whereas there have been greater discrepancies on effectiveness of TBF when used with patients who were on hypertensive medications.[58,59] Great care must be taken in monitoring the effectiveness of a BF program with this patient population.

KINESIOLOGIC EMG

Muscle function can be characterized in different movement situations by utilizing kinesiologic EMG. **Kinesiologic EMG** utilizes the electrical signals from the muscles being monitored and provides information related to normal and abnormal muscle recruitment during active movement and functional activities. This information can be used for therapeutic evaluation and interventions.

Quantification of EMG Data

EMG Signal Demodulation.[2,60,61]   The raw EMG signal is difficult to utilize for therapeutic purposes, so it is *demodulated* (altered) to be more understandable to the patient and therapist. With surface electrodes, the detail on each MU is minimal and not of great clinical significance for training purposes; therefore, the overall level of muscular activity is what is provided. **Figure 29–5A** displays raw EMG (measured in μV or mV) that contains a combination of positive and negative phases. This raw EMG is difficult to interpret quickly except for determining onset and cessation of muscle activation and gross changes in strength of contraction. Various methods of demodulation, or processing the EMG signal, change it into an easily understood visual display. **Figure 29–5B** displays full-wave rectification of the EMG signal (measured in μV or mV), where the raw signal is changed to a single polarity by either eliminating one polarity of the signal (half-wave rectification) or by inverting one polarity (full-wave rectification). Full-wave rectification is preferred because it preserves all the signal energy. A linear envelope (**Figure 29–5C**) is used to provide a window of activity that represents a profile of the EMG signal (measured in μV or mV) over a period of time. The signal rises above the baseline when the EMG signal begins, and it will remain elevated as long as an EMG signal is produced. As the EMG signal lessens, the display moves toward the baseline. It reaches baseline as the signal stops. The information obtained from the linear envelope includes the onset, duration, and overall pattern of the muscle contraction. Integration (**Fig. 29–5D**) refers to the total amount of EMG activity (measured in μV • seconds) occurring during a specific time interval, and integration is represented by the area under the curve of the visual display. Equipment that integrates the EMG signal usually indicates the timespan during which the integration continues; then the

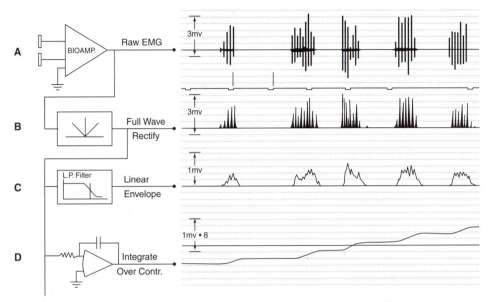

FIGURE 29–5   EMG demodulation. (A) Raw. (B) Rectified, full or half wave. (C) Linear envelope. (D) Integration. (*Reprinted with permission from Winter DA: Biomechanics of Human Movement, New York, NY, John Wiley & Sons, Inc. 1979, Fig. 7.10, p. 140.*)

processor resets back to zero and resumes integration to display the next time segment. For example, a visual display unit might integrate the EMG signal every 50 microvolt-seconds (ms), thereby displaying 20 data points per second. Each data point is a measurement of the total EMG activity for that 50-ms period. The time (ms) for each reset should be included in any documentation.

Demodulated EMG signals provide excellent information on control and overall performance of the muscle being monitored. The therapist and the patient will know the timing of muscle activation, its level of activity, and the quality of neuronal control. Other interpretations available, if displayed on a monitor, include the following:

- *Rise time of EMG activity* (**Fig. 29–6C**), which provides information on the relative speed of activating the muscle to the desired *amplitude* (see **Fig. 29–6C**). An isokinetic term for rise time is *time rate of tension development.*

- *Ability to relax after a contraction* (see **Fig. 29–6C**), which is especially problematic in patients with coactivation of muscles. These patients are often delayed in the rise time as well as more delayed in the time it takes to turn off a muscle for performance of a reciprocal activity. It is important for the therapist to focus not just on amplitude but also on a level of muscle activation necessary for the functional movement being trained. Patients

may cocontract the antagonist muscle to provide more resistance to the agonist, which increases amplitude in the target muscle. However, *this is not the goal of training.* Be aware of this possibility when training patients.

- *Ability to perform isolated movement* (**Fig. 29–6B**), which can be monitored when using a one- or two-channel unit. If only one channel is available and if your goal is to work on improving isolated control, then the channel should be used to monitor a pathologically activated muscle that you are training the patient to inhibit. Keep the FB down or absent while performing the desired movement. When two channels are available, one channel can monitor the prime mover while the other channel (or both channels) monitor one or more antagonist muscles.

- *Speed of smooth, reciprocal movements* (**Figs. 29–6A or C**), which is easily displayed with computer monitor types of visual feedback. The patient performs reciprocal movements and looks for a pattern showing only one channel active at a time while the movements are performed.

- *Fatigue* (**Fig. 29–6D**), which will be represented by an obvious decrease in the peak of the EMG display. This should trigger a rest period for the patient. Fatigue may result in an increase of coactivation and/or decreased coordination of the overall movement.

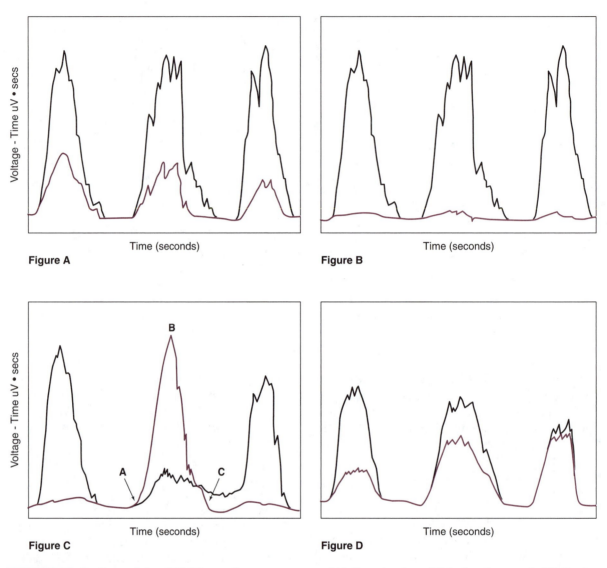

FIGURE 29–6   Demodulated EMG waveform parameters. (A) Coactivation. (B) Isolated control. (C) Reciprocal movements—rise time shown between A and B, force decay rate between B and C, amplitude at B, or the peak of the display. (D) Fatigue, as shown by the decrease in amplitude of one channel and the increase in coactivation due to loss of control.

Normalization of EMG

The myoelectric signal is used as an indirect measure of muscle force production. A standard of reference must be established for any intrasubject or intersubject comparisons during various activities. Such a process is referred to as *normalization*. This can also serve as a means of calibration prior to each session. Methods of normalization include the following:

- *Isometric maximal voluntary contraction* (**Fig. 29–7A).** This is the most commonly used method for normalizing EMG signals. The patient is asked to perform a maximal voluntary contraction in an isometric mode, and the maximal EMG signal is measured. This amplitude is then used to compare against all other measurements taken. Normalization is appropriate only for comparing isometric contractions. During isotonic contractions, the EMG production varies over changes

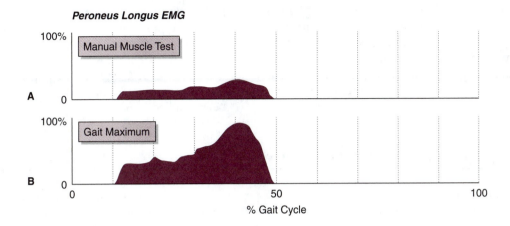

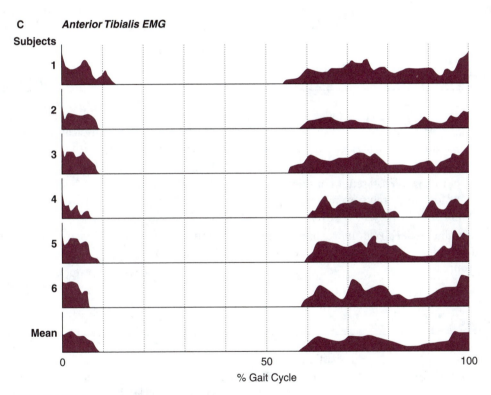

FIGURE 29–7   Normalization of EMG. (A) Isometric maximal voluntary contraction. (B) Normalization to the task. (C) Time adjusted. (*Source: Gait Analysis, Normal and Pathological Function, by Jacquelin Perry. Used with permission from Slack Publishers, Inc., Thorofare, NJ*).

in length of the muscle and is different with eccentric versus concentric contractions.

- *Normalization of the task* (**Fig. 29–7B**). This type of normalization has been used in gait analysis. The maximum output of a muscle during an activity is determined, and then output throughout the entire cycle of the activity is determined as a percentage of that maximal output. This method better accounts for the range of functional output required of a specific muscle.

- *Time adjusted average* (**Fig. 29–7C**). This step provides a comparison of the EMG activity for a specific muscle or for groups of muscles in relation to the time sequence of a specific activity.

For example, the unit often used for gait analysis employs a time-adjusted display that indicates when the muscle became activated during a cyclic activity; when there are changes in the amplitude throughout the active cycle of the muscle; and when the muscle ceased activity. This type of display is excellent for determining whether a muscle is being recruited during the normal timing of a functional activity, and whether activation is occurring too early, is prolonged, or is totally absent. This method of normalization is best when it is compared with the output required of a muscle for the same activity being studied.

SUMMARY AND FUTURE IMPLICATIONS

The reliability and validity of biofeedback devices is high, as long as patient setups are consistent and the equipment is used as described. Biofeedback is presently used in various modes for patient evaluation and training. Devices that patients can use independently or that help a patient to achieve optimal recovery will continue to be important in the armament of patient care. Biofeedback devices can also serve as objective measurement tools, even when not part of the daily intervention program. Continued research supporting the use of these devices in patient care is necessary to justify the patient effort and fiscal compensation provided.

REVIEW QUESTIONS

1. How is the raw EMG signal adapted for use in biofeedback?

2. Electromyographic feedback (EMG BF) can be used to reeducate the muscles in the leg of a patient with foot drop. What setup considerations are important for the therapist to produce an optimal session?

3. When is auditory feedback more appropriate than visual feedback? When is visual feedback more appropriate?

4. What are some ways in which EMG BF can be incorporated into a physical therapy intervention program for a patient with hemiplegia?

5. What are the stages of training that a patient must proceed through to obtain functional gains from a therapy program?

6. What are some good examples of the need to train a patient to improve weight transfer?

7. What is a clinical example of a disorder in which thermal feedback is appropriate?

KEY TERMS

biofeedback (BF)
electromyographic (EMG)
   feedback
volume conduction

spasticity
coactivation
galvanic skin response (GSR)

thermal feedback
temperature feedback (TFB)
kinesiologic EMG

NOTES FOR BIOFEEDBACK SYSTEMS

a. Thought Technology Ltd., 2180 Belgrave Ave., Montreal, Canada H4A 2L8.

b. J+J Engineering Inc., 22797 Holgar Ct. NW, Poulsbo, WA 98370.

c. SRS Medical Systems, Inc., 14950 NE 95th, Redmond, WA 98052.

d. Motion Lab Resources, 817 Maplewood Dr., Oxford, MS 38655.

e. Motion Control, 3385 West 1820 South, Salt Lake City, UT 84104.

f. Autogenic Systems (available through GE Miller, Yonkers, NY 10701).

g. Sensormedics, 22704 Savi Ranch Parkway, Yorba Linda, CA 92887 (800-231-2466).

h. J+J Engineering Inc., 22797 Holgar Ct. NW, Poulsbo, WA 98370.

i. Motion Control, 3385 West 1820 South, Salt Lake City, UT 84104.

j. Krusen Researach Center, Moss Rehabilitation Hospital, Philadelphia, PA 19141.

k. ForceGuard Weight-Bearing System, 1430 Nelson Road, Longmont, CO 80501.

l. NeuroCom International Inc., 9570 Lawnfield Rd., Clackamas, OR 97015.

REFERENCES

1. Cran HR, Kasman GS, Holtz J: *Introduction to Surface Electromyography*. Gaithersburg, MD: Aspen Publications; 1998.

2. Basmajian JV, Deluca CJ: *Muscles Alive: Their Functions Revealed by Electromyography*. 5th ed. Baltimore: Williams & Wilkins; 1985; 187–200.

3. Soderberg GL: *Kinesiology: Application to Pathological Motion*. 2nd ed. Baltimore: Williams & Wilkins; 1997.

4. Edgerton VR: Mammalian muscle fiber types and their adaptability. *Am Zoology* 18:113, 1978. In: McArdle WD, Katch FI, Katch VL, eds. *Exercise Physiology*. 3rd ed. Philadelphia: Lea & Febinger; 1991: 367–83.

5. Goodgold J, Eberstein A: *Electrodiagnosis of Neuromuscular Disease*. 3rd ed. Baltimore: Williams & Wilkins; 1983.

6. Basmajian JV, ed: *Biofeedback, Principles and Practice for Clinicians*. 3rd ed. Baltimore: Williams & Wilkins; 1989.

7. Goodgold J: *Anatomical Correlates of Clinical Electromyography*. Baltimore: Williams & Wilkins; 1984.

8. Pollock D, Sell H: Myoelectric control sites in the high-level quadriplegic patient. *Arch Phys Med Rehabil* 1978; 59:217–20.

9. Soderberg, GL: Recording Techniques. In: Soderberg GL, ed. *Selected Topics in Surface Electromyography for Use in the Occupational Setting: Expert Perspectives*. U.S. Department of Health and Human Services, NIOSH publication #91–100, 1992: 24–41.

10. Krasilovsky G: Surface electrode placement and its effect on the amplitude of EMG response. Unpublished paper, 1976.

11. Türker K: Electromyography: Some methodological problems and issues. *Phys Ther* 1993; 73:698–710.

12. Basmajian JV, Regenos EM, Baker MP: Rehabilitating stroke patients with biofeedback. *Geriatrics* 1977; 32:85–88.

13. Gianutsos JG, Eberstein A, Krasilovsky G, Ragnarsson KT, Goodgold J: Visually displayed EMG feedback: Single case studies of hemiplegic upper extremity rehabilitation. *Central Nervous System Trauma* 1986; 3:1, 63–76.

14. Wolf SL, Binder-Macleod SA: Electromyographic biofeedback applications to the hemiplegic patient. *Phys Ther* 1983; 63:9, 1404–13.

15. Burnside IG, Tobias HS, Bursill D: Electromyographic feedback in the remobilization of stroke patients: A controlled trial. *Arch Phys Med Rehab* 1982; 63:5, 217–22.

16. Mathieu PA, Sullivan SJ: Changes in the hemiparetic limb with training. I. Torque output. *Electromyogr Clin Neurophysiol* 1995; 35:8, 491–502.

17. Mathieu PA: Changes in the hemiparetic limb with training. II. EMG signal. *Electromyogr Clin Neurophysiol* 1995; 35:8, 503–13.

18. Brudny J, et al.: EMG feedback therapy: Review of treatment of 114 patients. *Arch Phys Med & Rehab* 1976; 57:2, 55–61.

19. Brudny J, Korein J, Grynbaum BB, Belandres PV, Gianutsos JG: Helping hemiparetics to help themselves. *JAMA* 1979; 241:814–18.

20. Basmajian JV: Biofeedback in rehabilitation: A review of principles and practices. *Arch Phys Med Rehabil* 1981; 62:469–75.

21. De Weerdt W, Harrison MA: The efficacy of electromyographic feedback for stroke patients: A

critical review of the main literature. *Physiotherapy* 1986; 72:108–18.

22. Wolf SL, Baker MP, and Kelly JL: EMG biofeedback in stroke: Effect of patient characteristics. *Arch Phys Med Rehabil* 1979; 60:96–102.

23. Wolf SL, Baker MP, and Kelly JL: EMG biofeedback in stroke: A 1-year follow-up on the effect of patient characteristics. *Arch Phys Med Rehabil* 1980; 61:351–54.

24. Sunderland A, Tinson DJ, Bradley EL, et al: Enhanced physical therapy improved recovery of arm function after stroke: A randomized controlled trial. *J Neurol Neurosurg Psych* 1992; 55:530–35.

25. Wolf SL: Electromyographic biofeedback applications to stroke patients: A critical review. *Phys Ther* 1983; 63:1448–55.

26. Wolf SL: Biofeedback. In: Gonzalez ER, Myers SJ, Edelstein, JE, et al, eds. *Downey & Darling's Physiological Basis of Rehabilitation Medicine.* 3rd ed. Boston: Butterworth Heinemann; 2001; 747–60.

27. Carr JH, Sheperd RB: *Movement Science.* 2nd ed. Gaithersburg, MD: Aspen Publications; 2000.

28. Sawner K, LaVigne J: *Brunnstrom's Movement Therapy in Hemiplegia.* 2nd ed. Philadelphia: Lippincott; 1992.

29. Davies, P: *Right in the Middle: Selective Trunk Activity in the Treatment of Adult Hemiplegia.* Berlin: Springer-Verlag; 1990.

30. Carr JH, Shepherd RB: *A Motor Relearning Programme for Stroke.* Heinemann: London; 1987.

31. Fields RW: Electromyographically triggered electric muscle stimulation for chronic hemiplegics. *Arch Phys Med Rehabil* 1987; 68:407–14.

32. Factor SA, Weiner WJ: Hyperkinetic Movement Disorders. In: Weiner WJ, Goetz CG, eds. *Neurology for the Non-Neurologist.* 3rd ed. Philadelphia: Lippincott; 1994; 121–45.

33. Greene P: Medical and Surgical Therapy of Idiopathic Torsion Dystonia. In: Kurlan R, ed. *Treatment of Movement Disorders.* Philadelphia: Lippincott; 1995; 153–82.

34. Brudny J, Grynbaum B, Korein, J: Spasmotic torticollis: Treatment by feedback display of the EMG. *Arch Phys Med & Rehabil* 1974; 55:405–08.

35. Korein J, Brudny J, Grynbaum B, Sachs-Frankel G, Weisinger M, Levidow L: Sensory feedback therapy of spasmodic torticollis and dystonia. Results in treatment of 55 patients. In: Eldridge R, Fahn S, eds. *Advances in Neurology.* New York: Raven Press; 1976; 375–401.

36. Cleeland CS: Biofeedback and Other Behavioral Techniques in the Treatment of Disorders of Voluntary Movement. In: Basmajian JV, ed. *Biofeedback: Principles and Practice for Clinicians.* 3rd ed. Baltimore: Williams & Wilkins; 1989; 159–68.

37. Motion Control, Inc. Videotape: Training the Client with an Electric Arm Prosthesis. Salt Lake City, Utah; 1995.

38. Wolfson LI, Whipple R, Amerman P, Kleinberg A: Stressing the postural response, a quantitative method for testing balance. *J Am Geriatr Soc* 1986; 34:845–50.

39. Shumway-Cook A, Anson D, Haller S: Postural sway biofeedback: Its effect on reestablishing stance stability in hemiplegic patients. *Arch Phys Med Rehabil* 1988; 69:395–400.

40. Bobath B: *Adult Hemiplegia, Evaluation and Treatment.* 3rd ed. Oxford, England: Heinemann; 1990.

41. deWeerdt, W, Crossley SM, Lincoln NM, Harrison MA: Restoration of balance in stroke patients: A single case design study. *Clin. Rehabil* 1989; 3:139–47.

42. Mack LA, Knotts SA: Weight-bearing limitation training: A comparison of traditional techniques with the use of electronic monitoring. Abstract presentation. Combined Sections Meeting of the APTA, Boston, MA, 1998.

43. Krasilovsky G: Weight-bearing feedback device. *Clin Management* 1991; 11:5, 64–66.

44. Dursun E, Humamei N, Dönmez S, Tüzünalp Ö, Cakei A: Angular biofeedback device for sitting balance of stroke patients. *Stroke* 1996; 27:1354–57.

45. *Taber's Cyclopedic Medical Dictionary*, Vol 18. Philadelphia: Davis; 1997.

46. Jacobs SC, Friedman R, Parker JD, et al: Use of skin conductance changes during mental stress testing as an index of autonomic arousal in cardiovascular research. *Am Heart J* 1994; 128:1170–77.

47. Panescu D, Cohen KP, Webster JG, et al: The mosaic electrical characteristics of the skin. *IEEE Trans Biomed Eng* 1993; 40:5, 434–39.

48. Cho SH, Chun SI: The basal electrical skin resistance of acupuncture points in normal subjects. *Yonsei Med J* 1994; 35:4, 464–74.

49. Scerbo AS, Freedman LW, Raine A, et al: A major effect of recording site on measurement of electrodermal activity. *Psychophysiology* 1992; 29:2, 241–46.

50. Grazzi L, Bussone G: Italian experience of electromyographic-biofeedback treatment of episodic common migraine: Preliminary results. *Headache* 1993; 33:8, 439–41.

51. Labbe EE: Treatment of childhood migraine with autogenic training and skin temperature biofeedback: A component analysis. *Headache* 1995; 35:1, 10–13.

52. Alien KD, McKeen LR: Home-based multicomponent treatment of pediatric migraine. *Headache* 1991; 31:7, 467–72.

53. Blanchard EB, et al: The role of home practice in thermal biofeedback. *J Consult Clin Psychol* 1991; 59:4, 507–12.

54. Osterhaus SO, et al: Effects of behavioral psychophysiological treatment on schoolchildren with migraine in a nonclinical setting: Predictors and process variables. *J Pediatr Psychol* 1993; 18:6, 697–715.

55. Saunders JT, Cox DJ, Teates CD, Pohl SL: Thermal biofeedback in the treatment of intermittent claudication in diabetes: A case study. *Biofeedback Self Regul* 1994; 19:4, 337–45.

56. Freedman RR: Physiological mechanisms of temperature biofeedback. *Biofeedback Self Regul* 1991; 16:2, 95–15.

57. Wittrock DA, Blanchard EB: Thermal biofeedback treatment of mild hypertension. A comparison of effects on conventional and ambulatory blood pressure measures. *Behav Modif* 1992; 16:3, 283–304.

58. Blanchard EB, Eisele G, Gordon MA, et al: Thermal biofeedback as an effective substitute for sympatholytic medication in moderate hypertension: A failure to replicate. *Biofeedback Self Regul* 1993; 18:4, 237–53.

59. Musso A, Blanchard EB: Evaluation of thermal biofeedback treatment of hypertension using 24-hour ambulatory blood pressure monitoring. *Behav Res Ther* 1991; 29:5, 469–78.

60. Gerleman DG, Cook TM: Instrumentation. In: Soderberg GL, ed. *Selected Topics in Surface Electromyography for Use in the Occupational Setting: Expert Perspectives.* U.S. Department of Health and Human Services, NIOSH publication #91-100; 1992; 44–68.

61. Perry J: *Gait Analysis: Normal and Pathological Function.* Thorofare, NJ: Slack; 1992.

30

Pelvic Floor Rehabilitation

MARILYN FREEDMAN, PT

LOUISE E. MARKS, MS, OTR

ELISE STETTNER, MS, PT

MARY WALSH, BS, RN

Chapter Outline

A working knowledge of pelvic floor muscle anatomy and function, along with bowel and bladder physiology, is essential when treating patients with **pelvic floor muscle dysfunction (PFMD).** This knowledge not only guides evaluation and intervention but also assists the therapist in deciding when a referral to another specialist is indicated. Physical therapists in the PFMD field work closely with other health care professionals, including colleagues experienced in myofascial and visceral mobilization techniques, gynecologists, urogynecologists, urologists, colorectal specialists, gastroenterologists, nurses, psychologists, and psychiatrists. It is recommended that PTs obtain some advanced training in applied psychophysiology and biofeedback, as well as urogynecological/colorectal anatomy and physiology. It is preferable to have at least a year of clinical experience in general physical therapy before treating patients with PFMD. Knowledge of excretory functions and sexuality, as well as a comfort in discussing these issues with patients, is an important asset in this field.

The Women's Health section of the American Physical Therapy Association (APTA) has ruled that the following three conditions must be met before the PT is allowed to either look at or touch a patient's perineum:[1]

1. Check state practice acts to see whether there are any exclusionary clauses.
2. Never treat the perineal area without a physician's signed order and a patient's signed consent.
3. Have completed clinical hands-on training at a recognized continuing education course, clinical affiliation, or academic setting.

A thorough review of the anatomy and neurophysiology of the urogynecological and colorectal systems is critical for clinicians who are treating conditions related to these areas.

Bladder, Bowel, and Pelvic Floor Dysfunction (Table 30–1)

Urinary Disorders

Storage Problems. **Stress urinary incontinence (SUI)** is defined by the International Continence Society as the involuntary loss of urine when the intravesical pressure exceeds the maximum urethral closure pressure in the absence of detrusor activity. Usually with stress incontinence, small amounts of urine are lost concurrent with the increased intra-abdominal pressure. Normally, the urethra is situated relative to the pelvic floor muscles so that when intra-abdominal pressure increases because of a cough, sneeze, or change of position, the amount of pressure exerted upon the bladder is equally transferred to the proximal portion of the urethra. This biomechanical transfer maintains urinary continence. However, if the pelvic floor muscles are weak, the proper urethral alignment is often lost, causing a transfer of pressure that results in insufficient closure and thus leakage. Aging, childbirth, disease, and muscle or nerve injury can result in pelvic floor muscle weakness. This muscle weakness can also cause pelvic organs to prolapse, creating additional mechanical difficulties by increasing the bladder neck angle, another cause of stress incontinence. A prolapse of the bladder into the vagina is called a **cystocele (Fig. 30–1).**

Urge urinary incontinence is the involuntary loss of urine associated with an uninhibited detrusor contraction that overwhelms the sphincter mechanism **(Fig. 30–2).** When the uninhibited bladder contraction arises from a neurologic condition such as multiple sclerosis, stroke, spinal cord injury, or spina bifida, the patient has detrusor hyperreflexia. On the other hand, **detrusor instability (DI)** presents with an uninhibited bladder contraction due to non-neurological conditions such as bladder or prostate cancer, bladder stones, or urethral obstruction. When there is no identifiable cause for the bladder contractions, the patient is said to have *idiopathic detrusor instability.* Episodes of idiopathic detrusor instability tend to occur when approaching a safe place to void (entering the home) or when hearing running water. The detrusor muscle has been conditioned to contract under these conditions, overriding normal inhibitory functions. Thus, a strong feeling of urgency is experienced, and control may be lost. This condition is sometimes referred to as "garage door" or "door key" syndrome.[2] Uninhibited bladder contractions associated with detrusor instability or detrusor hyperreflexia can cause leakage with or without symptoms of urgency (motor urge) or symptoms of urgency without incontinence (sensory urge).[3]

Urinary frequency related to storage difficulties can come as a result of the following: detrusor instability or hyperreflexia, poor bladder capacity (often from a learned behavior of frequent voidings), excessive liquid intake, interstitial cystitis, or bladder irritants. Bladder irritants are substances found in foods that cause detrusor contractions, urgency, and frequency. Such substances include caffeine, spicy foods,

TABLE 30–1 Intervention Options in Pelvic Floor Dysfunction (PFD)

	Education	Pelvic Floor Strengthening	Massage Myofascial Release	Synergy Training	Neuromuscular Relaxation with or without BFB	Dietary Counseling	Bowel or Bladder Retraining	Surface EMG	Electrical Stimulation	Ultrasound	Transelectrical Nerve Stimulation	Urge Suppression Techniques	Musculo skeletal	Cones	Dilators	Electrical Stimulation
Stress incontinence	X	X						X	X					X		X
Urge incontinence	X	X			X	X	X	X	X			X				X
Mixed incontinence	X	X			X	X	X	X	X			X		X		X
Urinary frequency or hesitancy with pelvic floor dyssynergia	X			X	X		X	X	X							
Fecal incontinence related to constipation	X			X	X	X	X	X								
Fecal incontinence related to pelvic floor weakness	X	X					X	X	X					X		
Constipation with pelvic floor dyssynergia	X			X	X	X	X	X								
Vulvodynia	X		X		X	X	X	X			X					
Painful episiotomy scar			X							X						
Levator ani syndrome	X		X		X		X	X	X		X		X		X	
Procalgia Fugax	X		X		X		X	X	X		X		X			
Interstitial Cystitis	X		X		X	X	X	X	X		X	X				
Irritable bowel syndrome, diarrhea dominant	X	X			X	X	X	X				X				
Irritable bowel syndrome, constipation dominant	X			X		X	X	X								
Descending perineal syndrome	X	X		X	X		X	X								

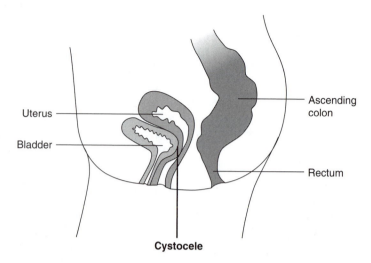

FIGURE 30–1   A cystocele is a hernial protrusion of the urinary bladder through the vaginal wall.

artificial sweeteners, and acidic foods or drinks. A stretched urethra, which can be due to fascial tightness from previous surgery or inflammation, can also increase sensory urgency and thus frequency of urination. Sometimes patients condition their bladders to empty frequently; fearful of urine leakage, they constantly empty their bladders to prevent accidents.

Mixed urinary incontinence is a condition wherein an individual has more than one type of incontinence, typically urge and stress urinary incontinence.

Emptying Problems.   **Overflow incontinence** results from either a noncontracting detrusor muscle, an obstruction to the bladder outlet, or both. An overfull bladder creates a pressure that overwhelms the sphincter mechanism. Causes of a weak or noncontracting bladder include effects of medication, nerve damage, or overdistention of the bladder. With overfilling, the detrusor becomes stretched and is no longer able to contract sufficiently to increase intravesical pressure for emptying. People engaged in work

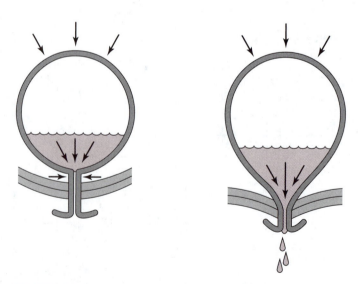

FIGURE 30–2   Urge urinary incontinence is the involuntary loss of urine associated with an uninhibited detrusor contraction that overwhelms the sphincter mechanism.

in which timely emptying of the bladder is inconvenient (eg, teaching) are more at risk for developing this condition.

Outlet obstruction can be caused by an enlarged prostate, prostate cancer, strictures, or bladder sphincter dyssynergia. Bladder sphincter **dyssynergia** occurs when the pelvic floor muscles contract simultaneously with a detrusor muscle contraction. Typically, a person with overflow incontinence experiences a constant dribbling resulting from an overfull bladder. If overflow incontinence is suspected by the therapist, an immediate referral to a physician would be appropriate to rule out organic causes and to prevent severe damage to the kidneys.

Urinary frequency relating to emptying problems can be caused by bladder sphincter dyssynergia and/or weak detrusor contractions. Since the bladder never completely empties, frequency often results. Urinary hesitancy, or "shy bladder," is common when attempting to void in a public restroom. The perceived lack of privacy inhibits the sphincter relaxation necessary to trigger the micturition reflex.

Anorectal and Gastrointestinal Disorders

Storage Problems.   **Fecal incontinence** is the involuntary loss of stool. Structural causes of stool leakage include weakness of the anal sphincter muscle resulting from injury to the pudendal nerve, weakness of the internal and/or external anal sphincter muscles resulting from muscle injury during childbirth or other

trauma, loss of ability to feel fullness in the rectum resulting from sensory nerve injury, and decreased compliance (elasticity) of the rectum from inflammation or other causes. **Functional fecal incontinence (FFI)** is defined as recurrent episodes of loss of control of stool for at least one month with no structural or organic cause. Functional fecal incontinence is often associated with constipation or diarrhea. Functional fecal incontinence associated with constipation is shown by fecal material filling the rectum, or evidence of megarectum or megacolon. Constipation is the most common cause of fecal incontinence in children. Loose fecal matter seeps around an impacted stool, and/or the pressure of stool upon the internal anal sphincter causes it to relax reflexively. Functional fecal incontinence can also be related to an elevated threshold for perception of rectal distention or a poorly functioning internal anal sphincter. Fecal incontinence associated with diarrhea is often found with **irritable bowel syndrome (IBS).** Watery stool, especially under explosive conditions, is difficult to hold back even with a strong sphincter muscle.

Emptying Problems.   Constipation can be caused by medication side effects, diabetes, hypothyroidism, painful anorectal disorders, depression, IBS, megarectum, megacolon, rectocele (**Fig. 30–3**), or colonic inertia. Pelvic floor dyssynergia is a functional cause of constipation for which the physical therapist may intervene. Pelvic floor dyssynergia presents with pelvic floor musculature that fails to relax or that actually

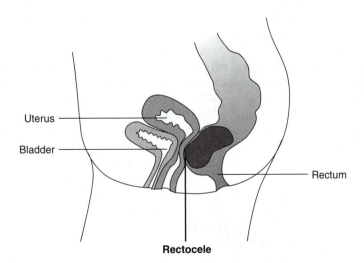

FIGURE 30–3   A rectocele is a hernial protrusion of part of the rectum into the vagina.

contracts during attempts to evacuate the bowel. Evidence of a nonrelaxing pelvic floor is show by surface electromyography (SEMG), manometry (pressure measurement), or defecography (X-ray study). With pelvic floor dyssynergia, there is no evidence of organic disease process. A rectocele is present, when part of the anterior rectal wall protrudes into the posterior vaginal wall, making it difficult to evacuate. Female patients can reduce it by placing their thumb inside the vagina and pressing posterior to support the posterior vaginal wall and to reduce the rectal bulge (vaginal splinting), thus helping the stool find a more direct exit through the anus. Chronic constipation can lead to fecal impaction, urinary incontinence, fecal incontinence (encopresis in children), dilation, and even perforation of the rectum.

Sometimes the pelvic floor muscles have been weakened and stretched over a period of time so that they descend below the ischial tuberosities when bearing down **(descending perineal syndrome).** Until the muscles have developed enough tone to position the pelvic floor and the rectum for optimal defecation, the patient can be shown how to support the pelvic floor manually (the index and middle fingers of each hand acts as a support of the pelvic floor on either side of the anus).[4]

Pain

Urogenital. **Vulvar dysesthesia,** also known as **vulvodynia,** literally means pain in the vulva. Itching, burning, stinging, or stabbing in the area around the vulva and the opening of the vagina characterizes this condition. Pain can be unprovoked, varying from constant to intermittent, or can occur only on provocation (eg, attempted vaginal penetration with sexual intercourse, or gynecological examination with a speculum). *Vulvar vestibulitis* syndrome or *vestibulodynia* are other names used to describe subcategories of vulvodynia. Symptoms of vulvodynia may range from mildly irritating to completely disabling. Although an open sore or area of redness may be visible, often the vagina shows no abnormalities or infections on gynecologic or dermatologic evaluation. It is common for women with vulvodynia to suffer the following symptoms: burning and pain with urination; throbbing, pain, and burning after defecation; and an inability to sit, wear tight clothing, or engage in sexual intimacy. Patients with vulvodynia often exhibit tense and unstable pelvic floor muscles as evidenced by SEMG.[5]

Clitorodynia presents with chronic burning pain in the clitoris, which could be neurological, glandular, vascular, or musculoskeletal in origin. Symptoms interfere with sexual arousal and may include an unprovoked and irritating low level of sexual arousal throughout the day. Ambulation can be difficult, as is sitting or moving from supine to a sitting position. This condition is sometimes described as pudendal neuralgia, because of the dorsal nerve innervation of the clitoris.

Interstitial cystitis (IC), is a condition characterized by oversensitivity of the bladder, whether or not inflammation of the bladder wall is present. It is a disease recognized by its symptoms. Although 90% of IC patients are women, this statistic may change in the future. Many men previously diagnosed with certain forms of prostatitis are now found to have IC. There are two different categories of IC. The classical ulcerated form is associated with red patches of inflammation, called Hunner's ulcers. This form is found in less than 10% of patients, and these patients tend to have more severe symptoms. There is a tendency to develop scarring of the bladder wall with a gradual diminishment of bladder capacity over time. In the nonulcerative condition that is seen more commonly, no specific lesions are noted upon routine bladder inspection. There is a wide range of severity with IC. Whereas many patients may awaken one or two times a night to urinate, others may need a bedside commode to deal with the urinary frequency. Some patients void as often as every 15 min. Patients frequently describe the pain as an uncomfortable pressure above their pubic bone that is somewhat relieved by urinating. Others are completely incapacitated by pain to the point where simply walking to the bathroom is a monumental effort.[6]

Urethral syndrome (US) involves burning and irritation of the urethra, especially at the urethral meatus, in the absence of an organic cause. The discomfort is often described as burning that may be present before, after, or during urination. In many instances the pain is constant. These symptoms are often accompanied by urgency and frequency of urination, pelvic pain, and pain with vaginal penetration. This condition sounds much like IC, and indeed most experts in the field consider US to be another form of IC, whether or not bladder complaints are present.[7]

Anorectal[8]. Trigger points in muscles of the posterior pelvic floor, including the sphintor ani, superficial transverse perineal, levator ani, piriformis, gluteus medius, and coccygeus muscles, refer poorly localized pain. Patients are often uncertain whether to call it tailbone, hip, or back pain. The pain centers in the region of the coccyx but often includes the anal area and the lower half of the sacrum. Both the levator ani and coccygeus muscles typically refer pain to the region of the coccyx. This referred pain pattern is often called **coccygodynia,** although the coccyx itself is usually normal and not tender. Several authors, however, insist that true coccygodynia results from traumatic injury to the coccyx.

Because the levator ani is the muscle most commonly involved, pain in the region of the coccyx is often called the **levator ani syndrome.** Levator ani spasm syndrome, chronic proctalgia, pelvic tension myalgia, piriformis syndrome, levator syndrome, puborectalis, and pelvic floor syndromes are other names for this condition. Pain may be located in the sacrum, the perineum, and the anal and gluteal region. Although bowel movements may not be painful, patients often report disturbed bowel function, constipation, or frequency. There is sometimes pain with sitting (especially on a hard surface) or when sitting down or standing up. Patients frequently experience a dull ache or discomfort in the rectum, lasting hours to days.

Proctalgia fugax is characterized by painful spasms of the muscles around the anus without known cause. Some patients experience pain from exaggerated or prolonged contraction of the pelvic floor muscles (eg, holding back elimination or after orgasm). Pain lasts for seconds to minutes and occurs infrequently, only a few times a year. Trigger points are sometimes found in the levator ani during a painful attack. Spasm of the internal anal sphincter, a smooth muscle, is thought by some to contribute to the pain in proctalgia fugax and levator ani syndromes.

In **obturator internus syndrome,** trigger points refer pain to the anococcygeal region and may have a spillover pattern to the upper portion of the posterior ipsilateral thigh. This syndrome causes pain and a feeling of fullness in the rectum. The thigh pain can also be caused by piriformis muscle involvement.

Irritable bowel syndrome (IBS) is characterized by abdominal pain that is relieved by defecation or associated with a change in frequency or constancy of stool. The following symptoms support a diagnosis of IBS: abnormal stool frequency (more than three times a day or less than three times per week); abnormal stool form (lumpy/hard or loose/watery); abnormal stool passage (straining, urgency, or feeling of incomplete evacuation); and passage of mucus and bloating or feeling of abdominal distension.[9] Patients with IBS have been found to have a lower pain threshold for bowel distention (bowel inflated in lumen of bowel). Anxiety and stress are believed to increase IBS symptoms along with a perceptual response bias. Sensations from the gut tend to be perceived as threatening and alarming. Patients can present with alternating bouts of diarrhea and constipation or can show symptoms consistently at the extremes of a diarrhea/constipation continuum.

It has been shown that patients with IBS and other forms of chronic functional GI disorders have extraintestinal dimensions to their bowel disorder. Common comorbid psychiatric conditions include anxiety, depression, and phobias. A history of sexual abuse is sometimes reported. Urinary symptoms of frequency, dysuria, urgency, nocturia, and incontinence are common complaints. Sexual dysfunction such as dyspareunia, decreased libido, and inhibited orgasms are common, as well as symptoms of fibromyalgia, Raynaud's syndrome, and other associated autonomic nervous systems disorders.

EVALUATION

The therapist does a general postural and musculoskeletal evaluation along with a complete medical history, detailing the onset and characterization of symptoms. It is helpful to have the patient fill out a bowel and bladder diary prior to the first visit. Salient information includes a daily recording of fluid intake, frequency of bladder and bowel emptying, frequency and volume of urine or stool leakage, situations that precede accidents, and time spent urinating or defecating, including frequency of straining.

An SEMG pelvic floor muscle evaluation is often done at the first or second visit. Surface electromyography is a minimally invasive procedure that objectively tests the pelvic floor muscles via vaginal, rectal, or externally placed sensors on the perineum. Functional characteristics are assessed, including muscle resting tension, speed of motor recruitment and relaxation, contractile strength, and muscle stability. The SEMG is both a diagnostic tool and an intervention modality (see Biofeedback in the modalities and agents section; see also **Chapter 29**).

A subjective test used for the purpose of grading is the **functional stop test.** It should be performed sitting on a toilet with the bladder partly emptied. This test is used for evaluation purposes only for persons with stress or urge urinary incontinence symptoms, and should not be performed as an exercise because of the potential to disrupt the voiding reflex. If the patient is always able to stop the urine flow midstream completely and quickly, the grade is 5/5. If the flow can be stopped 80% of the time, the grade is 4/5. When the flow can be stopped only sometimes, or partly stopped, it is a 3/5. The patient being able to deflect the stream a little grades 2/5, whereas if only the slightest change in stream is noticed, it is a 1/5.[10]

Some other evaluative, but more subjective, tools are grading the muscle tone, function, and strength by utilizing patient history and activity level (how many jumping jacks or coughs cause leaks). Another method is to palpate the **pelvic floor muscle (PFM)** contraction and relaxation in a window between the coccyx and ischial tuberosity. With anterior palpation, the deeper layers of the anterior PFMs can be felt. With posterior palpation, more of the puborectalis, ileococcygeus, and pubococcygeus are examined. The diagnosis, history, postural and musculoskeletal assessment, PFM evaluation, and bowel/bladder diary will together determine the intervention plan.

MODALITIES AND AGENTS

Patient education is an essential aspect of intervention to gain maximum patient cooperation and compliance. Basic pelvic floor anatomy, as well as bowel and bladder functioning, are explained with the assistance of simple illustrations.

Therapeutic Exercise

Strengthening, endurance training, stretching, coordination training, core stabilization, **proprioneuromuscular facilitation (PNF),** neuromuscular relaxation, eccentric, concentric, and open and closed chain exercises all form the foundation of PFM rehabilitation programs. There are many choices of instruction for PFM exercise. Teaching the patient how to isolate a PFM contraction minimizes substitution of accessory muscles.

Biofeedback

Biofeedback (electromyographic feedback, or EMG) is the process of measuring a physiologic function with sensitive instruments, amplifying the measured signal, and then displaying the physiologic variable to the patient, usually by visual or auditory means.

Various biofeedback modalities can be helpful in treating pelvic floor dysfunction (eg, thermal, respiration, heart rate, heart rate variability, skin conduction, EMG, and EEG). However, EMG feedback is the mainstay. Typically, when biofeedback is used as a modality, an SEMG pelvic floor muscle evaluation is performed at the beginning of each intervention session. It is standard to use two channels of EMG initially, one for the pelvic floor and the other for an accessory muscle (usually abdominal), in order to teach patients how to isolate a PFM contraction. A broadband EMG filter is used for the pelvic floor placement in order to capture a wide range of muscle activity, whereas for accessory muscles, a narrow bandwidth is selected to minimize artifact. The ongoing assessment serves to measure gains made throughout intervention. Areas requiring training are easily identified by both the therapist and the patient (who usually becomes highly motivated to produce a more normal EMG reading). Normal PFM function includes the ability to maintain low pelvic floor muscle resting tension prior to and following exercise; produce a rapid, strong, coordinated, isolated PFM contraction; return quickly to baseline readings (latency); and demonstrate a sustained contraction without the use of accessory muscles (eg, abdominals, gluteals, hip adductors, internal and external rotators). It is standard to test and prescribe home exercise programs for both fast- and slow twitch fibers by having the patient contract PFMs for both short (0.5–1.0 second) and sustained durations (5–10 seconds).

Tests for dyssynergia and endurance are usually performed. Endurance assessments require the patient to attempt to contract pelvic floor musculature up to 30–60 seconds. With dyssynergia testing and training, the patient is asked to simulate an attempt to have a bowel movement by bearing down or pushing out while maintaining a relaxed pelvic floor. This procedure is first performed while sitting in a chair in a biomechanically efficient toileting position. However, in order to approximate a real-life situation, the patient can be progressed to doing the biofeedback training while on a commode or toilet. A barrier such as a chuck can be placed between the toilet and bowl to prevent the sensor from falling into the bowl if it is pushed out. Often the patient is able to demonstrate a coordinated push out while in the office but not while seated on a toilet. Pelvic floor dyssynergia can be highly conditioned to circumstances (bathroom, public restroom).

Surface EMG pelvic floor muscle evaluations can be done with therapists prompting, as well as with

Samples of Surface EMG Biofeedback Displays

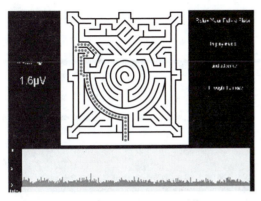

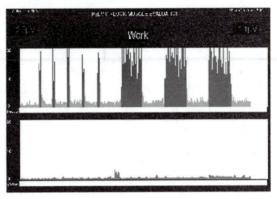

This biofeedback training screen reinforces pelvic floor muscle relaxation. When the rectal EMG reading is below an adjustable threshold, music turns on and advances are made through the maze. Good for use with a pediatric population.

A standard 2 channel sEMG line graph display. The pelvic floor EMG tracing changes color when the microvolt level exceeds an adjustable threshold. Used for pelvic floor muscle assessment and neuromuscular reeducation.

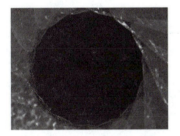 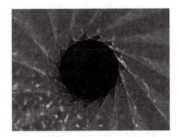 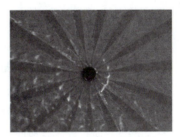

As the patient contracts or relaxes pelvic floor muscles, the sphincter animation mirrors in real time the motor activity. This animation is useful for relaxation, coordination, and strength training.

FIGURE 30–4   Samples of surface EMG biofeedback displays. (*Courtesy of Marks Software Tools for Pelvic Floor Dysfunction.*)

computerized protocols that are provided with EMG feedback instruments. The computerized protocols provide a consistence-standardized sequence and timed work/rest evaluation (**Figs. 30–4, 30–5A and B**).

Training for relaxation, coordination, strengthening, and endurance is usually done in a less structured fashion, using biofeedback displays that are appropriate for each patient. For example, if the patient has difficulty relaxing pelvic floor musculature, a training screen, which reinforces relaxation rather than strengthening, would be selected (**Fig. 30–6**). The therapist should be well-versed in operant conditioning that involves the strengthening of a response by offering a reward or positive reinforcement following the occurrence of the response. Biofeedback Units (**Fig. 30–7**) with auditory and visual events serve as positive reenforcers, as do the responses of the therapist upon viewing the appropriate motor responses indicated by the biofeedback. The therapist works as a coach to the patient, offering strategies to reach the desired objective.

Biofeedback is a powerful tool that can provide information on muscle activity that is outside sensory awareness. It can augment sensation and raise the patient's sensory and motor awareness. However, biofeedback is rarely used alone. Relaxation methods such as diaphragmatic breathing, progressive muscle relaxation, autogenic relaxation phrases, and guided imagery are often employed. For strengthening and coordination training, the principles of shaping, imagery, and verbal cueing for recruitment are used in conjunction with biofeedback. Thermal, respiration,

sEMG Tracings

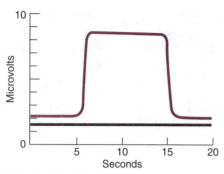

Isolated tonic pelvic floor muscle contraction: good motor recruitment and release, low pre and post baseline readings

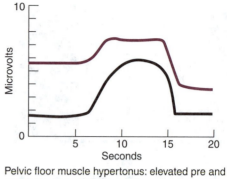

Pelvic floor muscle hypertonus: elevated pre and post base-line readings, weak contractions with abdominal substitution (pelvic floor myalgia)

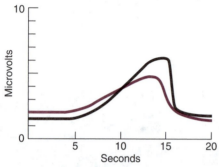

Weak and poorly isolated contractions with abdominal substitution (stress incontinence)

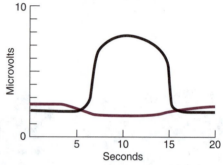

Good relaxation of pelvic floor muscles with bearing down.

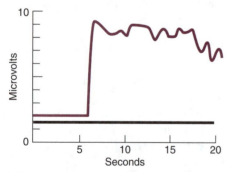

Good motor recruitment and strength with elevated and unstable readings following contraction: delayed and poor return to baseline (vulvodynia)

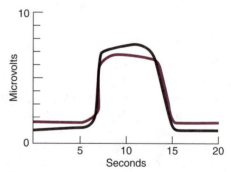

Co-contraction of pelvic floor and abdominal muscles when attempting to bear down (pelvic floor dyssynergia, constipation, urinary frequency and hesitancy)

—— Vaginal or Rectal   —— Abdominal

FIGURE 30–5   Surface EMG tracings. (*Courtesy of Marks Software Tools for Pelvic Floor Dysfunction.*)

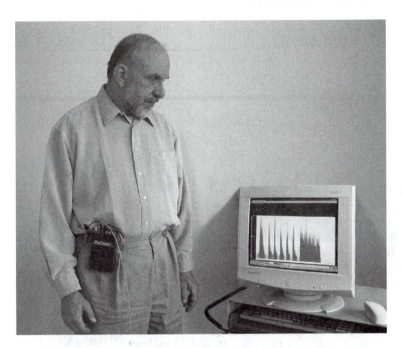

FIGURE 30–6 Eight-channel multimodality biofeedback instrument with fiberoptic cabling that allows for EMG measurements in a variety of positions, during and following ambulation. The self-insertable internal sensor makes it possible to provide intervention in a noninvasive fashion. (Used with pemission of Louise E. Marks, MS, OTR, and Marilyn Freedman)

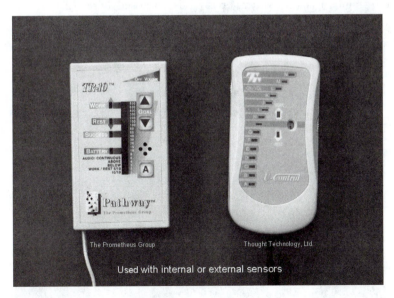

FIGURE 30–7 Surface EMG instruments for home training. (Used with permission of Louise E. Marks, MS, OTR, and Marilyn Freedman)

heart rate, heart rate variability, and EEG biofeedback modalities are frequently utilized for relaxation training involving conditions in which autonomic hyperarousal aggravates a presenting condition (eg, defensive muscle bracing, urinary hesitancy, urge incontinence, and pain syndromes).

Surface EMG sensors for internal vaginal, anal, or rectal use are devices that are easily inserted by the patient (**Fig. 30–8**). This feature offers the advantage of privacy, since the patient, following instruction, is left alone for self-insertion and can remain clothed during intervention. The therapist needs to develop procedures to prevent environmental contamination, such as directing the patient to use latex gloves. The tip of the sensor is lubricated, and if the patient is allergic or sensitive to one lubricant, there are alternatives (eg, petroleum jelly, natural oils). Proper orientation of the sensor within the vagina or anal canal should be reviewed in detail (refer to manufactures instructions). If too much lubricant is used, a bridge between the electrodes can occur that will generate false low readings. If this problem happens, the sensor should be removed, cleaned, and reinserted. Very high readings usually indicate artifact from electrical activity in the environment, in which case the patient needs to check whether the sensor is positioned properly.

The disadvantages of these internal surface sensors are initial higher cost ($25 to $75) and, periodically, a patient's reluctance to use an internal sensor. Sometimes the vagina is too fragile, has varicosities, or is just too dry, painful, or small for the vaginal sensor. In this instance, a smaller rectal sensor can be used in the vagina, or external electrodes can be used (see later). The anus or rectum may present similar challenges, in which case the choice is to place electrodes externally. The therapist places the two active electrodes on either side of the anal opening and places the ground electrode on the gluteals or bony landmarks nearby. With children, external sensors are often used in order to avoid vaginal or rectal penetration. However, external sensors are more invasive in the sense that the therapist must view and touch the patient's perineum because the patient would have great difficulty in accurate self-placement. Therefore, the authors' preference is the use of self-insertable vaginal or rectal sensors, except when working with young children. Parents can easily be trained to place the external surface sensors on their child's perineum.

Electrical Stimulation

If the patient does not have sufficient awareness and cannot isolate the contraction, PFM exercises can be taught using **electrical stimulation (ES)** to help the patient identify the muscle location, provide proprioception, and assist the contraction. Occasionally a patient with weak muscles (grades 0 to 2), and/or lack of sensation, proprioception, and awareness has difficulty learning how to contract the muscles using the methods discussed here. Electrical stimulation (especially

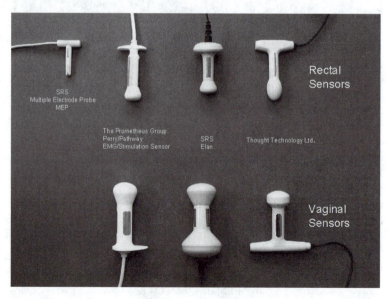

FIGURE 30–8   Internal surface EMG sensors. (Used with permission of Louise E. Marks, MS, OTR, and Marilyn Freedman)

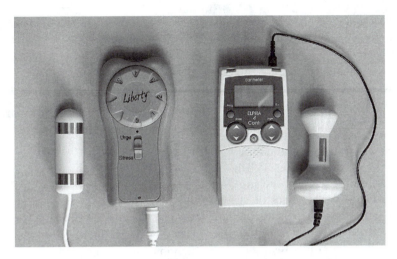

FIGURE 30–9   Electrical stimulation units. (Used with permission of Louise E. Marks, MS, OTR, and Marilyn Freedman)

with intact sensation) then may be the method of choice. Portable electrical stimulation units (**Fig 30–9**) can be used to simultaneously pinpoint the musculature involved, providing proprioception and the sensation of pelvic floor excursion. In situations where the patient has unstable bladder contractions, electrical stimulation is used at a different frequency to achieve autonomic dampening of these bladder contractions by augmenting sympathetic dominance.

Electrodes.   There is a great variety of both internal and external electrodes on the market today. External electrodes are mainly the standard ones used for TENS but can be of any size (even customized for the patient). When possible (and it almost always is, except in conditions of severely atrophied skin or an abnormally hypervascularized introitus), an internal electrode is preferred. Both patient and therapist place these correctly much more easily, and this method facilitates home self-intervention where appropriate. The silicone-filled, dumbbell-shaped type appears to be the most user friendly, both in feel (it is softer and warmer than metal counterparts) and in ability to be used in all positions (ie, it stays in position even with the patient standing, as long as the vagina/rectum is not too large for the electrode used). Electrodes are mostly customized for a vaginal or an anal fit (an anal electrode sometimes being the one of choice for a smaller or more atrophied vagina). Today, almost all electrodes are single-user.

Current.   The most comfortable currents are delivered by circular electrodes, which are able to disperse current over large surface areas. The frequency used for stimulating varies widely (5–50Hz.). Some practitioners prefer 50Hz, whereas others feel that 20Hz is more effective. Upper motor neuron input is not necessary, although total, or at least partial, innervation of the PFM must be intact for neuromuscular electrical stimulation (NMES) to be used this way. It is generally agreed that a higher frequency of 50Hz is most amenable to innervated muscle, and it works well to teach muscle contraction, proprioception, and awareness. To help treat detrusor instability and urgency, a lower frequency of 5–20Hz, with the average being 12Hz, is a more effective current choice.

The authors generally suggest protocols requiring minimal equipment, to facilitate patient independence, decrease cost, and maximize home compliance. In a situation of poor patient compliance—it requires more effort, energy, concentration, and will to initiate and follow through a program of voluntary contractions—using electrical stimulation becomes a means to an end.

Biofeedback-triggered electrical stimulation may be the most desirable combination of active and passive strengthening. The patient contracts muscles to a set threshold before electrical stimulation is triggered. Specific internal vaginal and rectal electrodes for this type of unit are currently in use.

Protocols.   Begin with the patient in an antigravity position (ie, relaxed hook lying or side lying with one or two pillows under the pelvis or between the legs), and slowly progress to standing. The use of 2 or 3 min of stimulation 1 to 3 times a day is a good beginning, gradually building up to 15 min 1 to 2 times a day. After the first few sessions, when the patient has been able to identify the contraction, ask the patient to contract with the current, relaxing in between. Once this technique is mastered, the patient can continue contracting after cessation of current, until the patient has learned how to self-initiate and gradually to build up endurance to 5–10 second contractions. Other agents like biofeedback and/or therapeutic exercise can be started as soon as good voluntary contractions have been established. **Note:** When the patient has a diagnosis of mixed (stress and urge) incontinence and when two different types of current are being used, it is important to separate the currents' applications by at least 8–10 hours. If the patient cannot manage this timewise, then different currents should be applied on alternate days.

Transcutaneous Electrical Nerve Stimulation (TENS)

Although TENS has been found to be useful in treating detrusor instability, it seems to be more effective in relieving pelvic and perineal pain. Related acupuncture points are useful—eg, spleen 6 (Sp 6), spleen 10 (Sp 10), and large intestine 4 (LI4). Electrodes can also be placed in a crossed fashion over the lower abdomen or lumbar sacral areas. Some patients respond better to a combination of acupuncture and abdominal or lumbar sites. Parameters are usually at a conventional setting using a submotor sensory amplitude and moderately high frequency of 60–100 Hz with a pulse duration of 100–150msec for 20–30 min duration, 1 to 5 times a day. Settings of continuous, burst, or modulated may be used according to patient preference. Low-rate (acupuncturelike) TENS is set at 2–10 Hz. according to patient tolerance for continuous stimulation as needed by the patient.[11–14]

Ultrasound

Physical therapists have found this modality to be clinically effective in treating a variety of pelvic floor conditions even though its use has not yet been satisfactorily documented statistically. Some examples of conditions treated are the following:

- *Damage to the pelvic floor muscles following a vaginal delivery.* More than 50% of women have an episiotomy or tear involving repair with stitches. As a result of the trauma, there is often swelling, bruising, and overstretching of the muscular and neurovascular tissues. The pain can interfere with a woman's ability to move around or to find

a comfortable position to breastfeed or care for her baby.
- *Scar tissue postepisiotomy* or *tear repair.* There can cause chronic pelvic pain.
- *Dysparunia.*
- *Difficulty in bowel and in urinary elimination.* These can occur because of pelvic floor dysfunction and spasm.

Application. Ultrasound is an effective way to treat this area. The authors prefer using a sleeve like a condom to cover the ultrasound head, making sure that contact medium covers both the area of the condom in contact with the perineum as well as the area of the condom in contact with the ultrasound head. This technique minimizes the interfaces between the ultrasound head and the patient, and it also allows better proprioception of the tissues involved. Where possible, it is preferable to use a small ultrasound head (eg, like one used to treat muscles around the TMJ). Be sure to use degassed water or ultrasound gel in order to minimize air bubbles.

Patient Position. Position the patient side lying (facing away from the therapist) with the lower leg straight and the upper leg bent and elevated on a pillow. The patient can help by separating and holding up the upper buttock.

Frequency. When tissue being treated is superficial, 3 MHz frequency is desirable. With chronic deep scarring, 1MHz is the frequency of choice.

Dosage. Select a dosage of 0.5–1.0 W/cm^2 for 3–5 min (1 min for every 10 cm^2 of surface covered). A lower dose is used for more acute superficial intervention (two to three interventions usually sufficing), whereas a higher dose is required to soften deeper scarring prior to soft-tissue release work (8–15 interventions may be required). If pulsed ultrasound or a fluid-filled bag is employed, the time of intervention needs to be increased accordingly.[15,16]

Bladder and Bowel Training

It is helpful to have patients fill out a bladder or bowel diary for 2 days (a weekday and a weekend day) prior to their initial visit (**Fig. 30–10**). Relevant information includes the average daily amount of liquid intake, type of liquids, time of intake, amount of fluid emptied, episodes of bladder or bowel emptying, and leaking or soiling events (indicating whether minor or major). Before the second visit, more detail may be

BLADDER DIARY

Name: _____

Date: _____

Day of Week: _____

Time	Urinated in toilet	Incontinent episode: small/ large	Activity or reason associated with incontinence	Fluid intake (type & volume)	Comments
6–8 am					
8–10 am					
10–12 am					
12–2 pm					
2–4 pm					
4–6 pm					
6–8 pm					
8–10 pm					
10–12 pm					
Overnight					

Number of pads used within 24 hour period. _____

Directions:
1. Check each time you urinated in toilet.
2. Note each incontinent episode, indicating small or large.
3. Describe activity or reason associated with inconti
4. Describe fluid intake for time interval, ex. 1 cup coffee, 1 glass water,
   1 cup of soup, etc.

FIGURE 30–10   Bladder diary.

included, like the activity of daily living (ADL) that precipitated an accident and the number of seconds it takes to excrete a measured volume of urine. With a problem of constipation, it would be useful to know the time spent in the bathroom and the appearance of the stool.

Manual Therapies

Manual therapies are often used to treat patients experiencing pelvic pain. Techniques vary from gentle massage, to myofascial techniques, visceral mobilization, and mobilization and manipulation, depending on the condition being treated and on musculoskeletal findings. With PFMD, the lumbar sacral spine, sacrum, and pelvis, with their concomitant viscera and soft tissue, are sometimes involved.

Diet and Medications

Both diet and medication play an important role in treating PFMD, and the therapist must be aware of their effect on the patient. Various medications affect the nervous system, enhancing or suppressing either sympathetic or parasympathetic dominance; some medications are diuretic in nature, whereas others can be constipating or laxative. Some foods and beverages are notorious bladder irritants. The fiber content of food may need to be modified according to the bowel dysfunction being treated. Therefore, a thorough history of patient medication as well as food and beverage intake is essential to plan a successful program.

Home Exercise Training Devices

Home units that provide electrical stimulation, biofeedback, or biofeedback-triggered ES are recommended when these devices are indicated. The authors have found that home units not only ensure better patient compliance but also result in fewer office visits while producing a desired outcome.

Vaginal or Rectal Weights

Vaginal and rectal weights, which are also known as **cones,** represent another option for patients. The patient must have a muscle grade of at least 3 for cones to be used (see stop test in the Evaluation section). These small cone-shaped devices are available in standard sets consisting of five identically sized but differently weighted cones (20–60 g). Other options include larger lighter-weighted, and smaller heavier cones. Cones are inserted vaginally or rectally. The patient then walks or stands while contracting the pelvic floor muscle sufficiently to keep the cone from falling out. The patient progresses from the lightest to the heaviest cone until able to retain the heaviest one for 5 min while walking. The patient then begins working to retain the cone while coughing, jumping, walking up and down steps, and engaging in any other activities that have caused urine/fecal incontinence. **Note:** The patient must learn how to release the muscles totally and to "deliver" the cones, as well as learning how much effort is required for continence with each activity. Standing, for example, requires rela-

tively little muscle strength, whereas jumping jacks need considerable strength.

Dilators

These diatlors are silicone, plastic, or glass dildos, which are made in various sizes to help teach PFM relaxation (while they are being inserted) and to allow accommodation by the vaginal and anorectal regions as those areas are being gently stretched. Dilators are especially useful when used in combination with biofeedback to help release muscle spasm and retrain the soft tissue so that the patient will be able to accommodate their emptying and sexual functions more comfortably. Dilators are relatively inexpensive and are therefore often used as an aid to home training. Once patients are able to relax their muscles sufficiently, dilators are lubricated with K-Y jelly (or the equivalent) in order to facilitate easier insertion. At first the patient will be able to tolerate only a few seconds but can gradually learn to leave the dilator in place for up to 10 min. Once comfortable with the procedure, progression is made by teaching the patient how to move the dilator in and out of the orifice, and to self-treat internal trigger points that are difficult to reach manually.

Heat

Application of moist heat has been found to be effective in relieving pain and spasm. Some patients have found it helpful to relieve pain and spasm by applying moist heat directly to the perineum. This procedure is usually done prior to working with a dilator, engaging in sexual intercourse, or moving the bowels. Heat can also be used after these activities or before/after intervention involving the perineum. A warm, moist facecloth, a condom filled two-thirds with warm water, a sitz bath, an electric pad, or a small rectangular hot pack made especially for this purpose can be used.[17]

Cold

The analgesic effect of cold on the perineum is useful in many of the pain conditions described previously. Mixing two-thirds water or ultrasound gel with one-third alcohol and then freezing the mixture in a condom can make a soft icepack. Freezing a moist, folded facecloth and then placing it in a sealed plastic bag provides a device that molds comfortably to the perineal area.[18]

CONCLUSION

Physical therapy is an integral part of the interdisciplinary team treating PFMD. The PT role in evaluating and treating muscle tone, strength, function, posture, and activities of daily living augments the diagnostic and intervention skills of other health professionals. Because incontinence, constipation, and pelvic floor dysfunction are multifaceted and complex, additional training and education are necessary, particularly the study of the anatomy and physiology of micturition, defecation, and pelvic pain syndromes. Expertise in exercise, posture, activities of daily living, myofascial mobilization, and physical agents makes the involvement of physical therapists in PFMD rehabilitation inevitable. The authors' goal in setting out the rudimentary knowledge of function, assessment, and intervention with PFMD is to emphasize the importance of using this awareness in the overall assessment and intervention with all patients.

REVIEW QUESTIONS

1. What three conditions should be met before a physical therapist is permitted to look at or touch a patient's perineum?

2. Explain the difference between urge, stress, and overflow incontinence.

3. Which parameters would you use when deciding whether to select internal or external (pelvic floor muscle) surface electrodes when training with biofeedback?

4. Describe how you would apply ultrasound to the perineum.

5. Which physical agents would be helpful in teaching patients how to address pelvic floor dyssynergia (eg, in fecal constipation)?

6. Which electrical stimulation currents have been found to be therapeutic in the intervention of urge incontinence?

7. Provide an outline of what should be included in the evaluation of an individual with PFMD.

8. Describe how biofeedback is used in the evaluation and intervention of individuals with PFMD.

9. Provide the rationale for the use of electrical stimulation in the rehabilitation of individuals with PFMD.

10. Provide an outline of the different types of exercises used in the rehabilitation of individuals with PFMD.

KEY TERMS

pelvic floor muscle dysfunction (PFMD)
stress urinary incontinence (SUI)
cystocele
urge urinary incontinence
detrusor instability (DI)
urinary frequency
mixed urinary incontinence
urge incontinence
overflow incontinence

dyssynergia
fecal incontinence
functional fecal incontinence (FFI)
irritable bowel syndrome (IBS)
descending perineal syndrome
vulvar dysesthesia, vulvodynia
clitorodynia
interstitial cystitis (IC)
urethral syndrome
coccygodynia

levator ani syndrome
proctalgia fugax
obturator internus syndrome
functional stop test
pelvic floor muscle (PFM)
proprioneuromuscular facilitation (PNF)
biofeedback
electrical stimulation (ES)
cones

RESOURCES

American Physical Therapy Association, Women's Health
PO Box 327
Alexandria, VA 22313
(800) 999-2782, ext. 3233

Association for Applied Psychophysiology and Biofeedback
10200 W. 44th Avenue, Suite 304
Wheat Ridge, CO 80033-2840
(303) 422-8436

International Foundation for Functional Gastrointestinal Disorders
PO Box 170864
Milwaukee, WI 53217-8076
(888) 964-2001

The International Pelvic Pain Society
Women's Medical Plaza, Suite 402

2006 Brookwood Medical Center Drive
Birmingham, AL 35209
(800) 624-9676

Society of Urologic Nurses and Associates
East Holly Avenue, Box 56
Pitman, NJ 08071-0056
1-888-TAP-SUNA or (856) 256-2335

REFERENCES

1. Herman H: The Gynecological Manual. Alexandria, VA: American Physical Therapy Association, Women's Health; 1997.

2. Blavis J: *Conquering Bladder Disorders and Prostate Problems.* New York: Plenum Trade; 1998; 48.

3. Kolton D, Monga A, Stanton SL: Does sensory urgency exist? *Neurourology and Urodynamics* 1985; 14:576–77.

4. Sapsford R, Bullock-Saxton J, Markwell S: *Women's Health.* Philadelphia: Saunders; 1998; 364–67.

5. Glazer H. Conversation, 2001.

6. Moldwin R: *The Interstitial Cystitis Survival Guide.* Oakland, CA: New Harbinger Publications; 2000; 5–8.

7. Op cit., p. 63.

8. Travell JG, Simons DG: *Myofascial Pain and Dysfunction,* Vol 2. Baltimore: Williams & Wilkins, 1999; 9, 120.

9. Ringel Y, Sperber A, Drossman D: Irritable bowel syndrome. *Ann Rev Med* 2001; 52:319–38.

10. Herman H: *The Gynecological Manual.* Ch 3. Alexandria, VA: American Physical Therapy Association, Women's Health. 1997; 76.

11. Brecker LR: Application of thermal and electrotherapeutic agents in obstetrics and gynecology. *Advance* 1993; 4:4–5.

12. Gersh MR: *Electrotherapy in Rehabilitation.* Philadelphia: Davis; 1992.

13. EMPI Inc: *The Fundamentals of Pelvic Floor Stimulation.* St. Paul, MN: author; 1994.

14. EMPI Inc: *Instruction Manual for TENS.* St. Paul, MN: 2001.

15. Sapsford R, Bullock-Saxton J, Markwell S: *Women's Health.* Philadelphia: Saunders; 1998; 296–99.

16. Shelly ER: *The Gynecological Manual.* Ch 6. Alexandria, VA: American Physical Therapy Association, Women's Health. 1997; 354–55.

17. Micklovitz SL: *Thermal Agents in Rehabilitation.* 2nd. ed. Philadelphia: Davis; 1990.

18. Cholhan HJ, Bent AE: Nonsurgical therapies. In: Benson TJ, ed. *Female Pelvic Floor Disorders.* New York: Norton; 1992; 199–209.

APPENDIX

CLINICAL PROBLEMS AND LABORATORY EXPERIMENTS

The practicing physical therapist must be able to evaluate a patient, comprehend the pathology being addressed, and decide on the best mode of intervention. This section addresses the role of physical agents within a total intervention plan. Physical therapists must learn the proper rationale for, and use of, modalities. The clinical problems presented in the appendix are designed to help the reader develop the skills needed to integrate physical agents into decision making. As the necessity for verifying the benefits of various physical agents becomes increasingly obvious, an effort must be make to focus on experimental research. With this in mind, several laboratory experiments that have been set up using a basic research design are included in this section. These experiments are designed to introduce clinical experimental procedures and can be performed easily and realistically. The interventions and experiments presented in this section must only be done with the approval and supervision of the course instructor and should follow the safety criteria and procedures for the academic or clinical facility in which they are carried out.

The aim of research in physical agents is to know that what we do is or is not beneficial. We must be able to validate why, as practitioners, we choose one method of intervention over another. Many therapists rely on the fact that a modality has been used in a certain way "for years" and that "it works." We do not want to minimize clinical evidence; however, we do wish to emphasize that experimental proof of the actual results of our techniques will validate our work to our colleagues and to the rest of the medical community. On the other hand, it may force us to let go of cherished beliefs. Eugene Michaels' comment remains timely for this second edition:

Expert opinion, private opinions, based upon physiological rationale are not enough to justify what we do. We must evaluate our intervention methods, and to do this we should establish standards for judging the value, importance, and usefulness of what we do. Among these standards should be one that calls for research evidence of the effectiveness of physical therapy methods. (Evaluation and reseach in physical therapy. *JAPTA* 1982; 62(6):828)

THERMAL AGENTS CLINICAL CASES

1. Question Related to Chap 13 Superficial Thermotherapy

Patient is 25 y/o obese male, employed as a furniture mover, c/o diffuse LBP for the past 2 wks. Pain is nonradiating and increases with strenuous lifting. How can one of the thermal agents be incorporated in his treatment program?

The patient was diagnosed with lumbosacral muscle spasms. Hot packs to L-S spine in combination with soft tissue mobilization, patient education (posture and proper body mechanics during lifting), and a graded exercise program is indicated.

The intervention position depends on the cause of pain or spasms. The prone position, with a pillow under the stomach, or side lying in the fetal position will put the lumbar area in a relaxed midrange, or flexed position. If one wishes to encourage passive extension, the prone position without pillows under the abdomen may be preferred. The supine position with the knees bent requires more towel layers and extra caution if a hot pack is placed under the back.

The rationale is to increase cutaneous circulation and produce analgesic and sedative effects that promote relaxation. Significant temperature changes will not occur in deep back muscles.

2. Question Related to Chap 13 Superficial Thermotherapy

Pt is a 45 y/o (R) hand dominant male, employed as a computer operator, sustained an injury to (R) hand 3 months ago. He presents with a progressive loss in (R) hand function. How can one of the thermal agents be incorporated in his treatment program?

The patient was diagnosed with a posttraumatic R hand soft tissue injury with diminished strength and range of motion. Paraffin in combination with P, AA, and AROM exercises and functional exercises is indicated.

The rationale for the paraffin is to decrease joint viscosity and increase soft tissue extensibility in the hand, prior to exercise. Paraffin contour to the hand is better then a hot pack. Fluidotherapy® or a whirlpool intervention can also be considered since both would allow the patient to move the hand while heat is being applied. Convenience and the patient's preference also must be considered. If evaluation indicates thermal sensory involvement, all three modalities should be used cautiously.

3. Question Related to Chap 13 Superficial Thermotherapy

A 58 y/o woman is admitted to the hospital for intervention of depression and anxiety neurosis. She complained to her physician of pain in her neck that radiated up the back of her head and into her forehead and temples. How can a superficial heating agent be incorporated in her treatment program?

The patient was diagnosed with head and neck pain related to stress and anxiety. An infrared intervention with soft tissue mobilization, EMG biofeedback, and patient education is indicated.

The rationale for using infrared is that it allows for an easier superficial heat application to the face. Hot packs can also be used on the neck, and EMG biofeedback can be used to make the patient more aware of excessive neuromuscular activity in the neck and face region.

4. Question Related to Chap 14 Cryotherapy

A 20 y/o female sustained an inversion sprain of the right ankle during a preseason scrimmage. She developed almost immediate pain and swelling over the anteriolateral and inferior aspect of the right lateral malleolus. What superficial thermal agent should be incorporated in her treatment program?

The RICE protocol was implemented for this individual. The intervention includes the following:

1. **R**esting the injured joint
2. **I**ce application
3. **C**ompression wraps
4. **E**levation of the injured part

The rationale for this intervention is that the rest prevented further injury; the ice reduced hemorrhage, edema, and secondary hypoxia; the compression increased the pressure gradient between the interstitial space and the capillary; and elevation allowed gravity to assist the return of fluid into the circulatory system. Early intervention is critical to minimize the effects of trauma.

5. Question Related to Chap 14 Cryotherapy and Chap 15 Ultrasound

A 25 y/o woman with chondromalacia patellae is referred to the clinic for physical therapy. She noticed pain and "puffiness" around the (R) patella about 1 week ago. She currently has pain when she rises from a sitting position and when she climbs stairs. She has mild crepitus and tenderness of the medial articular facet of the (R) knee. She has been resting and icing the knee for the past week. How can the thermal agents be integrated in her treatment program?

The knee is placed in a neutral position so that the patella could be mobilized in the medial direction. A graded exercise program of SLRs and proximal leg strengthening exercises are employed prior to and after patella mobilization. The thermal agents are integrated in the following sequence:

1. Ultrasound to provide pain relief and nonthermal effects. Intensity is continuous-wave mode, $0.5-W/cm^2$; or pulsed-wave mode, $1-1.5\ W/cm^2$, at 50% duty cycle.
2. Ice massage to provide pain relief and reduce risk of postexercise inflammation (a cold pack can also be used).

If weakness exists in the VMO, a combination of NMES and biofeedback could be used in this patient's treatment program.

6. Question Related to Chap 13 Superficial Thermotherapy

A 25 y/o woman involved in a car accident sustained a whiplash injury 2 weeks ago. Her X-rays were negative for any vertebral fracture or derangement. She has pain in her neck and trapezius area, and reduced range in all neck motions. She has headaches and pain when she attempts to move her neck and holds her head stiffly while walking. How can the thermal agents be integrated in her treatment program?

The patient is placed in a position of comfort and treated with a hot pack to the cervical area to decrease pain and promote relaxation. Manual cervical traction and soft tissue mobilization of the upper back, neck, and facial muscles are used to assist in increasing cervical ROM.

7. Question Related to Chap 15 Ultrasound

A 52 y/o man presents with limited ROM in the left shoulder following immobilization for a mid humeral fracture. How can the thermal agents be integrated in his treatment program?

The patient is placed in a supine position, and the shoulder elevated to the available end range of motion. Ultrasound is applied during passive stretching, and a cold pack is used following passive stretching and active exercises.

The rationale for the ultrasound is to increase extensibility in the periarticular structures of the shoulder during stretching. A continuous US of 1 MHz and 1.5 wts/cm^2 is applied as the shoulder is being stretched. The cold pack is used following stretching, joint mobilization, and active exercise to minimize postintervention inflammation.

8. Question Related to Chap 16 Diathermy

A 30 y/o man with chronic LBP is referred for evaluation and treatment. How can one of the thermal agents be incorporated in his program?

The patient presents with paraspinal muscle spasms and pain radiating into the (R) buttock. Inductive SWD followed by postural education, appropriate stretching and strengthening exercises are integrated into this individual's treatment program.

The SWD is used to reduce paraspinal pain and muscle spasm by increased thermal input and blood flow to the treatment area. Positional traction in a (L) side-lying position can also be used if it reduces the pain radiation into the (R) buttock.

THERMAL AGENTS LAB EXPERIMENTS

The purpose of these experiments is to establish the effects of thermal agents or to compare the effectiveness of different techniques of application. To enhance the accuracy of the data, observe the following:

1. Note the room temperature—because the ambient temperature can affect experimental results. Try to maintain the room at about the same temperature for all stages of the experiments.
2. Ensure that, whenever possible, the same researcher measures the same variable (eg, skin temperature, respiratory rate, pulse rate, range of motion, manual muscle test) before, during, and after application. Use a skin thermometer when measuring the temperature of the part being treated.
3. Record all measurements immediately after taking them.
4. Repeat the treatment and measurements on several individuals, using similar equipment for all subjects in each experiment.
5. Compile the data.
6. Compare the data: note individual and group differences, and determine the average for each individual and for each group. Realize that the results indicate effects only for the subjects or groups tested. The greater the number of subjects, the more the results apply to a larger population of young healthy subjects.

For **safety,** all the experiments should be performed under the conditions described in earlier chapters. All indications, contraindications, and precautions should be carefully noted.

I. Effect of Hot Pack Treatment on Respiratory Rate, Pulse Rate, and Skin Temperature

EQUIPMENT AND MATERIALS

1. Stopwatch.
2. Skin thermometer.
3. Hot water tank thermostatically controlled.
4. Hot packs that have been soaked in Hydrocollator® for 30 min.
5. New hot pack covers (envelopes).
6. Towels.
7. Pencil and paper for recording data.

PROCEDURES

1. Record the room temperature and the temperature of the water in the hot-water tank.
2. Position and drape the subject for treatment to the low-back area.

3. Instruct the subject to report any pain or discomfort, in which case the treatment will be discontinued.
4. Measure and record the respiration rate, pulse rate, and skin temperature in the area of the application of the pack.
5. Measure the temperature of the hot pack.
6. Apply the hot pack with eight layers of toweling (or an envelope cover and extra toweling) between the pack and the subject's skin.
7. Measure and record the respiration rate, pulse rate, and skin temperature again 10 minutes into the treatment. (Momentarily remove the pack to remeasure the temperature at the treatment site.)
8. Remove the pack after 20 minutes, and repeat the measurement procedures for respiration rate, pulse rate, and skin temperature.
9. Remeasure the temperature of the hot pack.
10. Record all final measurements
11. Compile and compare the data for individual subjects, and determine the average.

II. Effect of Infrared Treatment on Respiratory Rate, Pulse Rate, and Skin Temperature

EQUIPMENT AND MATERIALS

1. Luminous infrared unit.
2. Stopwatch.
3. Skin thermometer.
4. Tape measure.
5. Towels.
6. Pen and pencil for recording.

PROCEDURES

1. Follow procedures 1–4 as in Experiment I.
2. Position the lamp so that the beam is directed perpendicular to the treatment area.
3. Select a distance between 30–36 inches, and measure and record the exact distance between the lamp and the treatment area on the subject.
4. Turn the lamp on and immediately begin timing a 30-min treatment.
5. Monitor the skin every 5 minutes, and using a towel, wipe away any perspiration.
6. Repeat the measurements of the subject 10 and 20 min into the treatment as in Experiment I, Procedure 4, and record them.

7. After 30 min, terminate the treatment, and repeat the measurements.
8. Record all measurements.
9. Compile and compare data as in Experiment I, Procedure 11.

III. Effects of Paraffin Treatment on Skin Temperature, Respiratory Rate, and Pulse Rate

EQUIPMENT AND MATERIALS

1. Paraffin unit with thermometer.
2. Paraffin solution at 127°F (52.8°C).
3. Plastic bags.
4. Towels.
5. Pencil and paper for recording.

PROCEDURES

1. Follow procedures 1–4, as in Experiment I, but position and drape for treatment to hand-forearm area.
2. Follow the procedures given in **Chapter 13** for the paraffin glove method. (Treatment time = 30 min.)
3. Measure and record the respiration and pulse rates 10 and 20 min into treatment.
4. Remove the paraffin after 30 min, and immediately measure and record the skin temperatures, respiration, and pulse rates.
5. Compile and compare the data.

Similar experiments can be done to compare the effects of deep heat modalities (shortwave diathermy, microwave diathermy, ultrasound) on vital signs. The results can be compared with the results of the superficial heat modalities experiments.

IV. Effects of Dry versus Moist Towel Spacing on the Thermal Conductivity of Hot Packs

EQUIPMENT AND MATERIALS

1. Hot water tank thermostatically controlled and hot packs.
2. Towels.
3. Skin thermometer.
4. Timer.
5. Pencil and paper for recording.

PROCEDURES

A. 1. Record the room temperature.
    2. Follow procedures 2–5 in Experiment I. (Omit measuring the respiration and pulse rates.)
    3. Apply a specific sized hot pack that has been heated for at least 1 hour and immediately wrapped in eight layers of fresh *dry* towels.
    4. Remove the pack momentarily to measure and record the skin temperature every 2 min for the duration of a 20-min treatment period.
    5. The experiment can be varied by comparing temperature changes using a different number of towel layers or by comparing changes using terrycloth spacing and the commercially made hot pack covers.

V. Effect of Duration of Soaking of Hot Packs on Skin Temperature

EQUIPMENT AND MATERIALS

Same as for Experiment III.

PROCEDURES

A. 1. Randomly divide the subjects into three groups.
    2. Apply hot packs to all subjects in the three groups as follows: *Group 1*, a hot pack soaked in hot water overnight; *Group 2*, a hot pack soaked in hot water for 30 min; *Group 3*, a hot pack soaked in hot water for 10 min.
B. 1. Follow procedures 2–5 in Experiment I, omitting measurements of pulse, respiration, and the temperature of distal skin area.
    2. Measure the temperature of the skin in the area treated after the pack is on for 10 min, then for 20 min (momentarily removing pack), and again immediately after terminating a 30-min treatment.
    3. Compare the changes in the skin temperature of the different groups.

The same experiment can be performed measuring respiratory rate, pulse rate, or both.

VI. Effect of Hot Pack Application on Local and Distal Skin Temperatures

EQUIPMENT AND MATERIALS

Same as for Experiment IV.

PROCEDURES

A. 1. Record the room temperature.
    2. Measure and record the skin temperature of the area to be treated and at a specifically designated distal location.
    3. Apply the hot pack to the area to be treated.
    4. Remove it after 20 min.
    5. Immediately measure the skin temperatures again at both the treated area and the distal site.
    6. Record these temperatures.
B. Compare the pre- and postintervention temperatures at both the treated and the distal sites.
C. This experiment can be varied by using infrared or a deep heat modality in place of the hot packs.

Similar experiments can be done to compare the effects of deep heat (shortwave diathermy, microwave diathermy, ultrasound) and superficial heat (hot pack, infrared) on local and distal skin temperatures.

VII. Effects of Applying Cold Packs Adjacent to a Hot Pack on Local and Distal Skin Temperatures

EQUIPMENT AND MATERIALS

1. Hot water tank thermostatically controlled unit and hot packs.
2. Cold pack unit (5°C) and cold packs.
3. Towels.
4. Skin thermometer.
5. Timer.
6. Pencil and paper for recording.

PROCEDURES

1. Repeat the procedures described in Experiment VI, Part A.
2. Repeat the procedures described in Experiment VI, Part B.

3. Twenty-four hours later, repeat the same procedures, but, in addition, place a cold pack in the areas both proximal and distal to the area being heated.

4. Compare the results of the hot pack alone with those of the hot pack applied simultaneously with cold packs on the skin temperature of the heated and the designated distal areas.

VIII. Effect of Ice Massage on Respiratory Rate, Pulse Rate, and Skin Temperature

EQUIPMENT AND MATERIALS

1. Ice cubes.
2. Towels.
3. Skin thermometer.
4. Pencil and paper for recording.

PROCEDURES

1. Record the room temperature.
2. Position and drape the subject for treatment to the low-back area.
3. Measure and record the respiration rate, pulse rate, and skin temperature in the area to receive the massage.
4. Perform ice massage to the lumbosacral area following the procedures described in **Chapter 14.**
5. Measure and record the skin temperature after 5 min of treatment.
6. Discontinue the ice massage after 10 min, and repeat the measurements, as in Procedure 3.
7. Compile and compare the data from individuals, and determine the average.

Similar experiments can be done to study the effects of chemical cold packs, vapocoolant sprays, or both, and to compare the results of the various modalities.

ELECTROTHERAPY CLINICAL CASES

1. Question Related to Chap 19 Electrophysiology

A 17 y/o female presents with (L) dorsiflexor paralysis and a resultant foot drop following an MVA. Manual muscle testing reveals 4+/5 strength in the (L) ankle plantar flexors, but no palpable contraction in the (L) ankle dorsiflexors. How can therapeutic electrical currents be used to evaluate possible peripheral nerve degeneration?

To examine dorsiflexor innervation, the R/D test was performed on the left anterior tibialis. A small electrode was placed on the anterior tibialis motor point and a large dispersive pad on the proximal thigh. During short-pulse duration stimulation (biphasic PC), there was no motor response as intensity was slowly raised to the expected motor threshold. Following short-duration stimulation, DC stimulation was used and created a sluggish motor contraction in the left dorsiflexors. A comparison with the contralateral extremity revealed that the right anterior tibialis displayed a brisk contraction with the biphasic PC, indicating that the peripheral nerve was intact on the noninvolved side.

The involved-side R/D test results indicate that the anterior tibialis may have lost innervation from the deep peroneal nerve, as evidenced by an inability to respond to PC. The response to DC implies that the muscle was intact for direct muscle stimulation with a long-duration current. If a response had been obtained with PC, the dorsiflexor paralysis might be traced to a CNS lesion (ie, TBI or SCI) in which the peripheral nerve is still intact. Further evaluation that includes EMG and NCV studies would be indicated for this patient.

2. Question Related to Chap 20 Clinical Applications of Electrical Stimulation

A 37 y/o male presents with quadriceps weakness and atrophy secondary to immobilization following a right ACL tear. The patient is cleared for strengthening in all ranges of knee motion. How can electrotherapy be incorporated in his treatment program?

The patient is positioned supine with the noninvolved leg flexed at the hip and knee so that the foot is flat on the support surface. The involved leg is kept extended as a cuff weight of appropriate poundage is placed around the ankle. The patient is instructed to perform a straight-leg raise as the stimulation comes on. If the patient has an inability to achieve terminal knee extension (extension lag), then the supine position is chosen with a roll placed under both knees. Augmenting active terminal knee extension exercises with strong motor stimulation will promote strength gains needed to achieve terminal knee extension.

Stimulation parameters and electrode arrangement for clincal case #2

Pulse amplitude	Strong motor intensity as tolerated by the patient.
Pulse frequency	Tetanizing (50 pps).
Pulse width	Wide (400 microsec).
Modulation	Interrupted (1:3 ie; 10 sec on 30 sec off).
	Ramping (2 sec to peak intensity).
Electrode placement	Combination of vastus lateralis and medialis motor points or femoral nerve stimulation in the upper thigh.
Rationale	Enhance quadriceps recruitment during active exercise and improved recruitment of fast twitch muscle fibers. Minimize disuse atrophy by electrically induced muscle activation.

Stimulation parameters and electrode arrangement for clinical case # 3

Pulse amplitude	Motor intensity sufficient to raise the ankle/foot.
Pulse frequency	Tetanizing (50 pps).
Pulse width	Wide pulse width (300 microsec).
Modulation	Interrupted modulation starting with a 1 (on):3(off) ratio with ramping (1 sec ramp up to peak intensity and 1 sec ramp down from peak intensity).
Electrode placement	Cathode (-) slightly inferior and posterior to the fibula head and anode on the anterior tibialis motor point.
Rationale	Enhance motor control as the patient works with the stimulation. Recipricoal inhibition of spastic plantar flexors by dorsiflexor activation. Maintain ankle ROM, and minimize disuse atrophy by electrically induced dorsiflexion.

3. Question Related to Chap 20 Clinical Applications of Electrical Stimulation

A patient with (L) CVA/(R) hemiparesis presents with paralysis in the (R) ankle dorsiflexors. How can electrotherapy be incorporated in their treatment program?

Dorsiflexor NMES is integrated in the intervention program to improve motor control, reduce plantar flexor spasticity, maintain dorsiflexion ROM, and be used during ambulation. The patient starts in the sitting position and is progressed to standing. Electromyographic (EMG) biofeedback can be interfaced with NMES so that the patient initiates the movement in order to trigger NMES-induced contractions that complete the motion that cannot be actively achieved. A hand switch may also be used that allows the patient stimulation control as they work to augment NMES induced contractions. If the stimulation is integrated into ambulation, a heel switch can be placed in the shoe of the paretic leg. Every time weight is removed from the paretic leg in preparation for the swing phase of gait, the dorsiflexors are stimulated to allow foot clearance. Similar multichannel stimulation can be used for patients that require muscle contractions in other muscles used for stabilization and motion during the gait cycle.

4. Question Related to Chap 20 Clinical Applications of Electrical Stimulation

A patient is seen postoperatively following a (R) total hip replacement and presents with venous stasis and increased postoperative edema in the (R) ankle and foot. How can electrotherapy be incorporated in their treatment program?

The patient is encouraged to elevate and perform active muscle contractions in the (R) ankle, knee, and hip musculature to promote venous return and edema reabsorption into the lymphatic ducts. Leg elevation and external compression can be used in conjunction with electrically induced contractions.

Stimulation parameters and electrode arrangement for clinical case # 4

Pulse amplitude	Motor intensity.
Pulse frequency	Tetanizing (50 pps).
Pulse width	Wide (300–400 microsec).
Modulation	Interrupted (1:3 ie; 10 sec on 30 sec off)
	Ramping (2 sec to peak intensity). If claudication pain occurs, the off time can be increased.
Electrode placement	Electrodes placed at the quadriceps, hamstrings, anterior tibialis, and gastrocnemius motor points. Stimulation can be alternated through the different muscle groups or delivered simultaneously to create cocontractions.
Rationale	Increase venous return by creating lower extremity muscle contraction.
	Mobilizing postoperative edema with the external pressure created with electrically induced contractions.

5. Question Related to Chap 20 Clinical Applications of Electrical Stimulation

A patient has a poorly healing ulceration on the plantar aspect of the first metatarsal. The wound has been present for over 6 months and appears as a deep, punched-out wound with pericallous formation. The individual has a neuropathic foot secondary to diabetes mellitus and requires pressure relief to initiate healing. How can electrotherapy be incorporated in the treatment program?

Total contact casting or other pressure relieving interventions are indicated to assist with wound healing. Electrical stimulation through a conductive dressing may hasten the healing process by attracting the cells involved in inflammation and proliferation. A hydrogel filler with an occlusive dressing can be used between stimulation sessions to create the optimal environment for healing.

Stimulation parameters and electrode arrangement for clinical case # 5

Current type	Monophasic pulsatile; high voltage galvanic stimulation with twin peak monophasic waveform (possible use of LIDC).
Pulse amplitude	Sensory stimulation intensity (as determined by stimulation to an adjacent intact area with sensation).
Pulse rate, width, and modulation	To lay down as much polarity per unit time, stimulation should be continuous at a fast frequency and wide duration (must avoid a motor response).
Electrode placement	Start initial interventions with either negative or positive electrode over the wound, then switch polarity as needed. The electrode placed over the wound should be dressed with a moist conductive dressing such as saline soaked gauze or hydrogel dressing. The other electrode should be made larger to create a dispersive pad that can be placed on the proximal thigh.
Intervention time	Two-hour periods of stimulation recommended 2–3 times a day/5 days a week.
Rationale	Trigger the healing process by adding in an electrical potential that may be absent.
	Attract the cells involved in the inflammatory and proliferative phases of healing with polarity. Create a bactericidal environment, and strengthen scar tissue with polarity.

6. Question Related to Chap 21 Transcutaneous Electrical Nerve Stimulation

A 33 y/o man sprained his lower back while playing tennis. He has had no relief from pain using a heating pad at home and has been admitted to the hospital for

Stimulation parameters and electrode arrangement for clinical case # 6

Current type	Biphasic pulsatile.
Pulse amplitude	Comfortable sensory stimulation intensity.
Pulse rate, width, and modulation	To provide constant sensory stimulation, stimulation should be continuous at a fast frequency and wide duration (avoid a motor response if electrodes are in an area of acute pain).
Electrode placement	Use two channels of stimulation with the electrodes covering the area of pain.
Intervention time	Variable based on need.
Rationale	Increase non-noxious sensory input (Gate Theory of Pain).

bed rest and conservative management of low-back pain. He is currently in the subacute stage. He has no other medical problems. How can electrotherapy be incorporated in his treatment program?

The integration of TENS is used to decrease the patient's pain and allow better tolerance for other rehabilitation interventions. The electrodes are placed at the areas of pain, and sensory levels of stimulation are used.

7. Question Related to Chap 22 Iontophoresis

A 33 y/o male with plantar fasciitis is referred for possible orthotic evaluation and modalities to decrease soft tissue inflammation. How can electrotherapy be incorporated in his treatment program?

Dexamethasone is an anti-inflammatory agent that can be used for soft tissue inflammation. The skin needs to be checked frequently, and the expected redness from the DC chemical reactions checked with the capillary refill test. The negative electrode tends to have very strong chemical reactions, and it should be large enough to sufficiently decrease current density. Rest, evaluation, and intervention of foot and lower-extremity posture, strength, and flexibility should be addressed to prevent the source of the plantar fasciitis.

Stimulation parameters and electrode arrangement for clinical case # 7

Current type	Direct current.
Current amplitude	1.5 mA × 30 min = 45 mA-min (lower intensity indicated for small electrodes, and for individuals with very light skin (can treat with 1.0 mA 45 min to maintain the same dosage).
Pulse modulation, duration, and frequency	A continuous DC is used, so pulse frequency and duration are not applicable (the pulse duration is equal to the intervention time).
Electrode placement	The negative electrode cover is saturated with the dexamethasone sodium phosphate (Decadron) and placed over the plantar problem area. The conductive positive electrode (no medication) completes the circuit and is placed on the back of the ipsilateral calf.
Rationale	The strong electrical polarity pushes the medication from the electrode to the skin to enhance absorption into the target tissue in which the anti-inflammatory effect is desired.

8. Question Related to Chap 23 Clinical Electroneuromyography

A 65 y/o male with a history of diabetes presents with progessive tingling in both lower extremities and weakness in the lower leg and foot musculature. How can the status of possible nerve degeneration be evaluated?

An EMG evaluation can be performed in the lower leg and foot muscles. Abnormal electrical potentials due to neuropathy can be assessed during; needle insertion, AT rest, minimal effort contraction, and maximal effort contraction. In addition, motor and sensory NCV's can be performed to further evaluate peripheral neuropathy severity. The evaluation should also include; sensory, motor, reflex, and functional testing in conjunction with the EMG/NCV studies.

ELECTROTHERAPY LAB EXPERIMENTS

The purpose of these experiments is to establish the effects of electrical stimulation or to compare the effectiveness of different techniques of application. To enhance the accuracy of the data, observe the following:

1. Note the room temperature—because the ambient temperature can affect experimental results. Try to maintain the room at about the same temperature for all stages of the experiments.
2. Ensure that, whenever possible, the same researcher measures the same variable (eg, skin temperature, respiratory rate, pulse rate, range of motion, manual muscle test) before, during, and after application. Use a skin thermometer when measuring the temperature of the part being treated.
3. Record all measurements immediately after taking them.
4. Repeat the treatment and measurements on several individuals using similar equipment for all subjects in each experiment.
5. Compile the data.
6. Compare the data: note individual and group differences, and determine the average for each individual and for each group. Realize that the results indicate effects only for the subjects or groups tested. The greater the number of subjects, the more the results apply to a larger population of young healthy subjects.

For **safety,** all the experiments should be performed under the conditions described in earlier chapters. All indications, contraindications, and precautions should be carefully noted.

I. Effect of Electrical Stimulation on Skin Temperature

EQUIPMENT AND MATERIALS

1. Electric stimulator with biphasic and electric stimulator with monophasic waveform stimulus output.
2. Four electrodes (3″ × 3″) and leads.
3. Surface (skin) thermometer.
4. Timer.
5. Pencil and paper for recording data.

PROCEDURES

A. 1. Record room temperature.
   2. Position the subject supine, and place a roll of toweling under each knee.
   3. Measure the skin temperature over the quadriceps in the area to be stimulated.
   4. Stimulate the right quadriceps, using the bipolar technique, with monophasic pulses at 30 pps and surged at 20/min. Increase the amplitude gradually to the minimal visible contraction (MVC).
   5. Stimulate for 5 minutes.
   6. Remove the electrodes, and immediately measure and record the skin temperature under each electrode.
   7. Note any other changes in the stimulated areas.
B. Using the same setup as in A, stimulate the left quadriceps with biphasic 30 pps and surged at 20/min. Increase the amplitude to MVC. Stimulate for 5 minutes. Measure and record the results as in A.
C. Compare the results with the results in A. Discuss the results of the experiment.

Similar experiments can be done to compare the effects of other electrical stimulators.

II. Effects of Electrical Stimulation on Hyperemia

EQUIPMENT AND MATERIALS

Same equipment and materials in Experiment I.

PROCEDURES

A. 1. Conduct the experiment in a well-lit room.
   2. Position the subject comfortably with the right arm supported.
   3. Observe the skin color and condition in bicep area of the arm before stimulating. Record these subjective observations.
   4. Using bipolar technique, stimulate the right biceps with monophasic pulses at 30 pps and surged at 20/min.
   5. Increase the amplitude until the MVC is observed.
   6. Stimulate for 5 minutes.

7. Remove the electrodes, and observe the reaction to the stimulation.

8. Rate the extent of skin hyperemia using a scale of 0–3, where 0 represents no change in skin color, 1 is minimal hypermia, 2 is moderate hyperemia, and 3 is marked hypermia.

9. Record the results.

10. Compare the results with the contralateral nonstimulated area.

B. Using the same procedure as in A, stimulate the left biceps with biphasic pulses at 30 pps and surged at 20/min.

C. Compare the results with those in A, and discuss the rationale for this reaction.

III. Tolerance to Electrical Stimulation

The objective of this experiment is to compare the tolerance of a subject to various types of electric stimulation.

EQUIPMENT AND MATERIALS

1. Electric stimulator with biphasic and electric-stimulator with monophasic waveform stimulus output.
2. Four small (2″ × 2″) electrodes.
3. Timer.
4. Pencil and paper for recording data.

PROCEDURES

A. Apply the electrical stimulation to two groups of subjects. Subjects should be randomly selected to each group.

   Group 1. Apply monophasic pulses at 30 pps first, followed by biphasic pulses, at 30 pps, as described later.
   Group 2. Reverse the order of stimulators used: apply the biphasic pulses first, followed by the monophasic pulses.

B. 1. Explain to the subject the scale of comfort or tolerance to be used. Use a scale of 1 to 4, where 1 is least comfortable and 4 is most comfortable.

   2. Position the subject comfortably in a supine position.

   3. Prepare the area to be stimulated.

4. Locate the motor point of the right anterior tibialis muscle, using the bipolar technique, with the monophasic pulses, and stimulate.

5. Increase the intensity until maximum muscle contraction and full dorsiflexion of the ankle occurs.

6. Repeat the stimulation 10 times.

7. Ask the subject to rate the comfort of this stimulation on the scale of 1–4.

8. Record the subject's response.

9. Remove the electrodes, and observe any change in the tissues stimulated.

Repeat the same procedures, but stimulate the *left* anterior tibialis with biphasic pulses at 30 pps. Increase the intensity until maximum contraction and full dorsiflexion occur. Have the subject rate the comfort of this stimulation, as described earlier. Again remove the electrodes and observe any change in the stimulated tissue.

C. Compare the tolerance levels for each form of electrical stimulation.

Similar experiments can be done to compare tolerance to stimulation of other electrical stimulators such as the high-volt pulse current and interferential current. These experiments can be done without letting the subject know which stimulator is being used.

MECHANICAL AGENTS CLINICAL CASES

1. Question Related to Chap 24 Spinal Traction

A 36 y/o male shipping-room clerk is referred to your office with a diagnosis of L5-S1 disc herniation with irritation of the right sciatic nerve. How can one of the mechanical agents be incorporated in his treatment program?

Four different traction techniques can be applied in this case: intermittent, sustained, manual, and positional. To determine which technique will be most effective, actual trials will be necessary. The most common technique used is intermittent traction because of the high forces, as much as 200 pounds, that can be applied. The use of unilateral traction might make this intervention even more effective.

The position of choice will ultimately be determined by the patient's comfort. If the patient can hyperextend his lumbar spine, the prone position should be considered first. In this position, the vertebrae apply forces on the disc that are directed anteriorly; thus, there is a tendency to reduce the herniation.

The poundage will be determined by the patient's weight and medical condition, the amount of friction that must be overcome, and the patient's tolerance. On the first visit, begin with less poundage, and observe the patient's reaction; then you might decide to go to the optimal level. For example, if the patient weights 150 pounds, begin with approximately 25–30 pounds of force, and then increase to 40–50 pounds with progressive interventions.

Positional traction can also be used with the patient in a left side-lying position and a pillow roll under the left side. The upper trunk is rotated to the right and knees and hips flexed in this position. If the position centralizes the patient's pain, it can be integrated with manual therapy, therapeutic exercise, and postural education.

2. Question Related to Chap 24 Spinal Traction

A 66 y/o female with DJD in the cervical spine is referred to PT for evaluation and treatment. X-Rays and MRI reveal moderate facet joint degeneration in the lower cervical spine. How can one of the mechanical agents be incorporated in her treatment program?

Cervical traction is indicated, provided that the patient does not present with any conditions that are considered contraindications. The patient can first be treated with a hot pack to decrease pain and promote relaxation. Manual cervical traction can be initiated to monitor the patient's response to cervical traction. If the response to manual traction is favorable, then mechanical cervical traction can be integrated in her intervention program.

The patient is positioned in supine with the head and neck flexed to 20 degrees. A traction unit with suboccipital pads (ie, Saunders device) is used to provide traction forces. An intermittent traction with 10–20 lbs of force is used prior to therapeutic exercise and postural reeducation to reduce pain and improve function.

3. Related to Chap 25 External Compression

A 50 y/o male with a venous stasis wound above the (R) medial malleoli is referred for evaluation and treatment. How can one of the mechanical agents be incorporated in his treatment program?

The patient presents with a large, shallow wound with a moderate amount of drainage. Edema and he-mosideran deposits are present throughout the right lower leg, ankle, and foot.

The patient is treated with a foam dressing to absorb drainage, and compression is applied with an unna boot to reduce edema and venous stasis. The pneumatic compression pump is used between unna boot applications. An intermittent mode with 40 mmHg can be used provided that there are no contraindications (ie, PAOD or thrombophlebitis). Once the wound is healed, the patient should continue with external compression by using compressive socks.

4. Related to Chap 25 External Compression

A 66 y/o female with chronic lymphedema in the (R) UE due to lymphatic dysfunction is referred for evaluation and treatment. How can one of the mechanical agents be incorporated in her treatment program?

The patient has a history of lymphatic stasis in the (R) upper extremitiy for many years and has required constant edema management. A compressive garment is used with a pneumatic pump to control edema and minimize infection, pain, skin damage, limited ROM, and dysfunction in the (R) UE. Following manual lymphatic drainage, the pump is used for two-hour periods in an intermittent mode with a pressure of 45 mmHg. The arm is elevated and active muscle pumping is encouraged during the pressure off cycles. The patient needs to continue with elevation, a compressive garment, and home exercise program to maintain (R) UE mobility and function.

5. Related to Chap 26 Hydrotherapy

A 67 y/o female with a long history of RA is having difficulty with standing and ambulating because of pain and stiffness in bilateral LE joints. How can hydrotherapy be incorporated in her treatment program?

The patient has limitations in bilateral hip and knee joints and proximal weakness in both lower extremities. The patient is treated in the therapeutic pool to eliminate the effects of gravity and reduce weight-bearing forces through the lower extremity joints. Pain-free ambulation is possible, and active exercise is assisted with the effects of buoyancy. A progressive ambulation and exercise program at different depths can be employed to improve overall strength, ROM, and endurance in both lower extremities.

A pool temperature of approximately 98°F is employed, and the patient is instructed in a graded exercise and ambulation program. Patient tolerance is closely monitored, and a home exercise program is provided. The patient is also instructed in the use of appropriate assistive and joint conservation devices.

6. Related to Chap 26 Hydrotherapy

A 49 y/o male with DM presents with a poorly healing wound on the heel of his (L) foot. How can hydrotherapy be incorporated in his treatment?

There is necrotic tissue in the base of the patient's wound that requires debridement. The mechanical agitation and softening effects of a lower extremity whirlpool or pulsatile lavage is used to assist with debridement.

A water temperature of 94°F is used to increase local circulation without producing overheating. The proper levels of antimicrobials are added without creating too much toxicity to the wound. Sharp debridement is used following the whirlpool intervention, and an appropriate wound dressing and pressure relief are maintained.

MECHANICAL AGENTS LAB EXPERIMENTS

The purpose of these experiments is to establish the effects of thermal and mechanical agents or to compare the effectiveness of different techniques of application. To enhance the accuracy of the data, observe the following:

1. Note the room temperature—because the ambient temperature can affect experimental results. Try to maintain the room at about the same temperature for all stages of the experiments.
2. Ensure that, whenever possible, the same researcher measures the same variable (eg, skin temperature, respiratory rate, pulse rate, range of motion, manual muscle test) before, during, and after application. Use a skin thermometer when measuring the temperature of the part being treated.
3. Record all measurements immediately after taking them.
4. Repeat the treatment and measurements on several individuals using similar equipment for all subjects in each experiment.
5. Compile the data.
6. Compare the data: note individual and group differences, and determine the average for each individual and for each group. Realize that the results indicate effects only for the subjects or groups tested. The greater the number of subjects, the more the results apply to a larger population of young healthy subjects.

For **safety,** all the experiments should be performed under the conditions described in earlier chapters. All indications, contraindications, and precautions should be carefully noted.

I. Effect of Different Water Temperatures on the Vital Signs of a Subject Who Is Immersed in a Hubbard Tank

EQUIPMENT AND MATERIALS

1. Hubbard tank with water level sufficient for full immersion.
2. Towels.
3. Oral thermometer.
4. Stop watch.
5. Blood pressure measuring equipment.

PROCEDURES

A. 1. Divide the subjects into three groups. Designate each group for immersion in one of the following water temperatures: *Group 1*, 93°F (33.9°C); *Group 2*, 99°F (37.2°C); *Group 3*, 104°F (40°C).
   2. Take the subjects' vital signs before immersion: oral temperature, blood pressure, and pulse and respiration rates.
   3. Have the subjects sit quietly in the tank, neck high in water, for 20 minutes.
   4. Have the subjects get out of the water after 20 minutes and wrap themselves in dry towels.
   5. Take vital signs again immediately.
B. 1. Compare changes in vital signs between individuals in the same group.
   2. Calculate the mean of each vital sign for each group.
   3. Compare the means for each vital sign between groups.

The same experiment can be varied by comparing changes in vital signs while doing various grades of activities rather than while at rest in the water. Similar experiments can be done while sitting in whirlpool tanks instead of Hubbard tanks, with the water at various temperatures, at various water levels, or both: for example, waist level water.

Note: Because changing the water temperature in a Hubbard tank is time consuming, it may be necessary to extend this experiment over three or more laboratory sessions, using a different water temperature each day.

II. Effect of Cervical or Lumbar Traction on Range of Motion

EQUIPMENT AND MATERIALS

1. Motorized traction unit.
2. Traction table.
3. Stool.
4. Head halter with TMJ protectors and lumbar traction harness.
5. Pillow.
6. Goniometer.
7. Pencil and paper for recording.

PROCEDURES

A. 1. Use a goniometer to measure and record the active range of motion of the cervical spine of all subjects, and select those who demonstrate a limited range.
   2. Divide the subjects randomly into two groups (experimental and controlled).
   3. Subject the experimental group to 15 min of cervical traction (line of pull, 30° flexion) in the supine position.
   4. Subject the control group to 15 min of rest in the supine position.
   5. Remeasure and record the active range of motion in all subjects.
B. Compare the pre- and posttreatment results in both groups, and statistically analyze these results.
C. Using the same methods and procedures, determine the effects of lumbar traction.

Similar experiments can be done to compare different techniques of traction (eg, sitting versus lying, prone versus supine position).

PHOTOCHEMICAL AGENTS CLINICAL CASE

1. Question Related to Chap 27 Ultraviolet Radiation

A 62 y/o woman with DM was admitted to the hospital 10 days ago with a large sacral pressure ulcer. She has been receiving hydrotherapy tank interventions for wound cleansing and debridement for approximately 1 week. How can one of the photochemical agents be incorporated in her treatment program?

The wound was evaluated as a nonhealing stage III sacral decubitus. Ultraviolet is incorporated in the wound care intervention because of its bactercidal effects. In addition, UVR is used to stimulate new cell production and increase superficial circulation.

A cold quartz lamp is used for a localized application to the wound. The minimal effective dose (MED) is determined in relation to the distance from the wound. At a distance of 1 inch, the MED is 12–15 seconds: E_1, 36–45 seconds; E_2, 72–90 seconds; E_3, 135–180 seconds. To treat this condition, E_1 or, at a maximum, E_2 should be used. Intervention on contact should be 55% of these dosages.

High-voltage or low-intensity direct-current (LIDC) electrical stimulation can be used instead of, or in addition to, UV, using the recommended dosage and techniques for wound healing (see Electrotherapy clinical case # 5). Cold laser (Chap 28) may also be integrated into this patient's treatment program if UVR is not used.

A wound filler with an occlusive dressing (if not infected) and pressure relief with positioning and proper pressure relieving devices are indicated to assist with the healing of this wound.

PHOTOCHEMICAL LAB EXPERIMENT

The purpose of this experiment is to study the effects of cold laser and compare the effectiveness of different application techniques. To enhance the accuracy of the data, observe the following:

1. Ensure that, whenever possible, the same researcher measures the same variable (eg, before, during, and after application).
2. Record all measurements immediately after taking them.

3. Repeat the treatment and measurements on several individuals using similar equipment for all subjects in each experiment.

4. Compile the data.

5. Compare the data: note individual and group differences, and determine the average for each individual and for each group. Realize that the results indicate effects only for the subjects or groups tested. The greater the number of subjects, the more the results apply to a larger population of young healthy subjects.

For **safety,** all the experiments should be performed under the conditions described in earlier chapters. All indications, contraindications, and precautions should be carefully noted.

I. Effect of Cold Laser Treatment on Pain

EQUIPMENT AND MATERIALS

1. Pain scale questionnaire.
2. Cold laser unit.
3. Treatment table.
4. Pillow.
5. Curtain.
6. Pencil and paper for recording.

PROCEDURES

A. 1. Select students who have experienced musculoskeletal pain for more than 24 hours.

2. Divide the subjects randomly into two groups (controlled and experimental).

3. Ask subjects to fill out the pain questionnaire.

4. Position each subject behind a curtain so that he or she cannot see the modality or benefit from any body language that the operator might inadvertently use.

5. Expose only the part of the body to be treated.

6. Treat all subjects with a cold laser in the way suggested in Chapter 28 (the cold laser device will be off for the control group).

7. Ask all subjects to fill out the questionnaire again immediately after the treatment.

B. 1. Compare the pre- and postintervention data.

2. Analyze the results statistically.

Similar experiments can be done to compare different treatment approaches (eg, treating acupuncture points versus pain areas).

PELVIC FLOOR REHABILITATION AND BIOFEEDBACK CLINICAL CASE

1. Question Related to Chap 29 Biofeedback and Chap 30 Pelvic Floor Rehabilitation

A postmenopausal female diagnosed with stress incontinence is referred for trial use with PF electrical stimulation and biofeedback. Present interventions include the use of estrogen therapy and Kegel exercises.

Electrical stimulation can be initiated to increase strength and reeducate contractions in the pelvic floor prior to biofeedback training. Stimulation can be provided with the following parameters:

Pulse amplitude	Motor intensity sufficient to create pelvic floor contractions.
Pulse frequency	Tetanizing (50 pps).
Pulse width	Wide (300 microsec).
Modulation	Interrupted (1:2 ratio, ie, 5 sec on 10 sec off).
	Ramping to increase patient comfort (2 sec to peak intensity).
Electrode placement	Surface electrodes placed between the genitalia and anal opening and perianal region overlying the pelvic floor. Also a vaginal probe electrode can be used.
Rationale	Increase pelvic floor muscle strength and awareness needed for more effective urethral closure.

As active contractions in the pelvic floor are achieved, SEMG evaluation can be performed on the pelvic floor and accessory muscles (ie, gluteals, abdominals, hip rotators, and adductors) to teach isolated muscle contractions. The biofeedback is used to train control of pelvic floor resting tension prior to and following exercise. In addition, fast, slow, and sustained contractions are integrated in the biofeedback sessions to target the different muscle fibers in the pelvic floor and accessory muscles. The sensor electrodes are placed externally for the accessory muscles and either internally (vaginal) or externally (peri-vaginal/peri-anal) for specific pelvic floor musculature. Sensitivity settings and threshold for feedback are adjusted in a graded fashion as the patient gains increased strength and control in the muscles being trained. The patient is instructed in a home exercise program to maintain the gains from the pelvic floor rehabilitation intervention.

BIOFEEDBACK LAB EXPERIMENT

Effect of Electrode Spacing on Recorded EMG Output during Wrist Extension Biofeedback

EQUIPMENT AND MATERIALS

1. EMG biofeedback unit.
2. Surface electrodes with conductive gel.

PROCEDURES

A. 1. A within-subject comparison is made on each individual as the sensor electrodes are placed:

(1) 2 cm apart, (2) 4 cm apart, (3) 6 cm apart, and (4) 8cm apart.

2. Each subject is placed in the sitting position with the forearm supported.

3. The skin on the dorsal forearm is lightly abraded prior to electrode application.

4. The two active electrodes are placed on the dorsal forearm (distal to the lateral) epicondyle, and the ground electrode is placed in between. The proximal active and ground electrode placements need to be standardized.

5. The subject is instructed to perform a maximal voluntary isometric contraction (MVIC) of the wrist extensors at the end range of wrist extension.

6. Each subject should perform 3 MVICs with a two-minute rest period between each contraction for each electrode spacing condition. The order of electrode spacing should be randomized.

7. The average peak level of SEMG activity should be recorded for each electrode spacing condition.

B. 1. Compare the differences in average peak SEMG activity for the different electrode spacing conditions.

2. Calculate the mean average difference (%) for all of the subjects when comparing the different electrode spacing conditions.

Similar experiments on other muscles can be done to compare the influence of limb position and skin preparation on recorded SEMG activity.

Index